Pediatric Dentistry

Pediatric Dentistry

A clinical approach

Second edition

Editors

Göran Koch

Sven Poulsen

WILEY-BLACKWELL

A John Wiley & Sons, Ltd., Publication

This edition first published 2009

Blackwell Munksgaard, formerly an imprint of Blackwell Publishing was acquired by John Wiley & Sons in February 2007. Blackwell's publishing programme has been merged with Wiley's global Scientific, Technical, and Medical business to form Wiley-Blackwell.

Registered office
John Wiley & Sons Ltd, The Atrium, Southern Gate, Chichester, West Sussex, PO19 8SQ, United Kingdom

Editorial offices
9600 Garsington Road, Oxford, OX4 2DQ, United Kingdom
2121 State Avenue, Ames, Iowa 50014-8300, USA

For details of our global editorial offices, for customer services and for information about how to apply for permission to reuse the copyright material in this book please see our website at www.wiley.com/wiley-blackwell.

Library of Congress Cataloging-in-Publication Data
Pediatric dentistry : a clinical approach / editors, Göran Koch, Sven Poulsen. -- 2nd ed.
p. ; cm.
Includes bibliographical references and index.
ISBN 978-1-4051-6100-8 (hardback : alk. paper) 1. Pedodontics. I. Koch, Göran. II. Poulsen, Sven.
[DNLM: 1. Pediatric Dentistry. 2. Dental Care for Children--methods. WU 480 P36983 2009]
RK55.C5P447 2009
617.6'45--dc22
2008030047

A catalogue record for this book is available from the British Library.

Set in 10.5/12.5 Minion and produced by Gray Publishing, Tunbridge Wells, Kent
Printed in Singapore by Fabulous Printers Pte Ltd

4 2012

Contents

To Anna-Lena Hallonsten

Preface to the second edition

Pediatric Dentistry: A Clinical Approach was first published in 2001 with the aim of providing a comprehensive review of pediatric dentistry with special emphasis on evidence-based oral health care for the child and adolescent. In this second edition of this textbook, we have built upon the earlier volume by thoroughly updating the text, as well as replacing chapters and adding new ones as necessary.

The sciences behind pediatric dentistry, as well as strategies of clinical approaches, have developed rapidly over the past few decades. These advances have been reflected in the considerable work undertaken by the many clinicians and scientists who have contributed to this textbook.

Pediatric dentistry aims to improve the oral health of children and adolescents through health promotion, prevention and systematic and comprehensive oral care. It is concerned with the expression of, and interventions against, the major dental diseases as well as with a number of dental and oral conditions specific to childhood and adolescence. These comprise all aspects of dental and occlusal developmental disturbances, traumatic injuries to the teeth, periodontal conditions, oral pathological conditions, pain control, dental need and treatment of handicapped and medically compromised children. Pediatric dentistry applies principles from other clinical disciplines, medical and behavioral sciences and adapts them to the special needs of the growing and developing individual from birth through infancy and childhood to adolescent late teens.

Our objective is that this book will serve not only as a basis for undergraduate training in pediatric dentistry but will also be of relevance to postgraduate students and dental practitioners who want to increase their knowledge and skills in order to deliver up-to-date pediatric dental care.

Göran Koch and Sven Poulsen
Editors

Contributors

Jens O. Andreasen
Department of Oral and Maxillofacial Surgery
Copenhagen University Hospital (Rigshospitalet)
Copenhagen
Denmark

Kristina Arnrup
Department of Pediatric Dentistry
Postgraduate Dental Education Centre
Public Dental Service
Örebro
Sweden
and
School of Health and Medical Sciences
Örebro University
Örebro
Sweden

Anders G. Broberg
Department of Psychology
University of Gothenburg
Göteborg
Sweden

Ivar Espelid
Department of Paediatric Dentistry and Behavioral Science
Institute of Clinical Dentistry
University of Oslo
Oslo
Norway

Göran Dahllöf
Department of Pediatric Dentistry
Department of Odontology
Karolinska Institutet
Huddinge
Sweden

Dorte Haubek
Department of Pediatric Dentistry
School of Dentistry
Faculty of Health Sciences
University of Aarhus
Aarhus
Denmark

Gro Haukali
Department of Pediatric Dentistry
School of Dentistry
Faculty of Health Sciences
University of Aarhus
Aarhus
Denmark
and
Municipal Child Dental Service of Aarhus
Aarhus
Denmark

Martti Helkimo
Department of Stomatognathic Physiology
The Institute for Postgraduate Dental Education
Jönköping
Sweden

Hanne Hintze
Department of Oral Radiology
School of Dentistry
Faculty of Health Sciences
University of Aarhus
Aarhus
Denmark

Ingeborg Jacobsen
Department of Paediatric Dentistry and Behavioral Science
Institute of Clinical Dentistry
University of Oslo
Oslo
Norway

Birgitta Jälevik
Department of Paediatric Dentistry
Sahlgrenska University Hospital/Mölndal
Mölndal
Sweden

Ann-Katrin Johansson
Department of Clinical Dentistry
Faculty of Medicine and Dentistry
University of Bergen
Bergen
Norway

Anders Juul
Department of Growth and Reproduction
Copenhagen University Hospital (Rigshospitalet)
Copenhagen
Denmark

Gunilla Klingberg
Department of Paediatric Dentistry
Faculty of Odontology
Malmö University
Malmö
Sweden
and
Mun-H-Center, National Orofacial Resource Centre for Rare Disorders
Gothenburg
Sweden

Göran Koch
Department of Paediatric Dentistry
The Institute for Postgraduate Dental Education
Jönköping
Sweden

Sven Kreiborg
Department of Pediatric Dentistry and Clinical Genetics
School of Dentistry
Faculty of Health Sciences
University of Copenhagen
Copenhagen
Denmark

Jüri Kurol
Department of Orthodontics
The Sahlgrenska Academy
University of Gothenburg
Göteborg
Sweden

Stefan Lundeberg
Department of Pediatric Anesthesia and Intensive Care
Astrid Lindgren Children's Hospital
Karolinska University Hospital
Stockholm
Sweden

Tomas Magnusson
Department of Stomatognathic Physiology
The Institute for Postgraduate Dental Education
Jönköping
Sweden
and
School of Health Sciences
Jönköping University
Jönköping
Sweden

Katharina M. Main
Department of Growth and Reproduction
Copenhagen University Hospital (Rigshospitalet)
Copenhagen
Denmark

Luc Martens
Department of Paediatric Dentistry and Special Care
University of Ghent
Ghent
Belgium

Lars Matsson
Faculty of Odontology
Malmö University
Malmö
Sweden

Ingegerd Mejàre
Department of Paediatric Dentistry
Faculty of Odontology
Malmö University
Malmö
Sweden

Bengt Mohlin
Department of Orthodontics
The Sahlgrenska Academy
University of Gothenburg
Göteborg
Sweden

June Nunn
Public and Child Dental Health
School of Dental Science
Trinity College Dublin
Dublin
Ireland

Sven Poulsen
Department of Pediatric Dentistry
School of Dentistry
Faculty of Health Sciences,
University of Aarhus
Aarhus
Denmark

Magne Raadal
Department of Clinical Dentistry
Faculty of Medicine and Dentistry
University of Bergen
Bergen
Norway

Ulla Schröder
Department of Paediatric Dentistry
Faculty of Odontology
Malmö University
Malmö
Sweden

Bengt Sjödin
Department of Periodontology
Postgraduate Dental Education Centre
Örebro
Sweden

Marit Slåttelid Skeie
Department of Clinical Dentistry
Faculty of Medicine and Dentistry
University of Bergen
Bergen
Norway

Irma Thesleff
Developmental Biology Research Program
Institute of Biotechnology
University of Helsinki
Helsinki
Finland

Svante Twetman
Department of Cariology and Endodontics
School of Dentistry
Faculty of Health Sciences
University of Copenhagen
Copenhagen
Denmark

Lill-Kari Wendt
Centre for Oral Health
School of Health Sciences
Jönköping University
Jönköping
Sweden

1

Pediatric oral health care: the perspectives

Sven Poulsen and Göran Koch

How it began: the historical perspective

The history of pediatric dentistry as we know it today is usually considered to have started in the latter part of the nineteenth century. However, in 1743, Robert Bunon published his book *Essay sur les Maladies des Dentes*, where he for the first time discussed at length dental problems during childhood. Bunon emphasized the connection between the diet and health of the pregnant mother and the mineralization of her child's teeth. He also studied the influence of infectious diseases on dental development and described the principles of serial extraction. The importance of good dietary habits for prevention of dental disease was repeatedly stressed in his book. Robert Bunon rightly deserves the title "the father of children's dentistry".

One of the first dentists who dedicated himself to providing regular dental care for children was John Greenwood, who practiced in New York in the 1780s. He advertised a reduced fee for children who signed up for regular dental treatment. It is also known that around 1800, C.F. Delabarre undertook dental treatment in overfilled Parisian orphanages in wartime France. The first known proposal for a regular dental care program for children was put forward in 1851 by A.-F. Talma, dentist to King Leopold I of Belgium, and was based on regular examination of all children between the ages of 5 and 12 years. Similar programs were proposed in many other countries.

In this early era, enthusiastic pioneers – often on their own initiative – organized dental care for children (Fig. 1-1).

Community responsibility: the population perspective

The growing interest in dental care for children at the end of the nineteenth century was partly caused by large epidemiological studies on caries in children published in 1893–1895. These studies showed that more than 80% of the children had carious teeth and that only a few per thousand had received any dental treatment. These results were thoroughly discussed at world dental congresses and led dentists in many countries to urge their societies to organize public dental health services for children. The first municipal dental clinic for children was opened in Strasbourg in 1902 under the direction of the Danish-born Ernst Jessen. This very first school dental clinic became a model for the development of children's dental clinics in a number of countries.

It is interesting to note that the arguments for better dental services for children were based on epidemiological data. Using epidemiological information to document a health problem is to adopt a population approach rather than an individual clinical approach. This indicates that in the Nordic countries, organized child dental care has for more than a century been considered a collective responsibility rather than the problem of the individual. Formal legislation and regulations concerning child dental care were passed by the parliaments of all Nordic countries several decades ago and dental services, including outreach preventive services, have been developed to serve the whole child population. The epidemiological starting point of child dental care in Nordic countries may also explain why the child dental services in these countries have collected valuable epidemiological information to monitor continually the level of disease in their target groups.

From birth to adolescence: the oral health perspective

As already mentioned, child dental services originally focused on school-age children, often being limited to extraction of diseased teeth and restorative care of the permanent teeth. This focus had no rational foundation,

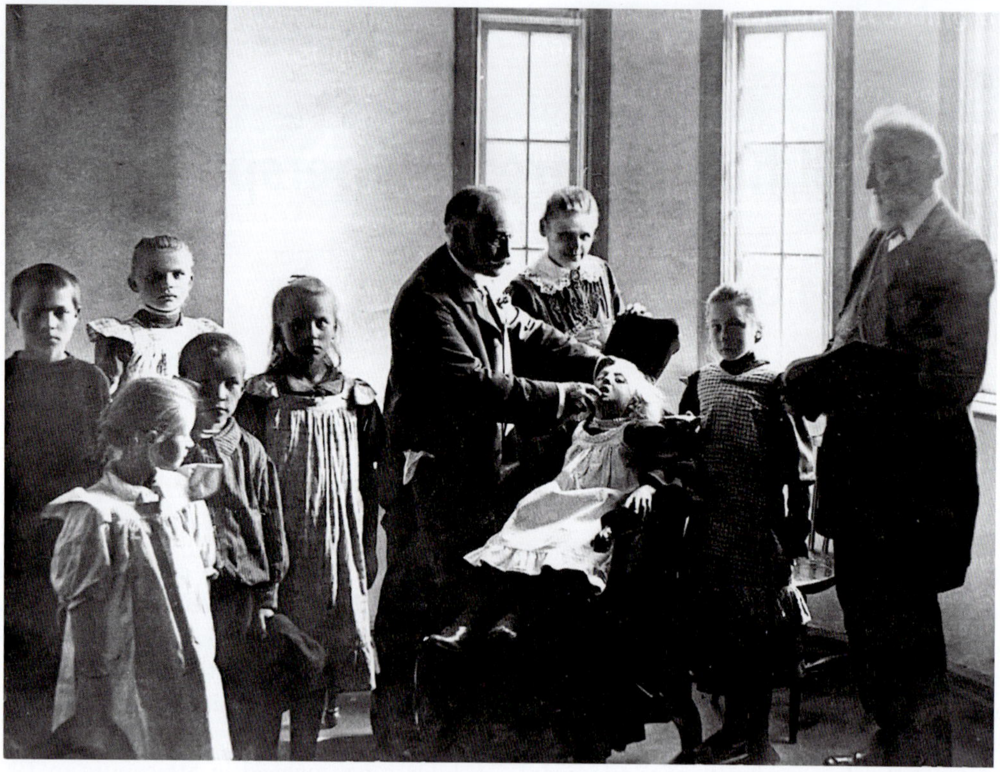

Figure 1-1 In Nordic countries, dental care for children was initiated by the end of the nineteenth century, often by oral health care pioneers. This 1898 photograph shows a private dental practitioner, Dr Marinus Kjær, performing one of his weekly screenings in a public school in Svendborg, a small provincial town in the southern part of Denmark.

but was merely due to the fact that children could easily be reached in schools. This philosophy is still prevalent in many countries in spite of the pain untreated dental disease and emergency care may inflict on the pre-school child with subsequent dental fear and anxiety. In this book we adopt the United Nations (UN) Convention definition of a child (every human being below the age of 18 years unless, under the law applicable to the child, majority is attained earlier). Thus, we see pediatric oral care as a continuous effort to secure good oral health as defined in Box 1-1 from birth to 18 years of age.

The World Health Organization (WHO) definition of health emphasizes that health cannot be isolated from the subjective experience of the individual (Box 1-1). In other words, a satisfactory definition of health needs to include somatic as well as nonsomatic dimensions. As oral health should be considered an integrated part of general health, a definition of oral health should also include not only sound teeth and oral structures, but also absence of dental fear and anxiety. This is consistent with recent research on patients' assessment of how their dental and oral conditions influence the quality of their daily life. Methods to measure oral health-related quality of life in children are now available, and it has been shown that dental conditions such as early childhood caries reduce children's oral health-related quality of life. It has also been shown that the oral health-related quality of life of children with a severe caries treatment need is improved after rehabilitation under general anesthesia (see Chapter 6).

Box 1-1 WHO definition of general health and an analogous definition of oral health

General health
A state of complete physical, mental and social well-being and not only the absence of disease or infirmity (1).

Oral health
A state of sound and well-functioning dental and oral structures as well as absence of dental fear and anxiety.

UN Convention on the Rights of the Child: the ethical perspective

Today, concern for the child's specific needs and rights is attracting increasing interest as reflected in the UN Convention on the Rights of the Child (2). This document is important to all professionals who relate to children – including pediatric dentists.

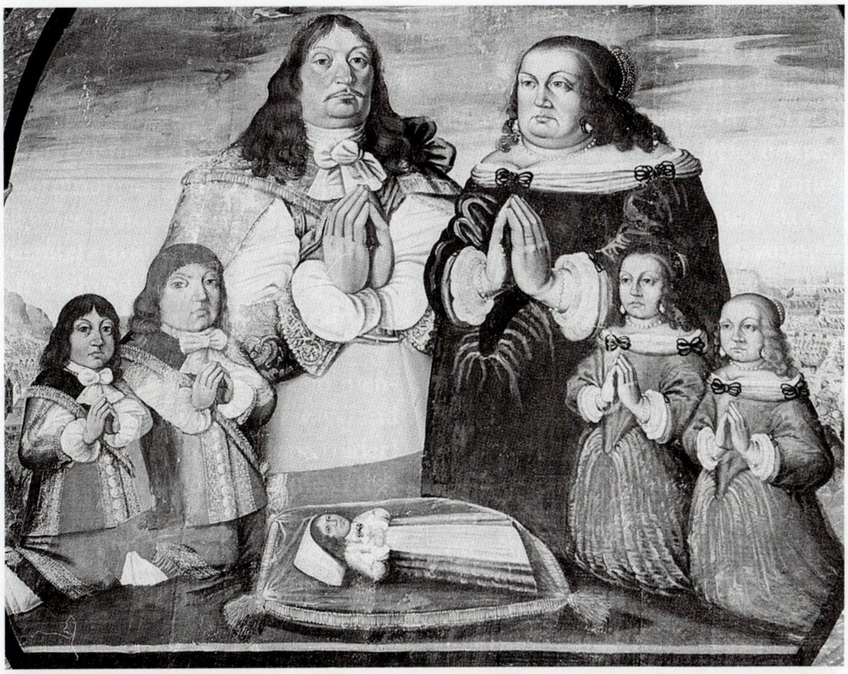

Figure 1-2 Until the eighteenth century children were considered to be small adults (sort of "miniature grown-ups").

One of the key items in this document is that children have rights as human beings and also need special care and protection, as often expressed by the saying that "children are not small adults" (Fig. 1-2). In order to secure children and adolescents high-quality oral health care, emphasis is now being placed on the concept of child competency (Box 1-2).

Box 1-2 Professionals should recognize that children are not "small adults", and that special competency (child competency) is needed, when meeting children

Children are different from adults in a number of ways:

- children are individuals in growth and development
  - physical
  - psychological
  - social
- oral health, including attitudes and behavior relating to oral health, is formed during childhood and adolescence
- children's situation is different from the situation of adults:
  - they are in the care of and dependent on adults
  - they are not able to foresee consequences of their own decisions and behavior.

Child competence is characterized by:

- a specific insight into the dental and oral health for the child and adolescent
- an ability to communicate effectively with children, adolescents, and their parents
- a positive professional attitude towards children, adolescents, and their parents.

The UN Convention on the Rights of the Child was adopted by the UN General Assembly on November 20, 1989, and has had a marked impact on the lives of children in a number of countries. The overriding point in the Convention is that children have *rights*. They have a right to be protected against bad or unfair treatment and they also have a right to be respected as individuals. Another principle is the "best interest of the child". Whenever we take a decision affecting children, their best interest should be a primary consideration. Further, the views of the child should be respected. The child should be free to express opinions and these should be given due weight "in accordance with the age and maturity of the child". In other words, children should have a say in matters of concern to them.

A number of the articles in the convention have obvious implications for pediatric dentists and the way we organize and deliver oral health care to children (Box 1-3).

Pediatric dentistry: the clinical perspective

Pediatric dentistry encompasses all aspects of oral health care for children and adolescents. It is based on basic knowledge from various odontological, medical and behavioral sciences that are applied to the unique situation of the developing child and young person. Starting prevention in early childhood makes it possible

Box 1-3 The UN Convention on the Rights of the Child (2)

The UN Convention on the Rights of the Child was adopted and opened for signature, ratification and accession by General Assembly resolution 44/25 of November 20, 1989. It entered into force on September 2, 1990, and contains important statements relevant to child oral health care, some of which are quoted below:

Article 3

In all actions concerning children, whether undertaken by public or private social welfare institutions, courts of law, administrative authorities or legislative bodies, *the best interests of the child* shall be a primary consideration.

States Parties undertake to ensure the child such protection and care as is necessary for his or her well-being, taking into account the rights and duties of his or her parents, legal guardians, or other individuals legally responsible for him or her, and, to this end, shall take all appropriate legislative and administrative measures.

States Parties shall ensure that the institutions, services and facilities responsible for the care or protection of children shall conform with the standards established by competent authorities, particularly in the areas of safety, health, in the number and suitability of their staff, as well as competent supervision.

Article 24

States Parties recognize the right of the child to the enjoyment of the highest attainable standard of health and to facilities for the treatment of illness and rehabilitation of health. States Parties shall strive to ensure that no child is deprived of his or her right of access to such health care services.

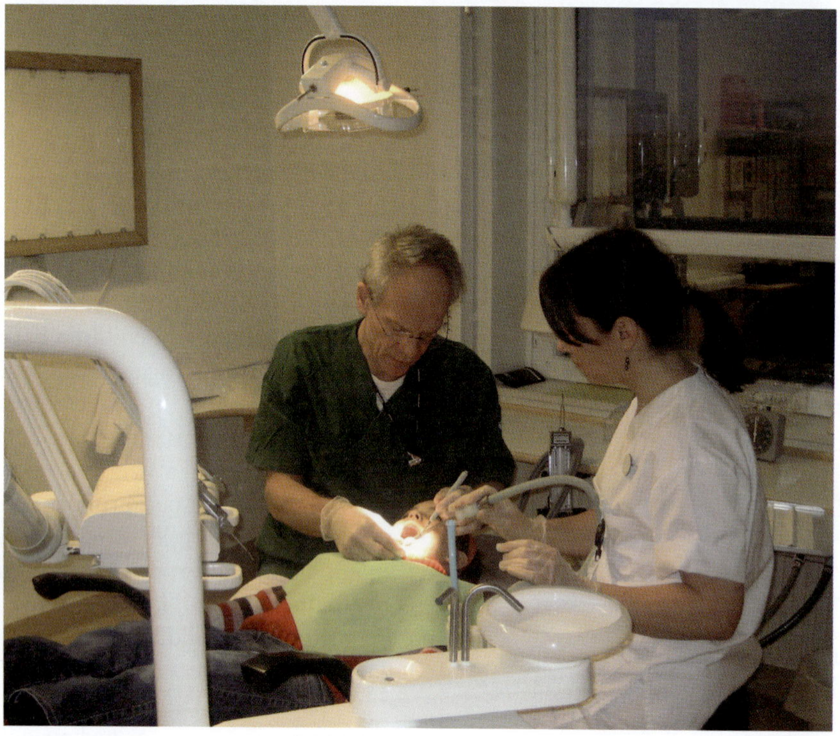

Figure 1-3 Today, comprehensive oral health care is delivered in a modern, well-equipped dental clinic by a dedicated team.

to preserve sound erupting teeth and keep oral structures healthy. Pediatric dentistry also implies early diagnosis and treatment of the multitude of oral diseases and conditions found in the child's and the adolescent's mouth, including caries, periodontal diseases, mineralization disturbances, disturbances in tooth development and tooth eruption, and traumatic injuries in otherwise healthy as well as sick and handicapped children (Fig. 1-3).

The quest for evidence-based interventions – preventive, diagnostic or rehabilitative – is urgent in pediatric dentistry as well as in all other fields of dentistry.

References

1. World Health Organization. *Basic documents*, 39th edn. Geneva: WHO, 1992.
2. UN Convention on the Rights of the Child. http://www.unicef.org/crc/ (accessed August 2008).

2

Growth and pubertal development

Anders Juul, Sven Kreiborg and Katharina M. Main

The evaluation of growth charts and pubertal development in children and adolescents is an important tool for any clinician in the assessment of health status. Optimal thriving and height attainment in accordance with family potential can only be achieved in an environment providing optimal socioeconomic conditions, health care, and psychosocial support. Thus, failure to thrive or to grow may be the first indication of an underlying problem that may need attention. In turn, treatment of children may need to consider the specific growth and developmental windows in order not to disturb this delicate balance.

Measurement of growth in different phases of life

The current concept of prenatal and postnatal growth suggests that there are distinct growth phases, which should be considered separately.

Prenatal growth

Prenatal growth is divided into three trimesters (by convention). The first trimester is characterized by organogenesis and tissue differentiation, whereas the second and third trimesters are characterized by rapid growth and maturation of the fetus. Fetal growth can be assessed by serial ultrasonography in the second and third trimesters. Abdominal circumference, head circumference, and femoral length of the fetus can be determined, and from these parameters fetal weight can be estimated using different algorithms (9). The fetal weight estimate should be related to normative data. Some reference curves for fetal growth are based on children born prematurely (11), and hence such curves therefore tend to underestimate normal fetal weights from healthy pregnancies. Alternatively, reference curves based on ultrasound studies of normal healthy infants exist (9) and should preferably be used. Based on the changes in fetal weight estimates over time, the fetus can be considered as having a normal fetal growth rate, or alternatively as experiencing intrauterine growth restriction (IUGR) (8). Children born at term (gestational age 37–42 weeks) are considered mature. Children born before 37 weeks of gestation are premature, and children born after 42 weeks of gestation are postmature. At birth, weight and length can be measured and compared to normative data correcting for gestational age at birth. Based on these comparisons, a newborn child can be classified as either appropriate for gestational age (AGA), small for gestational age (SGA), or large for gestational age (LGA).

IUGR fetuses will often end up being SGA at birth, but not necessarily so. Thus, IUGR infants may end up lighter than their genetic potential but remain within normal ranges (i.e., AGA). Therefore, IUGR and SGA are not synonymous entities, although they are often referred to as such in the literature (Fig. 2-1). Height velocity *in utero* is higher than at any time later in life, leading to an average birth length of 50–52 cm and birth weight of 3.5–3.6 kg after 37–42 weeks of gestation. It is therefore not surprising that growth disturbances during this phase may have long-lasting effects on growth and health later in life. Whereas the first trimester is dominated by tissue differentiation and organ formation, the second and especially third trimesters show a rapid gain first in length and then in weight. Fetal and placental endocrinology is highly complex and hormones such as insulin, leptin, placental growth hormone, insulin-like growth factor (IGF)-2, and thyroid hormone are only some of the many growth factors involved in the regulation of fetal growth.

Postnatal growth

Postnatally, height can be determined by measuring length in the supine position the first 2–3 years of life. After 2–3 years of age standing height can be measured

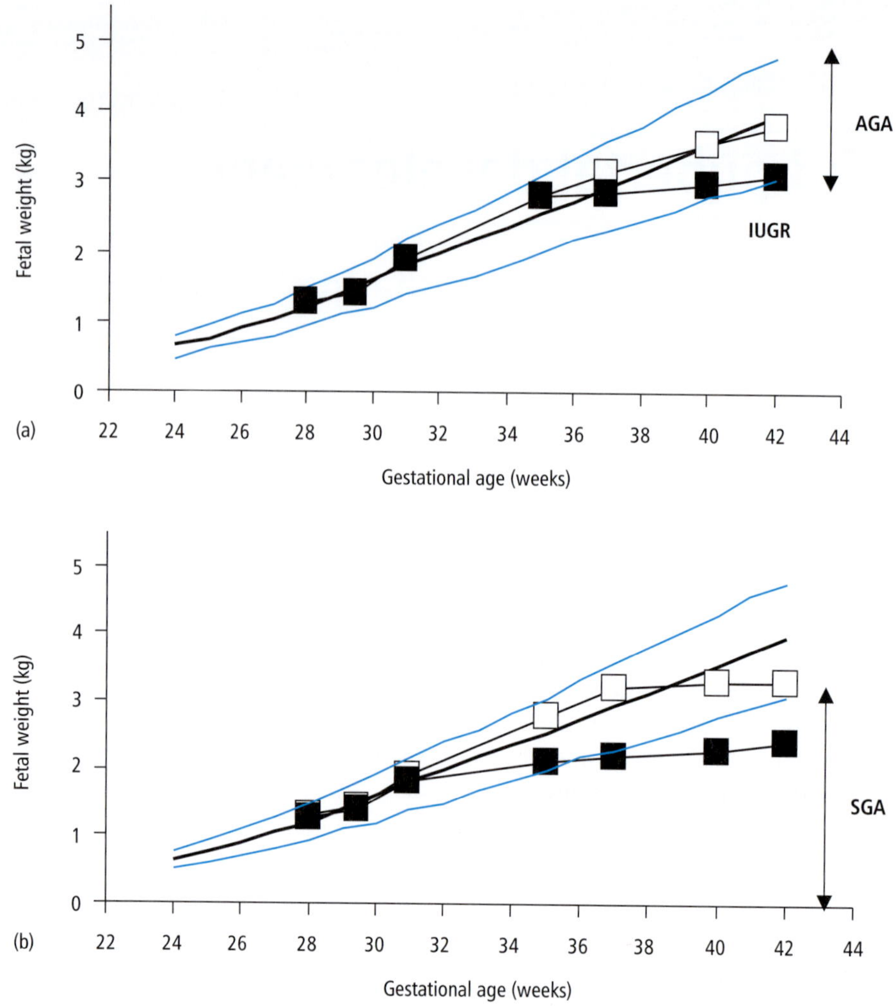

Figure 2-1 Reference ranges for fetal weight according to gestational age during pregnancy denoted by the blue lines (10th, 50th, and 90th percentiles) (8). Panel (a) shows examples of children with normal birth weights at term; a normally growing fetus ending with a birth weight which is appropriate for gestational age (AGA) and (■) a fetus with third trimester intrauterine growth restriction (IUGR) ending with a birth weight below the genetic potential but within normal limits (AGA). Panel (b) shows examples of fetuses with intrauterine growth retardation (IUGR) ending up AGA (□) or SGA (■).

preferably using a wall-mounted stadiometer. Height is determined without shoes, shoulders towards the wall, arms hanging down, and the face straight forward (Fig. 2-2). The eyes should be horizontally aligned with the external ear opening. The means of three measurements are recorded. The stadiometer should be calibrated on a daily basis.

Importantly, the body proportions (such as head circumference, facial appearance, sitting height, and arm span) may be helpful in the differential diagnosis of growth disorders (Fig. 2-1). This can simply be done by assessing the sitting height with subsequent calculation of the sitting height to standing height ratio. This enables quantification of whether or not a growth failure is proportional or disproportional (such as in hypochondroplasia). Reference ranges for this ratio exist (5).

Changes in height can be separated into infant, childhood, and pubertal growth phases according to the infancy–childhood–puberty (ICP) model described by Karlberg (7). The majority of children will follow the distinct growth patterns of these phases.

Infancy

After a brief initial weight loss of up to 10% of the birth weight, growth during the first months postnatally follows to a large extent fetal growth rate during the third trimester with 30 g/day and 3.5 cm/month. After that a rapid decline in growth rate occurs, in both weight and height. However, this period still represents a major growth phase during the lifetime with a three-fold increase in weight over 6 months. Very little is known about the regulatory factors of growth during this period

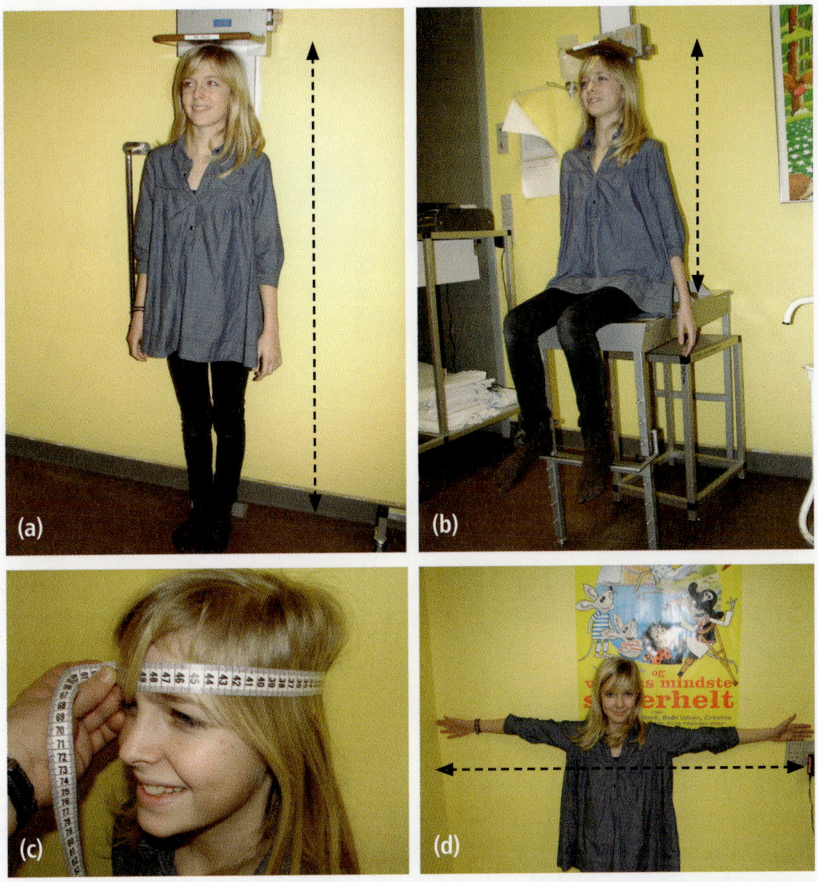

Figure 2-2 Standing height determined by a wall-mounted stadiometer (a). Height is recorded as the mean of three measurements. Sitting height is determined by a specifically designed chair (b). Head circumference is determined using a measuring tape (c). Armspan length is determined by measuring the distance from fingertips to fingertips (d).

of life, but nutrition and living conditions play a major role. Recently, the World Health Organization (WHO) published a new growth chart reference for infancy based on breastfed infants from different countries and ethnic origins living under optimal socioeconomic conditions. This chart did not find significant differences in growth patterns between these children, which indicates that genetic differences may first become evident later in life (14).

Childhood

In this phase growth is relatively constant, with a gradual decline in growth velocity over time. From 2 to 4 years children grow approximately 7 cm and 2 kg/year. Beyond 5–6 years of age this rate has decreased to approximately 5 cm/year. This growth phase is highly dependent on growth and thyroid hormones.

Puberty

During the pubertal growth spurt, which typically stretches over 4–5 years, total height gain is on average 20–25 cm for girls and 25–30 cm for boys with large interindividual variations. There is some tendency that early maturers obtain a higher peak height velocity compared to late maturers (Fig. 2-3). Sex steroids increase the pulsatile growth hormone secretion, which in turn increases IGF-1. Weight gain is highly individual and may occur both before and after peak height velocity.

In girls, the onset of the growth spurt is early and may even precede the development of secondary sexual characteristics in some. Typically, breast buds appear before pubic hair at 10–11 years of age, but occasionally this succession may be reversed (9). Both breast development and pubic hair attainment are graded into five stages (B1–B5 and PH1–PH5) according to Tanner and Whitehouse (13). The first menstruation, menarche, is a sign of adult level estradiol production and follicle maturation and occurs late during the growth spurt at approximately 13 years of age. Height attainment after menarche is small, with 4–8 cm over 1.5–2 years.

In boys, the pubertal growth spurt occurs relatively late during development. Puberty commences with enlargement of testis size from 3 to 4 ml at 11–12 years of age, and this very first sign of pubertal onset is usually

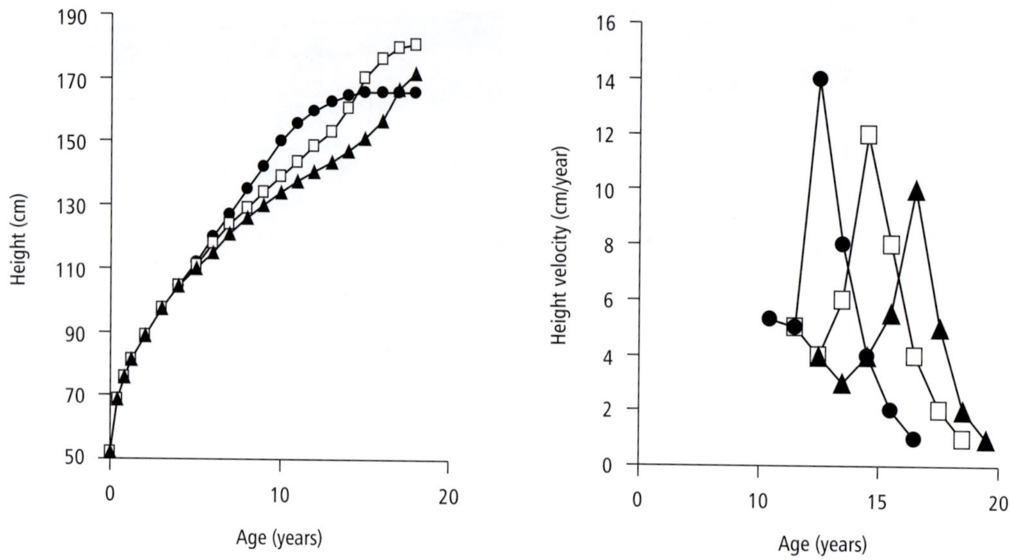

Figure 2-3 (a) Three examples for height curves and (b) height velocity curves from children with early puberty (●), normally timed puberty (□) and delayed puberty (▲). Note that final height is almost the same (a) and that peak height velocity is higher in earlier puberty (b).

not noticed by the boy or even less so by the parents. Pubertal development in boys is graded into five genital stages (G1–G5) according to Tanner and Whitehouse (13). Testis growth continues and within 6–12 months pubic hair can be seen. Testicular volume can be determined by the use of an orchidometer to which the size of the testes is compared. Maximum height velocity often occurs at a testis size of 10–12 ml at around 14 years of age, at the time when the voice breaks and facial hair appearance occurs. Thus, boys are already relatively virilized at the time of the adolescent growth spurt (10). In midpuberty, many boys develop physiological gynecomastia, which usually disappears within 6–12 months.

The onset of puberty is approximately a year earlier in girls than boys, which consequently results in earlier growth arrest in girls than boys (14–15 versus 16–17 years of age). The timing of puberty may also differ by 1–2 years according ethnicity and nationality.

Growing pains

A significant number of children and adolescents experiences intermittently pains, localized to the shins or legs when going to bed after a physically active day. The etiology of this phenomenon is unknown, but local warmth, gentle massage, and mild pain medication, if the child is in real discomfort, can normally ameliorate the problem, which resolves spontaneously.

Evaluation of growth charts

Growth evaluation should be based on observations over time by applying longitudinal measurements of height and weight on an age- and gender-specific growth chart. These charts are available for many populations and also for a variety of growth disorders and syndromes. Due to the secular trend in height, country-specific reference ranges should be constructed at regular intervals (6). Repetitive measures of growth will result in a trajectory of growth, which then can be evaluated against family potential (parental stature, growth of siblings). As some children show considerable seasonal variation in growth, follow-up periods of 6–12 months may be necessary. In children approaching puberty, pubertal staging (13) will additionally be necessary for adequate assessment.

Growth charts are usually based on cross-sectional data from children and adolescents, covering 95% of the population (±2 standard deviations). Charts may depict centiles or standard deviation lines. Per definition, 2.5% of the population will be below or above the outer limits (Fig. 2-4). In contrast, height velocity curves are based on longitudinal follow-up studies of healthy children (Fig. 2-5).

In the evaluation, both the position within the growth chart in relation to the parental potential and the trend of the individual growth curve are important. Deviations from the expected may represent two separate pathological conditions. In populations with a significant secular trend in height attainment due to recently improved socioeconomic conditions, the growth of siblings in comparison to the patient may be helpful as well. The simplest method to determine the family growth potential is based on calculation of midparental height (Box 2-1).

During childhood, most children will follow their trajectory of growth, which ideally should follow the

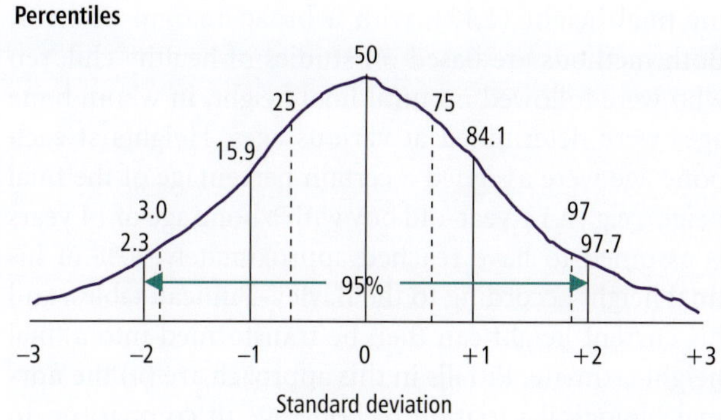

Figure 2-4 Normal (Gaussian) distribution of heights illustrating the 95% reference interval by percentiles or standard deviations (SDs).

> **Box 2-1** Calculation of family growth potential (equal to target height or genetic height potential)
>
> **Girls**
>
> [Maternal height (cm) + paternal height (cm)]/2 – 6.5 cm
>
> **Boys**
>
> [Maternal height (cm) + paternal height (cm)]/2 + 6.5 cm
>
> To allow for growth variation within a family, the target height range is calculated as midparental height of ± 6.5 cm for both genders.
>
> Potential pitfalls of this approach are: (a) the parents differ considerably in height centiles and (b) one of the parents is not of normal stature.

family potential. There are, however, two phases in life where this trajectory may not be followed without necessarily representing pathology: (a) during the first 2 years of life, children may "catch up" or "slow down" depending on their intrauterine growth and size at birth, a phenomenon also called regression towards the mean, and (b) during puberty, early maturation will lead to a growth spurt above average (vice versa for late maturation) and the individual child will therefore almost always deviate upwards (or downwards) compared to the mean on the growth chart (due to the cross-sectional design of the growth charts). In general, tall children have a tendency to enter puberty early, short children to enter puberty later.

Acute diseases during childhood and adolescence will often only result in a temporary weight loss with rapid catch-up after recovery. In contrast, height attainment will often get compromised in long-term or serious illness. These children may show considerable catch up growth after recovery, if their bone age allows further

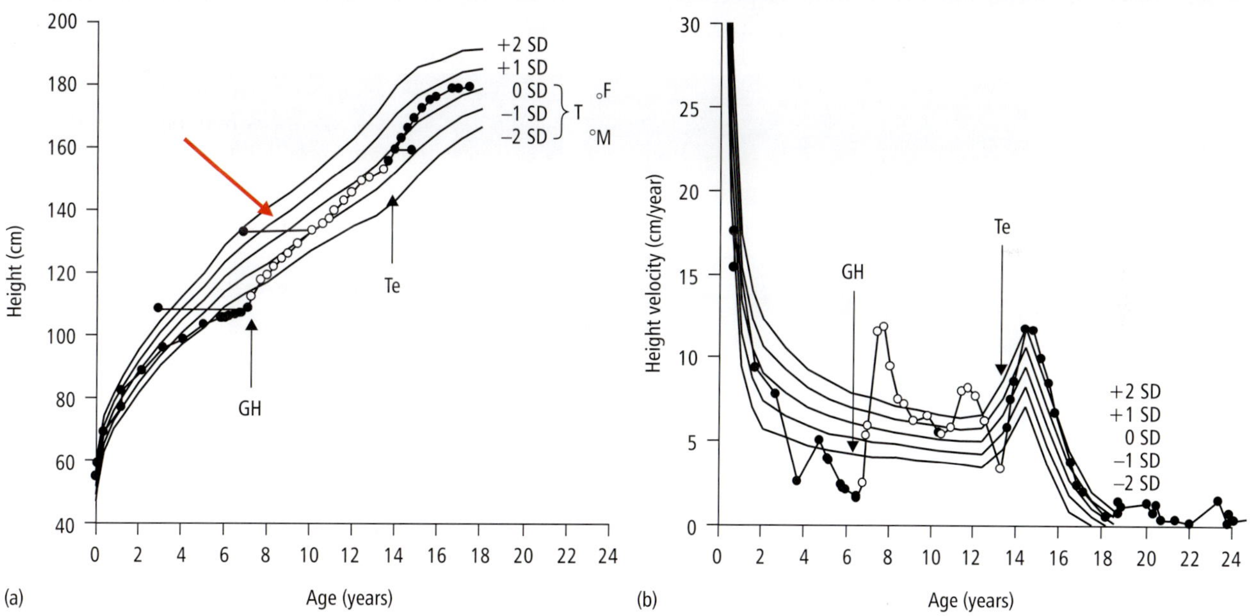

Figure 2-5 Normal height curve (a) based on healthy children. Lines denote mean ±1 standard deviation (SD) and ±2SD. One individual patient is depicted on the curve (●) before and after operation for a pituitary tumor (craniopharyngeoma) resulting in growth hormone deficiency. A typical deceleration is seen prior to diagnosis. Horizontal lines (red arrow) denote bone age. Following operation the child suffers from pituitary insufficiency and is substituted with L-thyroxine, hydrocortisone growth hormone, (GH) (arrow), and testosterone (Te) (arrow). This results in a final height well within target height. T = target height range, F = father's, and M = mother's height expressed as SDs. (b) Normal height velocity curve based on Tanner's longitudinal study of healthy children. The same child (●) is depicted on this curve illustrating the marked growth acceleration following GH therapy, as well as the acceleration when puberty is initiated.

growth potential. Thus, growth deceleration is seen commonly in the year(s) prior to diagnosis of severe chronic disease (e.g., brain tumors or malignancies) which is often first noticed in retrospect.

Detailed evaluation of growth includes bone age determination and final height predictions.

Bone age determination

Linear growth continues until the fusion of the ossification centers. Thus, determination of bone maturation may help to assess the growth potential in an individual, as many disorders of growth are associated with either delayed or accelerated bone age. Bone age is mostly measured with a radiograph of the left hand and wrist and a comparison of the epiphyseal growth plates with age- and gender-specific references (Fig. 2-6). Two main systems are used clinically: (a) the Greulich–Pyle method (3) and (b) the TW method (12). Computer-based automated bone-age assessments are currently being developed and will help to reduce interobserver variation and time expense.

Final height prediction

Both methods of bone-age determinations (Greulich–Pyle and TW methods) can be employed in prediction models (Bayley–Pinneau and TW method, respectively) for final height (1,12), with a broad margin of error. Both methods are based on studies of healthy children who were followed up until final height, in whom bone ages were determined at various ages. Heights at each bone age were assigned a certain percentage of the final height, e.g., a 13-year-old boy with a bone age of 14 years is assumed to have reached approximately 90% of his final height according to the Bayley–Pinneau tables, and his current height can then be transformed into a final height estimate. Pitfalls in this approach are (a) the normal biological variation of bone age in comparison to chronological age which is ±1 year and (b) the fact that prediction models are based on normally growing children and may therefore both underestimate and overestimate final height in pathological conditions.

Dental age determination

Dental age or dental maturity may be assessed in different ways. The simplest method is to record the teeth erupted and compare to normative data. A more precise method is to judge the development of the teeth from radiographs. Haavikko (4) has given normative data for individual permanent teeth, while Demirjian (2) has developed a scoring system based on assessment of all lower left permanent teeth (except the third molar) from an orthopantomogram. Demirjian's method has

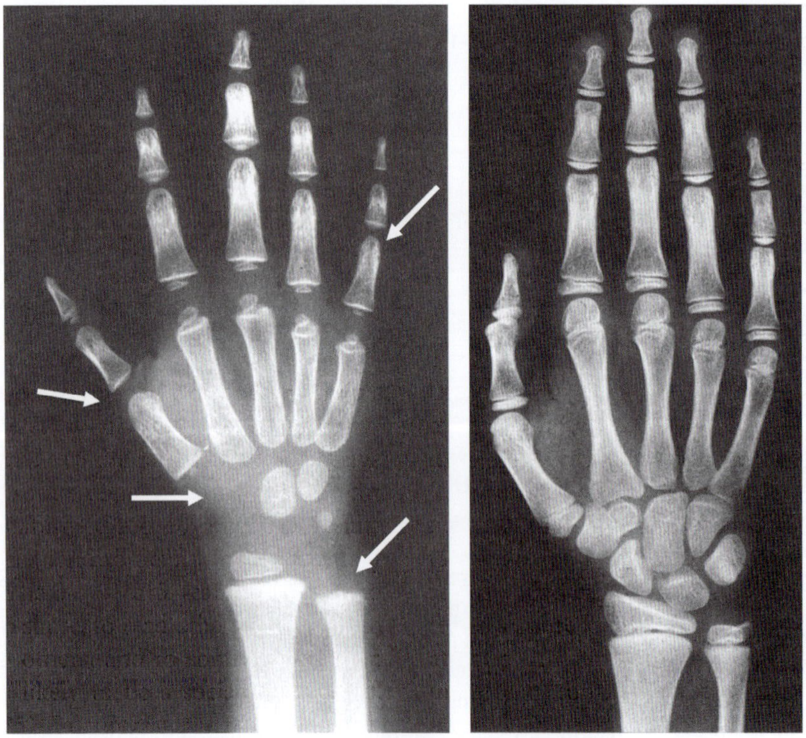

Figure 2-6 Two radiographs of the left hands of two healthy children. Note that the mineralization of the small bones has not yet occurred in the younger child (left).

gained general recognition as the most precise. In general, the correlation between dental age and bone age is, however, relatively low (Fig. 2-7).

Disorders of growth and puberty

Intrauterine growth restriction

Many adverse conditions can lead to impairment of intrauterine growth and development. Infections, medications, environmental chemicals, exposure to tobacco, maternal diseases, and uteroplacental insufficiency may cause early or late growth restriction. A fetus may follow a growth trajectory below normal throughout pregnancy and be born SGA, or growth restriction may have its onset during the third trimester and lead to IUGR.

Over the past few decades research has revealed that antenatal and early postnatal growth patterns may have health consequences in adult life, which may be caused by fetal programming to accommodate adverse conditions. Links have been established to cardiovascular disorders, dyslipidemia, diabetes mellitus, pubertal timing, and reproductive function. The majority of children born SGA or IUGR (80–85%) will show spontaneous catch-up growth after birth, typically within the first 2–3 years of life. Thus, the remaining 10–15% of IUGR/SGA children do not show catch-up growth and remain short in childhood and end up as short adults. These children respond well to treatment with biosynthetic growth hormone. Silver–Russell syndrome is associated with prenatal as well as postnatal growth failure, and children typically respond with significant improvement of final height despite the fact that they generally have no evidence of growth hormone deficiency.

Postnatal growth failure

Today, being of short stature is less well accepted by many societies than being tall. Therefore, many children are presented in the clinic (Fig. 2-8). In the majority of cases a growth curve evaluation will reveal that the child is within its family potential. A typical growth curve of a child with familial short stature is shown in Fig. 2-8(a). These children are typically growing at a normal growth rate and thus following their growth trajectory. These families need reassurance, as there is today no convincing treatment schedule available that will reliably and significantly increase final height. If, however, the child's position on the growth curve does not correspond to the familial potential or the growth trajectory deviates downwards due to low growth velocity, the child should be investigated further. Many chronic and systemic diseases (e.g., asthma, sleep apnea, malabsorption, and metabolic diseases) and systemic steroid treatment may lead to growth disorders. In rare cases even large doses

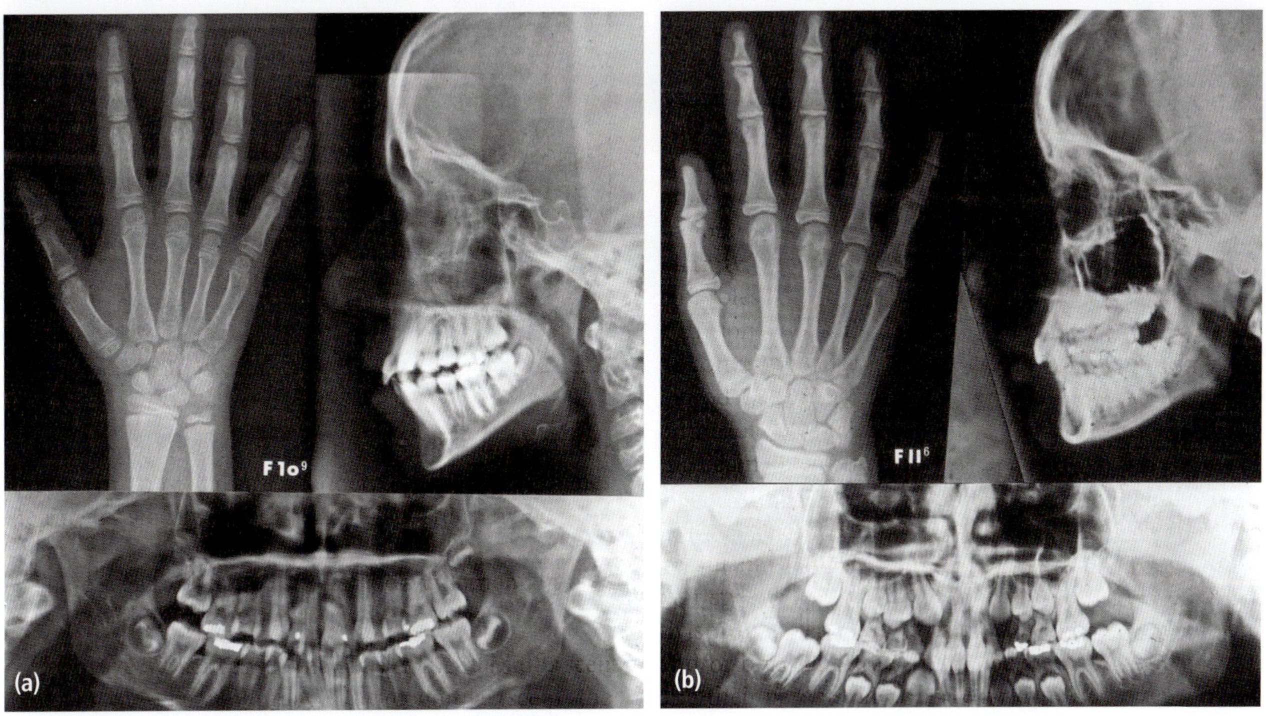

Figure 2-7 Illustrative examples showing low correlation between bone age and dental age. (a) A healthy girl, aged 10 years 9 months, with advanced dental maturity (nearly complete permanent dentition: DS4, M1) compared to the skeletal maturity (prepubertal hand–wrist radiograph). (b) A healthy girl, aged 11 years 6 months, with delayed dental maturity (early mixed dentition: DS2, M1) compared to the skeletal maturity (postpubertal hand–wrist radiograph).

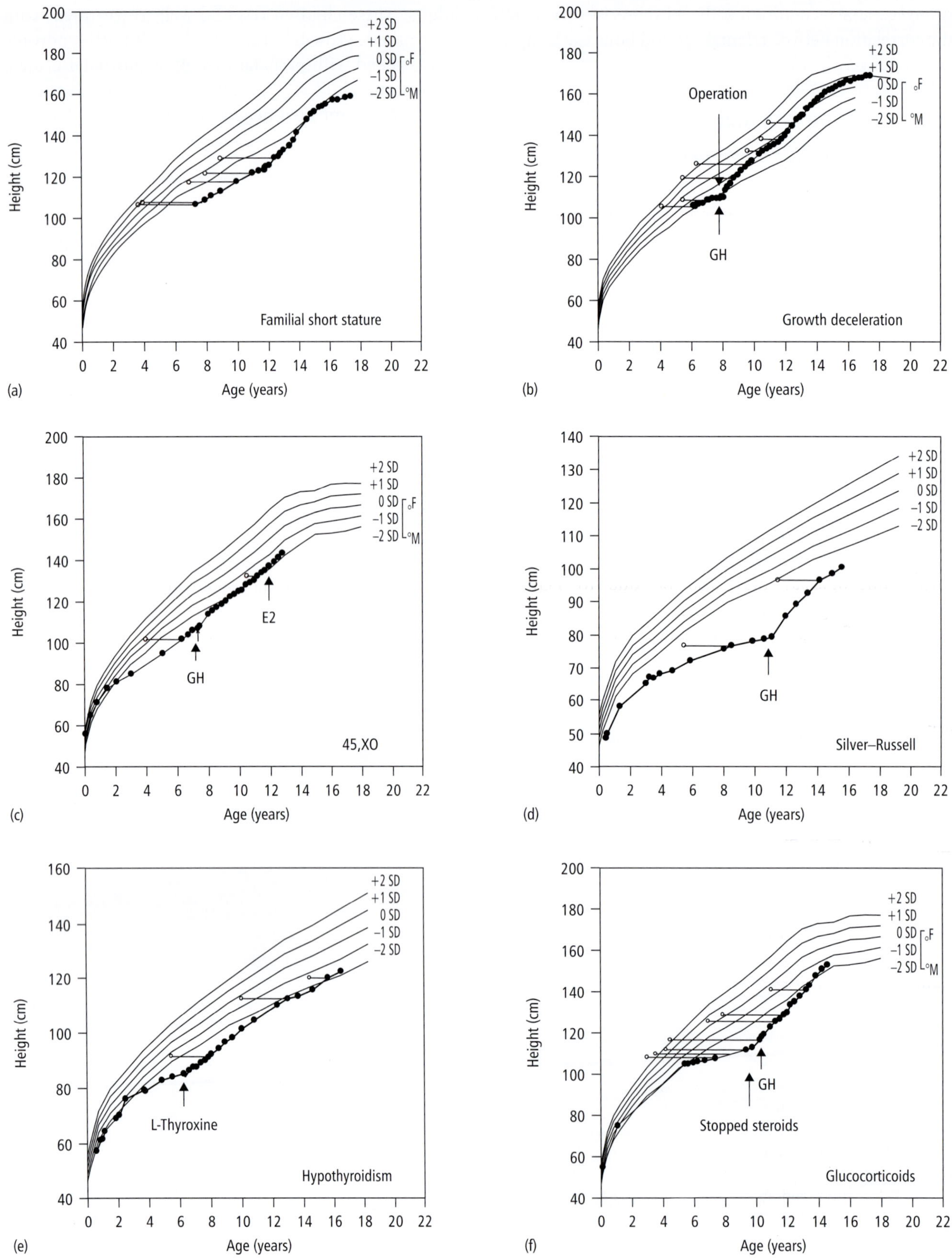

(a)
Height (cm)
Age (years)
+2 SD
+1 SD
0 SD
−1 SD
−2 SD
F
M
Familial short stature
(b)
Height (cm)
Age (years)
Operation
GH
Growth deceleration
(c)
Height (cm)
Age (years)
GH
E2
45,XO
(d)
Height (cm)
Age (years)
GH
Silver–Russell
(e)
Height (cm)
Age (years)
L-Thyroxine
Hypothyroidism
(f)
Height (cm)
Age (years)
GH
Stopped steroids
Glucocorticoids

Figure 2-8

of inhaled steroids may have a growth inhibitory effect (Fig. 2-8f).

Hormonal insufficiencies such as growth hormone deficiency (Fig. 2-8b) or hypothyroidism (Fig. 2-8e) and Cushing's syndrome typically present with stunting of growth. Likewise, chromosomal aberrations such as Turner syndrome in girls (45,X) (Fig. 2-8c), genetic syndromes such as Silver–Russell syndrome (Fig. 2-8d) or Noonan syndrome are well-known etiologies for postnatal growth failure. Also severe neglect or abuse may induce growth retardation (psychosocial dwarfism).

Importantly, skeletal dysplasias can cause severe stunting of growth. In this case, body proportions are skewed as in the typical case of achondroplasia. Achondroplasia is the most frequent form of short-limb dwarfism. Affected individuals exhibit short stature caused by rhizomelic shortening of the limbs, characteristic facies with frontal bossing and midface hypoplasia, exaggerated lumbar lordosis, limitation of elbow extension, genu varum, and trident hand. Achondroplasia is caused by mutation in the fibroblast growth factor receptor-3 gene (FGFR-3). There is some evidence to suggest that a minor fraction of the milder forms of skeletal dysplasias (hypochondroplasia) may also be due to FGFR-3 mutations. A large number of different skeletal dysplasias can be classified according to clinical and radiological criteria (Table 2-1).

Table 2-1 Short-limbed conditions and adult height (cm)

Condition	Adult height (cm)
Achondroplasia	106–142
Hypochondroplasia	132–147
Diastrophic dysplasia	86–122
Pseudoachondroplasia	80–130
Metaphyseal dysplasia	
McKusick type	105–145
Schmid type	130–160
Chondrodysplasia punctata	130–160
Chondroectodermal dysplasia	106–153
Acromesomelic dysplasia	97–123
Pyknodysostosis	130–150

Tall stature and growth acceleration

Tall stature is today socially more accepted, and some studies indicate that tall people may have higher social success and better job prospects. However, for some individuals, extreme tall stature may still present a major disadvantage and give numerous practical problems (Fig. 2-9).

Most cases are familial (Fig. 2-9F), but rare diseases may also be the underlying cause. Supernumerary sex chromosomes, such as Klinefelter syndrome (47,XXY) (Fig. 2-9a), the most common sex chromosome abnormality (1:660 newborns), triple X (47,XXX) and double Y syndrome (47,XYY) (Fig. 2-9b) are all characterized by increased growth compared to the reference population, as well as compared to their genetic target. Endocrine disorders, such as gigantism (growth hormone hypersecretion because of pituitary tumor) (Fig. 2-9c), are extremely rare, but should be excluded. Other genetic conditions such as Marfan syndrome (long limbs with narrow hands and long slender fingers, and arm span greater than height), Soto syndrome (prominent forehead, large ears and mandibles, and coarse facial features) and homocysteinuria may be found among patients referred because of tall stature.

Tall stature must be distinguished from conditions with temporary growth acceleration that do not lead to increased final height, such as obesity (Fig. 2-9d) in childhood, hyperthyroidism, and early sexual maturation (Fig. 2-9e). These children will deviate upwards on their growth chart, but their accelerated bone maturation will at the same time lead to premature fusion of the growth plates.

If the estimated final height is unacceptable to the child and family, gender-specific treatment with sex hormones to accelerate closure of the epiphyseal plates is an available option. This can be done either by induction

Figure 2-8 (opposite) Illustrative growth curves of children with growth failure. (a) A child with familial short stature who has a subnormal predicted adult height in accordance with the short genetic height potential and retarded bone age. (b) A child with growth deceleration due to the development of a benign brain tumor, which was diagnosed and operated upon. Following the operation, growth hormone (GH) therapy was started and a normal final height was obtained. (c) A girl with Turner syndrome diagnosed in late childhood because of growth failure and a height at diagnosis below genetic height potential. Growth hormone treatment results in growth acceleration, and at age 12 years puberty induction was initiated by low-dose estradiol treatment. (d) Prenatal and postnatal growth failure in a girl diagnosed with Silver–Russell syndrome before and after initiation of growth hormone therapy which results in marked catch-up growth. (e) A girl with deceleration of growth from 2 to 3 years of age concomitantly with constipation. She was diagnosed with acquired hypothyroidism and substituted with L-thyroxine which normalized growth. (f) Marked stunting of growth from 5 years of age and delayed bone age in a girl who was erroneously treated with high-dose inhalation steroids despite the fact that she no longer had asthma. Cessation of therapy accompanied by growth hormone therapy resulted in marked catch-up growth.

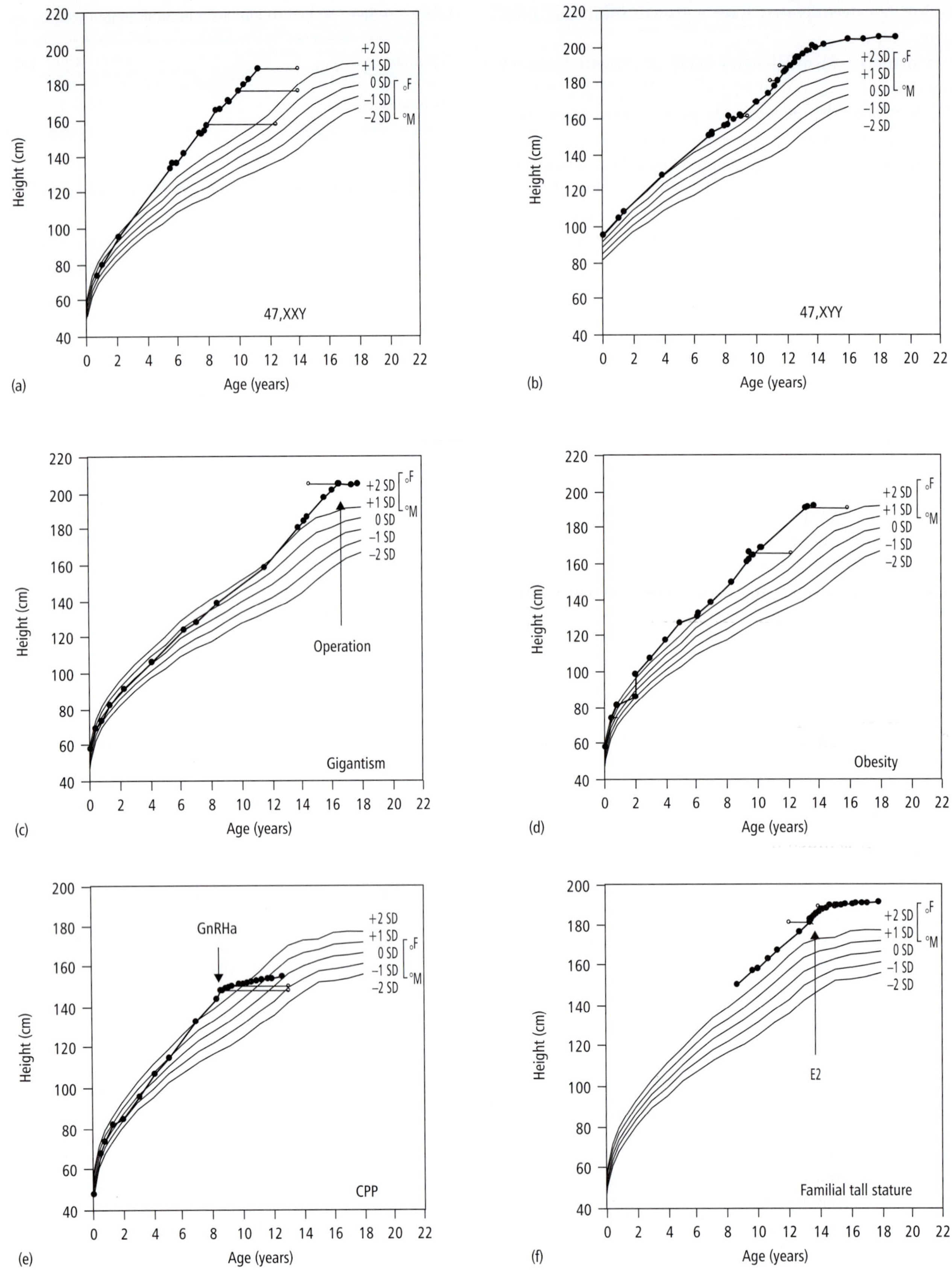
(a)
Height (cm)
Age (years)
+2 SD
+1 SD
0 SD
−1 SD
−2 SD
F
M
47,XXY
(b)
47,XYY
(c)
Operation
Gigantism
(d)
Obesity
(e)
GnRHa
CPP
(f)
E2
Familial tall stature

Figure 2-9

of early pubertal maturation or by addition of sex hormone during spontaneous puberty to shorten the pubertal growth spurt.

Early puberty

Early pubertal maturation is much more frequently seen in girls than boys. There are indications that true precocious puberty before the age of 8 years in girls and before the age of 9 years in boys is becoming more frequent in many populations. Foreign adopted children seem to be at greatest risk. There also appears to be a genetic component, as some families present with early puberty over several generations. In girls, early puberty often presents as an idiopathic premature activation of the hypothalamus–pituitary axis and is rarely caused by diseases. Conditions such as intracranial tumors, hydrocephalus, autonomous sex hormone production (gonadal tumors), and disorders of steroid biosynthesis such as congenital adrenal hyperplasia need to be excluded, especially in boys. It is possible to postpone further pubertal development until a more appropriate age by treatment with long-acting gonadotropin agonists. This treatment can be useful for children who have difficulties in coping with the psychological effects of early maturation or in very short children, in whom predicted final height is extremely low. Paradoxically, these children are usually referred at a time of pubertal growth acceleration, and therefore present with a height in excess of their peers. Parents are usually unaware of the fact that they may end up being very short (Fig. 2-9e).

Late puberty

Late puberty is much more frequently seen in boys than girls as an extreme of the natural gender dimorphism. In most cases, it is a simple delay of maturation without any underlying pathology. Family history may reveal inheritance from one or both parents as a constitutional delay of growth in puberty. These children usually present with short stature compared to their age-matched friends, lack of secondary sexual characteristics, a growth curve that shows deviation downwards with time and delayed bone age. In rare cases, delayed puberty is caused by endocrine disorders such as gonadotropin or pituitary insufficiency or developmental disorders of the gonads. Excessive sporting activities and eating disorders can also cause significant delay in physical maturation. In girls, delayed puberty may be caused by a chromosomal disorder, such as Turner syndrome (45,X).

If no pathology is found, simple reassurance may be the only treatment necessary. Delayed puberty itself does not lead to short final height. If puberty is delayed beyond acceptable limits for the child, treatment with low-dose sex hormones for 6–12 months may help to 'kickstart' the process.

Disorders with deviations in dental maturity

Many children with postnatal growth failure also show delay in dental maturity, e.g., growth hormone deficiency. Likewise most patients with Soto syndrome show advanced dental maturity. Thus, the dentist should be aware of the oral manifestations of general diseases and, thereby, contribute to early diagnosis (see Chapter 22).

Conclusion

Prenatal and postnatal growth reflects the general health status of an individual. Growth charts are easy to obtain, noninvasive, and cheap. Many countries offer health services that allow the longitudinal follow-up of height and weight attainment, together with an evaluation of puberty progression in teenage years. Pathological growth charts and a bone age that deviates significantly from chronological age can be the first indicators of a serious underlying condition that needs attention. Thus, knowledge about normal and abnormal growth patterns in children and adolescents is necessary for all medical personnel that are involved in their health care. In addition, the pediatric dentist should be aware of the fact that marked deviations in dental maturity could be part of a general growth problem.

Figure 2-9 (opposite) Illustrative growth curves of children with tall stature and growth acceleration. (a) A boy with marked growth acceleration from early childhood who was diagnosed with Klinefelter syndrome (47,XXY). He will end up above his target height despite advanced bone age. (b) A boy with growth acceleration from early childhood who was diagnosed with YY syndrome (47,XYY) who will end up with increased final height. (c) A boy with growth acceleration from 10 to 12 years of age who was diagnosed with gigantism and operated on for his growth hormone-producing pituitary adenoma. (d) A boy with growth acceleration and who was obese (simple obesity) who will end up with a final height within his target range, probably because of his advanced bone age. (e) Increased growth in a girl who presented with precocious puberty (regular menstruation at the age of 9 years), and markedly advanced bone age. She will end up with a final height at the lower end of her target range. (f) A girl with familial tall stature and delayed puberty who was treated with high-dose estrogen to accelerate epiphyseal fusion. Despite this, she reached a final height above target range.

References

1. Bayley N, Pinneau S. Tables for predicting adult height from skeletal age. *J Pediatr* 1952;**14**:423–41.
2. Demirjian A. Dentition. In: Falkner F, Tanner JM, eds. *Human growth.* London: Baillière Tindall, 1982.
3. Greulich WW, Pyle SI, Waterhouse AM. *A radiographic standard of reference for the growing hand and wrist.* Chicago, IL: Case Western Reserve University, 1971.
4. Haavikko K. Tooth formation age estimated on a few selected teeth. A simple method for clinical use. *Proc Finn Dent Soc* 1974;**70**:15–19.
5. Hertel T, Scheike T, Juul A, Main KM, Holm K, Bach-Mortensen N, *et al.* Body proportions of Danish children. Curves for sitting height ratio, subischial length and arm span. *Ugeskr Laeger* 1995;**157**:6876–81.
6. Juul A, Teilmann G, Scheike T, Hertel NT, Holm K, Laursen EM, *et al.* Pubertal development in Danish children: comparison of recent European and US data. *Int J Androl* 2006;**29**:247–55.
7. Karlberg J. A biologically-oriented mathematical model, (ICP) for human growth. *Acta Paediatr Scand Suppl* 1989;**350**:70–94.
8. Marsal K. Intrauterine growth restriction. *Curr Opin Obstet Gynecol* 2002;**14**:127–35.
9. Marshall WA, Tanner JM. Variations in the pattern of pubertal changes in girls. *Arch Dis Child* 1969;**44**:291–303.
10. Marshall WA, Tanner JM. Variations in the pattern of pubertal changes in boys. *Arch Dis Child* 1970;**45**:13–23.
11. Niklasson A, Ericon A, Fryer JG, Karlberg J, Lawrence C, Karlberg P. An update of the Swedish reference standards for weight, length and head circumference at birth for given gestational age (1977–1981). *Acta Paediatr Scand* 1991;**80**:756–62.
12. Tanner JM, Whitehouse RH, Cameron N, Marshall WA, Healhy MJR, Godtstein H. *Assessment of skeletal maturity and prediction of adult height,* 2nd edn. London: Academic Press, 1983.
13. Tanner JM, Whitehouse RH. Clinical longitudinal standards for height, weight, height velocity, weight velocity, and stages of puberty. *Arch Dis Child* 1976;**51**:170–9.
14. WHO Multicentre Growth Reference Study Group. Child growth standards based on length/height, weight and age. *Acta Paediatr Scand* 2006;**450**:76–85.

3

Child and adolescent psychological development

Anders G. Broberg and Gunilla Klingberg

Evidence has been accumulated over the past few decades to show that if dentists have a basic knowledge of children's cognitive and socioemotional development, then they will be much better prepared for any difficult situations that may emerge. The aim of this chapter is to provide the reader with an overview into the essentials of developmental psychology. It will describe those aspects of normal development that are useful for dentists treating "normal" children of different ages. We use the term children for the age range 0–12 years, and the term adolescents for children between 13 and 18. For the 0–12 range we make a further division into infancy (0–1), toddlerhood (2–3), preschool years (4–5) and the school years (6–12).

The chapter starts with an overview of how to conceptualize psychological development, it then follows with more focused aspects relating to cognitive, emotional, and social development in preschoolers, school-aged children, and adolescents. Finally, we present those aspects of the field of *developmental psychopathology* that we find most useful to pediatric dentistry.

Perspectives on psychological development

Long before developmental psychologists began to use scientific methods to study age-related changes, philosophers proposed explanations of development based on everyday observations. Many of their questions and assertions about the nature of human development continue to be central to modern-day developmental science.

The argument about nature versus nurture is one of the oldest and most central theoretical issues within both psychology and philosophy. Recently, biology in general and molecular biology in particular have made great progress. This has led to a heated debate with regard to how psychological development, and especially individual differences, can be explained by genetic differences (i.e., nature) rather than by environmental input from family, peers, and the society at large (i.e., nurture). In the section "Developmental psychopathology" we will return to the current way of addressing this issue.

A biopsychosocial approach

Human life is produced by the interaction and modification of three major systems: biological, psychological, and social. It is the integration of these systems that leads to a complex, dynamic portrait of human thought and behavior.

The *biological system* is made up of all the processes necessary for the psychological functioning of the organism. Biological processes develop and change as a consequence of genetically guided maturation, environmental resources, exposure to environmental toxins, encounters with accidents and diseases, and lifestyle patterns of behavior.

The *psychological system* consists of mental processes central to a person's ability to make meaning of experiences and take action. Emotion, motivation, memory, perception, problem solving, language, symbolic abilities, and our orientation to the future, all require the use of psychological processes. The psychological system provides the resources for processing information and navigating reality.

The *social system* is composed of processes through which a person becomes integrated into society. Societal influences include family organization; social support; culture; social roles; ethnic and subcultural influences; patterns of economic prosperity or poverty; and exposure to racism, sexism, and other forms of discrimination, to name only a few. The impact of the social system on psychological development results largely from interpersonal relationships, often relationships with significant others.

The biopsychosocial approach seeks to understand the internal experiences that are the product of interactions among biological, psychological, and social processes. Changes in one of the systems generally bring about changes in the others. At each period of life, children and adolescents spend much of their time mastering a unique group of *developmental tasks* that are essential for social adaptation. Solutions of developmental tasks will set children on different developmental trajectories with consequences for how future tasks will be solved. The importance of introducing time as a powerful ingredient in the interaction between the biological, psychological, and social systems has called for a new concept, the *transactional model of child development*.

Meaning is created out of efforts to interpret and integrate the experiences of the biological, psychological, and social systems. A primary focus of this meaning-making is the search for identity. Children and adolescents establish categories that define who they are connected to or not, who they care or do not care about, and who they admire or reject or deny.

With this broad introduction to developmental science as the psychologist sees it, we now turn to more narrow aspects of child and adolescent development.

Aspects of psychological development

Child development is most often described using either a variable- or a person-based approach. A variable-based approach divides child development into components: cognitive, emotional, social, etc., and describes the development of each component through childhood and adolescence. The person-based approach describes what is typical for a child of a certain age, whether preschooler, school-aged child, or adolescent, using a number of components simultaneously. Both approaches have their advantages and disadvantages and the choice is more a matter of taste. No matter what, a child's development is not divided into tidy packages labeled "physical development", "social development", and "language development" but is instead a coherent, integrated process. Nevertheless we will start by taking a look at particular processes and end with a more holistic approach.

Cognitive development

Cognition is the process of organizing and making meaning out of experience. Cognitive developmental theory focuses specifically on how knowing emerges and is transformed into logical, systematic capacities for reasoning and problem solving. Perhaps the most widely known and influential of the modern cognitive theorists is Jean Piaget (20). Recent interest in the social framework within which cognition develops has been stimulated by the work of Lev Vygotsky (28).

Cognitive development according to Jean Piaget

According to Piaget (1896–1980), every organism strives to achieve equilibrium: a balance of organized structures (motor, sensory, or cognitive). When structures are in equilibrium they provide effective ways of interacting with the environment. Equilibrium is achieved through adaptation; a process of gradually modifying existing ways of organizing knowledge in order to take into account changes and discrepancies between what is known and what is being experienced. Adaptation is a two-part process in which continuity and change interact. *Assimilation*, the tendency to interpret new experiences in terms of existing mental structures (schemas), contributes to the continuity of knowing, and it is balanced by *accommodation*, the tendency to modify familiar schemas in order to account for new dimensions of the object or event that are revealed through experience.

Piaget described cognitive development in terms of four stages, each of which is characterized by a unique capacity for organizing and interpreting information. At each new stage competencies of the earlier stages are not lost but are integrated into a qualitatively new approach to thinking and knowing.

The first stage, *sensorimotor intelligence*, is characterized by the formation of increasingly complex sensory and motor schemas that allow infants to organize and exercise control over their environment.

During the second stage, *preoperational thought*, children develop the tools for representing schemas symbolically through language, imitation, imagery, symbolic play, and symbolic drawing. Knowledge is, however, still very much tied to the child's perceptions.

During the third stage, *concrete operational thought*, children begin to appreciate the logical necessity of certain causal relationships. They can manipulate categories, classification systems, and hierarchies in groups. They are more successful at solving problems that are clearly tied to physical reality than at generating hypotheses about purely philosophical or abstract concepts.

The final stage of cognitive development according to Piaget is *formal operational thought*. This level of thinking permits a person to conceptualize many simultaneously interacting variables. It allows for the creation of systems of laws, or rules that can be used for problem solving. Formal operational thought reflects the quality of intelligence on which science and philosophy are built.

Piaget's theory has had an enormous influence on our understanding of cognition and the way we think about the reasoning capacities of children and adolescents. Some of this can be summarized as:

- Cognition has its base in the biological capacities of the human infant: knowledge is derived from action. Knowledge is constructed rather than passively absorbed.
- Discrepancies between existing schemas and contemporary experience promote cognitive development. Encounters with all types of novelty, especially experiences that are moderately distinct rather than widely different from what is already known, are important for advancing new ideas and new ways of organizing thought.
- Preschoolers and school-aged children (not to mention infants and toddlers) think in different ways, and the ways they think are different from the ways (older) adolescents and adults think. This does not mean that their thinking is unorganized or illogical, but the same principles of logic that typically govern adult thought do not govern the thinking of young children.
- Children can approach problems using many of the principles that are fundamental to scientific reasoning. They can also begin to reason about their reasoning (e.g., explain how they arrived at a specific conclusion), but it takes formal operational thought to grasp and make use of meta-cognition (i.e., thinking about thinking) in its more eloquent aspects.

Appearance and reality

The child's movement away from egocentrism during the preschool years seems to be part of a much broader change in his/her understanding of appearance and reality. Flavell (16) has studied this in a variety of ways. In one procedure the experimenter shows a child a sponge that has been painted to resemble a rock. After the child has felt the sponge/rock and has answered questions about what it looks like and what it "really" is, a researcher might ask something like this:

> "John [one of the child's play-mates] hasn't touched this, he hasn't squeezed it. If John just sees it over here like this, what will he think it is? Will he think it is a rock or will he think it is a sponge?"
>
> "A sponge" says 3-year-old Minnie, who thinks that the playmate will believe the object is a sponge, because she herself knows it is a sponge.
>
> "A rock" says 4-year-old Ken, who realizes that, because John hasn't felt the sponge, he will have a false belief that it is a rock.

Investigators have also asked whether the child can grasp the *false belief principle.* Individuals who understand the false belief principle can look at a problem or situation from another person's point of view in order to discern what kind of information can cause that person to believe something that is not true. In the past, a number of developmentalists have examined a theoretical notion known as *theory of mind*, or a set of concepts that explain other people's ideas, beliefs, desires, and behavior (16). Adults and adolescents have a much more fully developed theory of mind than have children. However, research also suggests that young children's degree of sophistication is greater than either Piaget or casual observers of children would expect, and that there are big individual differences with regard to when and how children's mentalizing abilities develop.

Children's development of a theory of mind shows that cognitive development is a relational process. The child learns to conceptualize the world around him or her by communicating with others. That cognitive development is an interpersonal endeavor is the hallmark of Vygotsky's theory.

Cognitive development according to Vygotsky

The Russian psychologist Lev Vygotsky (1896–1934) argued that development can only be understood within a social framework. New levels of understanding begin at an interpersonal level as two individuals, initially an infant and an adult, coordinate their interactions. Further, Vygotsky claimed that cognitive development can only be understood in the context of culture, and that high-level mental functions begin in external activity that is gradually reconstructed and internalized. He gave the example of pointing.

Initially, an infant will reach toward an object that is out of reach, stretching the hand in the direction of the object and making grasping movements with the fingers. As soon as the caregiver recognizes that the child wants the object and is able to satisfy the child's request, the child begins to modify the reaching and grasping movement into a socially meaningful gesture – pointing. The individual grasping has become an interpersonal communication gesture, and the child has internalized an understanding of the special relationship between the desired goal, the caregiver as mediator, and pointing as a meaningful sign.

According to Vygotsky, a child's learning of new cognitive skills is guided by an adult (or a more skilled child, such as an older sibling), who models and structures the child's learning experience, a process later called *scaffolding.* Vygotsky (28) offered the concept of the *zone of proximal development,* which is the discrepancy between how difficult a problem (e.g., in math) a child can solve on his or her own relative to solving a problem under adult guidance or in collaboration with capable peers. Learning within the zone of proximal development sets into motion the reorganization and internalization of existing developmental competencies, which then become synthesized at a new, higher intra-mental level.

Several specific implications of Vygotsky's work can be inferred (15), of which at least three are of relevance for understanding child development in relation to dentistry:

- The mental structures and functioning of people raised in a specific culture will be different from those of people raised in other cultures. In contrast to Piaget, who viewed the emergence of logical thought as largely a universal process, Vygotsky considered the nature of reasoning and problem solving as culturally created.
- Individuals can promote their own cognitive development by seeking interactions with others who can help draw them to higher levels of functioning within their zone of proximal development.
- Teachers, whether formal or informal (like parents or dental personnel), must navigate their "lessons" so that they can scaffold the child's learning within his or her zone of proximal development.

Adaptation, according to Piaget, or learning, according to Vygotsky, is effective only when the input is new (i.e., different from existing knowledge) but related enough to existing knowledge (i.e., within the zone of proximal development) to permit accommodation rather than assimilation (Piaget) and the building of more elaborate mental structures (Vygotsky) (Box 3-1).

Box 3-1

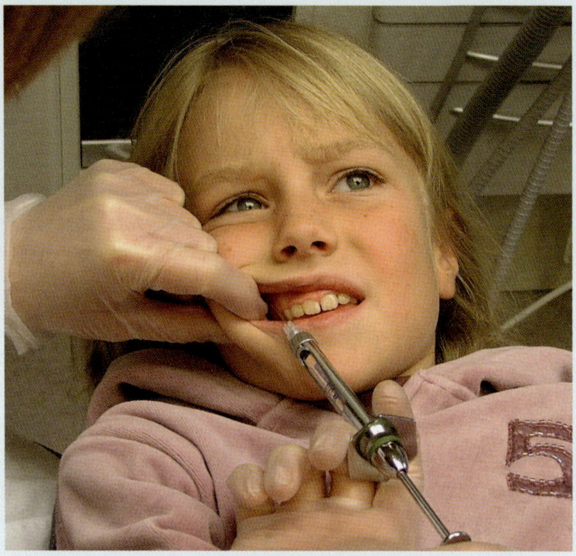

Children's understanding of the concept of pain and the need for local anesthesia varies considerably with age and cognitive development. First of all both are abstract phenomena. The preschool child's connotations to pain could be punishment or guilt. He or she does not understand the physical background of the pain. Also, local anesthesia is hard to grasp and the child is not capable of deciding whether to have an injection or not. Even if a preschool child receives good and age-appropriate information about these concepts and then declines local anesthesia when asked, he or she is not able to understand the cause and effect if feeling pain during treatment. While an adult would reason "I have to blame myself for experiencing pain as I did not want the local", the child understands this differently. He or she will probably just blame the dentist for hurting him or her. Because of this, it is obligatory when treating young patients that the dentist makes sure treatment is as free from pain as possible, and to use local anesthesia on proper indications. Since dental treatment implies some level of stress, the child needs to master more advanced reasoning to fully understand pain and how to prevent it during dental treatment. Therefore, as a rule of thumb, the decision whether to have local anesthesia or not should only be left to teenagers. It is not until adolescence, and being able to think at the level of formal operations, that the child can take full responsibility for pain if declining an injection.

Language development

Somewhere between 16 and 24 months, after an early period of very slow word learning (12–18 months typically), most children begin to add new words rapidly, as if they have figured out that things have names. For the majority of children, the naming explosion is not a steady, gradual process; instead, a vocabulary spurt begins once the child has acquired about 50 words. Noun learning precedes verb learning because infants lack the ability to associate words consistently with actions until about 18 months of age. During the preschool years, children continue to add words at a remarkable speed. At age 2½, the average vocabulary is about 600 words, about a quarter of which are verbs (2), and most children at this age are equipped with a language capacity that also enables them to begin to communicate verbally with unfamiliar adults, provided that (a) the adult adapts his or her way of speaking to the child's level of cognitive understanding, and (b) the emotional contact is such that the child feels free to talk. By age 5 or 6, total vocabulary has risen to perhaps 15,000 words – an astonishing increase of 10 words per day. The momentous shift in the way children approach new words happens around the age of 3 years. Understanding the categorical nature of words helps children develop what we might think of as mental "slots" for new words. Once the slots are in place, children seem to organize automatically the linguistic input they receive from parents, teachers, peers, books, television programs, and other sources to extract new words and fill the slots as quickly as possible.

Even though most children are reasonably fluent in their first language by the age of 3 or 4 years, there are still many refinements to be made. Soon after young children have figured out inflections and basic sentence forms, such as negation and questions, they begin to create remarkably complex sentences, using conjunctions such as *and* and *but* to combine two ideas or using embedded clauses. During middle childhood, children become skilled at managing the finer points of grammar, such as understanding various ways of saying something about the past (I went, I was going, I have gone, I had gone, I had been going, etc.).

Children use language not only for communication with others, but also for "internal purposes" – to help control or monitor their own behavior. Such *private speech*, which may consist of fragmentary sentences, muttering, or instructions to the self, is detectable from the earliest use of words and sentences (Box 3-2).

Box 3-2

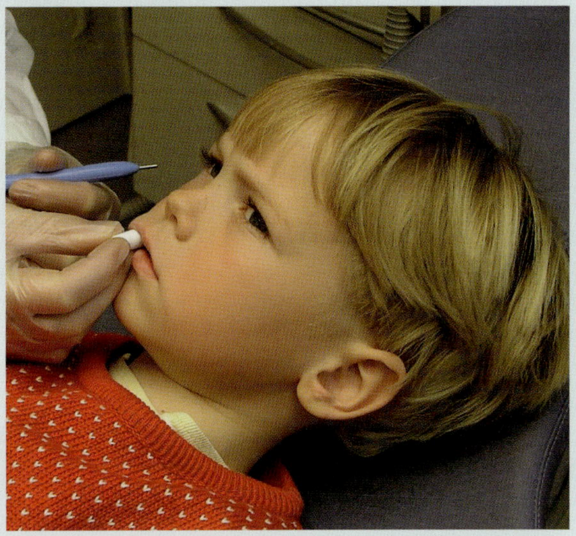

Peter, 7 years old, is having fissure sealants placed on his first permanent molars. This is the first real treatment for Peter and he is a bit cautious. At the previous appointment the dentist told him what was going to happen today and also promised to show everything step by step as the treatment progresses. The first tooth is fixed satisfactorily. And when the dental team is about to isolate the second tooth with cotton roles Peter says to himself: "lie still and open wide, this will not take long".

Emotional development

Emotions, for example, fear, sadness, anger, and joy, are part of a complex set of interconnected feelings, thoughts, and behaviors. Plutchik (21) conceptualized emotions as part of a feedback system; a stimulus, which could be an internal experience, such as pain, or an external stimulus, such as a looming object, is perceived and given some meaning. The meaning is associated with a feeling and with its accompanying physiological state. These combine to create an impulse for action that, if expressed, is observed in behavior. Two aspects of emotions that are of special interest for this chapter are temperament and emotional regulation.

Temperament

Temperament is a theoretical construct that refers to relatively stable characteristics of response to the environment and patterns of self-regulation (22). Theorists have offered different views about the specific features of temperament and what accounts for the stability of these features. However, they all tend to agree that a primary feature of temperament is the child's positive or negative reaction to environmental events, and that the stability of this reaction leads to a patterned reaction by others (27).

As early as the 1950s Thomas *et al.* (26) studied temperament and were able to classify infants into three temperamental groupings: *easy*, *slow to warm up*, and *difficult*. Roughly 35% of the sample could not be classified into any of these categories (Table 3-1).

Later work on temperament identified activity level, sociability, and negative emotionality as traits with a substantial genetic influence (7). Kagan and co-workers (17) have identified *behavioral inhibition* as a relatively

Table 3-1 Different types of early temperaments according to Thomas *et al*. (26)

Type	Description	Percentage of sample
Easy	Positive mood, regular body functions, low to moderate intensity of reaction, adaptability, positive approach rather than withdrawal from new situations	40
Slow to warm up	Low activity level, tendency to withdraw on first exposure to new stimuli, slow to adapt, somewhat negative in mood, low intensity of reactions to situations	15
Difficult	Irregular body functions, unusually intense reactions, tendency to withdraw from new situations, slow to adapt to change, generally negative mood	10

Adapted from (26).

stable temperamental trait which has been shown to be a vulnerability factor for the development of shyness and anxiety problems later in childhood.

Rothbart and Posner (23) have identified three broad temperamental factors in 3–7-year-old children: surgency/extraversion, negative affectivity, and effortful control. *Surgency* is primarily defined by positive emotionality and approach (including sensation-seeking, activity level, impulsivity, smiling and laughter, and low shyness). *Negative affectivity* involves shyness, discomfort, fear, anger/frustration, sadness, and low soothability. *Effortful control* is defined by high inhibitory control, attentional focusing, low-intensity (non-risk-taking) pleasure, and perceptual sensitivity.

To summarize, it makes sense to think of temperament as two basic processes:

- *Reactivity* – how easily aroused the child is, either positively or negatively. Both the very inhibited and the very impulsive child are highly reactive to environmental stimuli although his or her reactions have different origins in the brain and take very different forms.
- *Control* – how able the child is to handle his or her activated nervous system.

Both aspects of temperament are important in the dental situation, which for some children is packed with fear-eliciting stimuli from which one wants to escape, and for others with a number of exciting things one wants to explore. In both cases it will be difficult for the child to sit still and follow instructions. Temperament is closely linked to the concept of emotion regulation to which we turn in a moment. Let us, however, conclude with the aspect of stability in childhood temperament.

Although temperament shows consistency over the period of infancy and toddlerhood, it is in no way written in stone. Temperament is in fact only modestly stable over longer periods of time – the level of stability depending on culture, measurement techniques, and methods of analysis. Temperamental characteristics are modified as they come into contact with socialization pressures at home and at school, as well as with new capacities to regulate behavior. Whether it is temperament itself (in terms of a biological propensity) that changes, or if the child simply learns to "hide" or "suppress" aspects of his or her temperament that are not culturally sanctioned, is a question of debate.

Tim is a typical example of shyness in a young child and how this can manifest during a dental visit (Box 3-3). Other examples of temperament are active, speedy children who jump into the chair right away, and are eager to have their teeth checked. These children are very restless and seem to have very little time for conversation, which is why it is difficult to get through with information or instructions. There are also children who get upset very easily when feeling uncomfortable, for example, when the dentist uses the water suction. But if just given some extra attention, these children are often able to feel a lot more at ease and to cooperate well.

Box 3-3

Tim is a 3-year-old boy visiting the dentist for the first time. He is very cautious and does not respond with eye contact nor does he answer questions. He refuses to sit in the dental chair and to let the dentist have a look at his teeth. Tim has a sister who is 2 years older and who is also a patient at the clinic. She acted very much the same way when she was 3, but after careful introduction she now cooperates well. Both Tim and his sister spend their days at a day-care center. They function well in their peer groups, and play and have fun with friends, but have difficulties making new acquaintances. They are shy when meeting new people and it takes them quite a while to feel at ease in novel situations. In this case it is recommended that the dental team identifies the shyness and decides to use the first appointment to establish a good rapport and relationship with Tim and the accompanying parent. Tim is a child who needs extra time in order to feel at ease. If he is met with understanding and empathy combined with stepwise introduction to the dental examination, and to all new dental treatment in the future, he will most likely cooperate well.

Emotion regulation

Emotion regulation refers to a variety of processes that allow infants to control the intensity of their emotional state and reduce feelings of distress. These abilities, which mature over the first 2 years of life, have important implications for a child's successful social participation in preschool and later in childhood (8). One of the most important elements in the earliest development of emotion regulation is the way caregivers assist infants in managing strong feelings. Caregivers can provide direct support when they observe that a child is distressed: cuddling, hugging, rocking, or swaddling like a baby. They may offer food or a pacifier to the baby, or nurse him or her as a means of comfort. Through words and actions, the caregiver may help the child interpret the source of the stress, or suggest ways to reduce the stress.

There is a dramatic development during the infancy and toddler periods in terms of the acquisition and display of emotion regulation skills and abilities: the relatively passive and reactive infant becomes a child capable of self-initiated behaviors that serve regulatory functions

(24). Because the lack of adaptive emotion regulation skills may contribute to adjustment difficulties characterized by undercontrolled (i.e., acting-out) or overcontrolled (i.e., inhibited) emotion expressions, failure to acquire these skills may lead to difficulties in areas such as social competence and school adjustment. Children who have difficulty managing emotion in a flexible, constructive way may be less successful in negotiating peer relationships, or in managing academic challenges. Thus, the acquisition of adaptive emotion regulation skills and strategies is considered a critical achievement of early childhood (6,9). Moreover these skills may be linked in important ways to other dimensions of self-control or self-regulation that are also developing during early childhood (Box 3-4).

Developmental tasks

So far we have discussed different facets of child development as if they were separable. In reality they are not, and this section will introduce the principal concept used today to describe and understand child development and competency more broadly: *developmental tasks* (19).

Box 3-4

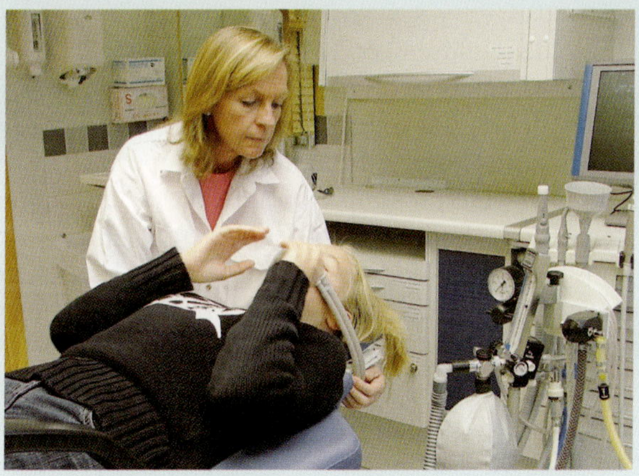

Dental treatment usually follows a well-known path, and most extractions of teeth are uneventful. However, from time to time things happen. The dentist may have just started to extract a tooth when suddenly the crown fractures and the dentist needs to do a small surgical treatment. Even though equally well informed in advance about the treatment procedure, children handle these new and unexpected situations differently. Some will just accept this as a matter of fact and cope well with what has to be done. Others can get very upset and the dentist will have to pay a lot of attention to the patient, comforting, informing, and so on, before treatment can be continued. In some cases it might even be impossible to proceed with the treatment right away or without use of sedation.

How do we know that a child is developing OK? There is a set of criteria common across many parents, communities, cultures, and measures that reflect major tasks of adaptation spanning development and the key criteria by which adjustment in society is assessed. Table 3-2 indicates psychosocial tasks of childhood and adolescence commonly found in textbooks on child development.

These developmental tasks reflect several broad domains of competence in the environment and, within each domain, a developmental progression. One fundamental domain is *conduct* (how well one follows the rules). Early in childhood, children are expected to begin controlling their behavior and complying with parental directives. Later, as they enter school, they are expected to learn and follow the rules for classroom conduct and refrain from striking out at people in a disagreement. By adolescence, they are expected to follow the rules of schools, home, and society without direct supervision. By middle childhood, *academic achievement* is an important domain of success for children in many societies; it continues to be important in adolescence, with the quality of expected performance continually rising. *Getting*

Table 3-2 Examples of developmental tasks

Age period	Task
Infancy to preschool	Attachment to caregiver(s) Language Differentiation of self from environment Self-control and compliance
Middle childhood	School adjustment (attendance, appropriate conduct) Academic achievement (e.g., learning to read, do arithmetic) Getting along with peers (acceptance, making friends) Rule-governed conduct (following rules of society for moral behavior and social conduct)
Adolescence	Successful transition to secondary schooling Academic achievement (learning skills needed for higher education or work) Involvement in extracurricular activities (e.g., sports, clubs) Forming close friendships within and across gender Forming a cohesive sense of self; identity

Adapted from (19).

along with other children becomes a salient domain by middle childhood, initially in terms of peer acceptance and later in terms of developing friendships and romantic relationships. Within the individual, the *self-domain* is the most common task arena, first in the form of differentiating one's self from the environment and later in terms of identity and autonomy.

Developmental tasks reflect both universal human phenomena in development, such as attachment to caregivers and language, as well as more culturally or historically specific tasks. School achievement, for example, is salient in many cultures, but not in all. Individual identity as a task may have more prominence in cultures that emphasize individualism and autonomy compared to those that emphasize community and belonging.

Deciding whether a child is competent can be difficult when a child lives in a cultural or community context that differs markedly from the larger society in which the community or ethnic group is embedded. Children may live in highly dangerous inner-city neighborhoods where survival could depend on behavior viewed as inappropriate in mainstream society.

Rapidly expanding knowledge about early child development indicates the importance of the early childhood years as a foundation for later competence. The early development of motor skills, language, self-confidence, play, and problem-solving abilities, for example, are highly relevant for understanding competence in the school years. Underlying these capabilities is a developing brain. Recent studies of humans and other species have made it clear that the brain is profoundly responsive to experience.

Motivational systems are also central to human competence. Babies are delighted by exercising new-found skills, like blowing bubbles, making sounds, or dropping food from the high chair, whereas older children find pleasure in activities like singing nonsense songs, making jokes, solving puzzles, or riding a bike. There is a *mastery motivation* system inherent in our species, which is readily observable in the inclination of young children to actively engage with the environment and to experience pleasure (feelings of efficacy) from effective interactions. It is clear that children's beliefs about their own success affect their behavior.

Man is a social animal

Without others we do not develop the different skills that make us into human beings. Personal relationships are central to children's and adolescents' ability to tackle developmental tasks and challenges. Some of these relationships are more important than others. Attachment relations come first (4), and they set the stage for later relations to siblings, peers, adults outside the immediate family, etc.

Attachment theory

Although extremely vulnerable and dependent, newborn babies arrive in the world equipped with a sophisticated array of inbuilt behaviors designed to maximize their survival. Two of these behaviors, and the systems that underpin them, are the *attachment* and *exploratory* behavior systems. Like the offspring of other nomadic mammals, human babies need to learn not *where* to flee in times of danger but to *whom*. The exploratory and the attachment systems work like communicating vessels; when one is active the other is downregulated. When the child feels safe and knows that his attachment figure is available, the child's exploratory system is turned up, and the child is free to interact with the world around him and to incorporate new aspects of the world around him. When the toddler or preschooler encounters something that is experienced as threatening the attachment system is immediately activated; exploration halts and the child instead focuses on reuniting with her attachment figure as soon as possible (12). Over the first years of life most children learn to use their parent or parents as a *secure base* from which to explore the surrounding environment, and as a *safe haven* to return to in times of stress or danger.

The older children get, the more capable will they be in handling mildly stressful situations on their own. It is, however, important to keep in mind that this does not mean that attachment becomes less important as the child grows older, it simply means that the attachment system is less often activated. However, when activated it is just as stressful for older children or adolescents not to have their attachment needs met properly as it is for young children.

Depending largely on the characteristics of the caregiving environment, children vary in their capacity to use the parent as a secure base/safe haven. Technically this is referred to as children developing different attachment patterns (secure, avoidant, resistant, disorganized) (1,18). The caregiving experiences children have with their attachment figures will be stored in the brain as mental representations, schemas or, as they are called in attachment theory, *internal working models* of the child interacting with important others. These internal working models carry within them important information with regard to the caregiver (as trustworthy and reliable or as unpredictable or even worse as dangerous) as well as the children themselves (as worthy of love and respect, as one who has to rely on themselves, as helpless, or in the worst scenario as someone used to being scoffed at or mocked).

The reason why internal working models are important for this chapter is that they are used as "filters". Later encounters with adults outside the immediate family will be experienced through the "lens" of these early working models. Remember Piaget's concepts of assimilation and accommodation? Children use their existing knowledge of social encounters (based to a high degree on their interaction with attachment figures) to predict how unknown people will interact with them, *and* how they should interact with these people. The more negative caregiving experiences the child has had, the more likely he or she is to treat nice strangers as if they were mean and unreliable. For similar reasons, encounters with medical personnel with unfortunate endings prime the child in a negative way (Box 3-5).

Social ecology

Since the 1970s there has been a strong push to widen the scope from the parent–child dyad to the family at large as well as to the child and his or her family in the context of the wider social network. Urie Bronfenbrenner (5) was one of the key people in launching this area of research. He emphasized that a child grows up in a complex social environment (a *social ecology*) with a distinct cast of characters: sibling(s), parent(s), grandparents, day-care workers, teachers, peers, etc. And this cast is in turn embedded within a larger social context. The parents may or may not have jobs, jobs that they may like or dislike. Day-care environments vary greatly in terms of organization and quality, the family's social support system (grandparents, neighbors, friends) may be thin and fragile or it can be dense and reliable. Depending on the family's financial and social situation they may live in a well-to-do suburb, or in an inner-city or suburban area stricken by ethnic violence and crime, or anywhere in between.

One of the most important aspects of Bronfenbrenner's research was his discussion of what he called *social addresses.* Social addresses are, for example, low socioeconomic status, working-class family, alcoholic parent, immigrant family. Much early research in clinical psychology and child and adolescent psychiatry had shown that psychological ill-health is much more common in children living in families with "negative" social addresses. But, as Bronfenbrenner repeatedly stressed, a child's psychological health is not influenced by the social address in itself. Most children in poor or immigrant families develop just as good psychological health as children from more well-to-do families. It is only when the social address impinges on the parent's caregiving capacity that we expect psychological consequences to follow. Thus, as Bronfenbrenner has warned us, the social address is only statistically, *not* causally, related to the psychological outcome (e.g., psychological health). The clinician should always have this in mind, trying the best he or she can to treat each new patient or parent as an individual and not as a representative of a social group (Box 3-6).

Box 3-5

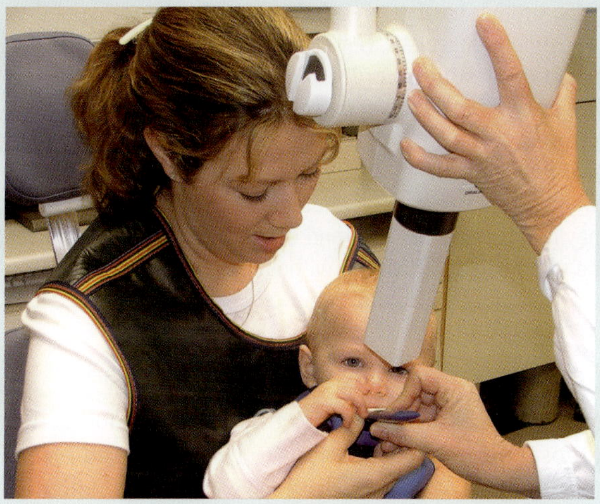

Typically children are cautious during their first dental visit and parents handle this in different ways. Many parents encourage their child to get acquainted with the novel situation by letting the child answer the questions from the dental team when possible; they praise the child's behavior, and make comforting comments. These parents function as a secure base from which the child makes expeditions. Other parents are quite the opposite. They answer all questions without giving the child even a chance, or they may literary cling to the child thereby restricting the possibility of the child being able to explore the dental operatory. Sometimes these different interaction patterns can already be observed when the child is in the waiting room. Some children are allowed to play freely, while others are more supervised, and sometimes even physically restrained, by their parents.

A holistic description of children of different ages

Let us end the description of normal development by trying to put the different pieces together. For the reader who wants to know more about children's psychological development there are a number of good textbooks in developmental psychology. The following holistic sketch of children of different ages is based on Helen Bee and Denise Boyd's *The developing child* (3).

The preschool years (3–5 years)

The main theme of the preschool period is that the child is making a slow, but immensely important shift in

Box 3-6

Ashif is a 6-year-old boy from an immigrant background who lives in a suburban area. He arrived as a refugee 2 years ago together with his mother, father, and two elder sisters. The family had to travel for quite a while and under hardship to get here but they now have a permit to stay. The parents have great difficulties understanding and speaking the language. The dentist expects to find a deteriorated oral health as she has seen before in many young patients with a background similar to that of Ashif. But the dental examination reveals healthy teeth and gums. Talking to Ashif and his accompanying parent she finds out that the family is very competent and motivated regarding oral hygiene and diet, and that they have very healthy habits.

balance with regard to how much and in which situations he or she depends on others, especially parents. The toddler, and later the preschooler, moves around easily, can communicate more (and more clearly), and has a growing sense of himself or herself as a separate person with specific qualities. He or she also has the beginning of cognitive and social skills that allow him or her to interact more fully and successfully with playmates. In these years, the child's thinking is decentering, to use Piaget's term: the child shifts from using himself or herself as the sole frame of reference and becomes less tied to physical appearances.

Among toddlers, newfound skills and new independence are often not accompanied by much impulse control. Two-year-olds in general are pretty good at doing, but they are terrible at *not* doing. If frustrated, they tend to hit things, and wail, scream, or shout. A large part of the conflict parents experience with children of this age arises because the parent must limit the child, not only for the child's own safety, but also to help teach the child emotional self-regulation. The preschool years also stand out as the period in which the seeds of the child's social skills and personality are sown (Box 3-7).

The attachment process that began in infancy continues to be formative, because it helps to shape the child's internal working model of social relationships. However, in the years from 2 to 6 the early model is continuously updated, for some children consolidated, for others revised and established more firmly. The resultant interaction patterns tend to persist into elementary school and beyond. The 3-, 4- or 5-year-old child who develops the ability to share, to read others' cues well, to respond positively to others, and to control aggression and impulsiveness is likely to be a socially successful, popular 8 year old (25). In contrast, the noncompliant, hostile preschooler is far more likely to become an unpopular, aggressive schoolchild (11).

Box 3-7

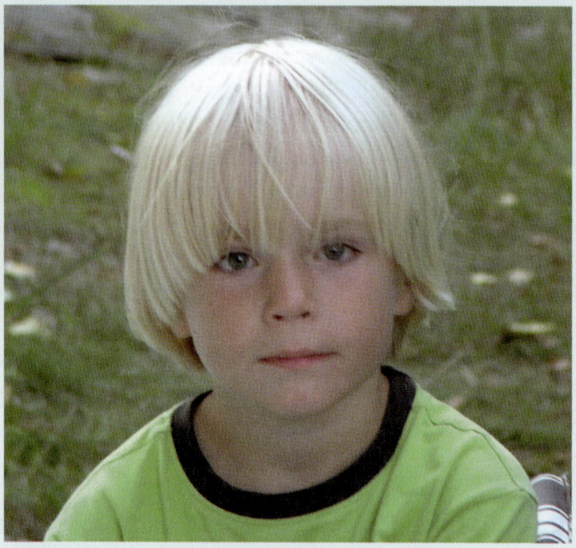

Joe is 4 years old and has just had a little sister. During weekdays he is at home with his mother, and usually sees children of his own age a couple of times every week. He likes playing with his friends, rides a three-wheeler and wants to have a two-wheel bike for his birthday. Becoming a big brother has been revolutionary; lots of jealousy and adjustment difficulties, but at the same time Joe is also very proud of his sister. In order to maintain his security and position with his mother he sometimes clings to her or wants to sit on her lap. During the dental visit he talks a lot and frequently asks for the names of the instruments and wants to know precisely what each is used for. He enjoys having his teeth checked, and cooperates well. His teeth can be examined and polished without any problems.

The elementary school years (6–12 years)

Some kind of transition into middle childhood is noted in most cultures. There seems to be widespread recognition that a 6-year-old child is somehow qualitatively different from a 4–5-year-old child: more responsible, and more able to understand complex ideas. The fact that schooling begins at this age in many cultures seems to reflect an implicit or explicit recognition of this fundamental shift. Cognitively, the child now understands, for example, conservation problems (that the amount of liquid is the same whether in a narrow and high container or in a wide and low). More generally, the child seems to be captured less by appearance, and instead focuses more on the underlying reality (i.e., pays less attention to surface properties of objects and more to underlying continuities and patterns). This can be seen not only in children's understanding of physical objects but also in their understanding of relationships and of themselves. In terms of self-concept, a global judgment

Box 3-8

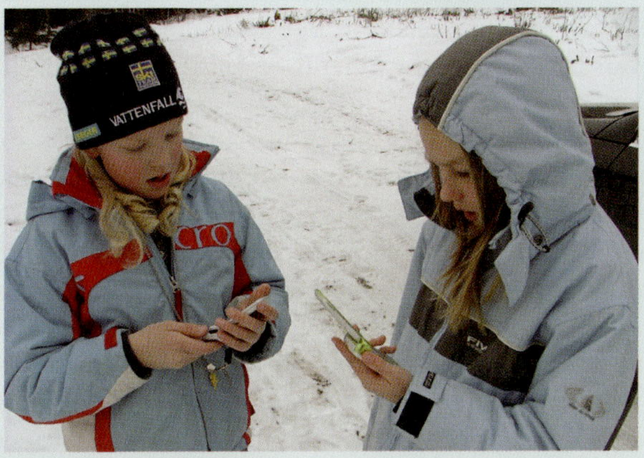

Sarah is 11 years old and spends most of her time with friends. When not together they chat on the Internet or send text messages to each other. She is doing all right in school, and is well aware of how her friends and classmates perform in different subjects. When seeing the dentist she is very talkative and eager to behave as she believes is expected of her. She has had a filling or two at a previous visit without any problems. Sarah has a deep cavity in a lower first molar. The filling therapy is carried out under local anesthesia without any problem and is much quicker than expected. As there is plenty of time left, the dentist suggests placing fissure sealants on two second upper molars that have just erupted. Sarah agrees to this. It turns out to be tricky to achieve good isolation for placing the sealants and suddenly Sarah is all in tears. In this case Sarah has already had a filling done, which was probably quite stressful. The filling was decided and agreed on beforehand, and was what Sarah had prepared herself for when she showed up. Sarah is typical of a child who wants to be a good patient, but not yet fully capable of saying no when the dentist suggests additional therapy even though she is not up to it. Apparently this was just too much for Sarah to handle. The dentist should not have suggested the sealant therapy. Instead the dentist should have stuck to the original agreement even though there was spare time for additional treatment.

of self-worth first emerges at about the age of 7 or 8 years. In most cultures gender segregation becomes the rule, especially in individual friendships, by age 6 or 7 years.

There seem to be two aspects of developmental processes at work in the elementary school years:

- Cognitive influences. Of the developmental shifts seen during middle childhood, the cognitive seem the most central, comprising a necessary condition for the alterations in relationships and in the self-scheme that also occur during this period. Similarly, the quality of a child's relationships with peers and parents seems to rest in part on a basic cognitive understanding of reciprocity and perspective taking. The child now understands that others read him or her as much as he or she reads them.
- Peer group influences. A great deal of a child's experiences at this age comes from social interactions with peers. Social relationships present the child with a unique set of demands, both cognitive and interactive, and have unique consequences for the child's social and emotional functioning. It is during the elementary school years, for example, that patterns of peer rejection or acceptance are consolidated, with reverberations through adolescence (and into adult life) (Box 3-8).

Adolescence (13–18 years)

Early adolescence, almost by definition, is a time of transition, of significant change in virtually every aspect of the child's functioning. Late adolescence is more a time of consolidation, when the teenager establishes a cohesive new identity, with clearer goals and commitments. Early adolescence is a time dominated by assimilation whereas late adolescence is primarily a time of accommodation, to use Piaget's terminology. The 12 or 13 year old is assimilating an enormous number of new physical, social, and intellectual experiences. While all this absorption is going on, but before the experiences have been digested, the child is in a more or less continuous state of disequilibrium. Old patterns, old schemes no longer work very well, but new ones have not yet been established. It is during this early period that the peer group is so centrally important. Ultimately, the 16, 17, or 18 year old begins to make the necessary accommodation, pulls the threads together, and establishes a new identity, new patterns of social relationships, new goals, and roles.

In some ways, the early years of adolescence have a lot in common with the toddler years. Many go through a period of negativism or sulkiness – from the parents' points of view strikingly similar to a 2 year old – right at the beginning of the pubertal changes. Many of the conflicts with parents center on issues of independence: to come and go when they please, listen to music they prefer (at maximum volume), and wear the clothing and hair style that are currently "in". As is true for the negativism of 2 year olds, it is easy to overstate the depth and/or breadth of the conflict between young teenagers and their parents. For the great majority there is no turmoil, but simply a temporary increase in the frequency of disagreements or disputes.

Drawing a parallel between young adolescents and toddlers also makes sense in that both age groups face

Box 3-9

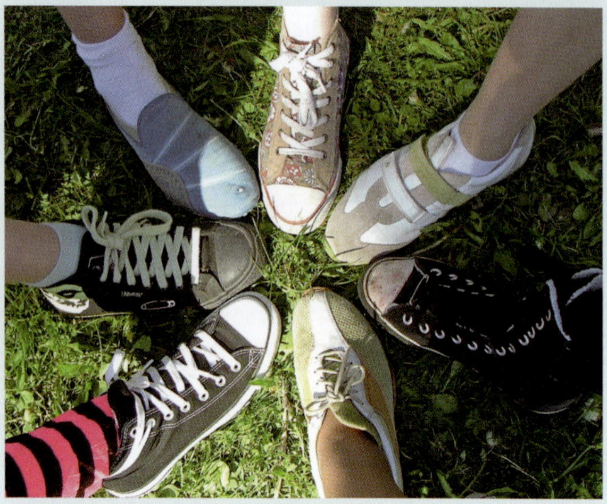

Mary is 14 years old and in blooming adolescence. She frequently misses her dental appointments, and is sometimes quite rude to the dental staff. Mary used to have a good oral health, but during the past couple of years she has developed several new cavities and her oral hygiene is poor. She has been assessed as a risk patient for oral disease and been on a recall system where she sees a dental hygienist every 4–6 months. This has not helped very much and when new radiographs are taken they disclose four new cavities needing conservative therapy and seven new incipient lesions. The dentist is concerned about Mary's well-being, but when asked about her health Mary is not very cooperative. The dentist loses patience and says he will have to contact her parents. When hearing this, Mary gets up and leaves the clinic without saying a word.

Mary wants to be both a child and a grown-up. Her behavior with missed appointments and rudeness indicates that she might be going through a stormy period of adolescence. It is often difficult to handle these patients in a good way. On the one hand the dentist is responsible for her dental care and the teenager is still legally under the care and supervision of her parents. Bringing the parents into the discussion, however, makes Mary feel patronized and looked upon as a young child. Allowing time for communication, and acknowledging the fact that oral hygiene and dental appointments are not among her top 10 priorities may help. It is important to show that you trust the patient, but also to make clear that you expect her to take responsibility for oral hygiene and to behave acceptably. Trying to reach an agreement with the adolescent so that she is involved in the decision, rather than told what to do, may help. It is suggested that parents are consulted only if this strategy fails.

the task of establishing a separate identity. Toddlers must begin to separate themselves from the relationship with their primary caregivers to make room for other important relationships (with other adults and with peers). Young adolescents must separate themselves from the identity as a child and begin to renegotiate their attachment relationships with the primary caregivers based on the fact that they will soon be adults too (Box 3-9).

Late adolescence is more like the preschool years, major changes have been weathered, and a new balance has been achieved. The physical upheavals of puberty are mostly complete, the family system has accommodated to allow the teenager more independence and freedom, and the beginnings of a new identity have been created. The task of forming emotionally intimate partnerships is a key task of late adolescence. How the society at large functions, in terms of welcoming the older adolescent into a meaningful community, is of great importance. If separating from the family of origin is not coupled with a new sense of belonging, not only in a peer group but also in the culture at large, adolescents will be left with a sense of betrayal and of rootlessness.

Caspi and Moffitt (10) made the more general point that any major life crisis or transition, including adolescence, has the effect of accentuating earlier personality or behavioral patterns rather than creating new ones. As one example, Caspi and Moffitt point out that girls who experience very early puberty have higher rates of psychological problems, on average, than do those who experience puberty at a more average age. Closer analysis, however, reveals that it is only the early-maturing girls who already had social problems before puberty, whose pubertal experience and adolescence are more negative. Not only do we "carry ourselves with us" as we move through the roles and demands of late adolescence and adult life, but existing patterns may be most highly visible when we are under stress.

With this we conclude our description of "normal development", and now end the chapter with an introduction into how most developmentalists currently conceptualize deviant development.

Developmental psychopathology

Our knowledge about psychological deviance has been enormously enhanced by an approach called *developmental psychopathology*, launched in the 1970s and 1980s by Norman Garmezy, Michael Rutter, Alan Sroufe, and others. It differs from traditional child and adolescent psychiatry (with its phenomenological psychiatric diagnoses) in several important ways. First of all psychopathology is conceptualized as normal development gone awry. Normal and abnormal development are both conceptualized as emerging from the same basic processes rather than being qualitatively different (13). Dental phobia is from this perspective quantitatively, not qualitatively, different from less severe forms of dental fear and anxiety.

Not only is a child's developmental status at any point in time seen as a result of an ongoing interaction between different biopsychosocial factors. Time itself is also an important aspect. Early care-giving experiences (as discussed earlier in the section on attachment) result in internal working models that the child carries with him or her to day-care, for example. The child's interaction with his or her care-providers and peers is thus affected by his or her earlier experiences with parents. In developmental psychopathology, the effect of earlier experiences is conceptualized as a result of a series of transactions between the child and his or her immediate environment. To every new transaction the child carries the result of previous transactions, that is how well he or she has resolved earlier developmental tasks, and how supporting the environment has been in helping with these accomplishments.

The biopsychosocial model

One outgrowth of the transactional model has been a growing acceptance of the viewpoint that neurobiological development and experience are mutually influencing. It has, for example, been demonstrated that just as gene expression alters social behavior, so do social experiences also exert actions on the brain by feedback to modify gene expression and brain structure, function, and organization. There is suggestive evidence that adverse early experiences inhibit structural plasticity via a hypersensivity to glucocorticoids and impair the ability of the hippocampus to respond adaptively to stress in later childhood, adolescence, and adulthood. Furthermore, it has been shown that alterations in gene expression induced by learning and by social and psychological experiences produce changes in patterns of neuronal and synaptic connections and, thus, in the function of nerve cells. Such modifications not only exert a prominent role in initiating and maintaining the behavioral changes, but also contribute to the biological basis of individuality, as well as to individuals being differentially affected by similar experiences (14).

The development of psychopathology is discussed not in terms of singular causes (whether environmental or genetic) but as the probabilistic development of abnormal development due to the cumulative effect of different vulnerability and risk factors. The concept of vulnerability is most often used to describe inborn (e.g., an inhibited or overactive temperament) or early acquired aspects of the child (e.g., disorganized attachment), while the term risk factor is more often used to describe aspects of the environment that are known to be associated with increased probability of developing psychopathology (e.g., various "social addresses"). Most research in developmental psychopathology shows that it is the number of vulnerability and risk factors, rather than any single factor, that will lead to a deviant outcome.

Resilience and protective factors

Developmental psychopathology emphasizes not only deviance but also health. The concept resilience is used to describe aspects that make some children able to stay well despite severe psychosocial hardship. Some of the aspects are part of the child's own make-up (such as intelligence and sociability), while others are aspects of the environment (e.g., grandparents who support the child's needs and make him or her able to endure severe parental shortcomings). The development of psychopathology is a transactional process, where the end result is the product of a balance over time among positive and negative influences on the child's development. Thus, it makes just as much, and sometimes more, sense to focus on the healthy aspects of the child and his or her environment, which promote positive development, as it does to focus on what does not work so well. By promoting protective factors, the impact of illness factors, which often are more resistant to change, will be less severe.

Developmental lines

Because of the multiplicity of interacting factors at different points in time, researchers and practitioners in developmental psychopathology focus not so much on psychiatric diagnoses which describe the patient's current status, as on the pathways (i.e., developmental lines) leading to both deviant and normal development, from infancy through childhood and into adult life.

How do different biopsychosocial influences interact in a given child's life? Some children follow continuously adaptive or maladaptive pathways, others may initially show a positive development that later turns maladaptive, and still other children show the reversed pattern of early maladaptation, which subsides over the years. The concept *equifinality* pinpoints the fact that different children can reach the same endpoint using different pathways. The developmental route leading up to dental anxiety or dental behavior management problems is certainly not the same for all children, thus it is more or less meaningless to search for the "one-and-only cause" of dental anxiety or dental behavior management problems. Instead the great individual variation in the development of these problems point to a multifactorial etiology. Psychological development and psychological psychopathology account for part of the explanation, where causes combine differently for individual children with dental anxiety or dental behavior management problems (see Chapter 4).

Similarly the concept *multifinality* is used to show that the long-term impact of a specific risk or vulnerability factor varies between children. To show a very inhibited temperament during toddlerhood is probably a vulnerability factor for the development of dental anxiety later in childhood, but most children with this early temperament do not develop dental fear. Some do develop other anxiety problems, but most children show no deviant development at all (see Chapter 4). Further, for some children other neurobiological and neuropsychiatric factors affect their abilities to cooperate and function in relation to dental treatment. This encompasses factors such as cognitive impairments/learning disabilities, and disorders involving social interaction and communication, e.g., autism and attention deficit hyperactivity disorder. However, these issues are not the scope of this chapter; instead they will be described in Chapter 23.

Summary

Children and adolescents differ greatly, not only in dental and physical development, but also with regard to psychological maturity. The psychological development from infancy through childhood and adolescence into adulthood is a long and fascinating journey. It guides the individual child when solving challenges that he or she encounters over the years. As dentists we need to be well orientated about this travel plan. Such knowledge and understanding are prerequisites for communication with children in the dental operatory: it helps when meeting, understanding, and treating them. The "embryo" for this travel plan is already outlined when sperm and egg cell unite, but from that point onwards it depends on a complicated interplay between biological and psychosocial factors. Cognitive development concerns reasoning and problem solving. The young infant already is able to explore and interact with the environment. These skills develop as the child learns from previous experiences, advances in physical activities, and interacts with other people. Cognitive and emotional development are intertwined from the very beginning when the child's first relationships with his or her primary caregivers form a base from which the world is explored. Temperamental factors are important and affect how the child reacts in novel situations, such as the first dental appointment. Every child has her or his own itinerary. The preschool child is still dependent on care-givers and the child's reasoning is usually on a preoperational level where it is difficult to understand the relationship between cause and effect. Starting school implies new challenges for the child, such as taking more responsibility and with peer relations becoming more important. Being a pupil also brings on new demands: functioning in the classroom, learning to read, and do math. The child's reasoning is more logical, but it is still concrete and it is therefore difficult for the young school-aged child to understand abstract phenomena. Adolescence is a time of transition. This period comprises both stormy and calm periods and its manifestations vary immensely between individuals. Peer relations are of core importance and the individual goes through a period of numerous physical, social, and intellectual changes. Reasoning advances and the individual starts grasping abstractions.

The dental appointment is perceived as stressful for many children and adolescents, which may make them not perform and reason at their best. The more they trust the dentist, the easier it is for them to perform in accordance with their level of maturity. Further, the young patient is part of a social context, and this should also be taken into account. As dentists we must tailor the dental appointment individually for every child and adolescent focusing on the individual's strengths, but also taking weaknesses into account.

References

1. Ainsworth MDS, Blehar MC, Waters E, Wall S. *Patterns of attachment: a psychological study of the strange situation.* Hillsdale, NJ: Lawrence Erlbaum, 1978.
2. Bates E, Marchman V, Thal D, Fenson L, Dale P, Reznick JS, *et al.* Developmental and stylistic variation in the composition of early vocabulary. *J Child Lang* 1994; **21**: 85–123.
3. Bee H, Boyd D. *The developing child,* 11th edn. Boston, MA: Pearson, 2006.
4. Bowlby J. *Attachment and loss,* Vol. 1, *Attachment,* 2nd edn. New York: Basic Books, 1982.
5. Bronfenbrenner U. *The ecology of human development: experiments by nature and design.* Cambridge, MA: Harvard University Press, 1979.
6. Bronson MB. *Self-regulation in early childhood: nature and nurture.* New York: Guilford Press, 2000.
7. Buss AH, Plomin RA. *A temperament theory of personality development.* New York: John Wiley, 1975.
8. Calkins SD. Early attachment processes and the development of emotional self-regulation. In: Baumeister RF, Vohs KD, eds. *Handbook of self-regulation: research, theory, and application.* New York: Guilford Press, 2004; 324–39.
9. Calkins SD, Hill A. Caregiver influences on emerging emotion regulation: biological and environmental transactions in early development. In: Gross J, ed. *Handbook of emotion regulation.* New York: Guilford Press, 2007; 229–48.
10. Caspi A, Moffitt TE. Individual differences are accentuated during periods of social change: the sample case of girls at puberty. *J Pers Soc Psychol* 1991;**61**:157–68.
11. Caspi A. The child is the father of the man. Personality continues from childhood to adulthood. *J Pers Soc Psychol* 2000;**78**:158–72.
12. Cassidy J, Shaver PR, eds. *Handbook of attachment: theory, research and clinical applications.* New York: Guilford Press, 1999.

13. Cicchetti D, Cohen DJ, eds. *Developmental psychopathology*, 2nd edn. New York: John Wiley, 2006.
14. Cicchetti D, Curtis WJ. The developing brain and neural plasticity: implications for normality, psychopathology, and resilience. In: Cicchetti D, Cohen, DJ, eds. *Developmental psychopathology*, Vol. 2, *Developmental neuroscience*, 2nd edn. New York: John Wiley, 2006; 1–64.
15. Davydov VV. The influence of L.S. Vygotsky on education theory, research and practice (Kerr ST, trans.). *Educational Researcher* 1995;**24**:12–21.
16. Flavell J. Theory-of-mind development: retrospect and prospect. *Merrill Palmer Q* 2004;**50**:274–90.
17. Kagan J, Snidman N. *The long shadow of temperament.* Cambridge, MA: Harvard University Press, 2004.
18. Main M, Hesse E. Parents' unresolved traumatic experiences are related to infant disorganized attachment status. In: Greenberg MT, Cicchetti D, Cummings EM, eds. *Attachment in the preschool years: theory, research and intervention.* Chicago, IL: University of Chicago Press, 1990; 161–82.
19. Masten AS, Coatsworth JD. The development of competence in favorable and unfavorable environments: lessons from research on successful children. *Am Psychol* 1998;**53**:205–20.
20. Piaget J, Inhelder B. *The psychology of the child.* New York: Basic Books, 1969.
21. Plutchik R. The nature of emotions. *Am Sci* 2001;**89**:344–50.
22. Putnam SP, Sanson AV, Rothbart MK. Child temperament and parenting. In: Bornstein MH, ed. *Handbook of parenting*, Vol. 1, *Children and parenting*, 2nd edn. Mahwah, NJ: Lawrence Erlbaum, 2002; 255–77.
23. Rothbart MK, Posner MI. Temperament, attention, and developmental psychopathology. In: Cicchetti D, Cohen DJ, eds. *Developmental psychopathology*, Vol. 2, 2nd edn. New York: John Wiley, 2006; 465–51.
24. Sroufe LA. *Emotional development: the organization of emotional life in the early years.* New York: Cambridge University Press, 1996.
25. Sroufe LA, Egeland B, Carlson EA, Collins WA. *The development of the person: the Minnesota study of risk and adaptation from birth to adulthood.* New York: Guilford Press, 2005.
26. Thomas A, Chess S, Birch H. The origin of personality. *Sci Am* 1970;**223**:102–9.
27. Vaughn BE, Bost KK. Attachment and temperament. In: Cassidy J, Shaver PR, eds. *Handbook of attachment: theory, research and clinical applications.* New York: Guilford Press, 1999; 198–225.
28. Vygotsky LS. *Mind in society.* Cambridge, MA: Harvard University Press, 1978.

4

Dental fear and behavior management problems

Gunilla Klingberg, Magne Raadal and Kristina Arnrup

The prevention and treatment of oral diseases in childhood and adolescence as the basis for good oral health throughout life is the aim of pediatric dentistry. There are two main, equally important, issues within this goal: (a) to keep the oral environment healthy, and (b) to keep the patient capable of using and willing to use the dental service. This chapter deals with the second of these issues, including how to help children to cope with dental treatment and how to prevent development of dental anxiety and odontophobia.

Children and adolescents show tremendous variation in maturity, personality, temperament, and emotions, leading to a corresponding variation in vulnerability and ability to cope with the dental treatment situation. As a consequence of this, the pediatric dentist needs a repertoire of strategies, in addition to the dental treatment techniques, to prevent behavior management problems and to manage children who display such problems. This repertoire should involve both *psychological* and *pharmacological techniques*.

Definitions and prevalence of dental fear and anxiety

Many children perceive a visit to the dentist as stressful. This can be expected since an appointment includes several stress-evoking components, such as meeting unfamiliar adults and authority figures, strange sounds and tastes, having to lie down, discomfort, and even pain. Uncooperative behavior and fear reactions are, therefore, common encounters in the daily dental clinical situation. The reported prevalence of dental fear/anxiety and behavior management problems varies from about 5% to nearly 20% and is shown in Table 4-1.

Table 4-1 Studies of the prevalence of dental fear and anxiety, and dental behavior management problems in children and adolescents

Country	Authors	Age (years)	Percentage
Dental fear and anxiety			
Canada	Murray *et al.*, 1989	12	9.4
Denmark	Wogelius *et al.*, 2003	6–8	5.7
Jordan	Taani *et al.*, 2005	12–15	10
Netherlands	ten Berge *et al.*, 2002	4–11	6
New Zealand	Thomson *et al.*, 1997	15	10.9
Norway	Skaret *et al.*, 1998	18	19
Russia	Bergius *et al.*, 1997	13–18	12.6
Scotland, UK	Bedi *et al.*, 1992	13–14	7.1
Singapore	Chellappah *et al.*, 1990	10–14	13.5
	Milgrom *et al.*, 1992	13–15	12.2
Sweden	Klingberg *et al.*, 1994	4–11	6.7
USA	Raadal *et al.*, 1995	5–11	19.5
Behavior management problems			
Sweden	Holst and Crossner, 1987	3–16	8
Sweden	Klingberg *et al.*, 1994	4–11	10.5

Adapted from Klingberg and Broberg (15), where full references to the included studies above are available.

Fear may be described as a natural emotion based on the perception of a real threat, while anxiety is associated with fear-reactions towards a situation of an anticipated, but not realistic, threat. Anxiety may therefore be looked on as a more disorder-like type of fear among those who have not been able to adapt to specific fearful situations. Phobia is a disorder that is diagnosed according to clinical criteria (Box 4-1). Based on these descriptions it is likely that dental fear as well as dental behavior management problems have their peaks at a young age followed by rather drastic decline while dental anxiety starts during

Box 4-1 Important concepts in the understanding of child behavior

Dental fear

- Relates to a specific object.
- Represents the reaction to a specific external threatening stimulus.
- A normal emotional reaction to threatening stimuli in the dental treatment situation.

Dental anxiety

- Not attached to an object.
- A more nonspecific feeling of apprehension.
- Represents a state where the person is evoked and prepared for something to happen.
- Associated with more abnormal conditions.

Odontophobia

- A severe type of dental anxiety.
- Characterized by marked and persistent fear of clearly discernible objections/situations.
- Results in people avoiding necessary dental treatment or enduring such treatment only with dread.
- Significantly interferes with daily routines and social life.

Dental behavior management problems

- Defined as uncooperative and disruptive behaviors resulting in delay of treatment or rendering treatment impossible.

early school age and then shows moderate increase. Dental phobia will probably affect fewer individuals, and show a more moderate increase as the individual grows older (Fig. 4-1). It is difficult to differentiate fear from anxiety in the clinical situation, and the terms dental fear and dental anxiety frequently are used interchangeably, as in this chapter.

A very relevant question to ask is: "is it possible to distinguish between dental fear and behavior management problems in the clinical situation?" (Box 4-2). There is no simple answer to this. In the clinical situation the dentist is not likely to miss a child presenting with behavior management problems. Clinicians may empirically recognize the child with inadequate understanding, maturity, or ability to cooperate. A child who is acting out by crying or physically resisting may be contrasted to a child whispering to his or her mother, making no eye contact with the dentist and distancing himself or herself from interaction. Children with dental fear and anxiety can be outgoing in their general behavior, but are sometimes more passive and silent during treatment. Thus, there is the risk of overlooking that a patient is anxious, which may increase the risk for harming him or her. It is important not to take cooperative behaviors alone as a sign of the child feeling comfortable. With increased knowledge about signs and causes of dental anxiety and behavior management problems, the dentist will become more attentive to these problems.

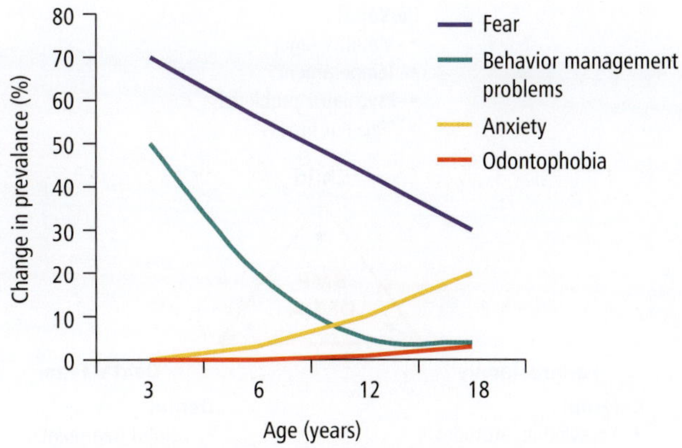

Figure 4-1 Estimated changes in prevalence of dental fear, dental anxiety, dental phobia and behavior management problems in children and adolescents.

Box 4-2 The relationship between dental fear and anxiety, and behavior management problems (drawing adapted from Klingberg, 14)

Behavior management problems are what the dentist observes, while dental fear and anxiety is what the patient feels – and the two things do not always correlate:

- Some children present behavior management problems without having fear and anxiety (the green area).
- Some children apprehend dental fear and anxiety, but are able to cope with the situation (orange area).
- Some children experience dental fear and anxiety and present behavior management problems (the overlapping area between the green and the orange areas).

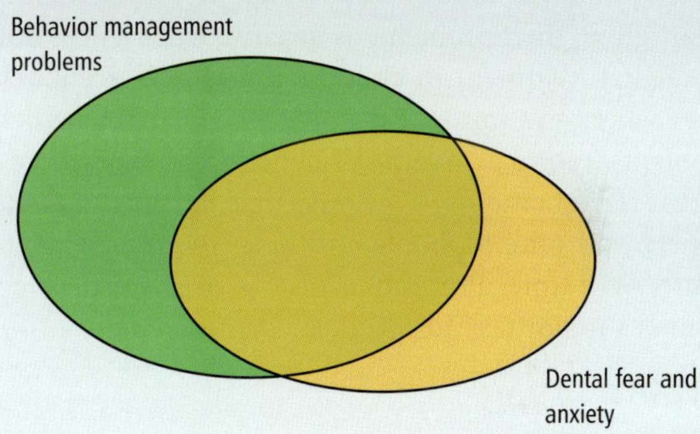

Etiology

Dental anxiety and behavior management problems in children are phenomena of multifactorial and complex origins. Three main domains of etiologic factors can be identified (Fig. 4-2). As the different components in each of the domains or groups vary in importance over

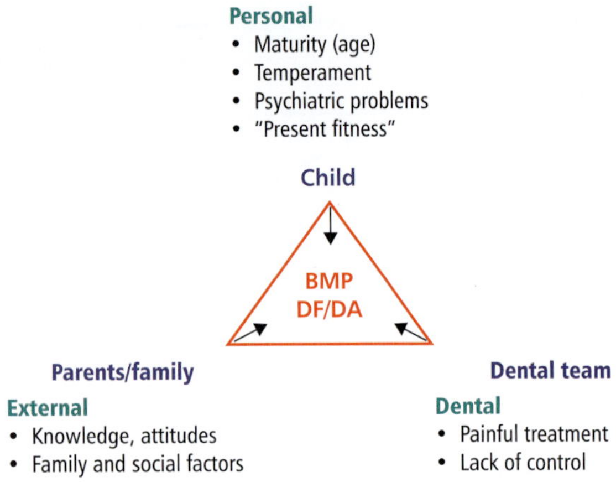

Figure 4-2 The reasons for dental fear/anxiety (DF/DA) and dental behavior management problems (BMP) are multifactorial and complex. Three groups of factors have been identified: personal, external, and dental factors. The impact and relative importance of the different factors vary between children and individually over time. If DF/DA and/or BMP lead to avoidance of dental treatment, there is a risk of entering and maintaining a vicious circle which may lead to odontophobia.

time, the patient's apprehension of anxiety as well as the behavior during dental treatments may vary. New aspects may be added leading to an increase in problems or, conversely, the child may learn to handle some of the anxiety-provoking components, leading to a decrease in problems. Thus, time is an important variable. The child patient we see today will grow to be an adult patient of tomorrow. From research about dental anxiety and odontophobia in adults we know that they often identify the origin of their problems as negative experiences during dental treatment in childhood and adolescence. In cases where the initial fear and behavior management problems lead to avoidance of dental treatment, there is a great risk of entering a vicious circle, leading to dental anxiety and odontophobia and deterioration of dental health over time. Prevention of this negative development is a major task for pediatric dentists.

Personal factors

The prevalence figures shown in Table 4-1 differ to some extent between different surveys. There are several reasons for this: different criteria for definitions of dental anxiety or behavior management problems, differences in selection and size of samples, differences in age, and probably also differences due to cultural factors or differences in the systems for dental care in various countries. However, one factor clearly emerges as important in explaining the occurrence of dental anxiety and behavior management problems, namely, *the age of the child.* Both dental fear and behavior management problems are more common in young children, reflecting the influence of a child's psychological development on his or her ability to cope with dental treatment (15). A young child may experience and understand the dental situation differently than older children. One major reason for this is that the process of understanding and having the motivation to comply with dental treatment differs depending on psychological development. The latter is also dependent on communication skills in the dental teams, for example. After all, dental treatment requires a great deal from a child: to lie down without moving; to tolerate discomfort; strange tastes; maybe even pain; and all this in an unfamiliar environment with strange people, etc.

All children go through developmental periods of obstinacy often coinciding with the crisis that the child is dealing with during the different phases in his or her socioemotional development. These normal, but trying, periods are sometimes revealed as behavior management problems in the dental treatment situation. When talking to the parents they often describe a sudden change in the mood of their child, from compliant and easy-going to showing and testing a behavior and stubbornness. This is a transient period that will pass in a couple of weeks or maybe a month or two.

Symptoms of fear and anxiety are normal developmental phenomena in children, and many children display a relatively high number of anxiety symptoms without having anxiety disorders. Young children show fear of more and of different stimuli than older children. Several studies have shown a clear and positive relationship between high *general fear level, emotional disorders*, or *general anxiety* on the one hand and dental fear and anxiety, or behavior management problems on the other (15). Associations between fear problems such as medical fears, fear of the unknown, and fear of injury on the one hand and dental fear and anxiety on the other have been reported.

In this context it is important to bear in mind the difficulties of distinguishing between dental fear and dental anxiety in children. The visit to the dentist could well be fearful to many children without giving rise to anxiety. Fearful reactions in young children are natural and this may explain the high prevalence in these age groups. Dental anxiety and phobia develop later in childhood and should be regarded as pathological phenomena.

Fear/anxiety/phobia of blood, injections, and injuries is a special type of anxiety that frequently seems to interact negatively with dental treatment, since most of these children are fearful of dental injections (blood–injection–injury phobia: BII phobia) (20). There is a strong tendency to faint or nearly faint when exposed to the fearful stimuli, which is unique to this type of phobia. The age of onset is thought to be early, which means that the prevalence is highest among young children. Positive relationships between BII and dental anxiety and dental avoidance have been shown, indicating that BII is a contributing factor.

Temperament is a personal emotional quality that is moderately stable over time and appears early in life. It is also believed to be under some genetic influence. Difficulties approaching novel situations and unfamiliar people have been reported to characterize children with dental fear and/or behavior management problems. Associations have also been reported with characteristics described as "negative mood", "unhappy child", "easily distressed", or "impulsiveness". Thus, dental fear and/or behavior management problems have been associated with aspects of children's temperament (Box 4-3) (15). One dimension of temperament is shyness, which is found in about 10% of children. Shy children need extra time to feel at ease with the situation. Another temperamental dimension, associated with dental fear as well as behavior management problems, is negative emotionality. Children with behavior management problems have also been reported to score higher on activity and impulsivity.

Looking at fear, temperament, and behavior together, different subgroups have been identified among children with dental behavior management problems. Among these subgroups are children with high dental and general fear, children with fear combined with inhibited temperamental profile (shyness, negative emotionality, and internalizing behavior), and children with less pronounced fear combined with impulsiveness and externalizing/outgoing behavior (1).

In the group of children with dental anxiety without uncooperative behaviors it seems likely to find children with pronounced shyness or an inhibited temperamental profile. These children are well aware of how they should behave during a dental visit and therefore cope well with the treatment despite their anxiety. These children require special awareness on the part of the dental team during treatment in order not to be forced beyond their coping abilities. As inhibited children do not have an outgoing behavior, the lack of uncooperativeness could be misinterpreted for agreeing with the treatment situation if the dentist is not aware of this temperamental trait.

Box 4-3 Some dimensions of temperament associated with dental fear and/or behavior management problems (temperamental dimensions according to the EASI temperamental survey, Buss and Plomin, 4)

Shyness	A tendency to be slow to warm up in novel situations or when meeting new people.
Negative emotionality	Easily aroused expression of irritability or aggression when frustrated.
Activity	Tempo and vigor, i.e., the tendency to hurry or speed and force in walking and talking.
Impulsivity	Impatience and lack of perseverance.

Uncooperative behavior in dental care situations may also be related to neuropsychiatric disorders such as attention deficit hyperactivity disorder (ADHD), autism, Asperger syndrome, Tourette syndrome, or to other psychological/mental disabilities. Recent studies have found dental anxiety and behavior management problems to occur more frequently in children with ADHD (3). Approximately 5% of children are expected to have some kind of neuropsychiatric disorder (9). ADHD represents a significant proportion with prevalence figures reported to vary from 3 to 7% (7).

External factors

It is well known that *parental dental anxiety* affects dental anxiety in children. Children may also acquire dental fear through social learning from siblings, other relatives, and friends. Apart from transmitting subtle feelings of fear and anxiety to their children, fearful parents sometimes also interfere with the dental treatment of their child, for example by questioning the need for injections or restorative treatments, or may give accounts from their own negative experiences. On these occasions they may serve as live and powerful negative models of dental anxiety for their children. Studies among adult odontophobic patients by Berggren and Meynert (2) and Moore *et al.* (21) have reported that negative family attitudes towards dental care and dental fear in the family were common reasons for the development of odontophobia. For many of these adult patients the problems with dental fear and anxiety started in childhood, often even before their first dental visit.

The *social situation* of the child is likely to be of importance. Children live under different circumstances in modern society, sometimes also on the margins of society in one aspect or the other. Dental fear problems have been reported to be more frequent in subpopulations such as immigrants. Groups with lower socioeconomic standards have also been reported to exhibit a higher prevalence of dental anxiety and behavior management problems. It is possible that these differences can be leveled out to some extent in countries where organized free dental care for children is provided. Hence, some studies from Sweden and Norway have failed to establish a relationship between socioeconomic variables and dental fear. One explanation might be that oral health is less affected by socioeconomic standards in these populations. A child who has good oral health runs a smaller risk of caries and filling therapy and thereby a smaller risk of encountering discomfort and pain in the dental situation. Family risk factors (for example, parents not living together and low socioeconomic status) *per se* are not presumed to influence children's fear and behavior, but rather to influence parents' attitudes and behavior, and thereby their ability to guide and support their children during dental treatment. A recent Swedish study among patients referred for specialized pediatric dental care because of dental behavior management problems reports that the referred children and adolescents more frequently have a "burdensome" life and family situation, including low socioeconomic status, and parents not living together (10).

Children in *refugee families* are in a vulnerable situation since the children and their parents generally bear traumatic memories and many have post-traumatic stress syndrome. The numbers of refugee families have increased over the years and it is important to remember that some of them have been involved in war, or have even been subjected to torture, etc. These parents can have problems functioning like adults or active parents in front of their children. A dental care situation, with its ingredients of intense lights from the operatory lamp, dental instruments in the mouth, strange tastes, and smells, can lead to flashbacks. In circumstances where the child's family is occupied with this kind of problem it might not function like a sound family and the risk of developing dental anxiety for these children is obvious.

Child rearing may also have an impact on how the child will comply with dental treatments. Dental teams often identify factors related to family or upbringing as a cause of problems. The situation for both children and parents has changed over the past few decades and continues to do so. In many countries this has led to an alteration of the role children play in society. Previously, the distinctions between childhood and adulthood were clearer. The adult, a parent, a schoolteacher, or dentist was more clearly the one setting the rules and leading the way. Today, children frequently question adult people's authority and this certainly affects the dental treatment situation. However, the cultural context of the child can imply great variation on this theme.

Dental factors

One of the most commonly mentioned causes of dental fear/anxiety and behavior management problems is *painful dental treatments.* Pain is defined by the International Association for the Study of Pain (17) as an unpleasant sensory and emotional experience associated with actual or potential tissue damage, or described in terms of such damage. It is important to acknowledge that the sensation is not necessarily dependent on tissue damage; it may also be generated by conditioned stimuli such as the sound of the drill or a gentle touch of the needle. Since painful stimuli normally bring about physiological and psychological reactions to protect the body from tissue damage, uncooperative behavior is a logical and relevant reaction when a child experiences pain or discomfort. Unfortunately, experiences of pain are not uncommon in child dental care, since it has been shown that many children have, for instance, restorative treatments carried out without local anesthesia (19,22).

Children's understanding of (and vulnerability to) pain varies considerably depending on cognitive abilities, and the reactions and thoughts concerning painful stimuli vary according to age and maturity (16). In addition to this, factors such as the child's socioemotional development, family and social situation, parental support, kind of rapport with the dental team, etc., affect how the child will cope with stress, pain, and discomfort. There is also a growing body of evidence showing that children who have been subjected to painful procedures without adequate anesthesia develop increased perception of pain about future procedures, despite adequate pain control (8). One strong painful dental stimulus could be enough to cause dental fear and anxiety in a vulnerable child patient. However, repeated exposure to dental treatments that are only somewhat discomforting or a little painful, or are perceived as such by the child, can have the same result. It is, therefore, not acceptable from an ethical point of view to withhold local anesthesia from children, especially as this is a documented way to reduce or even prevent pain.

Perceived lack of control has been shown to be another major triggering factor for behavior management problems and dental fear/anxiety (24). This may imply that the child patients have not been properly informed about the treatment (informational control), or that they have deprived influence of their own behavior (behavioral control), or even that they are not given sufficient information after the treatment (retrospective control). Painful dental treatment in situations when the child feels lack of control has been shown to be particularly harmful (18).

Discomfort goes hand in hand with pain and children frequently have problems distinguishing between the two. Discomfort can represent a psychological comprehension of a stressful situation. This is often experienced in novel situations, if the child is frightened about what will happen, or feels lack of control, etc.

Again, when looking at the prevalence figures in Table 4-1 it seems possible to assume that a large proportion of the behavior management problems and refusal to go along with treatment reflects the fact that children are fearful, particularly when they perceive pain, discomfort, or stress. These are normal and fully adequate reactions, especially in young children lacking experience of their own coping ability. However, it is still an important task for the dental team primarily to prevent these adverse reactions and, if they occur, to handle them properly in order to prevent future dental anxiety.

The *dental team* has a delicate task when treating child patients. They represent authority and can, if perceived in this way, imply a threat or something frightening to some children. The attitudes towards children among dentists and other members of the team are important as to how they behave and interact when treating children. As attitudes also include cognition it is important that dental personnel working with children have a good knowledge not only of dentistry, but also of children, child development, and child psychology. Child competency is a concept grounded in the United Nations (UN) Convention on the Rights of the Child. It encompasses the knowledge and competencies we need to have in order to fulfill the requirements that the convention states regarding personnel within the health sector. In order to provide high-quality comprehensive care including communication with the child patient and his or her family we as dentists need to ensure that we acquire and maintain child competency.

Principles of management

This section deals with the use of psychological techniques for the prevention of behavior management problems and dental fear/anxiety/phobia, as well as how to manage children displaying such problems. Knowledge of the multiple and interacting etiologic factors of fear, anxiety, and behavior management problems is necessary in order to be successful in these tasks. As explained in the previous section, etiologic factors can be described within three domains:

- personal factors
- external factors
- dental factors.

The first two of these determine how vulnerable the child is when entering the dental clinic. Irrespective of age, some children are very robust and tolerate a lot, while others are vulnerable and respond negatively even to minor stress stimuli. The dental staff has no influence on this, but they must be sensitive and adapt their behavior and treatment strategy to it. Dental factors are those that the dental staff are able to control. The prevention of pain and discomfort combined with the establishment of a good psychological relationship with the child and his or her parents on the one hand, and the dental team on the other, are the major issues.

A complex network of interactions arises between the child, parent, dentist, and dental assistant when uncooperative or fearful children are treated. The behavior of the dentist has been shown to have a clear impact on the behavior of the child. Each attempt to treat must be preceded by diagnosis and planning, which, for children, also involves the parent to a varying degree. The concept of informed consent, parental permission, and assent from the child has been adopted from pediatric care, and the parent's involvement during treatment has become standard. Thus, in addition to being a source of information, the parent is participating in a shared decision-making and treatment-planning process and is more likely to comply and adequately support their child when actively involved and informed. A relationship built on trust, empathy, and mutual respect gains patient cooperation.

The suggested treatment techniques are based on the principles of cognitive behavioral therapy (CBT) (12) and are basically the same as used for prevention (behavior shaping) and treatment (desensitization) of dental fear/anxiety and behavior management problems. CBT seeks to identify the child's beliefs that generate fear and avoidance in the clinical situation, and to produce a cognitive change in these beliefs. This is combined with behavioral exercises in which the child is helped to test his or her threat beliefs.

The practice of CBT in pediatric dentistry involves two basic issues:

- creating a safe environment for the child
- exposing the child to fearful stimuli in a controlled way.

Creating a safe environment for the child

When a child is accompanied by his or her parents, it is necessary to establish an equally good and respectful communication with both the child and the adult (Box 4-4). This is an absolute prerequisite for founding the platform on which the diagnosing, treatment planning, and shared decision-making have to take place. Time used for rapport building at the beginning of a treatment should be seen as a necessary investment in the relationship, which can be assumed to "repay" itself many times over during a child's dental care career. If for some reason it is difficult to establish a good rapport and relationship with the child and/or parents, it is usually a good idea to have another dentist involved.

Small children should not be separated from their parents during this initial phase, since the separation anxiety may increase their general stress levels and decrease their possibility for communication. More mature children and adolescents must not be treated in

Box 4-4 Communication

- Must be adapted to age and maturity of the child.
- Should include the parents.
- Includes sending as well as receiving messages.
- A message is not communicated until it has been received.
- Can be verbal and nonverbal.
- Nonverbal communication is at least as important as spoken words to anxious patients.

a patronizing way, even if their behavior and attitudes frequently are provocative. They must feel a reasonable level of equity in the situation. Keeping these very simple strategies in mind when taking the history in the beginning of a dental visit, as well as during the subsequent oral examination and dental treatment, is the key to the establishment of a good psychological environment in the treatment situation (see also Chapter 3).

Most anxious children fear that some kind of catastrophe may occur, e.g., that the dentist suddenly will do something painful. It is therefore important to establish reliable confidence between the dentist and the child that information will be given and consent obtained before anything happens. Establishing confidence is a prerequisite for a successful result of exposure treatment of fearful patients, since the exposures create unpleasant fear reactions.

It is, further, important that the child patient has a number of pain-free appointments without any adverse events prior to experiencing treatments that could include discomfort or pain. Repeated successful and pain-free dental visits can "vaccinate" or protect the child against dental anxiety. This process is termed "latent inhibition" and may protect individuals who experience painful or traumatic events during later treatment sessions (6). The latent inhibition phenomenon is supported by several studies and constitutes a powerful argument for providing regular dental visits and care to all children, preferably focusing on the maintenance of good oral health. Finally, dentists should realize that some treatment could be perceived as painful, e.g., injection of local anesthesia. Prior to any possibly painful events the dentist must, apart from using techniques to reduce the pain, inform the child about what can be expected and suggest strategies to cope with it. This will, by decreasing surprise and increasing predictability and control, lead to lower immediate feelings of fear and possibly have the same effect in a longer perspective.

It has been reported by Weinstein *et al.* (23) that there are some effective and ineffective interactions between the dental personnel and preschool patients. Generally, it is important to provide specific guidance to the child, using terms that are easily understood. Clear and concise directives, such as "Open your mouth a bit more, please" instead of "Could you open your mouth?" were more effective. Also when giving feedback, it is important to be specific, for example, by saying "You are doing a great job by holding your head so still" instead of "You are doing perfectly". Coercion (threats) and coaxing (pleas) are ineffective behavior management procedures, while questioning for feelings tends to be followed by reduced fear. Further, the clinicians should focus on what they want the child to do, and thereby prevent problematic behaviors, instead of trying to stop or slow down such behaviors when they emerge.

When treating dental fear and anxiety in children it is important to bear in mind that the etiology is both multifactorial and complex. Often the case history of the child indicates that explanatory factors can be found in all three domains of etiological factors (personal, external, and dental factors). However, many patients focus the cause of their problems on anticipations or experiences in the dental setting. The dental profession is limited to work within the field of dentistry. Therefore, it is usually wise to start with and concentrate on the dental situation and the stimuli perceived as stressful. This treatment may have positive side-effects on the patient's general well-being as well as on the psychosocial situation. If the treatment repertoire available to the dentist for some reason turns out to be inadequate, the dentist should be prepared to consult a specialized pediatric dentist or a specialist in child psychology or child psychiatry.

Behavior shaping

Behavior shaping of children implies training in how to cope with dental instruments and procedures that they will meet. All children need behavior shaping in the dental chair, irrespective of their dental vulnerability and potential treatment need. However, while some children are very difficult to shape and need a lot of time for this, most are easy and quick to familiarize with dental treatment.

Behavior shaping in dentistry may be based on the principles of CBT. After having disclosed the child's dental experience and beliefs about feelings and coping ability, the procedure is explained to him or her in a comprehensive way. Then the child is exposed step by step to potential anxiety-provoking instruments and procedures where each step creates a moderate increase in stress and fear, and the patient is kept in this exposure situation until he or she experiences a decrease in fearful reactions (Fig. 4-3). A feeling of ability to cope with the stimuli is thereby created. If the exposure is interrupted before the fear decreases, for example by avoiding or

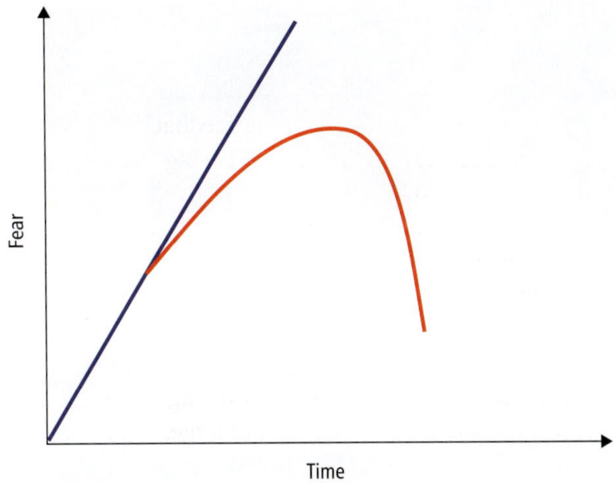

Figure 4-3 Exposure curve. If a patient is kept long enough in an exposure situation perceived as moderately stressful, the fear reaction will eventually decrease. This will create a feeling of ability to cope with the stimulus (red curve). If, however, the exposure is interrupted before the fear reaction decreases, the feelings of defeat and lack of coping usually increase the anxiety (blue curve).

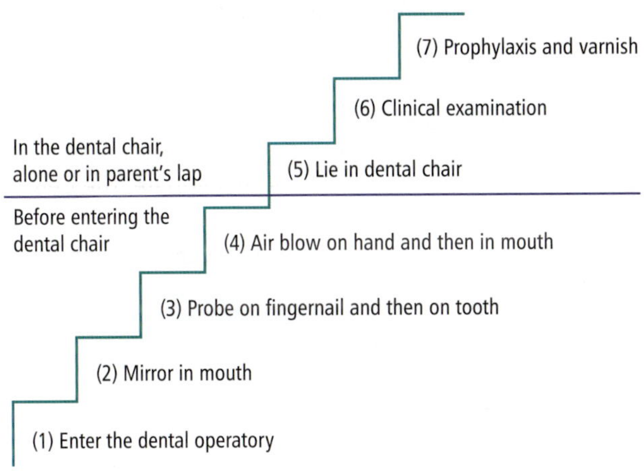

Figure 4-4 Behavior shaping based on the exposure technique. Introductory steps to the dental situation as suggested by Holst (13) for the first dental visit for young children.

interrupting the exposure, the level of fear increases and creates a feeling of defeat and lack of coping.

The different steps and order in the behavior-shaping staircase must be adapted to the individual situation. The one illustrated in Fig. 4-4 has been suggested by Holst (13) for the first dental visit of young children. During each step or exposure the "tell–show–do" technique is used. The child is first told what will happen, then shown, and finally exposed to the procedure (Fig. 4-5). If the child positively accepts the procedure, his or her impression of coping must be reinforced by making the child aware of his or her capability (feedback). If the acceptance is negative, the child should be met with empathy and given more training on the previous step. The first exposures may be performed before the child is seated in the chair. If the child is reluctant to get into the chair alone, he or she could be seated on the parent's lap. After the oral examination and prevention steps, the individual treatment need will determine the next exposure steps. If invasive dental treatment is needed, such as restorative or surgical therapy and local anesthesia, exposure steps must comprise all of the procedural steps of the relevant treatment (see the next section).

The behavior-shaping procedure is the basis for future compliance with dental treatment. Most kinds of behavior management problems are prevented if enough time and consciousness are invested. In terms of time, this is the most cost-efficient in the long run. This type of behavior therapy is quick and demands minor use of time for most children. However, there are some vulnerable children for whom this part of the dental treatment may be more time consuming. Examples of such risk groups are children from refugee and immigrant families, medically or socially compromised children who have a long history of previous pain and suffering, children who for other reasons are sensitive to procedural pain, very shy children, and children with a strong gag reflex. These children may even be extremely sensitive to negative experiences, and unless in a definite emergency situation, there is no excuse for omitting the behavior shaping before the dental treatment.

The behavior-shaping procedure may, in general, be performed by any kind of dental personnel. It is probably cost-efficient to have a dental hygienist or dental assistant do the routine introduction to dentistry among the youngest children who come for their first visit, since most of them have no restorative treatment need. However, it must be pointed out that when children are trained for the most stressful procedures, such as restorative care and surgery, the compliance is dependent on the child's relationship to the operator, and not to any other person.

Desensitization

This section deals with methods to be used when children for some reason are unable to cope with dental treatment, e.g., that they have developed dental anxiety or odontophobia. Since there are so many types of dental anxiety among children, the first step will be to evaluate the nature of the problem and to identify the most anxiety-provoking procedures, and particularly to unveil types of catastrophic thoughts.

The method of choice for desensitizing a child for invasive dental treatment is based on the theory of CBT, in which cognitive restructuring is combined with

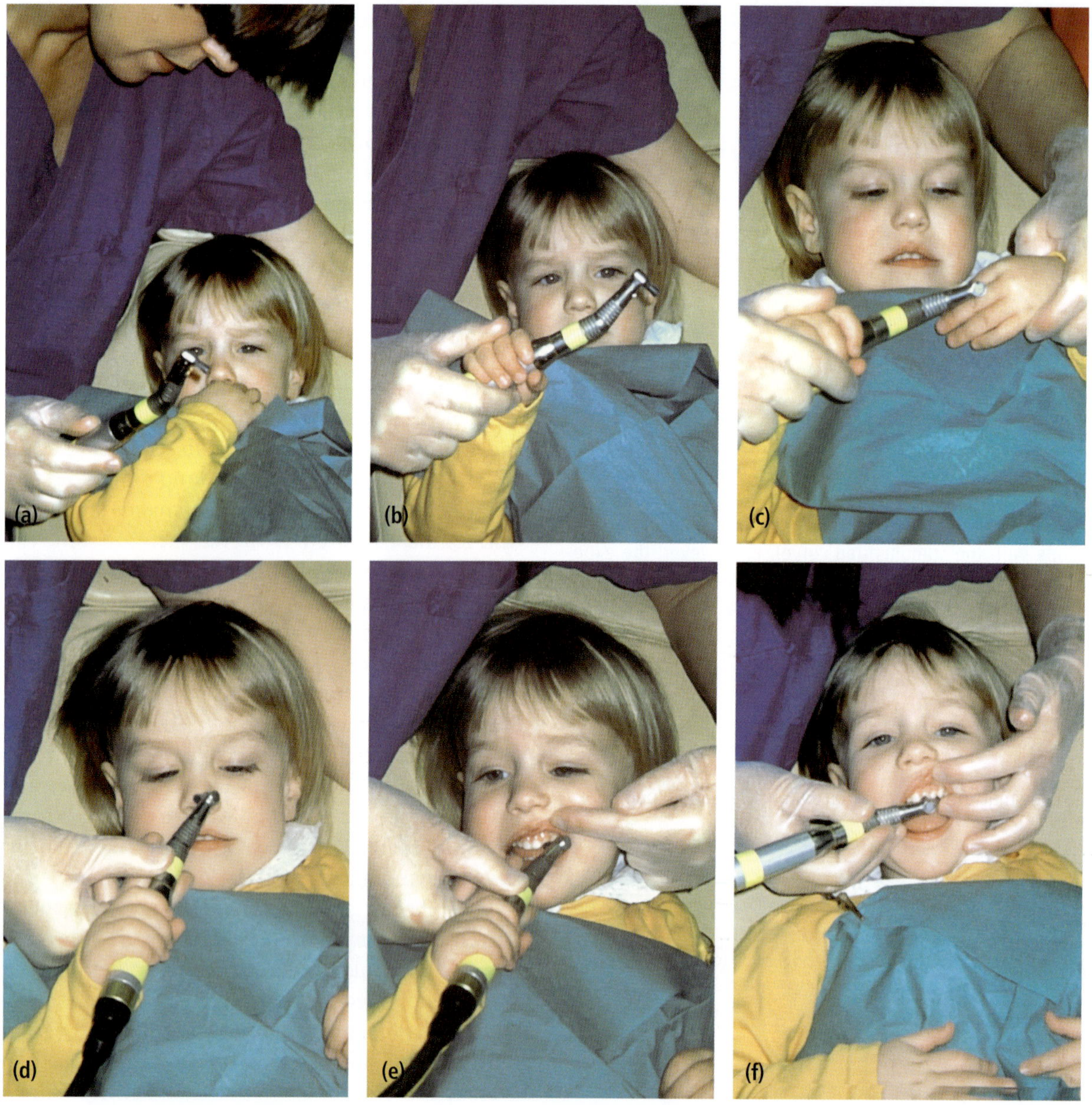

Figure 4-5 A 3-year-old girl at her first dental visit. Behavior shaping by use of the exposure technique to introduce low speed for prophylaxis. (a) After telling the child what will happen (polishing the teeth) the low-speed polisher is demonstrated to her. (b) The child experiences the vibrations from the low speed. (c) The low-speed polisher is exposed closer to her, polishing a finger nail, (d) polishing tip of nose, (e) polishing the teeth while the child is still keeping a hand on the polisher to sense control. (f) The child feels safe and able to control the situation and rests her hands on her stomach.

behavioral exposure. The procedure is similar to the behavior-shaping technique, as described for the introduction of local anesthesia (Fig. 4-6), for example. The steps in the staircase constitute a hierarchy of anxiety-provoking stimuli aiming at gradually exposing the child to the fearful objects or procedures.

As previously stated, the child needs to feel safe in the dental clinic before unpleasant procedures are initiated. The most important consideration during the first treatment phase is therefore not the type of dental treatment achieved, but giving the child a set of positive experiences during subsequent dental visits and thereby a sense of coping ability. A number of previous positive experiences with dental treatment are beneficial for compliance, while negative experiences are destructive (Box 4-5). In cases of severe anxiety or phobia, this procedure may sometimes be extremely time consuming, and it may be helpful for dentists to view themselves more as psychologists than dentists during this phase of treatment. Investing time at this point pays off.

Many children are fearful of dental injections, occasionally as a symptom of BII phobia. Nevertheless, the

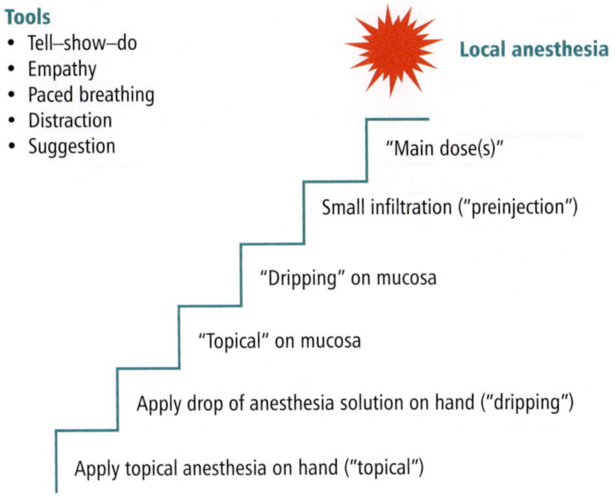

Figure 4-6 Example of exposure steps in desensitization for children who are unfamiliar with or fearful of local anesthesia. The words in parentheses are used to make the child familiar with the procedures of the steps.

Box 4-5 Dental treatment for children is like keeping a bank account

Positive experiences represent savings, while negative experiences are synonymous with withdrawals. When the day comes that the child must face an unpleasant experience in the dental chair, his or her coping ability depends on the "account status".

use of local anesthesia is of utmost importance for painless dental treatment. The first issue is, therefore, to get the child to accept this part of the treatment. An example of behavior shaping related to use of local anesthesia is illustrated in Fig. 4-6. The stepwise procedure ensures that the child has substantial knowledge about what is going on, minimal pain stimulation, and a certain sense of control ("tell–show–do"). Only small steps must be taken at each exposure. The "toolbox" comprises techniques that may be used during the exposure to help the child control any fear reaction before proceeding to the next step. How these techniques are applied depends on the age and maturity of the child. Paced breathing, which is an extremely effective technique for bringing fear reactions down by generating parasympathetic stimulation, may, for example, be applied with small children by having them blow a windmill toy, blow up a balloon, etc. A relaxation exercise implies focusing on special muscles or body parts, alternately contracting and relaxing them. In addition to making the muscles more relaxed and thereby feeling that the whole body becomes less tense, the method is also effective for distraction. Other methods of distraction are story telling, imagery of television programs, having the child play with the vacuum or saliva ejector, etc. It must, however, be realized that these techniques are mostly effective in reducing stress during painless procedures and are not a substitute for the use of local anesthesia during invasive procedures. The use of hypnotherapy may also be useful in children who are disposed for this and where the therapist is familiar with these kinds of techniques. The combined use of relaxation, distraction, and monotony bring many children easily into a light trance, which may be useful in reducing pain and discomfort.

It should be noted that children who are fearful of injections due to BII phobia may display a unique diphasic autonomic nervous reaction as described by Dahllöf and Öst (5). This phenomenon is characterized by an initial sympathetic stimulation followed by a massive parasympathetic (vagal) reaction, which makes the patient faint or at least feel dizzy. This reaction is extremely unpleasant for many children, and should be prevented. It should be pointed out that the use of relaxation techniques is contraindicated in these situations, while Hellström *et al.* (11) have shown applied tension of the muscles to be useful.

Similar behavior-shaping and desensitization procedures can be applied to several kinds of therapy, e.g., restorative treatment, where the potential fear-provoking stimuli (steps in the staircase) are the sight of the drill, the sound of the drill, the feeling of the drill rotating on a tooth, the rubber dam, the matrix system, etc.

During such rehearsals in coping with the different clinical procedures, the child must not be subjected to any nociceptic pain stimuli until he or she is familiar with the procedures. After that, when they have acquired a certain level of confidence in their own coping ability, most children are able to cope with small and short-lasting pain stimuli.

Behavioral techniques in combination with sedatives

The use of sedatives and pain-relieving pharmaceuticals is discussed in Chapter 5. However, since the use of these methods normally must be in combination with the behavioral methods, they are briefly discussed here as well.

The major goal of sedative use in children's dentistry, such as nitrous oxide and benzodiazepines, is to provide a light (conscious) sedation, which makes the child more easily influenced by the behavioral techniques. The goal is usually not to have them so deeply sedated that they are unable to cooperate during the treatment, because deep sedation may be accompanied by loss of the protective reflexes and thereby increased risks for aspiration. Conscious sedation, where the children are able to keep their mouth and eyes open as well as to communicate and cooperate, usually increases the effectiveness of the behavioral techniques previously described, and should therefore be applied in cases where dental treatment is expected to be particularly stressful. Typical examples of such indications are emergency cases, small children with complicated treatment need, and children with generally low coping ability (e.g., children with learning disabilities).

After having achieved a suitable level of sedation, a similar exposure therapy as described above could preferably be adapted, using tell–show–do as the basic tool. However, it must be realized that a child's memory may have been reduced by the medication, and that he or she will therefore very quickly forget what was experienced. The child's attention should be kept all the time, even though it is usually easy to distract. Paced breathing reduces the stress reactions, and is also valuable for the control of the breathing capacity. Since benzodiazepines usually create a certain degree of amnesia, it should be realized that the child's lasting memory of what was experienced may have been reduced. This may be both positive (for negative experiences) and negative (for positive experiences) for a child's future coping ability.

Emergency situations

Emergency situations are the most troublesome with respect to the prevention of dental fear and anxiety, since children frequently have to undergo painful and unpleasant procedures without having the necessary coping ability. These are the typical dental treatment situations where children are exposed to pain without having the feeling of control. It is, therefore, of utmost importance that dentists, before carrying out such treatment, evaluate the degree of emergency of the situation and explore possible treatment alternatives. Toothache itself is not a definite reason for exposing a reluctant child to painful treatment under restraint, since toothache usually passes and can be treated by analgesics. Even infection in a pulp or jaw is not in itself a reason, since it may decrease with antibiotics. Whenever an emergency situation occurs that involves a child who is unable to cope with the optimal treatment, one should look for alternative treatment methods which postpone the unpleasant or painful procedure until the child is behaviorally conditioned to tolerate it. Keeping in mind the basic principle of having the patient's or parents' informed consent before doing any kind of treatment, different alternatives must be presented to them before a decision is taken.

However, there are certainly many emergency cases in pediatric dentistry that demand immediate intervention. Before treatment, these are some issues to consider: (a) the use of sedation combined with a gradual exposure technique reduces the child's perception and memory of pain and stress, and (b) involving the accompanying parent in the preparation as well as, if necessary, in restraint of the child will certainly increase the child's feeling of control and decrease its feeling of being offended. In the treatment decisions it is essential, from an ethical point of view, that the treatment itself as well as the modes of treatment are beneficial to the child in a long-term perspective. If the dentist has to choose between two alternatives, the alternative that gives positive long-term effects should be given priority before alternatives that may be efficient in a shorter perspective, but counterproductive in the long run.

Specialized pediatric dentists

Dental anxiety and behavior management problems are the most frequent reasons for referral to specialized pediatric dentists, at least in Sweden. It may be reasonably asked whether these dentists should have a particular responsibility for the treatment of children showing fear/anxiety or behavior management problems, thus being a resource for high-quality dental care for those needing special attention. However, it is our opinion that all dentists treating child patients must have substantial knowledge of and engagement in how to prevent behavior management problems and dental anxiety as well as in how to identify and handle children with these problems. The specialized pediatric dentist should be able to take care of individual cases of high complexity, as well as being a source of up-to-date knowledge and competency for other dentists in a region. By collaborating with those in charge of the evaluation and supervision of the dental health programs and strategies for children in the region, the specialized pediatric dentist may contribute as an instance of quality assurance in this field.

Quality assurance can be handled from several different aspects depending on who or what you represent. It is possible to identify several perspectives regarding dental anxiety. There are the patients' expectancies of oral health and quality in dental care; society's request that high-quality care is provided to all citizens at a low cost; care-givers', primarily dentists', wishes to carry out dental treatment of good quality with little or no side-effects, etc.

In order to ensure that children are treated according to high clinical standards, specialized pediatric dentists should, because of their knowledge of children, be included in the working groups that plan dental care within public dental health systems. This planning should include strategies aimed at preventing anxiety and cooperation problems. Specialized pediatric dentists also have an important role when evaluating such programs and strategies. Unfortunately, almost all descriptions of satisfaction, success in treatment, etc., consist of information compiled by professionals. The children are rarely asked. Therefore, it is important that specialized pediatric dentists also support a strategy where the viewpoints of children are asked for and are considered throughout the work. This is in line with the UN Convention on the Rights of the Child. In cases where children cannot be involved, specialized pediatric dentists should represent the child patients' points of views in that they try to take their perspectives and substitute for the autonomy of children when necessary.

References

1. Arnrup K, Broberg AG, Berggren U, Bodin L. Lack of cooperation in pediatric dentistry – the role of child personality characteristics. *Pediatr Dent* 2002;**24**:119–28.
2. Berggren U, Meynert G. Dental fear and avoidance: causes, symptoms, and consequences. *J Am Dent Assoc* 1984;**109**: 247–51.
3. Blomqvist M, Holmberg K, Fernell E, Ek U, Dahllöf G. Oral health, dental anxiety, and behavior management problems in children with attention deficit hyperactivity disorder. *Eur J Oral Sci* 2006;**114**:385–90.
4. Buss AH, Plomin R. *Temperament: early developing personality traits.* Hillsdale, NJ: Lawrence Erlbaum, 1984.
5. Dahllöf O, Öst LG. The diphasic reaction in blood phobic situations: individually or stimulus bound? *Scand J Behav Ther* 1998; **27**:97–104.
6. Davey GC. Dental phobia and anxieties: evidence for conditioning processes in the acquisition and modulation of a learned fear. *Behav Res Ther* 1989;**27**:51–8.
7. Faraone SV, Sergeant J, Gillberg C, Biederman J. The worldwide prevalence of ADHD: is it an American condition? *World Psychiatry* 2003;**2**:104–13.
8. Fitzgerald M, Howard R. The neurobiologic basis of pediatric pain. In: Schechter NL, Berde CB, Yaster M, eds. *Pain in infants, children, and adolescents,* 2nd edn. Philadelphia, PA: Lippincott Williams & Wilkins, 2002; 19–42.
9. Gillberg C. Epidemiological overview. In: Gillberg C, ed. *Clinical child neuropsychiatry.* Cambridge: Cambridge University Press, 1995; 4–11.
10. Gustafsson A, Arnrup K, Broberg AG, Bodin L, Berggren U. Psychosocial concomitants to dental fear and behavioural management problems. *Int J Paediatr Dent* 2007;**17**:449–59.
11. Hellström K, Fellenius J, Öst LG. One versus five sessions of applied tension in the treatment of blood phobia. *Behav Res Ther* 1996;**34**:101–12.
12. Hollon SD, Beck AT. Cognitive and cognitive-behavioral therapies. In: Lambert MJ, ed. *Bergin and Garield's handbook of psychotherapy and behaviour change,* 5th edn. New York: John Wiley, 2004; 447–92.
13. Holst A. Behaviour management problems in child dentistry. Frequency, therapy and prediction. Thesis. Malmö: Faculty of Odontology, University of Lund, 1988. *Swed Dent J* 1988; Suppl 54.
14. Klingberg G. Dental fear and behavior management problems in children. A study of measurement, prevalence, concomitant factors, and clinical effects. Thesis. Gothenburg: Faculty of Odontology, Göteborg University, 1995. *Swed Dent J* 1995; Suppl 103.
15. Klingberg G, Broberg AG. Dental fear/anxiety and dental behaviour management problems in children and adolescents – a review of prevalence and concomitant psychological factors. *Int J Paediatr Dent* 2007;**17**:391–406.
16. McGrath PA, Miller LM. Modifying the psychological factors that intensify children's pain and prolong disability. In: Schechter NL, Berde CB, Yaster M, eds. *Pain in infants, children, and adolescents,* 2nd edn. Philadelphia, PA: Lippincott Williams & Wilkins, 2002; 85–104.
17. Merskey H, Bogduk N. *Classification of chronic pain; descriptions of chronic pain syndromes and definitions of pain terms,* 2nd edn. International Association for the Study of Pain, Task Force on Taxonomy. Seattle, WA: IASP Press, 1994; 209–14. Also via http://www.iasp-pain.org (accessed August 2008).
18. Milgrom P, Vignehsa H, Weinstein P. Adolescent dental fear and control: prevalence and theoretical implications. *Behav Res Ther* 1992;**30**:367–73.
19. Milgrom P, Weinstein P, Golletz D, Leroux B, Domoto P. Pain management in school-aged children by private and public clinic practice dentists. *Pediatr Dent* 1994;**16**:294–300.
20. Milgrom P, Mancl L, King B, Weinstein P. Origins of childhood dental fear. *Behav Res Ther* 1995;**33**:313–19.
21. Moore R, Brodsgaard I, Birn H. Manifestations, acquisition and diagnostic categories of dental fear in a self-referred population. *Behav Res Ther* 1991;**29**:51–60.
22. Murtomaa H, Milgrom P, Weinstein P, Vuopio T. Dentists' perceptions and management of pain experienced by children during treatment: a survey of groups of dentists in the USA and Finland. *Int J Paediatr Dent* 1996;**6**:25–30.
23. Weinstein P, Getz T, Ratener P, Domonto P. The effect of dentists' behaviors on fear-related behaviors in children. *J Am Dent Assoc* 1982;**104**:32–8.
24. Weinstein P, Milgrom P, Hoskuldsson O, Golletz D, Jeffcott E, Koday M. Situation-specific child control. A visit to the dentist. *Behav Res Ther* 1996;**34**:11–21.

5

Pain, pain control, and sedation

Magne Raadal, Stefan Lundeberg and Gro Haukali

In clinical dentistry and medicine, pain is synonymous with significant discomfort. However, it is important to remember that pain has a necessary and purposeful function. Pain signals tissue damage, and thereby alerts the individual to take action in alleviating such damage.

Pain may be acute or chronic and associated with trauma, diseases, postoperative healing, and treatment. In this chapter the main focus will be on acute pain associated with dental procedures (procedural pain). Painful procedures experienced during childhood have proved to be one of the most important factors behind fear, anxiety, and behavior management problems in connection with dental treatment (11,12) (see also Chapter 4).

Pain is defined as a subjective sensory and emotional experience, which may or may not be associated with tissue damage (Box 5-1). This implies that only the child patient himself or herself can decide whether a clinical procedure is painful or not (21). This may be difficult to understand for the clinical dentist who will tend to relate the level of pain to the level of tissue damage. There are several reasons for this discrepancy between pain perception and tissue damage that we observe (38).

During the past 20 years there has been more focus on children's perception of pain in different health-care situations, based on the fact that children's pain was underestimated and not sufficiently treated. It was believed that the newborn child's central nervous system (CNS) was immature and not able to register pain as in adults. More recent research has, however, shown that both neonates and small children are at least as pain sensible as the adult, based on less developed functions that inhibit or modify pain responses in their CNS (3). It has also been shown that children may be hypersensitive for pain when exposed to painful stimuli in early life, particularly children with chronic diseases and those who have been critically sick. Such children may show signs of hyperalgesia, either general or local, and their behavior may be affected by it.

Box 5-1 Definitions

- *Pain* is an unpleasant sensory and emotional experience associated with actual or potential tissue damage or described in terms of such damage.
  Note: pain is always subjective. Each individual learns the application of the word through experiences related to injury in early life (21).
- *Analgesia* literally means without pain, while *anesthesia* means without feeling. The term local analgesia is, therefore, more correct than local anesthesia as only pain, not all sensations, is removed by this procedure.
- *Local analgesia* is defined as a reversal temporary cessation of painful impulses from a particular region in the body.
- *General analgesia* is a state of reduced pain perception in a conscious patient.
- *Sedation* is described as a depressed level of consciousness, which may vary from light to deep. At a light level of sedation (conscious sedation) the patient retains the ability to independently maintain an open airway and respond appropriately to verbal commands. The protective reflexes are normal or minimally altered, and the patient may have amnesia. At a deep level of sedation some depression of the protective reflexes occurs but, although more difficult, it is still possible to arouse the patient.
- *General anesthesia* describes a controlled status of unconsciousness accompanied by partial or total loss of protective reflexes including the inability to independently maintain an airway or respond appropriately to verbal commands.

Evidence also exists that children who have experienced painful dental procedures, particularly at young ages, are more pain sensitive and display more behavioral problems during dental treatment than those who have not. The risk for this increases potentially if the painful stimuli have been experienced in combination with a feeling of lack of control. A typical clinical situation is when the child is being exposed to painful procedures under restraint (behavioral control), or when the painful stimulus comes suddenly without having prepared the child for it (informational control).

Another reason that children may perceive pain in situations without tissue damage is based on classical conditioning. If a child has undergone a painful procedure based on tissue damage (e.g., drilling into dentin) during a dental procedure, and this stimulus (unconditioned stimulus) is combined with other stimuli such as the sound and the water spray of the drill (conditioned stimuli), it may result in pain perception when the conditioned stimuli are presented alone (Fig. 5-1).

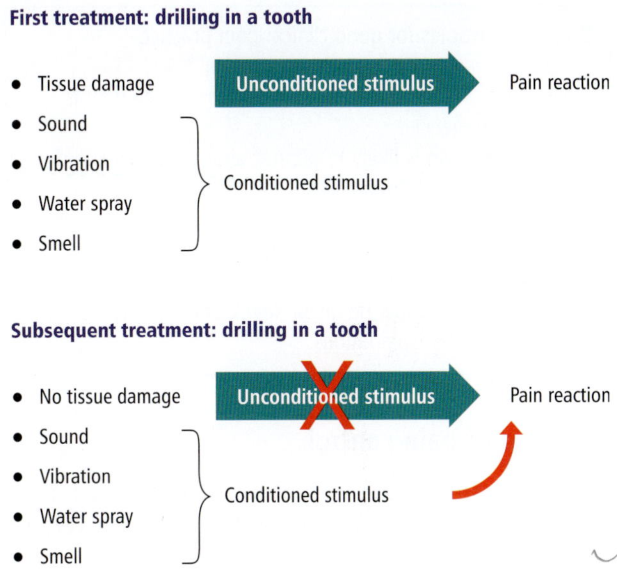

Figure 5-1 Pain perception based on classical conditioning: a painful procedure based on an unconditioned stimulus (e.g., tissue damage when drilling into dentin), combined with other stimuli such as the sound and the water spray of the drill (conditioned stimuli), may result in pain perception when the conditioned stimuli are presented alone.

There are a number of additional factors known to affect the individual perception of pain, such as peripheral and central sensitization, biological variation, previous pain experience, context, and a variety of psychological factors. The complexity of pain perception can explain the lack of correspondence between the degree of noxious stimuli and the intensity of pain experience. From the neurophysiological point of view a noxious stimulus creates both a local sensitization in the damaged area and changes within the CNS which amplify the ingoing signaling to pain areas. This plasticity within the nervous system can alter the pain signaling for an extended time, long after healing has occurred in the affected area (physiological pain memory) (9,42). The transmission of pain impulses does not only target the sensory cortex. A complex system with signaling from the sensory cortex as well as direct impulses from lower brain structures reaches the limbic system. The limbic system accounts for the affective reaction to a pain stimulus and plays a major part of a pain perception. Previous pain experiences (psychological pain memory) and fear are two of the most important factors contributing to the affective component of pain perception.

A simplified illustration of the frequently observed lack of correspondence between the degree of tissue damage and pain reaction is illustrated in Fig. 5-2.

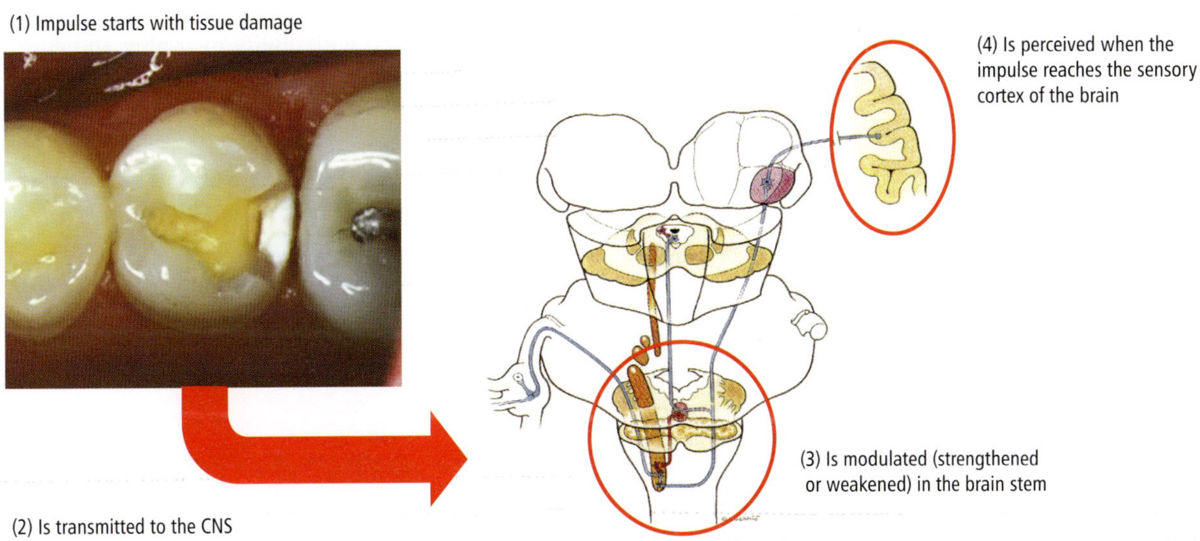

Figure 5-2 The perception of procedural pain due to tissue damage (nociceptive pain) depends on a variety of factors, owing to the fact that the stimuli are modulated in the central part of the brain before reaching the sensory cortex. Previous pain experiences (psychological pain memory) and fear are the most important factors contributing to the affective component of pain perception.

Box 5-2 Principles for good clinical pain practice

- Only the child in pain can really tell how much pain is being experienced.
- Whenever pain is likely to occur it should be measured and targeted for intervention.
- It is better to prevent pain than to treat it once it occurs.
- When painful procedures are impossible to avoid:
  - If possible, parents should accompany their children.
  - The children must be given developmentally appropriate explanations.

Box 5-4 Principles for the prevention and treatment of procedural pain

Child-centered approaches:
- cognitive behavioral methods, including exposure therapy
- muscle relaxation
- paced breathing
- distraction
- modeling.

Disease-centered approaches:
- local analgesia
- analgesic drugs, including inhaled nitrous oxide
- conscious sedation.

Methods of pain control

The complexity of pain perception is a challenge for the dental practitioner when treating children. However, the prevention and alleviation of pain is a basic human right that exists regardless of age, which demands some basic principles for good clinical pain practice to be maintained in pediatric dentistry (Box 5-2).

Measuring pain is an important factor to improve care in children. The aim is to provide acceptable pain levels for the child undergoing dental treatment and therefore we as caregivers have to find ways to assess the pain experience in the individual child. Pain assessment puts pain on the treatment agenda, and can help us to identify pain under treatment and to evaluate new pain treatment strategies. Since pain is personal and subjective, age-appropriate self-report scales should be used when possible (e.g., visual analogue scale, faces pain scale, colored analogue scale, Box 5-3). In children with limited communication skills indirect measurement can be used as observation of behavior (e.g., behavior rating scales) and physiologic reactions (e.g., heart rate, sweating). In clinical practice these methods must be adapted to the cognitive and linguistic skill of the individual child and easy to use.

Both the prevention and treatment of procedural pain should be based on a preoperative judgment of factors that may be assumed to affect the child's perception of pain. These factors may be divided into *child-centered approaches* and a *disease-centered approach*, and examples are given in Box 5-4.

The child-centered approaches are based on the great plasticity of pain perception in children, meaning that environmental and psychological factors may be powerful in influencing their perception of pain. The most basic techniques are described in Chapter 4. The selection of methods should be based on a clinical judgment of how vulnerable the child may be, which must be done in collaboration with the child itself and its parents. Among factors to be taken into consideration are age and maturity, temperament, previous pain experiences, and family/social network.

The need for disease-centered approaches must be estimated based on both the nature and extent of tissue damage and the vulnerability of the child. Robust and experienced children with ability of coping and control are able to undergo considerable dental treatment with minimal use of pharmaceutical agents. On the other

Box 5-3 Assessment of pain intensity (6,10,13,24,30,31)

Pain can be assessed through self-reported measures (e.g., faces scale, visual analogue scale, pain diaries), behavior measures (e.g., facial expression of infants, behavioral rating scales), and physiological measures (e.g., heart rate, transcutaneous oxygen, sweating, and electroencephalogram).

An example of a self-reported faces scale used in children 3–7 years of age (20):

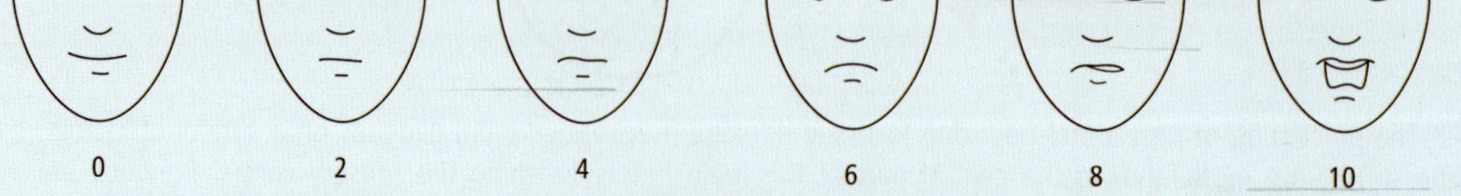

0 2 4 6 8 10

hand, the vulnerable child with low coping ability and previous negative experiences with painful procedures must be taken care of by extensive use of both psychological and pharmaceutical methods.

Local analgesia and pain control

Local analgesia is an efficient and safe method for controlling pain in pediatric dental care. The rate of success, however, depends on both the technique and the operator. Some methods of injections produce minimal discomfort, as will be described in the following. Furthermore, the operator's attitude and confidence in administrating local analgesia influence the success rate, and it has been shown that some dentists find it stressing to give a mandibular block to children below school age (36,44).

In addition to pain control, local analgesia can be used as a diagnostic tool and in the control of hemorrhage.

Intraoral topical analgesics

Topical local analgesic agents are extremely important in reducing pain during intraoral injections and should be used routinely. They are available as spray, gel, ointment, and solution. The most commonly used are lidocaine (5 or 20%) and benzocaine (20%) as ointment or gel. Topical analgesic agents will anaesthetize the surface tissue in a depth of 2–3 mm if used properly. The ointment or gel is applied on dry mucosa for 2–5 minutes depending on the concentration of the agent. For many children the use of topical analgesics will be connected with their first experience of intraoral pain control, and it is of great importance that it is given sufficient time to be effective. The child must also be informed about the strong taste of the agent. The application is most practically made with a cotton bud over a limited area. It is important to limit the amount used (Fig. 5-3a). The uptake from the mucosa is rapid and it is important to remember that the concentration of the active agent in the topical solution often is high.

Topical application of 5% lidocaine solution for mouthwashing before taking an impression can be of help for children with pronounced gag reflexes.

Local analgesic solutions

There are a number of local analgesics available for injection, both with and without vasoconstrictors, and with variable duration. The efficiency of the drug is increased and prolonged by the addition of vasoconstrictors, while the toxicity is decreased. Most commonly used in Scandinavian pediatric dental care are lidocaine (20 mg/ml) with adrenaline (12.5 μg/ml) and articaine (40 mg/ml) with adrenaline (5 μg/ml). Both have an intermediate analgesic duration on the pulp of approximately 60 minutes. More rarely there may be indications for a local analgesic with long duration, e.g., pulpal analgesia for 90 minutes and more, which can be obtained by bupivacaine with adrenaline.

Methods of administration

Infiltration

Infiltration is the application of a local analgesic solution around the nerve ends. The aim is to deposit the solution as close as possible to the apex of the tooth. The maxillary and mandibular bone plate in children is generally less dense than in adults, which permits a more rapid and complete diffusion of the analgesic solution through the bone. Infiltration can therefore be used with great success in the primary as well as the permanent dentition. Buccal infiltration of 0.5–1 ml solutions is sufficient for pulpal analgesia of most teeth in the maxilla of a child. There can be some difficulties anaesthetizing the maxillary first permanent molars by the infiltration technique due to the zygomatic process which is closer to the alveolar bone in children than adults. Infiltration close to the apices of the maxillary central incisors should be performed carefully, as it can be very painful. In the mandible, buccal infiltration of 0.5–1 ml will often be sufficient for pain control in the primary dentition, although the effect on the second primary molar will not always be sufficient.

Technique

After penetrating a stretched and topically anesthesized mucosa the needle is directed towards the apex of the tooth. The injection is done very slowly supraperiostally. Deposition under the periost can be very painful and should be avoided; at least before the periost itself has been anesthetized. Applying finger pressure to the area of injection prior to the injection may distract the patient's attention. Thin (30 G) or standard (27 G) needles are recommended, and the solution should have room temperature – never be used directly from the refrigerator.

In principle, infiltration can be done anywhere in the oral cavity including the palate. However, in order to prevent painful injection in the palate, transpapillary injection is preferred (Fig. 5-3). All injections must be done *very* slowly (25).

Blocks

By far the most used block analgesia in children is the mandibular foramen block (Fig. 5-4). Prior to the injection it is of great importance to prepare the child for the procedure in a way that is adjusted to its age and maturity (see Chapter 4). The patient should open

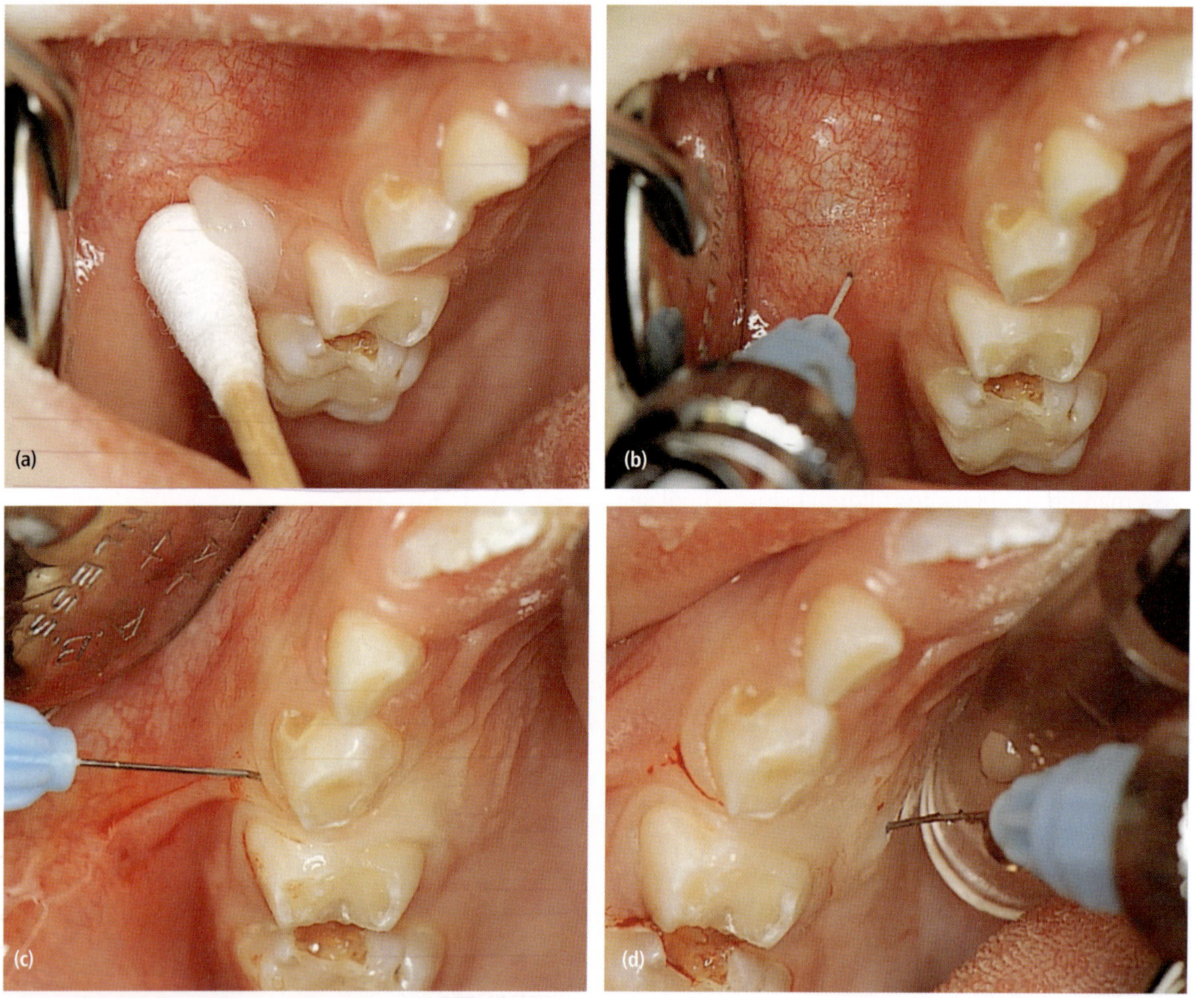

Figure 5-3 (a) Topical application of local analgesia ointment on a cotton bud at the injection spot. (b) Infiltration analgesia followed by (c) a transpapillary injection started from the buccal and (d) continuing to the palatal mucosa. Note blanching of the palatal papilla and mucosa in (c).

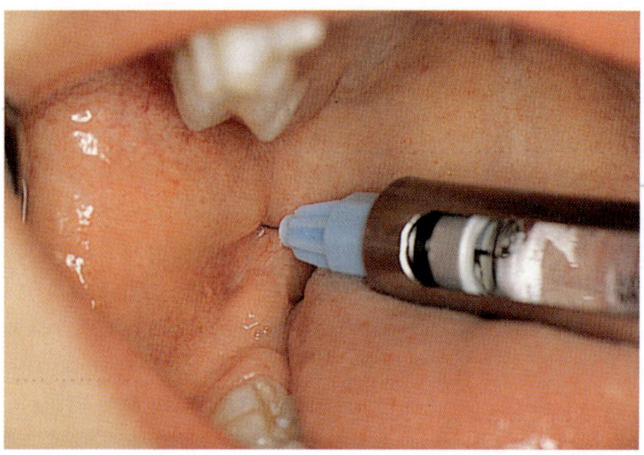

Figure 5-4 Mandibular block analgesia in a preschool child.

maximally and the needle be introduced just laterally to the pterygomandibular fold at its deepest point (the pterygoid notch). In children, the direct injection from the opposite primary molar region is recommended. This technique requires less needle movement after tissue penetration. To secure a good block, the needle should be introduced into the tissue without any resistance. If resistance is felt, the needle is slightly withdrawn and redirected. The most common reason for resistance is the strong medial tendon from the temporal muscle along the temporal crest.

The foramen of the mandibular nerve lies below the occlusal plane on a line where the ramus is narrowest, two-thirds of the way back from the anterior concavity (Fig. 5-5). Palpation of the mandibular ramus will give the point of insertion, the direction in the horizontal and vertical planes, and the depth.

The needle is inserted between the pterygomandibular raphe and the ascending border of the mandibular bone. Inject a small amount of solution before advancing the needle into the deeper tissues. In young children bone will be reached after about 15 mm and a 25-mm needle can be used. However in older children a depth of penetration up to 25 mm may be necessary, thus requir-

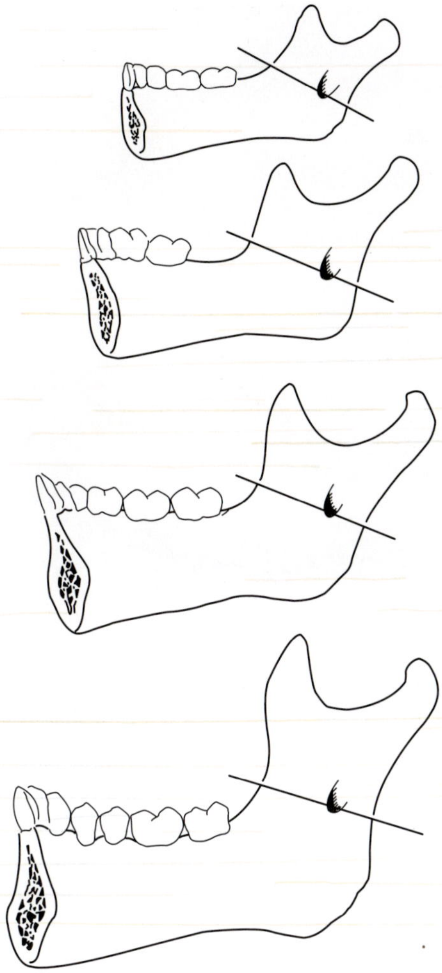

Figure 5-5 The position of the mandibular foramen changes during growth. However, the mandibular foramen is below the occlusive plane in children. The foramen is always situated on the line, where the ramus is narrowest, two-thirds of the way back from the anterior concavity.

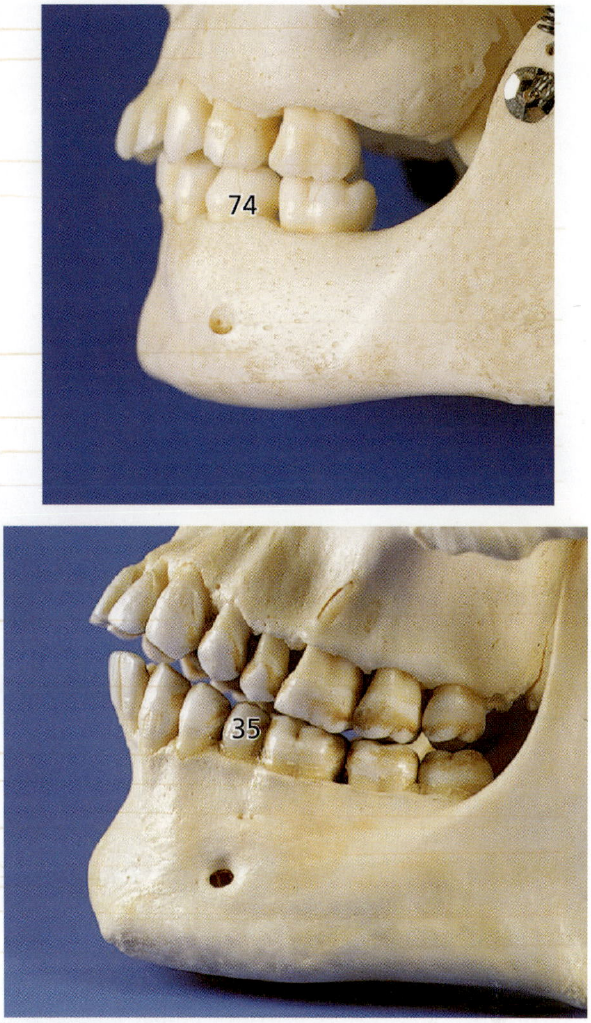

Figure 5-6 Pictures of skulls. The mental foramen is located closer to the primary mandibular first molar in children and the permanent second premolar in adults.

ing a 35-mm needle. When contact with the bone is obtained the needle is slightly withdrawn to avoid periost. Aspiration is performed and 1.2–1.5 ml of the solution is deposited. The lingual nerve is blocked when withdrawing the needle halfway and depositing a little of the remaining solution here. A chair-side dental assistant is necessary when delivering a mandibular block for preventing sudden movements of hands and head in a comfortable way (35).

A mental block may be the result of an infiltration close to the primary mandibular first molar (Fig. 5-6). Use of the regional maxillary block technique is seldom if ever required in a young child.

Computerized delivery systems

During recent years, computerized delivery systems (e.g., the Wand®) have become part of the equipment for many dental practitioners treating children (Fig. 5-7a). These systems deliver the analgesic solution with a constant and very slow speed which minimizes the pressure to the tissue and thereby the pain from the injection (34). They can be used for all types of injections, both infiltration and blocks (33), but the great advantage is to be found in the "new palatal block procedures" and in the modified periodontal ligament (PDL) injection. When using these techniques the child does not experience the soft tissue analgesia which often is difficult to accept especially for young children. A disadvantage is that the anesthetic solution may leak into the child's mouth and produce a bitter taste. Therefore it is important that the chair-side assistant is aware of the problem and uses a cotton bud to assemble the solution.

The lightweight handpiece held like a pen enables the dentist to manipulate the needle placement with fingertip accuracy, rotating the needle when penetrating the mucosa and deliver the local analgesic with a foot-

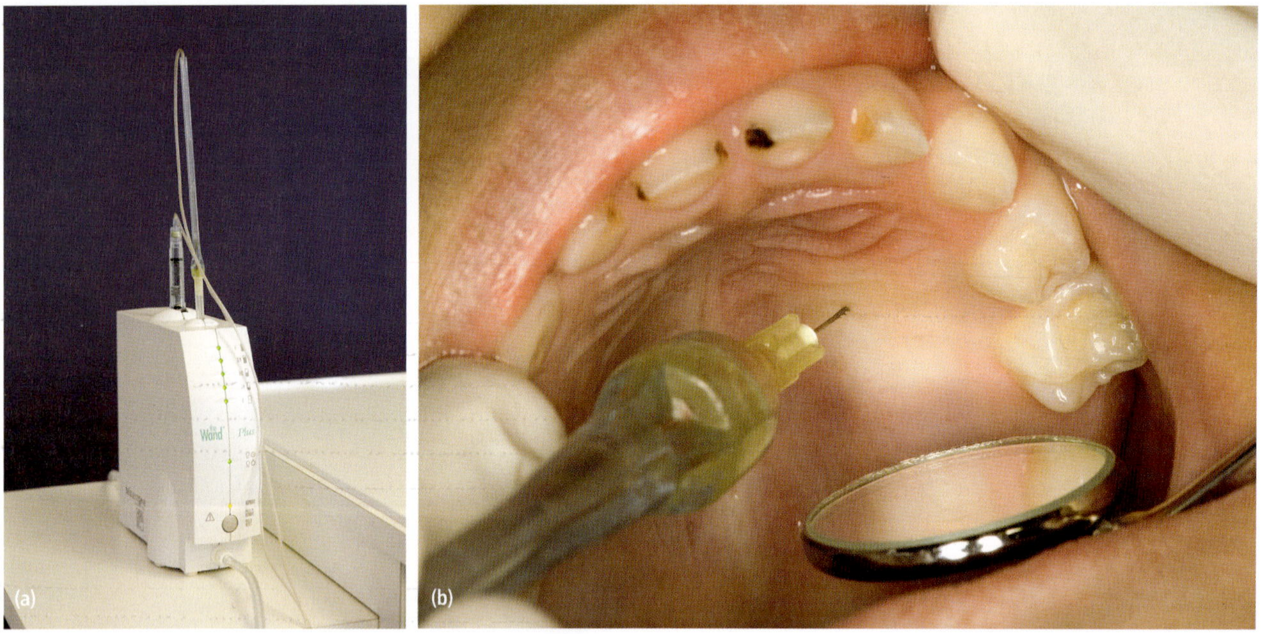

Figure 5-7 (a) The Wand® is an example of a computerized system that delivers the analgesic solution with a constant and very slow speed which minimizes the pressure to the tissue and thereby the pain from the injection. (b) The AMSA injection technique.

activated contact. The flow rate is computer controlled and remains constant irrespective of variations in tissue resistance.

By using the computerized delivery systems, two "new palatal block procedures" plus a modified PDL injection are now possible:

- Anterior middle superior alveolar (AMSA) injection technique. The AMSA provides pulpal analgesia to the upper primary molars and canines, the surrounding palatal tissue and mucoperiosteum without any numbness of the lip, cheek, and muscles. For some children this gives a greater comfort and makes it easier to accept. A 30-gauge extra-short needle is oriented midway between the upper primary molars and midway between the free gingival margin and the palatine suture (Fig. 5-7b). The suggested dosage should be delivered at a slow flow rate.
- Palatal anterior superior alveolar (P-ASA) injection technique. This is a modified injection technique for the anterior maxilla and provides bilateral analgesia of the maxillary incisors and partially of the canines with a single-needle penetration without involving lip and face. A 30-gauge extra-short needle is inserted adjacent to the incisive papilla. Topical ointment is applied in advance and it is critical to use only a slow flow rate.
- PDL injection technique. This is a good alternative to the mandibular block when treating lower primary and first permanent molars. The technique is not recommended for teeth with active periodontal inflammation. The modified PDL technique employs two injection sites (mesial and distal) while the traditional PDL are performed with four. A 27- or 30-gauge extra-short needle is oriented with the bevel toward the tooth. The bevel should follow the surface of the tooth. The needle is advanced until resistance while the slow flow rate is activated. Approximately half the cartridge is deposited at each side of the tooth.

General techniques

The administration of a pain-free or an almost pain-free injection depends primarily on the operator and factors that can be controlled by the operator: equipment, materials, and techniques (see Box 5-5).

Box 5-5 Attaining painless local analgesia

One of the most important factors in attaining painless local analgesia is slow injection. In addition the pediatric dentist should:

- dry the mucosa prior to application of topical analgesic in order to get optimal effect
- apply topical ointment in a small and accurate amount
- let it stay in place for 2–5 minutes
- dry the mucosa again
- apply finger pressure to the area
- stretch the mucosa
- insert the needle
- if bone contact is obtained, withdraw the needle
- aspirate.

Topical ointments with different tastes are available, and some children may find some of them more preferable than others. Only sharp needles, thin (30 G) or standard (27 G), should be used. Some authors mention that aspiration through a 30-gauge needle can be difficult, although possible. A narrow needle is more likely to penetrate blood vessels than a needle with a wider gauge. When using a 35-mm long needle, the deflection is larger in narrow compared with wide-gauge needles. It is suggested that the syringe is self-aspirating. The analgesic solution should have room temperature. The acidity of the analgesic solution is a factor provoking discomfort during injection, and the pH of solutions with vasoconstrictor is generally lower than those without (approximately 5.5 vs 4.5).

Contraindications

A child's unwillingness or inability to cooperate is one of the few contraindications to local analgesia used alone (e.g., without sedation). Local analgesia is also contraindicated in the case of genuine allergy to the agents, although this is actually very rare. It is also not advisable to inject into deep tissues in patients with bleeding and coagulation disorders due to the risk of uncontrollable hematoma. In such cases, the patient's physician has to be consulted before local analgesia is given. Medical conditions such as severe liver disease or poor blood supply to a tissue may also be contraindications.

Local analgesia with adrenaline is *not* contraindicated for patients being treated with tricyclic antidepressants if injected slowly, and if the aspiration is performed before injection. Neither is local analgesia with adrenaline contraindicated for patients with hypertension or cardiac arrhythmia, if the same precautions are taken. In these patients, it is actually the amount of endogenously produced adrenaline, due to stress and pain, that is the problem.

Complications

In general, there are few side-effects and complications following local analgesia in children and adolescents. The most common problem is without doubt that the efficiency of the procedure may be less than desired. The most common systemic side-effect is syncope or fainting, a loss of consciousness due to decreased blood supply to the brain. This may be due to a genetic anxiety disorder (blood–injection–injury phobia: BII phobia), which is rather frequent in children and adolescents as is discussed in Chapter 4. If the patient faints, he or she should be placed in a recumbent position with elevated legs. The airways should be secured by tilting the head backwards and forcing the mandible forward. General allergic reactions to local analgesia solution are very rare and consist of skin eruptions, occasionally bronchial constrictions, and a drop in blood pressure. In the case of proven allergy, another product should be tested. Most complications or side-effects are of local origin, such as self-inflicted bites of anesthetized tissue (Fig. 5-8), which are best treated with chlorhexidine gel 1%. Blanching of the cheek after local analgesia injection is a sympaticus reaction (Fig. 5-9) and will last in a few patients for up to 10 minutes. Hematoma sometimes arises during injection, and in these cases the patient and the parents should be informed about its nature. The effusion of blood into extravascular spaces can result from inadvertently nicking a blood vessel during the injection of a local analgesic. It should be explained that swelling and discoloration will appear.

Toxicity

Toxic reactions from local analgesia can be caused by accidental intravascular injection, excessively rapid

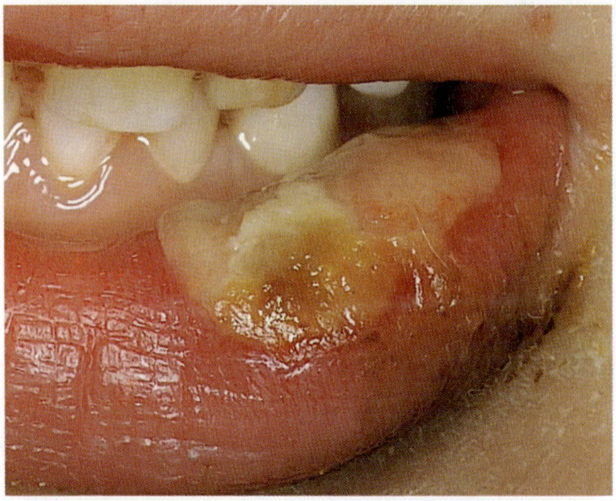

Figure 5-8 Side-effect of local analgesia. Bite wound.

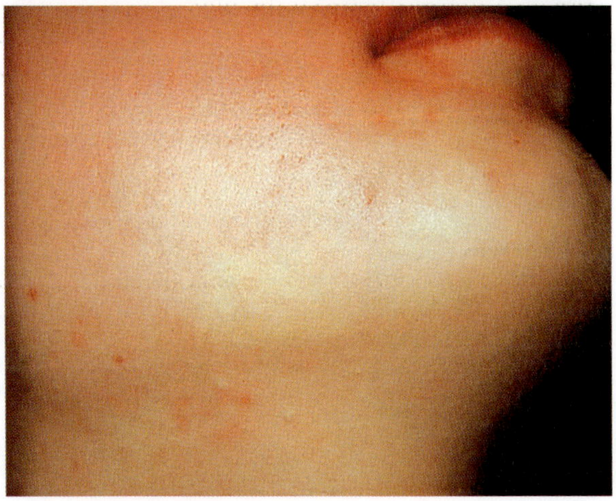

Figure 5-9 Blanching of the cheek (sympaticus reaction) after local analgesia injection in a child.

injection, or drug overdose. Patients may complain of slight dizziness and visual or hearing disturbances. They may become agitated, confused, and have difficulties in breathing. There may be a cardiovascular system reaction, with an increased heart rate and blood pressure and – in the second phase of local analgesic toxicity – a drop in blood pressure. Dentists who treat children should always be mindful of local analgesia toxicity and the recommended maximum safe dose of local anesthetic for each child should be calculated (Box 5-6).

Box 5-6 Recommended doses of local analgesia for children

The recommended child dose can easily be calculated from the listed formula, when the adult dose is known.

$$\text{Child dose} = \text{adult dose} \times \frac{\text{Age in years}}{\text{Age in years} + 12}$$

Examples: recommended maximum dose in mg of local analgesia with and without vasoconstrictor:

	Adult	*Child of 3 years*
Lidocaine		
without vasoconstrictor	300	60
with vasoconstrictor	500	100
Articaine		
with vasoconstrictor	500	100
Mepivacaine		
without vasoconstrictor	400	80
with vasoconstrictor	400	80
Prilocaine		
without vasoconstrictor	400	80
Bupivacaine		
with vasoconstrictor	90	18

Preparation of the patient

Children of all ages should be given some kind of preparation before an oral injection, adapted to their age and maturity (Fig. 5-10). The preparation must be preceded by establishing a good relationship between the operator and the patient and consists of giving the child a feeling of control during the situation (see Chapter 4). It may be advisable to announce the injection in a session prior to the treatment session. In young children of 3–6 years, a simple statement that local analgesia will be used should be made along with an adjusted explanation. A more elaborated introduction can be given just prior to the injection, taking into account that the child should only be given information that he or she can handle. A young child can become more nervous when faced with too much detailed information. Whether the needle should be shown to the child before injection should also be considered from the same point of view. When the child is older (6–7 years old) he or she will be able to handle more detailed information, and the dentist has to give the child more control. It may also be necessary to teach different coping techniques, e.g., relaxation and paced breathing. Children with tendency to faint should be encouraged to tighten their muscles (applied tension) instead of relaxing in order to maintain blood pressure (for more details about fear of injections, see Chapter 4). However, children vary quite considerably in their

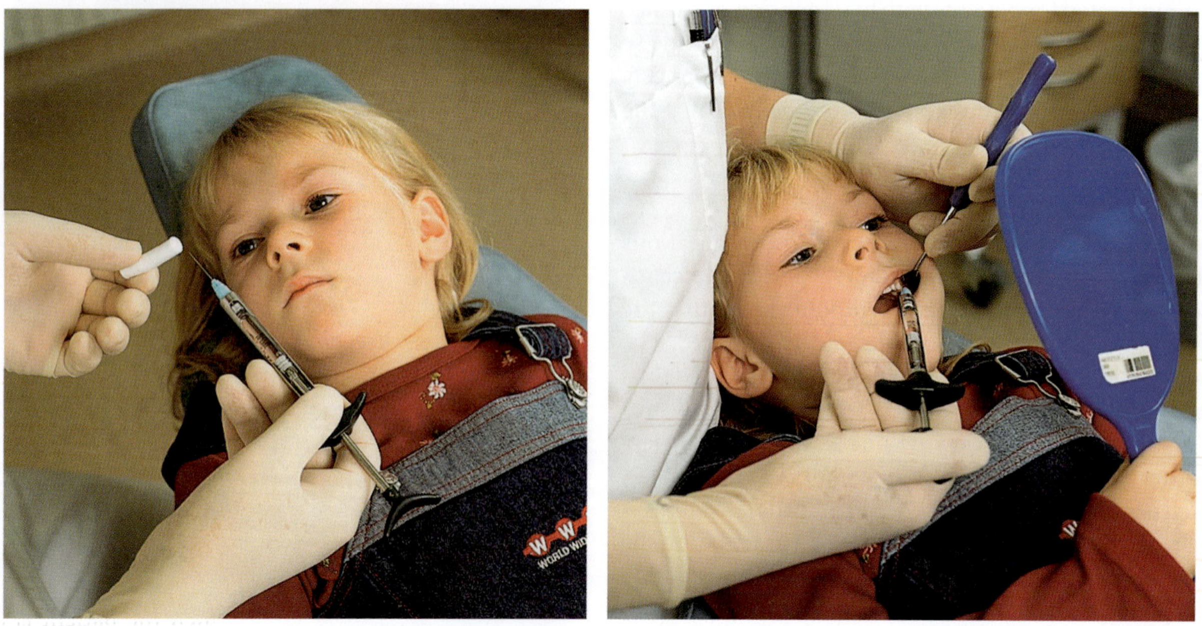

Figure 5-10 Instruments should always be open and displayed. In the right-hand picture the local analgesia procedure is demonstrated by sham operation observed by the girl in the hand mirror.

coping abilities; some benefit greatly from watching and viewing every step, in other cases it is better to pamper and distract the child at the actual moment of the injection. When children develop the ability of abstract thinking at about 12 years, their reaction to pain is more like that of an adult. Most children at this age will also be able to take full responsibility for whether local analgesia should be used or not. Before that age, the dentist has the responsibility to make the decision. The dental assistant plays an important role in preventing the child from making sudden movements during the administration of local anesthesia (Fig. 5-11).

General analgesia

The most commonly used and recommended general analgesics for children are paracetamol and nonsteroidal anti-inflammatory drugs (NSAIDs). Paracetamol (acetaminophen) is a central-acting drug, as compared with NSAIDs, which exert their analgesic effect mostly in the peripheral tissue. Both paracetamol and NSAIDs reach their maximal analgesic effect after about 2 hours when administered orally, which is the preferred route. The rectal uptake of paracetamol is more erratic as compared with the oral route and the maximum analgesic effect is reached as late as 3–4 hours after administration. The initial starting dose or single dose of paracetamol should be higher than the maintenance dose used in the postoperative phase (4). NSAIDs also have an effect on platelets which could have a negative effect on coagulation. An alternative to nonselective NSAIDs is to use cyclooxygenase (COX)-2 inhibitors, as celecoxibe, if bleeding is a concern during the procedure or in the postoperative phase. A combination of paracetamol and NSAIDs is recommended for optimal pain relief, and

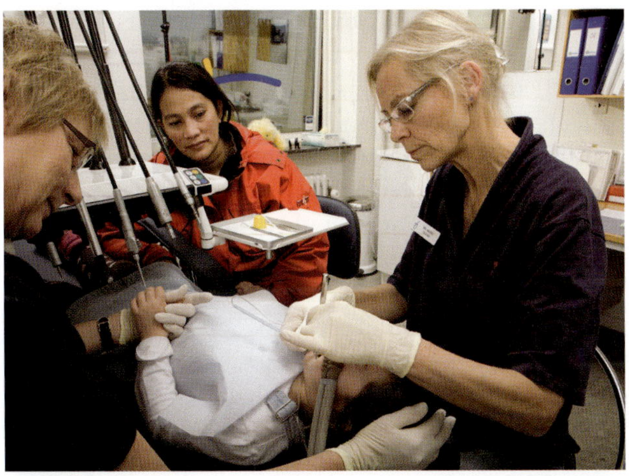

Figure 5-11 During an injection, the assistant can support the child by holding a hand and also keep the other hand on the child's head to be sure the child does not make a sudden movement.

Box 5-7 Oral doses of general analgesics for short-time use (maximum 3 days) for children >1 year

Paracetamol	30–40 mg/kg (single or initial dose), followed by 60–90 mg/kg/24 h, divided into four daily doses (15–20 mg/kg)
Diclofenac	3 mg/kg/24 h, divided into two to three daily doses
Naproxen	10–15 mg/kg/24 h, divided into two daily doses
Ibuprofen	20–40 mg/kg/24 h, divided into three to four daily doses
Celcoxibe	2–4 mg/kg/24 h, one dose daily

they should be administered about 2 hours before the treatment in order to assist in the prevention of procedural pain. If pain is expected during the postoperative phase it is recommended to give the patient an analgesic on a regular basis especially during the first 1–2 days (26–28). Acetylsalicylic acid (aspirin) should be avoided for postoperative pain due to its anticoagulant effect and possible toxicity.

Box 5-7 presents oral doses for short-time use of some general analgesics for children.

In patients where the use of a sedative drug is indicated, it is a good practice to combine the sedative with an analgesic. The alpha-2 receptor agonists, clonidine and dexmedetomidine, represent an interesting profile of drugs which both have a sedative and an analgesic effect without the risk of ventilatory depression found with opioid use. Clonidine can be administered orally or rectally. Dexmedetomidine has a limited oral uptake but transmucosal (buccal) administration has been described as effective. It should be remembered that most sedatives commonly used for procedures are lacking analgesic effect. The use of analgesics is mandatory in procedures where pain is anticipated.

Conscious sedation

The term *conscious sedation* is defined as a medically controlled state of depressed consciousness that allows protective reflexes to be maintained, retains the patient's ability to maintain a patent airway independently and continuously, and permits appropriate response by the patient to physical stimulation or verbal command, e.g., "open your mouth" (17). This can be achieved by different drugs administered either by the oral, rectal, or intravenous routes, or by inhalation. The term *deep sedation* denotes a deeper state of depressed consciousness or unconsciousness from which the patient is not easily aroused. This may be obtained by the same drugs as for conscious sedation when used in higher doses. It

Box 5-8 Goals of using conscious sedation during dental treatment of children and adolescents

General goal

- Prevent the development of behavior management problems and dental anxiety due to unpleasant dental experiences.

Specific goals

- Increase effect of behavior management techniques.
- Reduce perception of pain and discomfort.
- Amnesia (possibly).

is acknowledged that deep sedation is accompanied with risks when administered by dentists alone during oral treatment procedures. This is due to the fact that deep sedation may be accompanied by a partial or complete loss of protective reflexes, including the inability to maintain a patent airway independently and to provide a purposeful response to physical stimulation or verbal command. Only conscious sedation is dealt with in this section, since this may be administered by the operating dentist alone without the necessity of being assisted by a specialist in anesthesiology.

Different guidelines for conscious sedation in dental care have been developed (1,8,17). The suggested main goals of using sedation during dental treatment of children and adolescents are listed in Box 5-8. It must be underlined that conscious sedation alone is frequently inadequate to make the very fearful child cope with dental treatment, as deep sedation or general anesthesia will do. Patients are awake and conscious of what is going on, but the anxiolytic and sedative effect makes them less sensitive to unpleasant stimuli and more accessible for behavioral techniques such as distraction and comforting. Even if the drug itself has no analgesic effect, the pain perception may also be reduced since this is dependent on the anxiety level.

Indications and contraindications

Conscious sedation is indicated when *both* patient and dental indications are present (Box 5-9). It is the combined assessment of these two types of indications that should be the basis for suggesting whether a certain type of oral examination or treatment should be done conventionally or under some type of sedation or general anesthesia. Children with low coping ability (e.g., immature children) or high dental anxiety, and with extensive or complicated treatment needs, should be treated under deep sedation or general anesthesia, which requires anesthesiology staff. This is probably most appropriate from the perspective of the child, parents, and dental staff, and may also be cost-effective since the majority of treatment may be done in one session.

Box 5-9 Indications for conscious sedation should be based on a combined assessment of patient and dental indications

Patient indications

- Patients with inadequate coping ability.
- Patients with high dental fear/dental anxiety/odontophobia (see Chapter 4).
- Need for reduction of patient's pain perception (prevent fear-induced pain).

Dental indications

- Oral examinations and treatments of *moderate* extent and complexity (extensive treatment needs should be accomplished under general anesthesia).
- Emergency treatment (e.g., extractions and emergency treatment of traumas).

Box 5-10 Physical status classification of the American Society of Anesthesiologists (ASA) (2)

Class	*Physical status*
I	A normal healthy patient
II	A patient with a mild systemic disease
III	A patient with a severe systemic disease that limits activity, but is not incapacitating
IV	A patient with an incapacitating systemic disease that is a constant threat to life
V	A moribund patient not expected to survive 24 hours with or without surgery

For the preoperative assessment of the patient, particularly whether there are any contraindications for use of sedation, the American Society of Anesthesiologists' (ASA) classification system of the patient's physical status should be used (Box 5-10). The dentist is expected to take the responsibility for treating patients in Classes I and II under conscious sedation, while treatment of patients in Classes III and IV should be decided on in consultation with a physician/anesthesiologist.

Sedation of children below 2 years of age is connected with increased risks and should therefore be done in collaboration with an anesthesiologist. Sedation of children with any kind of acute general disease should also be avoided. Other contraindications are allergy to any of the drugs, neuromuscular diseases, and if an interaction with other medications is suspected.

Oral and rectal administration of benzodiazepines

Although it has been stated that a definitive conclusion on which drug is the most effective for sedation of anxious children (29), the benzodiazepines are the drugs of first choice, possibly beside nitrous oxide. The benzodiazepine group contains a variety of chemical variations, where the most frequently used in dentistry in the Scandinavian countries are diazepam, midazolam, and flunitrazepam (22,23). Their clinical effects are anxiolytic, sedative/hypnotic, and muscle relaxing, and the toxicity is low (5). A certain degree of depressed respiration and anterograde amnesia must also be expected. The amnesia may have a positive or negative effect depending on whether it is valuable for the child to remember the clinical session or not. The site of action of the benzodiazepines is in the CNS where they increase the effect of the inhibiting neurotransmittor gamma-aminobutyric acid (GABA) (32). Diazepam, midazolam, and flunitrazepam have similar pharmacological properties, but different duration time, and the choice between them may therefore be based on how long a time sedation is needed. *Diazepam* has a long working time due to long elimination half-life and active metabolites, and it is therefore most suitable for reducing preoperative anxiety and preventing sleep disturbances prior to treatment. It is available in both tablets and rectal solutions. *Midazolam* has the shortest working time because of fast elimination and is therefore most suitable for perioperative sedation under treatments of short duration. The drug is available only in ampoules for intravenous injection (tablets available in some countries), but the solution can also be used for rectal and oral administration. Since the taste of midazolam is very bitter, it must be mixed with some kind of juice or other additives to taste in order to have children drink it. The working time of *flunitrazepam* lies between diazepam and midazolam, and it is available in tablets with no particular bad taste. It may be either swallowed as a whole, placed underneath the tongue (absorption through the mucosa), or crushed and dissolved in some kind of drink.

Routes and doses

Intravenous sedation is the most effective regarding fast response, effect, and possibility to adjust the dosage to an optimal level of effect, but this is usually not practicable in small, anxious children. Oral administration is generally preferred from a practical point of view, but some children are unable or unwilling to take an oral medication. The alternative routes are rectal and nasal, but there are drawbacks with both of these. Rectal administration is connected with ethical problems and only applicable in very young children in collaboration with their parents. Nasal administration is effective, but very unpleasant for the child due to irritation of the nasal and pharyngeal mucosa, and may counteract the goal of establishing a positive relationship between dentist and child. The oral route may, however, be used in children who are unwilling to drink from a cup by placing the solution in the retromolar area from a needleless syringe (Fig. 5-12).

The suggested doses of benzodiazepines for conscious sedation are given in Table 5-1. The doses as well as the time to onset of desired effect are dependent on the administration route. The fastest and most effective absorption of the drug is through the nasal mucosa, which means more rapid onset and slightly lower dosage than for the rectal and oral routes. The absorption through the rectal mucosa is also rather fast and more effective than the oral route, due to the fact that a portion of the drug is metabolized in the liver after absorption from the ventricle/intestines. However, whatever route, there are extremely large individual variations in degree of absorption and time until maximum plasma

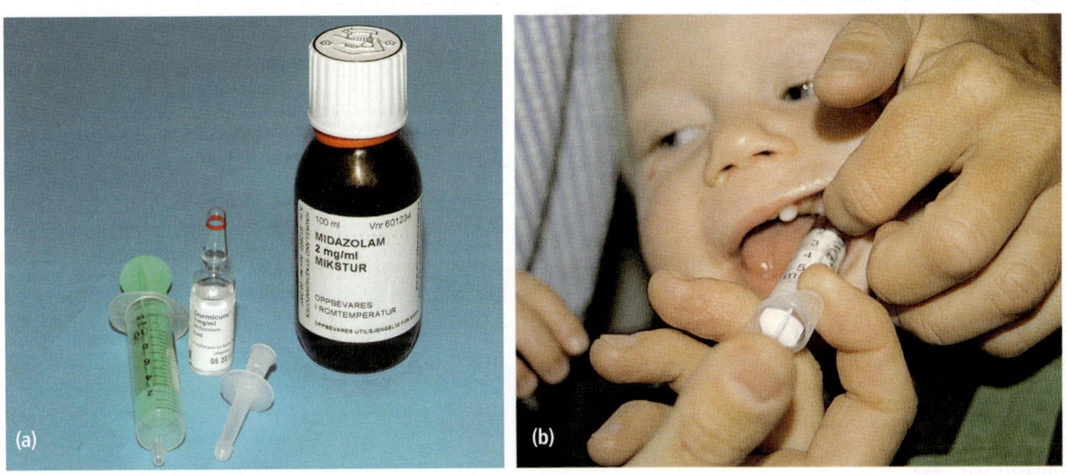

Figure 5-12 (a) Examples of material and applicators for rectal and oral administration of midazolam. (b) Oral sedation with needleless syringe in a 2-year-old child.

Table 5-1 Suggested doses of benzodiazepines for perioperative sedation (17)

Drugs and routes	Dosage (mg/kg)	Maximum dose (mg)
Midazolam, oral	0.4–0.5	12
Midazolam, rectal	0.3–0.4	10
Flunitrazepam, oral	0.02–0.025	20–40 kg: 0.5 >40 kg: 1.0
Diazepam, oral	4–8 years: 0.5–0.8 >8 years: 0.2–0.5	15 15
Diazepam, rectal	0.7	15

concentration is obtained. Combined with the fact that there are also large individual variations in dose response, there is considerable unpredictability about the effect of an individual dosage. Generally it may be estimated that the time from administration to onset of effect varies between 15 and 30 minutes, and that the maximum effect is obtained after about an hour.

Sedation with benzodiazepines should be used with special caution in patients who are using other medications, particularly other substances with depressing effect on the CNS, such as antipsychotics, antidepressants, antiepileptics, and opioids. Interactions may also be important for the dosage, e.g., the absorption of midazolam is enhanced by erythromycin and grapefruit juice. Drug interactions may be found in national databases.

Clinical considerations

Since the use of sedation in dentistry is associated with increased risks for the patients and responsibility for the operator, the practitioners should estimate their own competency within the framework of their authorization (8,17). The competency must include sufficient knowledge about the drugs, their effects, side-effects, and interactions, as well as the national regulations relating to them. The operator must have knowledge about and be able to practice preoperative considerations based on the ASA classification system, and also be able to handle possible complications. This includes also appropriate equipment for airway protection, oxygen delivery, and drugs for emergency use.

Prior to conscious sedation it is recommended that the child should fast in order to prevent possible aspiration in case of nausea and vomiting. The suggested rules are given in Box 5-11. For the emergency patient, where proper fasting has not been assured, the increased risk of sedation must be weighed against the benefits of the treatment, and the lightest effective sedation should be used. If possible, such patients may benefit from delaying the procedure.

Box 5-11 Suggested rules for fasting before conscious sedation (17)

- No clear liquids 2–3 hours before sedation.
- No solid foods or nonclear liquids 4 hours before sedation.

Clear liquids are nonfruity juice, water, tea, and coffee. All milk products (nonclear liquids) are considered as solid foods. Children under school age should drink a sugar-containing clear liquid up to 2 hours before treatment in order to avoid a low blood sugar level.

The patient must continuously be monitored during the treatment, both by the operating dentist and by an assistant. Keeping verbal contact with the patient is most important, thereby estimating the depth of the sedation. If the patient is not able to maintain verbal contact, with a tendency to fall asleep, not being able to keep the mouth open and not react to physical stimulation, the sedation stage may be too deep. This implies reduced reflexes and increased risks for aspiration during oral treatment, and one should aim to cancel such treatment and concentrate on securing the patient's airways. The use of pulsoximetry in order to be able to disclose possible blood desaturation is also suggested to increase safety.

After the treatment, the child must also be monitored and not dismissed until the sedative effect is definitely reduced and the child has regained normal psychomotor abilities. The child must be accompanied back home and be under observation by adults for the rest of the day. Preoperative and postoperative instructions in writing must be given in advance of the procedure to the child and the parent or guardian.

Inhalation sedation: nitrous oxide–oxygen sedation

For inhalation sedation, nitrous oxide–oxygen is the method most commonly used and its high success rate and safety are well documented (18). There are even studies that indicate the possibility that nitrous oxide–oxygen sedation prevents further development of anxiety (41).

Nitrous oxide–oxygen sedation is defined as a state of sedation with a varying degree of analgesia induced by inhalation of a mixture of nitrous oxide and oxygen while retaining an adequate laryngeal reflex. Nitrous oxide is always administered with oxygen to safeguard the patient's supply of oxygen. The sedation procedure starts by giving the patient 100% oxygen for 2–3 minutes. The nasal mask is adjusted to prevent leakage and the gas flow is regulated. Nitrous oxide is then administered in increasing concentrations until a suitable stage of conscious sedation (usually requiring 30–50% nitrous oxide) has been achieved (Fig. 5-13). After completion of the dental treatment, 100% oxygen is given for 5 minutes. Although the patient is able to leave the chair after the first 5 minutes, he or she is not ready to leave the surgery for about another 20 minutes.

Nitrous oxide has anesthetic, sedative, and analgesic effects, but the individual susceptibility varies. Even if the anesthetic effect is rather poor, some patients may lose consciousness breathing a 50% mixture of nitrous oxide. This requires slow induction (increasing concentrations of nitrous oxide) in patients who are given the gas for the first time in order to establish a suitable concentration for conscious sedation of the individual. The peak alveolar concentration is attained within a few minutes of inhalation, which implies that the sedative effect of a specific concentration of the gas can be assessed very shortly. Nitrous oxide–oxygen sedation is therefore a method that gives the operator an excellent opportunity to adjust the dose of the medication to a suitable level during the treatment with almost immediate effect, which increases the safety of the procedure. Since the analgesic effect is limited, it should be combined with local analgesia during invasive operative procedures.

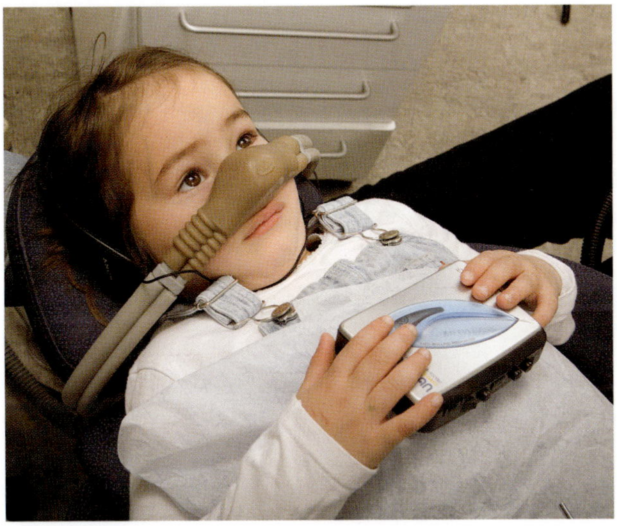

Figure 5-13 Nitrous oxide–oxygen sedation supported by audio-analgesia.

After uptake in the lungs, nitrous oxide gas is transported by the blood to the CNS, which is its site of sedative and analgesic actions. The exact mechanisms are, however, not known. The gas does not bind to body fluid or tissue and has little or no effect on respiration, blood circulation, and metabolism. The gas is eliminated quickly after termination of administration.

Side-effects of nitrous oxide, as described by patients, are excitation (oversedation), nausea, vomiting, dysphasia, sweating, restlessness, anxiety, panics, headache, nightmares, tinnitus, and urinary incontinence. In a study carried out in Sweden in 1982, of 823 patients given nitrous oxide–oxygen sedation during dental treatment, 8.3% exhibited side-effects, 0.1% due to oversedation (18).

Chronic exposure to low doses of nitrous oxide has been reported to be connected with occupational health hazards, causing an increased risk of spontaneous abortion, liver and kidney disease, and neurological conditions in dental staff (14,37,39). The gas interferes with the metabolism of vitamin B_{12} (43), a discovery that is probably without importance for the patient, but may explain the side-effects occurring in dental staff if chronically exposed to low concentrations of excess of gas owing to inadequate scavenging or leakage.

The administration of nitrous oxide–oxygen sedation requires special equipment. The machine must always supply not less than 20% oxygen (Scandinavia 40%) in the gas mixtures. Rebreathing or addition of air is not permitted and the tubes must have low breathing resistance. The gas flow must be continuous and the apparatus equipped with a failsafe device, i.e., if the oxygen pressure falls, the supply of nitrous oxide automatically stops. If the gas supply is disconnected, the patient must be able to breathe air via an emergency air-valve. Excess gas and exhaled gas must be effectively eliminated by scavenging (15,16,19).

Indications for nitrous oxide–oxygen sedation are generally the same as for the benzodiazepines. However, the fact that the gas has additional analgesic properties and is administered by inhalation makes the method a suitable alternative for a number of specific cases (see Table 5-2).

Inhalation sedation is contraindicated for patients belonging to ASA anesthesia risk Classes III and IV (Box 5-10), and these patients must eventually be treated only in collaboration with a responsible doctor or anesthetist. Also among patients in risk groups I and II there are

Table 5-2 Indications for conscious sedation and type of sedation used in children (++ = very good, + = good)

	Benzodiazepines		
	Oral	Rectal	N_2O/O_2
Too immature for treatment, e.g., low age or mental disability (mental age <3–4 years)	++	++	
Fear/anxiety	++		++
Medically compromised patients	+		++
Muscular tone disturbances			++
Pronounced gag reflexes			++
Treatment stress	+		++
The nature of the dental treatment (e.g., oral surgery)	+		++
Facilitates sleep the night before treatment	++		

some contraindications specific for nitrous oxide–oxygen sedation: partial obstruction of the respiratory airways, psychosis, recent otological operation, sinusitis, porphyria, or a history of malignant hypothermia in the family.

Nitrous oxide–oxygen sedation can be used in combination with benzodiazepines, which implies that the two types of sedatives have additive effect. A frequently applied approach is that the patient is given an initial dose of benzodiazepine preoperatively, which is supplemented with nitrous oxide–oxygen if an additional sedative/analgesic effect is needed during the treatment.

Box 5-12 Indications for dental treatment under general anesthesia

- Treatment of severely mentally and/or physically handicapped children who lack the ability to cooperate during treatment.
- Severe management problems in patients with a genuine psychiatric disorder.
- Extensive and/or complicated treatment need in children and adolescents with lack of coping ability (e.g., due to immaturity, dental anxiety/odontophobia, disability, etc.).

General anesthesia

Some patients lack the physical or mental ability to cooperate during treatment. Dental treatment under general anesthesia may then be the only solution (Box 5-12). Moreover, some surgical procedures are so extended in time and tiring that no other methods of pain control can be considered.

The prevalence of serious complications in association with dental treatment under general anesthesia is very low when performed in a hospital setting (Fig. 5-14). General anesthesia is probably safer than giving deep sedation to a patient in a normal dental setting. The indication for dental treatment under general anesthesia, however, must be restricted because anesthesia itself can exert physical and mental stress compared with the alternative methods (7). It should be the last resource when all efforts to treat a child in the conventional manner have failed.

In Scandinavia, dental treatment under general anesthesia requires the assistance of a registered anesthetist who selects the method of anesthesia according to the child's condition and the nature of the treatment to be performed. Postoperative pain should be a concern in the same way as described earlier in this chapter. After major dental surgery more potent analgesics may be required in the first postoperative period. The hospital setting makes this a possibility as compared to outpatient management. In a study from a Swedish county with good access to sedation, the number of children

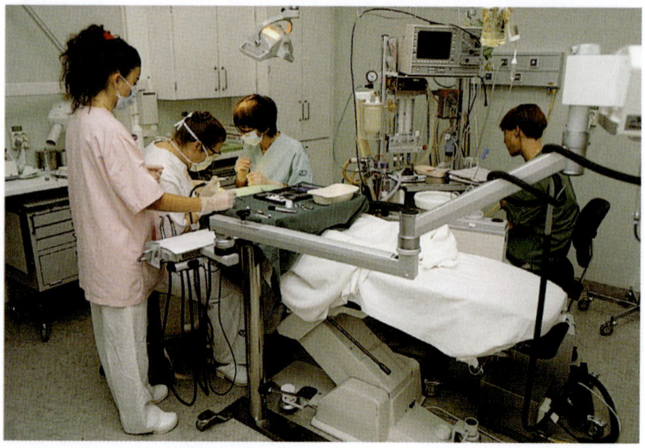

Figure 5-14 Dental treatment under general anesthesia in a hospital setting.

aged 0–19 years in need of dental treatment under general anesthesia was 0.7–2.2/1000 per year (40).

Every possible effort should be made to return the child to routine therapy in the future. After dental treatment under general anesthesia, adequate prophylactic dental care should start as soon as possible.

References

1. American Academy of Pediatric Dentistry. Clinical guideline on the elective use of minimal, moderate, and deep sedation and general anesthesia in pediatric dental patients. *Pediatr Dent* 2004;**26**:95–103.
2. American Society of Anesthesiologists. ASA standards, guidelines and statements, 2006. http://www.asahq.org (accessed August 2008).
3. Anand KJ, Hickey PR. Pain and its effects in the human neonate and fetus. *N Engl J Med* 1987;**317**:1321–9.
4. Arana A, Morton NS, Hansen TG. Treatment with paracetamol in infants. *Acta Anaesthesiol Scand* 2001;**45**:20–9.
5. Berthold C. Enteral sedation: safety, efficacy, and controversy. *Compend Contin Educ Dent* 2007;**28**:264–71; quiz 72, 82.
6. Bieri D, Reeve RA, Champion GD, Addicoat L, Ziegler JB. The Faces Pain Scale for the self-assessment of the severity of pain experienced by children: development, initial validation, and preliminary investigation for ratio scale properties. *Pain* 1990;**41**:139–50.
7. Blain KM, Hill FJ. The use of inhalation sedation and local anaesthesia as an alternative to general anaesthesia for dental extractions in children. *Br Dent J* 1998;**184**:608–11.
8. Department of Health. Conscious sedation in the provision of dental care. Report from an expert group on sedation for dentistry. Department of Health, 2003, http://www.dh.gov.uk (accessed August 2008).
9. Fitzgerald M, Howard R. The neurobiologic basis of paediatric pain. In: Schechter N, Berde CB, Yaster M, eds. *Pain in infants, children, and adolescents.* Baltimore, MD: Williams & Wilkins, 2002; 19–42.
10. Gaffney A. How children describe pain: a study of words and analogies used by 5- to 14-year-olds. In: Dubner R, Gebhart GF, Bond MR, eds. *Pain research and clinical management.* Amsterdam: Elsevier, 1988; 341–7.
11. Gaffney A, Dunne EA. Developmental aspects of children's definitions of pain. *Pain* 1986;**26**:105–17.
12. Gaffney A, Dunne EA. Children's understanding of the causality of pain. *Pain* 1987;**29**:91–104.
13. Gaffney A, McGrath PJ, Dick B. Measuring pain in children. In: Schechter N, Berde CB, Yaster M, eds. *Pain in infants, children, and adolescents.* Baltimore, MD: Williams & Wilkins, 2002; 128–39.
14. Girdler NM, Sterling PA. Investigation of nitrous oxide pollution arising from inhalational sedation for the extraction of teeth in child patients. *Int J Paediatr Dent* 1998;**8**:93–102.
15. Hallonsten AL. Nitrous oxide scavenging in dental surgery. I. A comparison of the efficiency of different scavenging devices. *Swed Dent J* 1982;**6**:203–13.
16. Hallonsten AL. Nitrous oxide scavenging in dental surgery. II. An evaluation of a local exhaust system. *Swed Dent J* 1982;**6**:215–23.
17. Hallonsten AL, Jensen B, Raadal M, Veerkamp J, Hosey MT, Poulsen S. EAPD Guidelines on Sedation in Paediatric Dentistry. European Academy of Paediatric Dentistry, 2006. http://www.eapd.gr/Guidelines/index.htm (accessed August 2008).
18. Hallonsten AL, Koch G, Schroder U. Nitrous oxide–oxygen sedation in dental care. *Community Dent Oral Epidemiol* 1983; **11**:347–55.
19. Henry RJ, Primosch RE. Influence of operatory size and nitrous oxide concentration upon scavenger effectiveness. *J Dent Res* 1991;**70**:1286–9.
20. Hicks CL, von Baeyer CL, Spafford PA, van Korlaar I, Goodenough B. The Faces Pain Scale-Revised: toward a common metric in pediatric pain measurement. *Pain* 2001;**93**:173–83.
21. International Association for the Study of Pain, 2007. http://www.iasp-pain.org (accessed August 2008).
22. Jensen B. Benzodiazepine sedation in paediatric dentistry. *Swed Dent J* 2002 (Suppl);1–45.
23. Jensen B, Matsson L. Benzodiazepines in child dental care: a survey of its use among general practitioners and paediatric dentists in Sweden. *Swed Dent J* 2001;**25**:31–8.
24. Johnston S, Stevens B, Boyer K, Porter F. Development of psychologic response to pain and assessment of pain in infants and toddlers. In: Schechter N, Berde CB, Yaster M, eds. *Pain in infants, children, and adolescents.* Baltimore, MD: Williams & Wilkins, 2002; 19–42.
25. Jones CM, Heidmann J, Gerrish AC. Children's ratings of dental injection and treatment pain, and the influence of the time taken to administer the injection. *Int J Paediatr Dent* 1995;**5**:81–5.
26. Krauss B, Green SM. Procedural sedation and analgesia in children. *Lancet* 2006;**367**:766–80.
27. Lönnqvist PA, Morton NS. Postoperative analgesia in infants and children. *Br J Anaesth* 2005;**95**:59–68.
28. Lundeberg S, Lönnqvist PA. Update on systemic postoperative analgesia in children. *Paediatr Anaesth* 2004;**14**:394–7.
29. Matharu L, Ashley PF. Sedation of anxious children undergoing dental treatment. *Cochrane Database Syst Rev* 2006; CD003877.
30. McGrath PA. Evaluating a child's pain. *J Pain Symptom Manage* 1989;**4**:198–214.
31. McGrath PA, Seifert CE, Speechley KN, Booth JC, Stitt L, Gibson MC. A new analogue scale for assessing children's pain: an initial validation study. *Pain* 1996;**64**:435–43.
32. Mohler H, Fritschy JM, Rudolph U. A new benzodiazepine pharmacology. *J Pharmacol Exp Ther* 2002;**300**:2–8.
33. Palm AM, Kirkegaard U, Poulsen S. The wand versus traditional injection for mandibular nerve block in children and adolescents: perceived pain and time of onset. *Pediatr Dent* 2004;**26**:481–4.
34. Primosch RE, Brooks R. Influence of anesthetic flow rate delivered by the Wand Local Anesthetic System on pain response to palatal injections. *Am J Dent* 2002;**15**:15–20.
35. Ram D, Peretz B. Administering local anaesthesia to paediatric dental patients – current status and prospects for the future. *Int J Paediatr Dent* 2002;**12**:80–9.
36. Rasmussen JK, Frederiksen JA, Hallonsten AL, Poulsen S. Danish dentists' knowledge, attitudes and management of procedural dental pain in children: association with demographic characteristics, structural factors, perceived stress during the administration of local analgesia and their tolerance towards pain. *Int J Paediatr Dent* 2005;**15**:159–68.
37. Rowland AS, Baird DD, Weinberg CR, Shore DL, Shy CM, Wilcox AJ. Reduced fertility among women employed as dental assistants exposed to high levels of nitrous oxide. *N Engl J Med* 1992;**327**:993–7.
38. Schechter NL, Berde CB, Yaster M. Pain in infants, children, and adolescents: an overview. In: Schechter N, Berde CB, Yaster M, eds. *Pain in infants, children, and adolescents.* Baltimore, MD: Williams & Wilkins, 2002; 3–9.

39. Sweeney B, Bingham RM, Amos RJ, Petty AC, Cole PV. Toxicity of bone marrow in dentists exposed to nitrous oxide. *Br Med J (Clin Res Ed)* 1985;**291**:567–9.
40. Varpio M, Wellfelt B. Some characteristics of children with dental behaviour problems. Five-year follow-up of pedodontic treatment. *Swed Dent J* 1991;**15**:85–93.
41. Veerkamp JS, Gruythuysen RJ, Hoogstraten J, van Amerongen WE. Anxiety reduction with nitrous oxide: a permanent solution? *ASDC J Dent Child* 1995;**62**:44–8.
42. Wall P, Melzack R. *Textbook of pain.* Edinburgh: Churchill Livingstone, 1999.
43. Weimann J. Toxicity of nitrous oxide. *Best Pract Res Clin Anaesthesiol* 2003;**17**:47–61.
44. Wondimu B, Dahllof G. Attitudes of Swedish dentists to pain and pain management during dental treatment of children and adolescents. *Eur J Paediatr Dent* 2005;**6**:66–72.

6

Dental caries in children and adolescents

Marit Slåttelid Skeie, Lill-Kari Wendt and Sven Poulsen

Dental caries is the most common chronic disease among children and adolescents (21), and thus the one most often affecting both oral and general health (17,49). The impact of caries on oral and general health depends on what age the lesions appear, the depth of the lesions, and where the lesions are located in the dentition. The impact of the disease is more serious in younger children, in children with chronic health conditions (CHC), and in children with poor access to adequate dental health services.

Childhood dental caries as a health problem

"Health is a state of complete physical, mental and social wellbeing, not merely the absence of disease and infirmity." This definition of health by the World Health Organization (WHO), which dates back half a century, although criticized for its shortcomings (60) (Chapter 1), has been a starting point for today's generally accepted holistic approach to health (49). As oral health is an integrated part of general health, it is natural to use this concept even when describing caries and its sequelae in children and adolescents (64).

Dental caries has impacts on both oral and general health (Box 6-1), and when left untreated, often leads to pain. An obvious impact of a painful tooth is the reduced ability to chew and eat (17). Limitations in the choice of foods, a loss of appetite, and a lessened enjoyment of eating (17) are some of the reasons why severe caries may be associated with reduced weight and delayed growth (1,9). However, after therapeutic intervention under general anesthetic, children with severe caries often gain weight rapidly (1). New research also indicates that dental treatment of young children under general anesthetic is often associated with considerable improvement in oral-health-related quality of life (38).

An Irish study concluded that almost half of all hospital dental emergencies were due to caries sequelae (22).

Box 6-1 Childhood dental caries has an impact on both oral and general health, including quality of life

Physical
- Pain and discomfort due to infection and abscess formation.
- Invasive dental treatment with risk of procedural pain.
- Disturbed development of permanent teeth.
- Negative impact on future oral health.
- Disturbed occlusal development with risk of future orthodontic problems.
- Retarded growth due to loss of appetite and reduced intake of food.
- Disturbed sleep.
- Special problems in children with CHC.

Psychological and emotional
- Dental fear and anxiety.
- Reduced aesthetics with lowered self-esteem as a consequence.
- Being teased by other children due to aesthetics or speech difficulties.

Behavioral
- Behavior management problems.
- Lack of regular attendance to dental care.

Social
- Interruption of daily function.
- Embarrassment while eating and speaking in front of others.

Candida, osteomyelitis, or sepsis due to infected teeth are reported in countries that have poor access to adequate dental or general health services (49). Even in the Western world for some children with CHC (i.e., those who have cardiac diseases, those who are immunocompromised by disease and/or therapy, those suffering from hemophilia, or children receiving irradiation of the jaws), dental infections, and to some extent the treatment of caries lesions, may represent a life threat (23).

Caries with onset early in life is synonymous with an increased risk of future caries development (5,26), a topic that will be covered in more detail later in this chapter. Insufficient oral hygiene around a tooth with caries also often induces additional gingival problems (77). Furthermore, deep caries lesions constitute a risk of endodontic complications and abscess development (61), which often leads swelling and to further pain and discomfort during chewing. Regarding infected primary teeth, there is a risk for potential injuries on the permanent tooth such as enamel opacities, hypoplasia, or incomplete development (23).

Treatment of caries lesions, although giving the patient relief from the immediate acute symptoms, may in the long term have negative consequences. Extractions of primary teeth at an early age may lead to reduced dental arch, tooth displacement, tilting, and rotations (58). If several teeth with important phonetical functions are extracted, normal language development may be interfered with or retarded (66). Having to perform operative restorative treatment of caries at an early age may similarly affect future oral health negatively. About one-third of fillings in primary teeth will need replacement during the age of 7–12 years (6). It has also been documented (37,55) that approximal cavity preparations may damage two-thirds or more of the neighboring sound surfaces, making them more susceptible to caries. As shown by a recent study, children with caries before the age of 6 years needed three and a half times more treatments (new restorations, replacement of a restorations, disking, or extraction) of primary teeth from 7 to 12 years than children without caries (i.e., without diagnosed caries lesions) at the age of 6 years (4). In addition, it has to be taken into consideration that early exposure to components from dental material may contribute, although only to a minor extent, to a potential for adverse allergic reactions (12).

A well-documented consequence of severe caries with pain is the reduction of the individual's quality of life. Disturbed sleeping, concentration problems (3,21,57), and interruption in play and schoolwork (17,70) may induce emotional stress with anger and irritability. Because of aesthetics and/or phonetic problems, there is also a risk that children will be teased, which again may negatively influence their self-esteem, resulting in the child acquiring a silent demeanor or avoiding smiling and laughing (36).

Experiences of pain during dental treatment during childhood are documented to increase the risk of developing behavioral management problems and dental anxiety later in life (32). A study has shown that for a group of children with more than 10 caries lesions at the age of 5 years, more than every third child acquired dental anxiety 5 years later (56), indicating that painful experiences during restorative treatment are a major risk factor for the development of dental anxiety. A higher prevalence of missed dental appointments among children who have had dental treatment in connection with toothache has also been documented (82). Neglected oral health may be the consequence, which also means increased economic treatment costs later in life.

Epidemiology of dental caries in children and adolescents

Epidemiology is defined as "the study of the distribution and determinants of health-related states or events in specified populations, and the application to control of health problems" (35). From this definition it is obvious that understanding and interpreting epidemiological data are an essential part of managing pediatric dental care. More specifically, epidemiology has two important applications in child dental care: to describe the distribution of caries in the population, and to describe changes in caries prevalence over time. It is important to define certain basic terms in order to understand epidemiological data on dental caries in children and adolescents, and these are given in Box 6-2. Epidemiological data can be used, for example, to provide information on:

- The prevalence of caries in the population, according to age, gender, and socioeconomic and ethnic background. This is important in order to determine the magnitude of the problem and the distribution of the burden of disease in the population.

Box 6-2 Important epidemiological terms used in describing occurrence of dental caries

Prevalence
The number of persons in a population with a disease or a condition at a specified point in time (*point prevalence*) or during a specified period (*period prevalence*).

Incidence
The number of new events, e.g., new cases, of a disease in a defined population within a specified period of time.

dmft/dmfs (defs)
Decayed, missing (extracted due to caries), and filled primary teeth (t) or tooth surfaces (s).

DMFT/DMFS
Decayed, missing (extracted due to caries), and filled permanent teeth (T) or tooth surfaces (S).

Box 6-3 Epidemiological data are important for *quality development* and *quality control* of child dental care

The following are goals proposed by the regional office of WHO for oral health in Europe by 2015 (noncavitated caries lesions not included) (83):

- 6 year olds: 80% or more will be caries free
- 12 year olds: DMFT shall be no more than 1.5, of which at least 1.0 shall be FT
- 18 year olds: no teeth missing due to caries (MT = 0)

Epidemiological data, if possible to collect, will give information on whether these goals are fulfilled.

- The incidence of caries in the population. This will give information as to the future level of disease in the population.
- Oral health strategic planning for caries control, e.g., how to use existent personnel resources efficiently, how to evaluate child dental care, and how to inform the dental health authorities responsible for financing health care.
- Formulation of goals and determining whether these goals are fulfilled or not (see Box 6-3).

Thus, epidemiological data are important in *quality development* and *quality control* of child dental care.

Epidemiological data on dental caries

During recent years increasing emphasis has been placed on the dynamics of the caries lesion as developing from a subclinical lesion through an initial, noncavitated lesion to a manifest lesion, eventually resulting in complete destruction of the tooth. It is now generally accepted that arrest and even reversal of initial, noncavitated caries lesions can occur (19). This has resulted in the development of interceptive strategies in children and adolescents in the management of these kinds of lesions (see Chapter 10).

Nordic countries have, for administrative purposes, established data collection systems to monitor the level of dental caries. The information collected in some of these systems is by and large data on already placed restorations or on the need for restorative treatment reported by dentists. Today's move to a more conservative treatment philosophy (24) may compromise valid comparisons between studies from different epochs.

However, there are exceptions to the scheme of collecting epidemiological data using cavitation or the need for restorative intervention as the diagnostic cut-off point. One exception is the system implemented by the National Board of Health in Denmark. Caries data are collected by this institution according to written

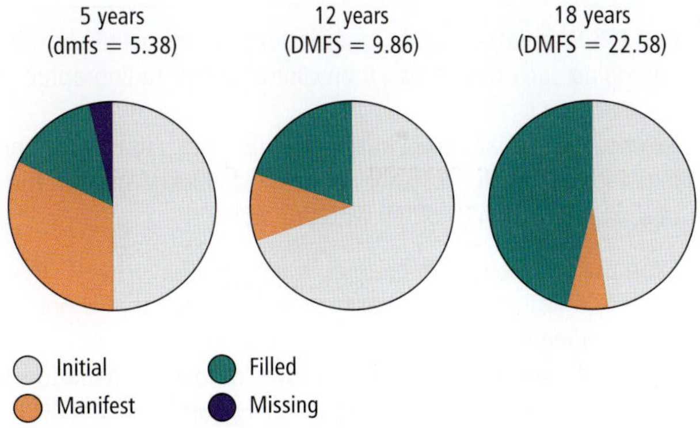

Figure 6-1 Contribution of initial and manifest lesions, filled and missing (due to caries) surfaces of the total caries index in Norwegian children (7).

epidemiological criteria, and noncavitated caries lesions are recorded as a separate caries diagnosis. Over the past few decades, several other epidemiological projects in Nordic countries have been carried out using similarly detailed diagnostic criteria. These studies have shown that noncavitated caries lesions constitute a large proportion of the total caries experience (Fig. 6-1). In teenagers, it is reported that approximal noncavitated caries lesions may make up as much as 80–90% of the total number of caries lesions (5,44). Consequently, some national reports will underestimate considerably the true prevalence (7). Thus, for a number of reasons it is very important to make explicit the criteria used for diagnosis, when presenting, interpreting, and making use of data on the occurrence of caries in children and adolescents (Box 6-4).

However, the different caries measurement systems capable of incorporating noncavitated caries lesions vary in detail, in the way they are used, and in terminology (Box 6-5). A common trait is ambiguity and incompat-

Box 6-4 The importance of using the initial, noncavitated caries lesion as a diagnostic cut-off point

It is important to differentiate between initial, noncavitated caries lesions and manifest caries lesions when collecting epidemiological data because:

- Early intervention can arrest or reverse the noncavitated caries lesion, and is more gentle to the child than restoration at a later stage of development of the lesion.
- Noncavitated caries lesions can be arrested or reversed through self-care. The parents should be informed about appropriate dental health care and an appropriate diet for the child.
- Initial, noncavitated caries lesions can be treated by other dental personnel than dentists.

Box 6-5 Diagnosis of early caries lesions has attracted considerable attention during recent years. Below are excerpts of references describing such criteria based on clinical and/or radiographic evaluation

Example 1. Initial caries in pits and fissures, clinical diagnostic criteria (33)
Initial loss of tooth substance appearing as chalky spots in the enamel surface layer without breakdown of the surface in the form of cavitation when explored with the probe.

Example 2. Changes in enamel in pits and fissures (ICDAS) (31)
Code 1: A visible carious opacity or discoloration that is not consistent with the clinical appearance of sound enamel, seen either after prolonged air drying *or* on wet enamel.
Code 2: A carious opacity and/or brown carious discoloration that is wider than the natural fissure/fossa and not consistent with the clinical appearance of sound enamel (tooth seen wet).
Code 3: In addition to the criteria of Code 2, and after dried once for approximately 5 s, a carious loss of tooth structure at the entrance to or within the pit or fissure/fossa, is seen. The dentin is *not* visible in the walls or base of the cavity/discontinuity.

Example 3. Diagnostic criteria, incorporating location of the caries lesions (45)
Criteria are described for:

- Pits and fissures
- Vestibular and lingual smooth surfaces
- Radiographic evaluation of proximal surfaces.

Type 1: Enamel surface contour is broken; a shadow between the enamel surface and a border not more than one-quarter through the enamel.
Type 2: Shadow has reached dentinoenamel junction.

Example 4. Diagnostic criteria for enamel approximal caries, radiographic diagnostic criteria (18)
Grade 1 (A1): Radiolucency in outer half of enamel.
Grade 2 (A2): Radiolucency in inner half of enamel.

Example 5. Initial approximal caries, radiographic diagnostic criteria (5)
$D_i a$: A caries lesion in the enamel that has not reached the dentinoenamel junction or a lesion that reaches or penetrates the dentinoenamel junction, but does not appear to extend into the dentin.

Example 6. Definition of precavitation caries ("iceberg model") (51)
D_1: Clinically detectable enamel lesions with "intact" surfaces.
D_2: Clinically detectable "cavities" limited to enamel.

Example 7. Diagnostic criteria, differentiating between active and inactive caries lesions at noncavitated levels (47)
Active caries with intact surface, active caries with surface discontinuity, inactive caries with intact surface, inactive caries with surface discontinuity.

ibility in caries diagnostic thresholds around the dentinoenamel junction. Although detailed caries diagnostic systems should be considered as a step forward in the field of epidemiology, measures of caries activity are still relatively poorly developed (52).

Table 6-1 shows various Nordic caries surveys of children and adolescents on which the caries description in this chapter is based. Epidemiological data from these surveys are not presented mainly owing to lacking a basis of data comparison as previously discussed.

Dental caries in the primary dentition of preschool children

Dental decay in infants and toddlers has a distinctive pattern. The definitions first used to describe this condition were related to etiology, with the focus on inappropriate use of nursing practices. "Nursing bottle mouth", "baby bottle tooth decay", "nursing bottle syndrome", and "nursing caries" were terms previously used. The current internationally accepted definition of caries with early onset is early childhood caries (ECC). This terminology encompasses a much broader meaning, better fitting the understanding that unfavorable feeding practice is not the only important cause of ECC. However, pediatric dentists have not yet succeeded in agreeing on a mutual and uniform definition of ECC, and inconsistencies in the case definitions and diagnostic criteria still exist (Box 6-6) (30). The definition of ECC used in this chapter is the occurrence of any sign of dental caries on any tooth surface during the first 3 years of life (29). A more virulent form of ECC, severe ECC (S-ECC), is defined according to age.

Table 6-1 Nordic caries surveys of children and adolescents on which the present caries description is based

Author and year of publication	Country	Age
Wendt *et al.* (1991)	Sweden	12–14 months
Grindefjord *et al.* (1993)	Sweden	1 year
Wendt *et al.* (1992)	Sweden	36 months
Petersen (1996)	Denmark	2–3, 7 years
Mattila *et al.* (2001)	Finland	3 years
Wennhall *et al.* (2002)	Sweden	3 years
Sundby and Petersen (2003)	Denmark	3, 5 years
Skeie *et al.* (2005, 2006)	Norway	3, 5 years
Hugoson *et al.* (2005)	Sweden	3, 5, 10, 15, 20 years
Grindefjord *et al.* (1995)	Sweden	42 months
Stecksén-Blicks *et al.* (2004)	Sweden	4 years
Vehkalathi *et al.* (1997)	Finland	5, 15 years
Amarante *et al.* (1995)	Norway	5, 12, 18 years
Poulsen and Pedersen (2002)	Denmark	5, 7, 12, 15 years
Wendt *et al.* (1999)	Sweden	Follow-up 3–6 years
Varpio (1993)	Sweden	Follow-up 3–8 years
Skeie *et al.* (2004, 2005)	Norway	Follow-up 5–10 years
Seppä *et al.* (1989)	Finland	Follow-up 6–13 years
Stenlund *et al.* (2002)	Sweden	Follow-up 11–13 years
Mejàre *et al.* (1998, 1999, 2000)	Sweden	Follow-up 6–12, 11–22, and 12–18 years
Alm *et al.* (2007)	Sweden	Follow-up 3–15 years

Dental caries during early childhood is a multifactoral disease, and has numerous biological, psychosocial, and behavioral risk factors, which vary from population to population and may combine in different patterns to result in a caries lesion. Patterns of behavior that affect dental health such as oral hygiene and dietary habits are established early in a child's life and persist during childhood (27) as well as during adolescence (8). Although ECC is among the most prevalent health problems of infants and toddlers from immigrant and from low-income families (81), little attention and few resources have been allocated to understanding why individuals from these groups develop dental caries and why some of them are so severely affected.

Box 6-6 Nomenclature and definition of ECC

Early childhood caries, Ismail (29)
Occurrence of any sign of dental caries on any tooth surface during the first 3 years of life.

Early childhood caries, National Institute of Dental and Craniofacial Research (NIDCR) 1999
Presence of one or more decayed (noncavitated or cavitated lesions), missing (due to caries), or filled surfaces in any primary tooth in a child <6 years.

Severe early childhood caries
Children with "atypical", "progressive", or "rampant" patterns of dental caries (described separately for each age group):

- < 3 years: any sign of dental caries in smooth surfaces
- 3–5 years: one or more cavitated, missing (due to caries), or filled smooth surfaces in maxillary teeth or a dmfs score of 4, 5, and 6 surfaces for ages 3, 4, and 5 years, respectively.

At 1 year of age some children already have developed caries lesions and at 3 years of age about 30% have caries (noncavitated caries lesions included). The first sign of dental caries in infants with ECC is the appearance of white demineralized areas on the cervical part of the buccal or lingual surfaces of the maxillary anterior teeth, while the mandibular incisors usually remain unaffected (80). The most frequently affected surfaces in older preschool children are the occlusal surfaces of the second primary molars and the distal surfaces of the first primary molars (25,75).

There is a strong correlation between ECC and later caries development in both primary and permanent dentitions. In one study, children with manifest caries lesions at 3 years of age experienced a mean caries increment of 4.5 tooth surfaces from 3 to 6 years, compared to 0.9 tooth surfaces for children who at the baseline had no manifest caries lesions (79). Furthermore, there is a strong relationship between caries in early childhood and caries development both in the primary dentition up to 10 years of age (69) and in the permanent dentition up to mid-teenage years (5). The dmft recorded at the age of 6 years seems to be better correlated to caries increment between 7 and 13 years of age than is caries in the permanent first molar (63). These facts make infants and toddlers an important target group for preventive dental care, and also point to the importance of early identification of children with ECC or, even better, with a high risk of developing ECC. The importance of informing parents or even pregnant women of preventive dental health practices, implemented from an early age for their children, cannot be emphasized enough.

The general trend of caries decline observed among children and adolescents in Nordic countries during the past few decades has been less marked for the primary dentition of preschool children. As an example, a series of cross-sectional epidemiological surveys carried out in the city of Jönköping in Sweden in 1973, 1983, 1993, and 2003 has shown that while mean dmfs in 3- and 5-year-old children decreased between 1973 and 1993, there has been no further decrease between 1993 and 2003 (28) (Fig. 6-2). This is in line with a study from Umeå, also in Sweden (71). Over a 30-year period mean dmfs of 4 year olds decreased from almost 8 to 2, but the decrease was largest at the beginning of the period. Since 1980 mean dmfs has been constant at about 2. A similar pattern has been observed in Denmark (54).

However, the distribution of dental caries among 4 year olds is characterized today by a marked positive skewness, as a small, but constant group up to this age has developed 10 or more dmfs. According to Vehkalahti *et al.* (76) 8% of 5 year olds accounted for 76% of the total number of teeth with current untreated caries in their age group. Thus, while dental caries is less of a burden than previously for most preschool children, it remains a significant problem for some individuals. Lorenz curves are useful to illustrate skewness in the distribution of caries within a population (53), but are also a graphical aid to discriminate skewness between groups (67) (Fig. 6-3). Such curves demonstrate the proportion of individuals who are responsible for a given burden of all caries lesions.

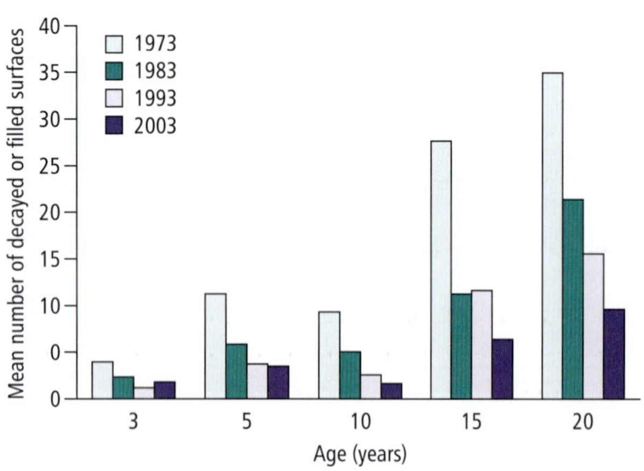

Figure 6-2 Mean number of decayed and filled tooth surfaces in the city of Jönköping, Sweden, according to age in 1973, 1983, 1993, and 2003. Only caries in primary teeth were recorded and examined for 3–5 year olds while only caries in permanent teeth were examined in subjects 10 years or older. Initial, noncavitated lesions were included. [After Hugoson *et al.*, 2005 (28).]

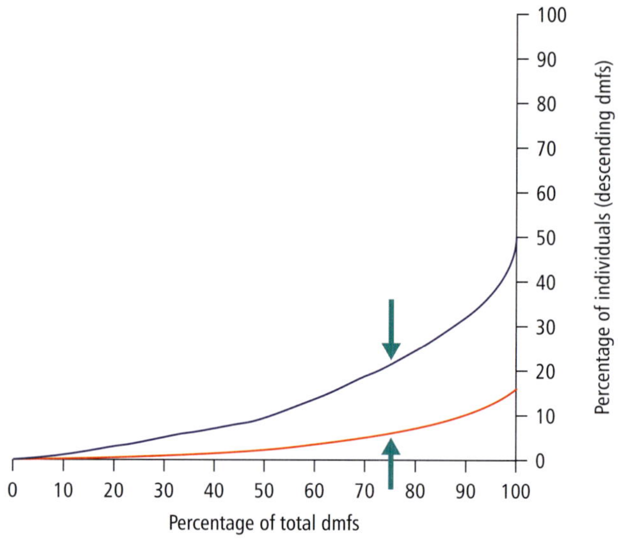

Figure 6-3 Lorenz curves used to give a graphical representation of the cumulative distribution of caries lesions in two populations of 3-year-old children, one of Western origin (red curve) and one with immigrant, non-Western background (blue curve) (67). Each point on the curves denotes the proportion of the population (*y*-axis) responsible for the proportion of the total burden of caries lesions (*x*-axis). The crossing-point of curves with the *y*-axis represents the caries prevalence (15.9% for the Western group, and 50.0% for the immigrant group). The arrows indicate that 6% of the Western group and 23% of the immigrant group carry about 75% of the total caries burden in their respective groups.

Caries in the permanent dentition

Caries in the permanent dentition has decreased considerably. As an example, the epidemiological surveys conducted in the city of Jönköping over 30 years have shown a decrease in DFS in all age groups (10, 15, and 20 years) between 1973 and 2003 (28) (Fig. 6-2). Other data, such as those reported for 15-year-old Danish children, revealed a marked shift to the left of the distribution according to DMFS (Fig. 6-4). A consistent finding in all Nordic countries is that the decrease in mean DMFS is followed by an increase in skewness of the distribution according to DMFS (Fig. 6-5). The majority of the caries lesions nowadays are located on specific teeth and tooth morphology types such as pits and fissures (occlusal surfaces). It has been described as a general pattern that when caries prevalence falls, the largest reduction is found on the least susceptible surfaces (proximal and free smooth surfaces) (10). Caries lesions on these surfaces in low-caries populations are thus an indication of a high risk of caries (10). The least susceptible of all sites in the dentition are on the lower anterior teeth and canines. Independent of age, such a location of the lesions indicates that an individual is extremely caries active.

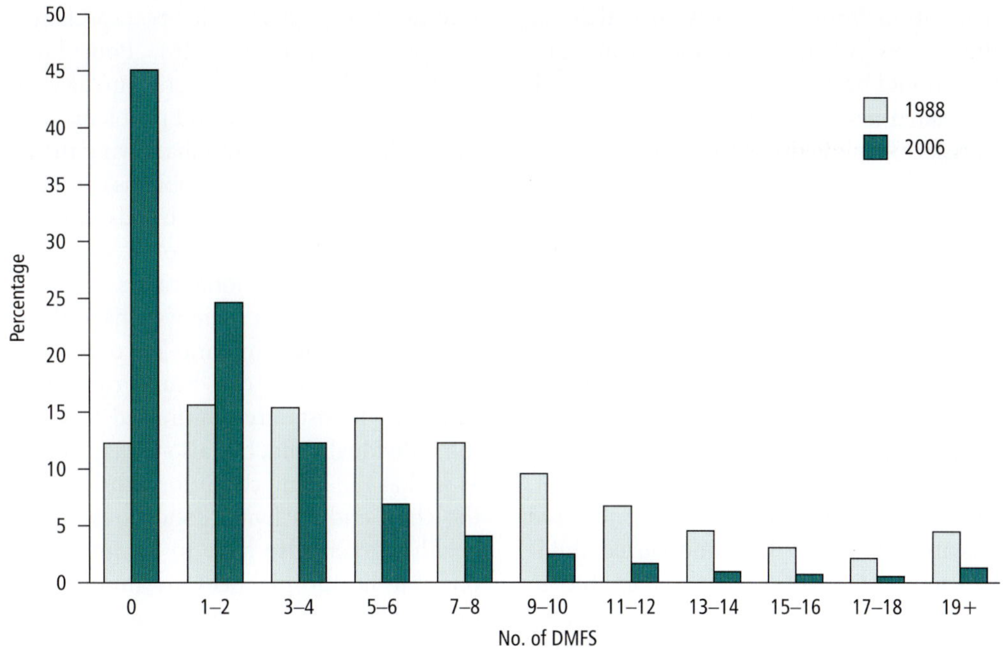

Figure 6-4 Distribution of 15-year-old Danish children according to DMFS (initial, noncavitated lesions not included) in 1988 and 2006. (Based on data collected by the Danish National Board of Health, 2007.)

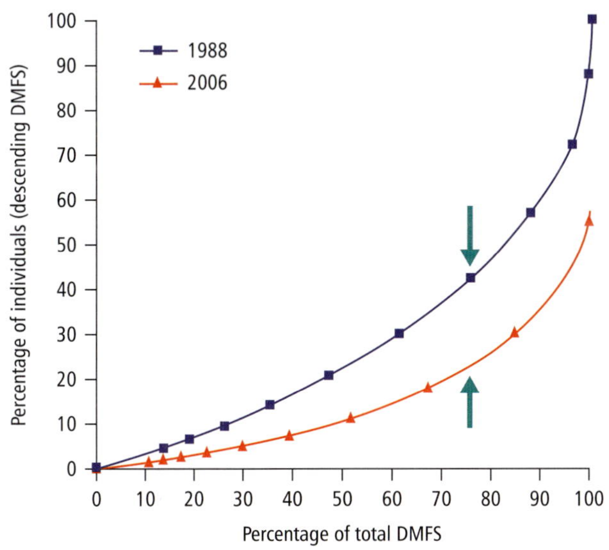

Figure 6-5 Lorenz curve describing the distribution of the burden of caries in 15-year-old Danish children (initial, noncavitated lesions not included). In 1988, 75% of the total number of DMF surfaces were found in the 43% of children with the highest DMFS. The corresponding number in 2006 was 13%. (Based on data collected by the Danish National Board of Health, 2007.)

In the young permanent dentition the permanent first molars constitute the most caries-susceptible teeth, and in line with what is described above, up to the age of 12 years pits and fissures are the most frequent sites for caries development. The caries rates decrease as the time after eruption increases, suggesting that the first 4–5 years after eruption constitute risk ages for new approximal caries (72). At the age of 12 years, the mesial surface of the first permanent molars accounts for the majority of approximal lesions (43), strongly correlated with past caries experience of the adjacent surface of the primary molar (74). At 21 years of age the occlusal, mesial, and distal surfaces of the first molar account for 60% of all restored surfaces (41). Above the age of 12 years caries progression in general is slower. One study found that caries progression (from inner half of the enamel to outer half of the dentin) on the mesial surface of the first permanent molar was almost four times faster in a young age group (6–12 years) than in an older group (12–22 years) (43).

It is also a general trait in Nordic countries that the rate of caries progression has become increasingly slower, especially in approximal enamel surfaces in permanent teeth (42). The morphology of the caries lesion has changed as well. In comparison with the previous situation, a clearly visually evident caries lesion is now often indicative of a considerable destruction of underlying tissue (51).

Caries in children and adolescents in a changing society

As caries distribution is skewed at population, individual, and dentition level (teeth/surfaces), so is the distribution of caries determinants (50). Furthermore, caries determinants, as with other health risks, cannot be considered in isolation from the society to which the individual belongs (59). All changes in the social situation for children should be monitored in order to search for possible associated new or changing caries determinants or caries risks (34). It is therefore obvious to pose the question: "Are there any structural society changes traceable in Nordic countries at the start of the new millennium?" Compared to the conditions today's generation of parents and grandparents lived through when they were young, children nowadays experience a different everyday life, in both pattern of family life and style of parenting (15). There are also reasons to believe that some of the traits of the modern lifestyle have led to caries-promoting behavior; such as irregular meals, "democratic negotiations" between child and parent, parental indulgence about children's bedtimes, increased intake of snacks and soft drinks, institutionalized childhood (kindergartens) with absent parents unable to control children's diet, and so on. Many of the same behaviors are also associated with lifestyle diseases such as being overweight and obesity (49) which today represent a common medical condition in children and adolescents (11). Focusing on diet for example, the common risk factor approach, described by Sheiham and Watt, addresses the mutual etiologic factors of both dental caries as well as being overweight and obesity (65).

Another trait in society is migration. During recent decades Nordic countries have had an influx of immigrants from the non-Western world, changing Nordic societies to multicultural societies (73). Immigrant children represent a major challenge to our oral health care, especially very young children (48). Dental health disparities between immigrant and nonimmigrant children have during the past decade been documented by many Nordic studies showing a considerably higher caries prevalence, caries of a more severe character, and with an earlier onset in immigrant children than nonimmigrants (67,73,79,80). The previously mentioned study from a low-economic status multicultural population in an urban area of Malmö, Sweden, found a caries prevalence (noncavitated caries lesions included) of 85% among 3-year-old children (81).

Immigrant children are not a homogeneous group, but with backgrounds from a wide range of countries. Danish authors described children of Turkish, Pakistani, ex-Yugoslavian, and Albanian origin as having a high caries prevalence (48,73), indicating that the culture of the country of origin may be used as a caries risk indicator. It has for long been accepted that cariogenic practices are culturally embedded (20). Also, parental dental attitudes towards children's oral health are considered to be affected by cultural and ethnic diversity (2,68). In some minority groups and cultures, dental care is therefore not always given priority, especially dental care of the primary dentition (46). Poor knowledge about dental health-related matters, language problems, surrounding stress factors, and problems with resettlement might all be barriers overshadowing the need for dental care (14,62,78). Besides problems caused by socially and culturally different backgrounds, immigrant families often live in low socioeconomic surroundings, thereby experiencing an additional caries risk factor (13).

As those factors in society we have already mentioned are important determinants for oral health in children, it is important that oral health care services as well as pediatric dentists are committed to consider not only the individual child, but also the entire child population as well as the living conditions and the network around the child and its living conditions (40). Public dental health workers also have to communicate information on oral health practices to immigrant groups in a manner that is sensitive to their cultural background (16). Lastly, the importance of good cooperation between professionals working in dental clinics and child health care centers must be stressed (39).

References

1. Acs G, Shulman R, Ng MW, Chussid S. The effect of dental rehabilitation on the body weight of children with early childhood caries. *Pediatr Dent* 1999;**21**:109–13.
2. Adair PM, Pine CM, Burnside G, Nicoll AD, Gillett A, Anwar S, *et al.* Familial and cultural perceptions and beliefs of oral hygiene and dietary practices among ethnically and socioeconomically diverse groups. *Community Dent Health* 2004;**21** Suppl 1:102–11.
3. Adulyanon S, Vourapukjaru J, Sheiham A. Oral impacts affecting daily performance in a low dental disease Thai population. *Community Dent Oral Epidemiol* 1996;**24**:385–9.
4. Alm A, Wendt L, Koch G. Dental treatment of the primary dentition in 7–12 year-old Swedish children in relation to caries experience at 6 years of age. *Swed Dent J* 2004;**28**:61–6.
5. Alm A, Wendt L, Koch G, Birkhed D. Prevalence of approximal caries in posterior teeth in 15-year-old Swedish teenagers in relation to their caries experience at 3 years of age. *Caries Res* 2007; **41**:392–8.
6. Alm A, Wendt LK, Koch G. Dental treatment in the primary dentition of 7–12 year-old Swedish schoolchildren. *Swed Dent J* 2003;**27**:77–82.
7. Amarante E, Raadal M, Espelid I. Impact of diagnostic criteria on the prevalence of dental caries in Norwegian children aged 5, 12 and 18 years. *Community Dent Oral Epidemiol* 1998;**26**:87–94.
8. Astrom AN, Jakobsen R. The effect of parental dental health behavior on that of their adolescent offspring. *Acta Odontol Scand* 1996;**54**:235–41.
9. Ayhan H, Suskan E, Yildirim S. The effect of nursing or rampant caries on height, body weight and head circumference. *J Clin Pediatr Dent* 1996;**20**:209–12.
10. Batchelor PA, Sheiham A. Grouping of tooth surfaces by susceptibility to caries: a study in 5–16 year-old children. *BMC Oral Health* 2004;**4**:2.

11. Berg IM, Simonsson B, Brantefor B, Ringqvist I. Prevalence of overweight and obesity in children and adolescents in a county in Sweden. *Acta Paediatr* 2001;**90**:671–6.
12. Blomgren J, Axell T, Sandahl O, Jontell M. Adverse reactions in the oral mucosa associated with anterior composite restorations. *J Oral Pathol Med* 1996;**25**:311–13.
13. Bolin AK, Bolin A, Jansson L, Calltorp J. Children's dental health in Europe. *Swed Dent J* 1997;**21**:25–40.
14. Chen M. Oral health of disadvantaged populations. In: Cohen LK, Gift HC, eds. *Disease prevention and oral health promotion: socio-dental sciences in action.* Copenhagen: Munksgaard, 1995.
15. Dencik L. Growing up in the post-modern age: on the child's situation in the modern family, and on the position of the family in the modern welfare state. *Acta Sociol* 1989;**32**:155–80.
16. Dhawan N, Bedi R. Transcultural oral health care: 6 The oral health of minority ethnic groups in the United Kingdom – a review. *Dent Update* 2001;**28**:30–4.
17. Edelstein BL. Disparities in oral health and access to care: findings of national surveys. *Ambul Pediatr* 2002;**2**:141–7.
18. Espelid I, Tveit AB, Mjör IA, Eriksen HM, Fjelltveit A, Øiestad V. Indekser for registrering av okklusalkaries og approksimalkaries. *Nor Tannlegeforen Tid* 1990;**100**:658–63.
19. Fejerskov O, Nyvad B, Kidd E. Clinical and histological manifestations of dental caries. In: Fejerskov O, Kidd E, eds. *Dental caries: the disease and its clinical management.* Oxford: Blackwell Munksgaard, 2003.
20. Feldens CA, Vitolo MR, Drachler Mde L. A randomized trial of the effectiveness of home visits in preventing early childhood caries. *Community Dent Oral Epidemiol* 2007;**35**:215–23.
21. Filstrup SL, Briskie D, da Fonseca M, Lawrence L, Wandera A, Inglehart MR. Early childhood caries and quality of life: child and parent perspectives. *Pediatr Dent* 2003;**25**:431–40.
22. Fleming P, Gregg TA, Saunders ID. Analysis of an emergency dental service provided at a children's hospital. *Int J Paediatr Dent* 1991;**1**:25–30.
23. Foster H, Fitzgerald J. Dental disease in children with chronic illness. *Arch Dis Child* 2005;**90**:703–8.
24. Gimmestad AL, Holst D, Fylkesnes K. Changes in restorative caries treatment in 15-year-olds in Oslo, Norway, 1979–1996. *Community Dent Oral Epidemiol* 2003;**31**:246–51.
25. Grindefjord M, Dahllof G, Modeer T. Caries development in children from 2.5 to 3.5 years of age: a longitudinal study. *Caries Res* 1995;**29**:449–54.
26. Grindefjord M, Dahllof G, Nilsson B, Modeer T. Prediction of dental caries development in 1-year-old children. *Caries Res* 1995;**29**:343–8.
27. Grytten J, Rossow I, Holst D, Steele L. Longitudinal study of dental health behaviors and other caries predictors in early childhood. *Community Dent Oral Epidemiol* 1988;**16**:356–9.
28. Hugoson A, Koch G, Gothberg C, Helkimo AN, Lundin SA, Norderyd O, *et al.* Oral health of individuals aged 3–80 years in Jonkoping, Sweden during 30 years (1973–2003). II. Review of clinical and radiographic findings. *Swed Dent J* 2005;**29**: 139–55.
29. Ismail AI. Prevention of early childhood caries. *Community Dent Oral Epidemiol* 1998;**26**:49–61.
30. Ismail AI, Sohn W. A systematic review of clinical diagnostic criteria of early childhood caries. *J Public Health Dent* 1999;**59**: 171–91.
31. Ismail AI, Sohn W, Tellez M, Amaya A, Sen A, Hasson H, Pitts NB. The International Caries Detection and Assessment System (ICDAS): an integrated system for measuring dental caries. *Community Dent Oral Epidemiol* 2007;**35**:170–8.
32. Klingberg G. Dental fear and behavior management problems in children. A study of measurement, prevalence, concomitant factors, and clinical effects. *Swed Dent J Suppl* 1995;**103**:1–78.
33. Koch G. Effect of sodium fluoride in dentifrice and mouth wash on incidence of dental caries in schoolchildren. *Odontol Rev* 1967;**18** Suppl 12.
34. König K. Implications of changes in caries prevalence on research. *Int Dent J* 1994;**44**:451–6.
35. Last JM. *Dictionary of epidemiology.* Oxford: Oxford University Press, 2001.
36. Low W, Tan S, Schwartz S. The effect of severe caries on the quality of life in young children. *Pediatr Dent* 1999;**21**:325–6.
37. Lussi A. [Damage to neighboring teeth during the preparation of proximal cavities. An *in-vivo* study]. *Schweiz Monatsschr Zahnmed* 1995;**105**:1259–64.
38. Malden P, Thomson W, Jokovic A, Locker D. Changes in parent-assessed oral-health-related quality of life among young children following dental treatment under general anaesthetic. *Community Dent Oral Epidemiol* 2007;**32**:108–17.
39. Mattila ML, Rautava P, Aromaa M, Ojanlatva A, Paunio P, Hyssala L, *et al.* Behavioural and demographic factors during early childhood and poor dental health at 10 years of age. *Caries Res* 2005;**39**:85–91.
40. Mattila ML, Rautava P, Ojanlatva A, Paunio P, Hyssala L, Helenius H, *et al.* Will the role of family influence dental caries among seven-year-old children? *Acta Odontol Scand* 2005;**63**: 73–84.
41. Mejàre I, Kallestal C, Stenlund H, Johansson H. Caries development from 11 to 22 years of age: a prospective radiographic study. Prevalence and distribution. *Caries Res* 1998;**32**:10–16.
42. Mejàre I, Kallestål C, Stenlund H. Incidence and progression of approximal caries from 11 to 22 years of age in Sweden: a prospective radiographic study. *Caries Res* 1999;**33**:93–100.
43. Mejàre I, Stenlund H. Caries rates for the mesial surface of the first permanent molar and the distal surface of the second primary molar from 6 to 12 years of age in Sweden. *Caries Res* 2000;**34**:454–61.
44. Moberg Sköld U, Birkhed D, Borg E, Petersson LG. Approximal caries development in adolescents with low to moderate caries risk after different 3-year school-based supervised fluoride mouth rinsing programmes. *Caries Res* 2005;**39**:529–35.
45. Möller IJ, Poulsen S. A standardized system for diagnosing, recording and analyzing dental caries data. *Scand J Dent Res* 1973; **81**:1–11.
46. Ng MW. Multicultural influences on child-rearing practices: implications for today's pediatric dentist. *Pediatric Dent* 2003; **25**:19–22.
47. Nyvad B, Machiulskiene V, Baelum V. Reliability of a new caries diagnostic system differentiating between active and inactive caries lesions. *Caries Res* 1999;**33**:252–60.
48. Petersen PE. Community-based oral health care for ethnic minorities – the example of Denmark. *Int Dent J* 1996;**46** Suppl 1: 271–6.
49. Petersen PE. The World Oral Health Report 2003: continuous improvement of oral health in the 21st century – the approach of the WHO Global Oral Health Programme. *Community Dent Oral Epidemiol* 2003; **31** Suppl 1: 3–23.
50. Pitts NB. Are we ready to move from operative to non-operative/preventive treatment of dental caries in clinical practice? *Caries Res* 2004;**38**:294–304.
51. Pitts NB. Diagnostic tools and measurements – impact on appropriate care. *Community Dent Oral Epidemiol* 1997;**25**:24–35.

52. Pitts NB. Modern concepts of caries measurement. *J Dent Res* 2004; 83 Spec No C: C43–7.
53. Poulsen S, Heidmann J, Vaeth M. Lorenz curves and their use in describing the distribution of 'the total burden' of dental caries in a population. *Community Dent Health* 2001;**18**:68–71.
54. Poulsen S, Malling Pedersen M. Dental caries in Danish children: 1988–2001. *Eur J Paediatr Dent* 2002;**3**:195–8.
55. Qvist V, Johannessen L, Bruun M. Progression of approximal caries in relation to iatrogenic preparation damage. *J Dent Res* 1992;**71**:1370–3.
56. Raadal M, Strand GV, Amarante EC, Kvale G. Relationship between caries prevalence at 5 years of age and dental anxiety at 10. *Eur J Paediatr Dent* 2002;**3**:22–6.
57. Ratnayake N, Ekanayake L. Prevalence and impact of oral pain in 8-year-old children in Sri Lanka. *Int J Paediatr Dent* 2005;**15**: 105–12.
58. Rönnerman A, Thilander B. A longitudinal study on the effect of unilateral extraction of primary molars. *Scand J Dent Res* 1977; **85**:362–72.
59. Rose G. *The strategy of preventive medicine.* New York: Oxford University Press, 1992.
60. Saracci R. The World Health Organisation needs to reconsider its definition of health. *BMJ* 1997;**314**:1409–10.
61. Schwartz S. A one-year statistical analysis of dental emergencies in a pediatric hospital. *J Can Dent Assoc* 1994;**60**:959–68.
62. Selikowitz HS. Acknowledging cultural differences in the care of refugees and immigrants. *Int Dent J* 1994;**44**:59–61.
63. Seppä L. Past caries recordings made in Public Dental Clinics as predictors of caries prevalence in early adolescence. *Community Dent Oral Epidemiol* 1989;**17**:277–81.
64. Sheiham A. Dental caries affects body weight, growth and quality of life in pre-school children. *Br Dent J* 2006;**201**:625–6.
65. Sheiham A, Watt RG. The common risk factor approach: a rational basis for promoting oral health. *Community Dent Oral Epidemiol* 2000;**28**:399–406.
66. Skaug I. *Norsk språklydlære.* Oslo: Cappelens akademisk forlag, 1996.
67. Skeie MS, Espelid I, Skaare A, Gimmestad A. Caries patterns in an urban, preschool population in Norway. *Eur J Paediatr Dent* 2005;**6**:16–22.
68. Skeie MS, Espelid I, Riordan PJ, Klock KS. Caries increment in children aged 3–5 years in relation to parents' dental attitudes; Oslo, Norway 2002 to 2004. *Community Dent Oral Epidemiol* 2008;**36**:441–50.
69. Skeie MS, Raadal M. Caries in primary teeth at 5 and 10 years of age: a longitudinal study. *Eur J Paediatr Dent* 2004;**5**:194–202.
70. Slade GD, Spencer AJ, Davies MJ, Burrow D. Intra-oral distribution and impact of caries experience among South Australian school children. *Aust Dent J* 1996;**41**:343–50.
71. Stecksen-Blicks C, Sunnegardh K, Borssen E. Caries experience and background factors in 4-year-old children: time trends 1967–2002. *Caries Res* 2004;**38**:149–55.
72. Stenlund H, Mejàre I, Kallestal C. Caries rates related to approximal caries at ages 11–13: a 10-year follow-up study in Sweden. *J Dent Res* 2002;**81**:455–8.
73. Sundby A, Petersen PE. Oral health status in relation to ethnicity of children in the Municipality of Copenhagen, Denmark. *Int J Paediatr Dent* 2003;**13**:150–7.
74. Vanderas AP, Kavvadia K, Papagiannoulis L. Development of caries in permanent first molars adjacent to primary second molars with interproximal caries: four-year prospective radiographic study. *Pediatr Dent* 2004;**26**:362–8.
75. Varpio M. Changes in comprehensive dental care of the primary dentition from 1979 to 1989. II. Restorative treatment of primary molars in a population treated at a university dental clinic. *Swed Dent J* 1993;**17**:35–42.
76. Vehkalahti M, Tarkkonen L, Varsio S, Heikkila P. Decrease in and polarization of dental caries occurrence among child and youth populations, 1976–1993. *Caries Res* 1997;**31**:161–5.
77. Wang NJ, Riordan PJ. Fluoride supplements and caries in a non-fluoridated child population. *Community Dent Oral Epidemiol* 1999;**27**:117–23.
78. Weinstein P, Domoto P, Wohlers K, Koday M. Mexican-American parents with children at risk for baby bottle tooth decay: pilot study at a migrant farmworkers clinic. *ASDC J Dent Child* 1992;**59**:376–83.
79. Wendt LK, Hallonsten AL, Koch G. Oral health in pre-school children living in Sweden. Part III – a longitudinal study. Risk analyses based on caries prevalence at 3 years of age and immigrant status. *Swed Dent J* 1999;**23**:17–25.
80. Wendt LK, Hallonsten AL, Koch G. Oral health in preschool children living in Sweden. Part II – a longitudinal study. Findings at three years of age. *Swed Dent J* 1992;**16**:41–9.
81. Wennhall I, Matsson L, Schroder U, Twetman S. Caries prevalence in 3-year-old children living in a low socio-economic multicultural urban area in southern Sweden. *Swed Dent J* 2002; **26**:167–72.
82. Wogelius P, Poulsen S. Associations between dental anxiety, dental treatment due to toothache, and missed dental appointments among six to eight-year-old Danish children: a cross-sectional study. *Acta Odontol Scand* 2005;**63**:179–82.
83. World Health Organization. *Health 21: the health policy framework for the WHO European region.* European Health for All Series No. 6. Copenhagen: WHO Regional Office for Europe, 1999.

7

Case history and clinical examination

Sven Poulsen and Lars Matsson

The purpose of the present chapter is to describe the case history and the clinical examination of children and adolescents. The chapter will not deal with details concerning signs and symptoms of specific conditions, such as caries and periodontal disease; these will be dealt with in subsequent chapters of this book. This chapter will merely describe the systematic approach necessary to collect data to arrive at a correct diagnosis for the individual patient.

A thorough case history and clinical examination is just as important for decisions on prescribing, for example, radiographic and laboratory examination and arriving at a proper diagnosis and an appropriate treatment plan in the pediatric dental patient as in the adult (Box 7-1).

Since child dental services in Scandinavia cover the entire child population, the dentist is in many cases the medical professional who sees the child most often. As an example, chronic illness in children is relatively frequent (Box 7-2) and dentists should be aware of signs and symptoms of the most common conditions and diseases in childhood and adolescence.

Furthermore, the case history and the clinical examination are often the initial and very important contact of a young child and its parents with the dental team and the clinical setting.

A thorough case history and clinical examination is not only mandatory at the child's first visit to the dentist, but just as important at the start of every new treatment period.

Box 7-1 Initial examination

A thorough case history and clinical examination of the child dental patient is important in order to:

- establish good contact with and knowledge of the child and its parents
- decide on prescription of radiographic and laboratory investigations
- identify possible signs of general conditions and diseases
- arrive at a proper diagnosis and subsequent appropriate treatment plan.

Box 7-2 Chronic illness in children (2)

The prevalence of chronic illness of all 6080 children aged 0–15 years in a defined geographical area in southern Sweden was studied. Information on the health status of the children was obtained from health and medical records, interviews with the district and school nurses, and questionnaires to the parents. Chronic illness was defined as a disability interfering with normal life and/or demanding treatment for at least 3 months during the year 1981 and was revealed in 510 children corresponding to the period prevalence 84/1000 with 95% confidence interval (CI) 60–108/1000. Boys predominated. 131 children suffered from more than one disease. Chronic illness caused severe disability in 40 children, moderate disability in 113 and mild disability in 357 children. Atopic disorders were the leading cause of chronic illness (34/1000 with 95% CI 29–39/1000). Mental and nervous system disorders and congenital malformations were the most frequent causes of severe disability.

Case history

In contrast to taking the case history in an adult patient, the case history in children and especially in young children has to be taken through another person, often one of the parents. This has two important implications.

First of all, the information obtained from the accompanying person may not necessarily reflect the situation of the child. Most often it does, but the dentist should keep in mind that the adult is talking on behalf of the child when evaluating pain, for example. In the case of traumatic injuries, the pediatric dentist should be especially aware of atypical lesions that do not seem to correspond with the information obtained in the history in order to identify cases of child abuse. Second, the dentist may tend to forget to communicate with the child, which occasionally leads the child to feel that he or she is being overlooked. The dentist telling the child that he is going to talk to the accompanying person for a short while, before he looks at the child's teeth, can avoid this.

During the first visit, children and parents form their opinions about the attitudes of the dentist and his or her team towards treatment of children. Thus, it is important that the examination of the child is performed in a friendly and relaxed atmosphere. The dental team should be fully aware of this and meet the parents with a warm and supportive attitude. It is important to focus on the child and parents as people and not primarily as patients. This also gives the dentist a good opportunity to form an impression of the general background of child and parents, their attitudes to dentistry, and their expectations.

The case history should start by obtaining the personal data of child and parents (name, age, etc.) and a description of the present complaint(s), if any, of the child.

At this point it may be advantageous if the dentist takes a quick look at the child's mouth and teeth. In practice, the case history should take the form of a relaxed conversation rather than an enquiry. Standardized forms to be filled in by the parents can be used to obtain part of the case history, but their use should always be followed by an interview.

The complete case history consists of a family history, a general medical history, and a dental history. Important information to be collected under each of these headings is shown in Box 7-3.

Box 7-3 Important elements in a case history

Personal data (name, age, etc.)
Present complaint(s)

Family history
- occupation of parents
- social status
- number of siblings
- attendance in day institutions

General medical history
- pregnancy
  - duration
  - mother's health during pregnancy
  - medication
- delivery
  - complications
  - breech presentation
  - birth weight
  - birth complications
- neonatal period
  - birth length
  - birth weight
  - icterus
  - respiratory problems
  - feeding problems
  - deformations
  - neonatal teeth
- child's health during first year of life
  - somatic development
  - psychomotor development
- childhood diseases and previous medical treatment
- medication including adverse reactions to drugs
- traumatic injuries
- disorders of the circulatory, respiratory, digestive, or nervous system
- sleeping disturbances

Dental history
- past dental care, including the child's reactions
- oral habits
- oral hygiene habits
- food habit patterns (dietary history)
- fluoride therapy

The family history

The purpose of the family history is to provide relevant information about the social background of the child and, most important, his or her family.

Such factors as the number of children in the family, the housing conditions, the parents' occupations, and the child's attendance at day institutions and schools, are important in selecting a realistic plan for preventive and restorative dental care.

The family history should also include the occurrence of any genetic diseases, oral or general. It should be emphasized that the information required for an adequate family history is considered confidential by many parents. Thus, the dentist should be very tactful in attempting to obtain it.

General medical history

Known disease or symptoms of unknown disease should be identified. The general medical history brings the oral and dental problems into a broader perspective of total patient care.

Congenital or acquired diseases or functional disturbances may, directly or indirectly, cause or predispose to oral problems (e.g., craniofacial syndromes, juvenile rheumatoid arthritis, diabetes, hematological diseases) or they may have effects on the delivery of care and treatment of oral disease in the individual child.

The general medical history includes information about pregnancy, delivery, the neonatal period, and early childhood. It should review hospitalizations, illnesses, traumatic injuries, and previous and current medical treatment. Information about infectious diseases (e.g., childhood diseases, otitis media), immunizations, allergies (including adverse reaction to drugs), and sleeping disturbances should be obtained.

Finally, current and past problems as well as any current signs and symptoms of disease in the head, respiratory, cardiovascular, gastrointestinal, neuromuscular, and skeletal systems should be included in the general medical history. When necessary this information should be supplemented with information from hospital records and the family physician.

Dental history

The child's past experience with dental services should be reviewed. The kind of dental treatment received, including pain-control measures and acceptance of earlier dental treatment, gives the dentist important background for evaluation of the child's past behavior in the dental situation and may reveal treatment procedures which have been especially trying for the child. Factors of importance for future dental health should be identified as part of the dental history, including day-to-day oral hygiene, dietary and sucking habits. The dental history also aims at identifying etiological explanations for such unusual conditions as rampant caries, erosion, atypical attrition, and gingival recession noted during the initial, brief inspection.

In addition, a survey of the previous dental records and radiographs, if available, may give important information for the treatment.

Clinical examination

General appearance

As mentioned earlier, the pediatric dentist is, in many cases, the medical professionals who sees the child most frequently. Thus, the dentist has the opportunity to identify medical and functional problems that may have gone unnoticed and can contribute to an improved health service by making appropriate referrals.

Assessment of general appearance should start before the child is seated in the dental chair. If the dentist personally meets the child in the waiting room and they walk together to the clinic, he or she has an excellent opportunity to form a first impression of the child's stature, proportions, posture, head, mouth, breathing, and gait. This assessment may indicate growth disturbances, central nervous system disorders, neuromuscular disorders, or orthopedic problems worthy of further examination.

Examination of the skin for color, pigmented lesions, bullae, scarring, dryness, and scaling may indicate the presence of systemic disease. The hands should be examined with emphasis on webbing, or syndactyly of fingers (indicative of a syndrome), and evidence of habits. The quality and the shape of the nails should be assessed. In ectodermal disorders the nails may be missing or be of poor quality. In chronic respiratory diseases or congenital heart disease, the fingernails may be markedly convex and the fingers clubbed.

Examination of the head and neck

If the family history, the patient's past history, or the gross clinical examination gives rise to suspicion of congenital or acquired craniofacial anomalies, a systematic examination of the head and neck should be carried out. This should include assessment of each anatomical structure for integrity, function, development, and pathology. Minor anomalies should also be assessed since such anomalies are present in many multiple congenital anomalous syndromes and since it has been shown that in newborns with three or more minor anomalies, 90% have a major anomaly. Even with early care and evaluation many anomalies and developmental problems are not identified until early childhood and the dentist should thus be aware of variations from the normal that may signify other problems.

The examination of the face should also include an assessment of the adequacy of the upper lip, the position of the lower lip, the presence of the supramental groove, and the activity of the mentalis muscle. Lip closure and the tonus of the muscles in lips and cheeks are often insufficient in handicapped children and may result in drooling.

The color, amount, and quality of the hair should be evaluated. In certain types of ectodermal dysplasia and various metabolic diseases the hair is missing or sparse and thin (Fig. 7-1).

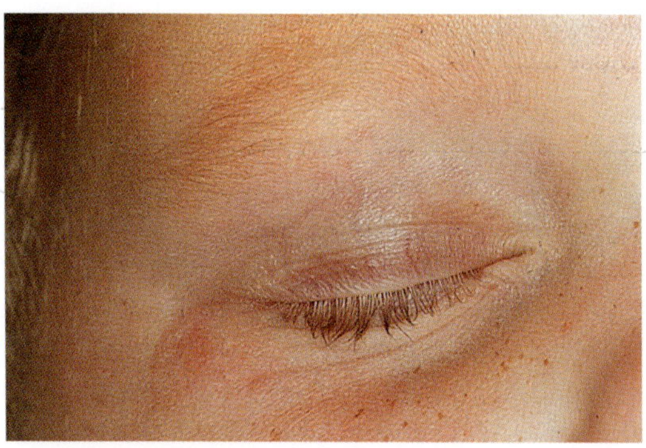

Figure 7-1 Sparse eyebrows in a 12-year-old boy with ectodermal dysplasia.

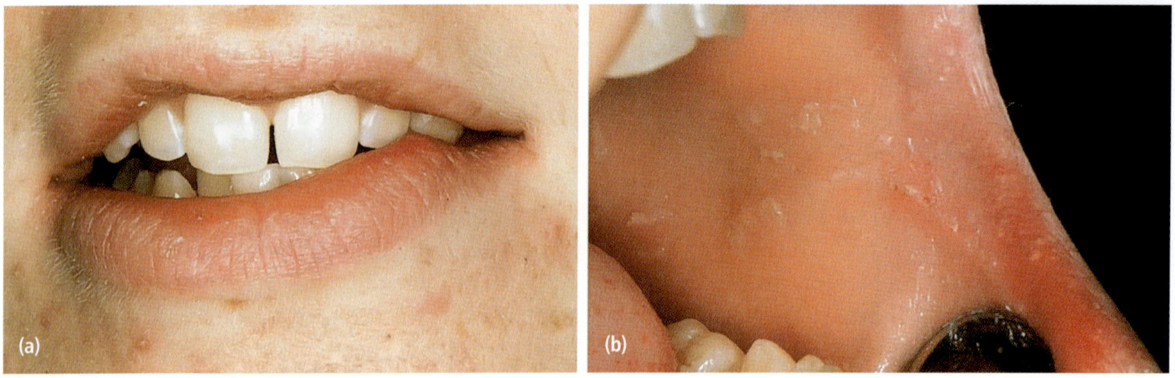

Figure 7-2 (a) Some children and adolescents may develop a habit of chewing the cheek. (b) This will result in hyperkeratinization of the mucosa of the cheek.

Intraoral examination

For the young child, the intraoral examination may be the first contact with dental instruments. For this reason the dentist should use simple intraoral examination procedures to accustom the child to manipulations with mirrors, probes, and other instruments in the oral cavity. A "tell–show–do" technique (as described in Chapter 4) should be employed to its full extent. During and after the intraoral examination, the dentist should take the opportunity to show parents what has been found. Most parents welcome explanations and discussions on their children's dental conditions.

The oral cavity should be examined in a systematic way in order to avoid omission of important conditions. The equipment needed for routine intraoral examination can be limited to a few instruments. The examination can almost always be performed with the child in the dental chair. In some cases, for example very small children, it may be an advantage to perform the examination with the child seated in the parent's lap.

Examination of the oral mucosa

The soft oral tissues are examined before the hard dental tissues. This part of the examination should also include an assessment of the tonsils (size and infection).

The oral mucosa should be examined – being wiped off if necessary – starting with the inside of the lips and continuing to the mucosa on the inside of the checks, including the upper and lower alveolar sulci (Fig. 7-2). The palate is inspected using a mirror. The mucosa of the tongue and the floor of the mouth are examined after careful retraction of the tongue (Figs 7-3 and 7-4).

During examination of the oral mucosa, which may include palpation and inspection, ulcerations, changes in color of surface, swellings, or fistulae are noted. When examining alveolar processes special attention should be given to any minor swellings or retraction of the gingival margin, which could be a sign of periapical or inter-radicular pathological processes and, especially in older children and adolescents, a sign of marginal periodontal disease. Such findings will often indicate the need for radiographic examination (Fig. 7-5).

The presence and attachment of frenulae should be examined with special emphasis on the possible complicating effects of high insertion of such frenulae on the periodontal tissues.

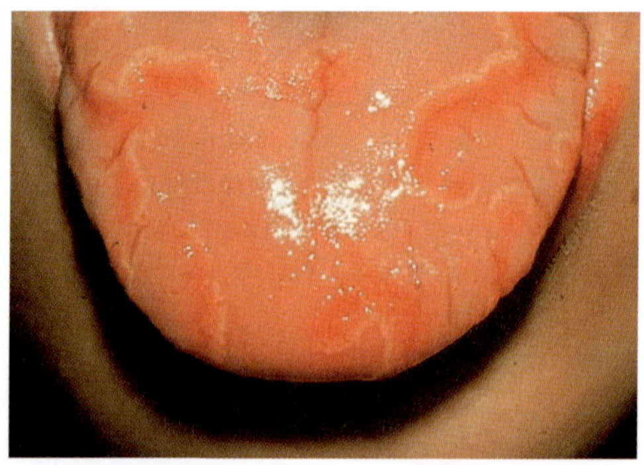

Figure 7-3 Geographical tongue is a relatively common condition found in children (courtesy of A.-L. Hallonsten).

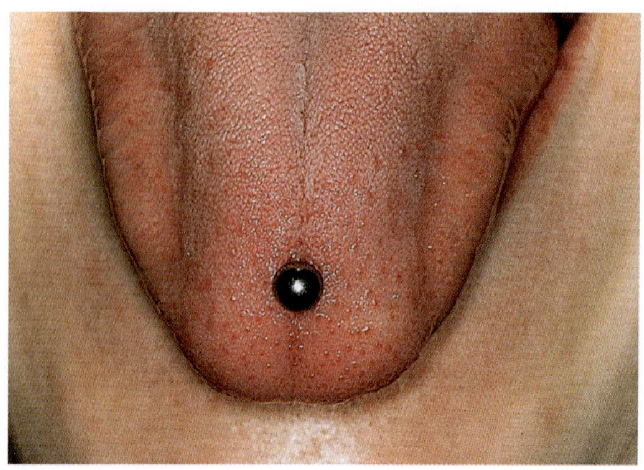

Figure 7-4 Piercing has become a part of teenage culture. Insertion of metallic objects in the tongue increases the risk of damage to the soft oral as well as the hard dental tissues.

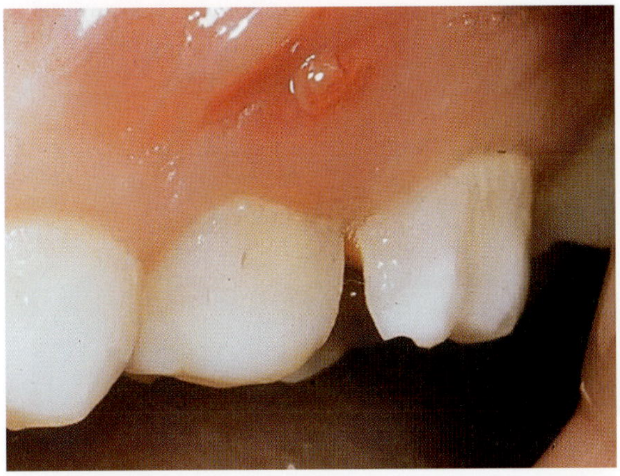

Figure 7-5 Fistula in the buccal mucosa of 64. A radiograph should be taken.

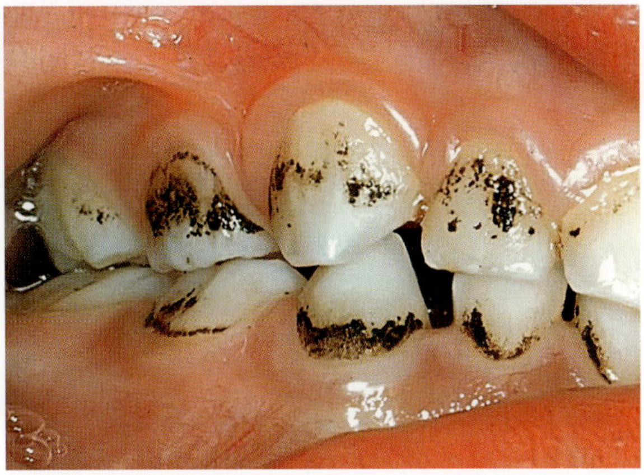

Figure 7-6 Black stains can be observed in children.

Examination of periodontal tissues

Periodontal tissues are examined for inflammatory changes. The gingival margin is gently checked with a blunt periodontal probe for areas with bleeding.

A complete periodontal examination of all teeth for loss of attachment is hardly feasible on a routine basis. There is little reason to recommend periodontal probing in the primary dentition unless radiographic signs of bone loss or general medical conditions motivate this. In the permanent dentition, loss of attachment may be seen during the teenage years. Thus, if periodontitis is not suspected from radiographs, it seems reasonable to postpone systematic periodontal probing until the age of 13–14 years.

Deposits on the teeth can be either hard or soft. Calculus is, however, not a common finding before the teens, although some cases of calculus in the primary dentition can be found on surfaces close to the orifices of the salivary gland ducts and occasionally on the proximal surfaces in the posterior region. The amount of deposits as well as the color should be noted (Fig. 7-6).

Examination of teeth

The number and types of erupted teeth, as well as any irregularities and asymmetries, are noted (Fig. 7-7).

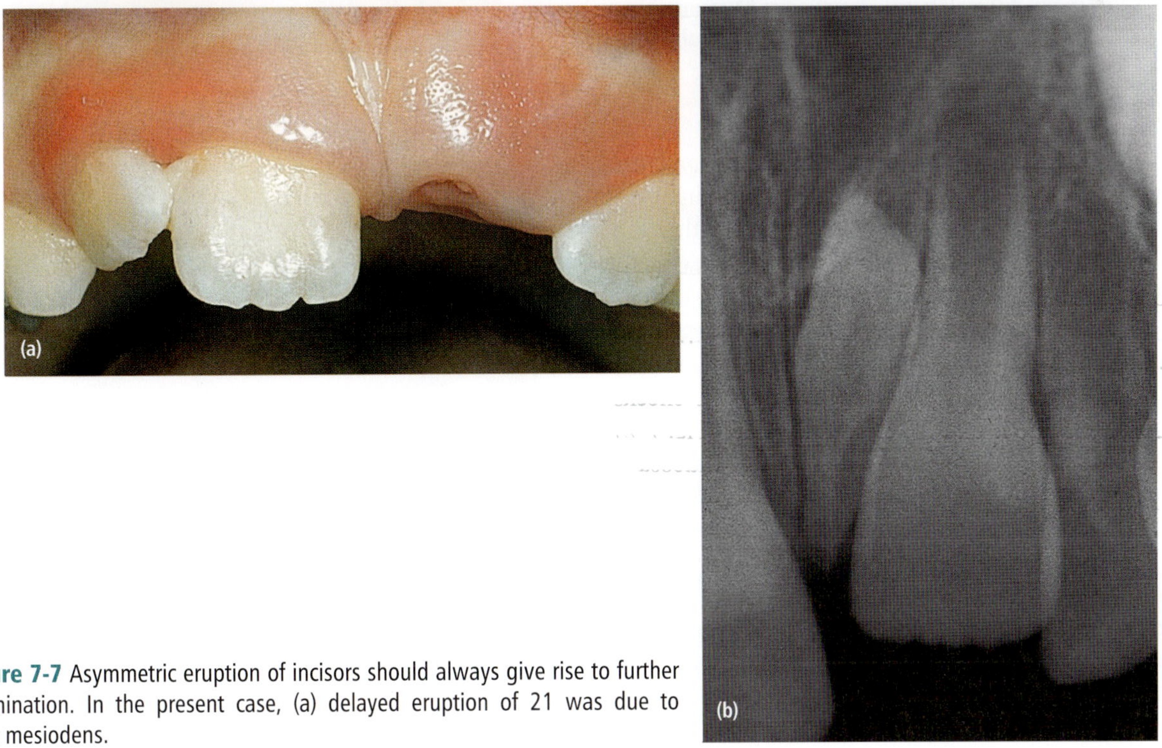

Figure 7-7 Asymmetric eruption of incisors should always give rise to further examination. In the present case, (a) delayed eruption of 21 was due to (b) a mesiodens.

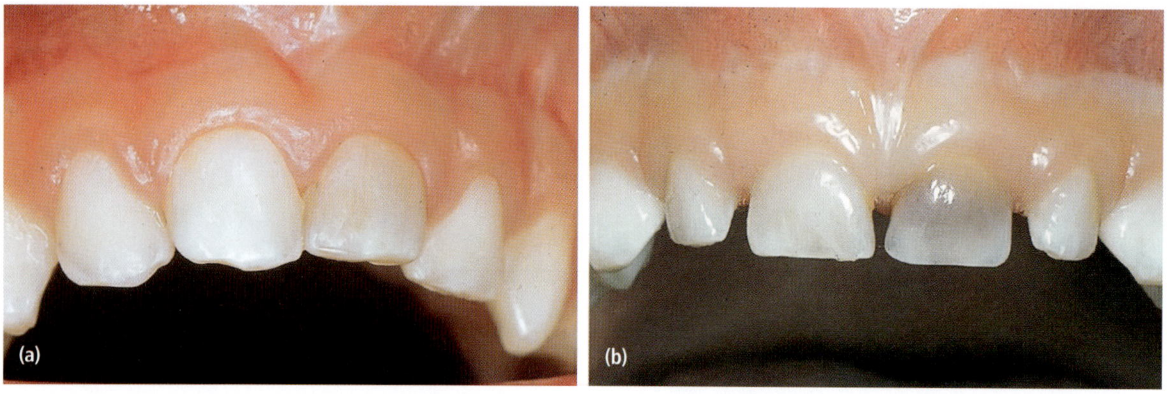

Figure 7-8 Examples of color changes in the primary dentition varying from (a) slightly yellow–gray to (b) darker gray.

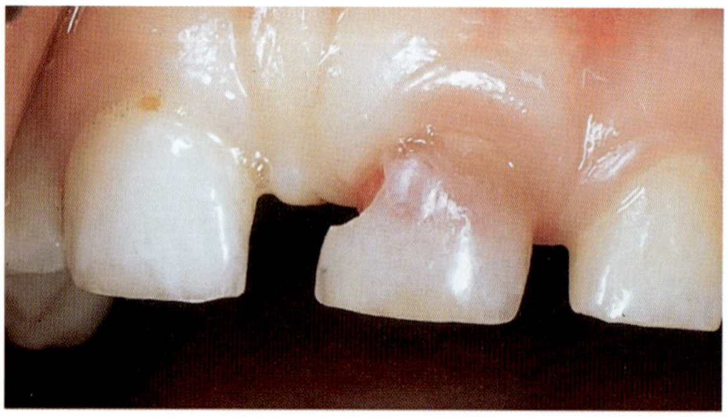

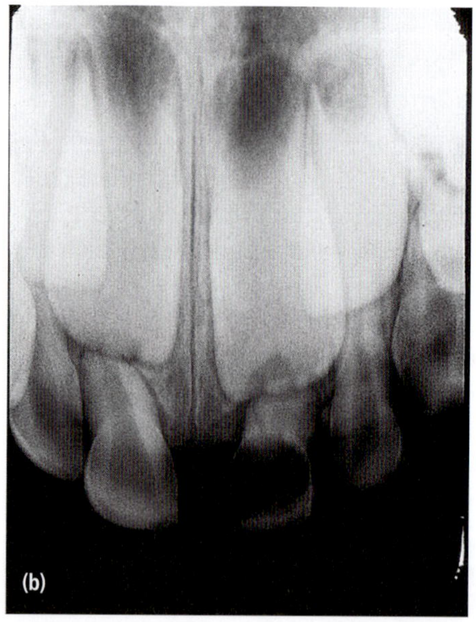

Figure 7-9 (a) Internal resorption of 61 resulting in pink color changes. (b) Radiograph shows the extent of the lesion.

Variations in number, morphology, color, and surface structure should be observed under good light and after careful isolation and drying. Cleaning of the teeth may have to be done to detect minor changes in the enamel surface. This is especially important in the case of very mild hypomineralization as in mild cases of dental fluorosis.

In the case of traumatically injured teeth, the color and translucency of the injured tooth or teeth should be evaluated carefully using both reflected and transmitted light (Figs 7-8 and 7-9). Slight color changes are often found as one of the first signs of early intrapulpal damage after trauma. Variation in the angulation of the light beam is often necessary to reveal minor changes in translucency.

Good diagnosis of erosive changes and mineralization disturbances requires careful inspection and good lighting (Figs 7-10–7-12).

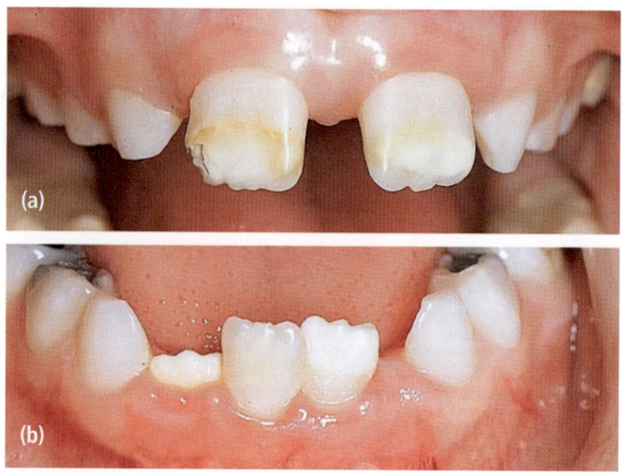

Figure 7-10 Severe hypomineralization of permanent maxillary and mandibular incisors complicated by posteruptive breakdown of the enamel on the distal corner of 11. Note the asymmetric pattern on the mandibular central incisors.

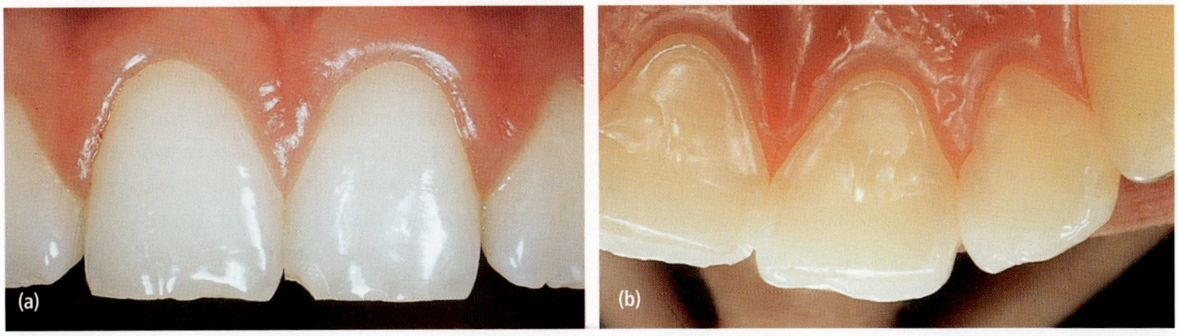

Figure 7-11 Erosions of the maxillary central incisors of a 15-year-old boy due to excessive intake of soft drinks. (a) Note the glass-like appearance of the buccal surfaces of 11 and 21, the concavity on the buccal surface of 21 and the chipping of the incisal edge. (b) Palatal view of the same teeth showing complete loss of the anatomy of the palatal surfaces of 11 and 21 with dentin exposure. Note the pseudo-chamfer contour along the gingival margin.

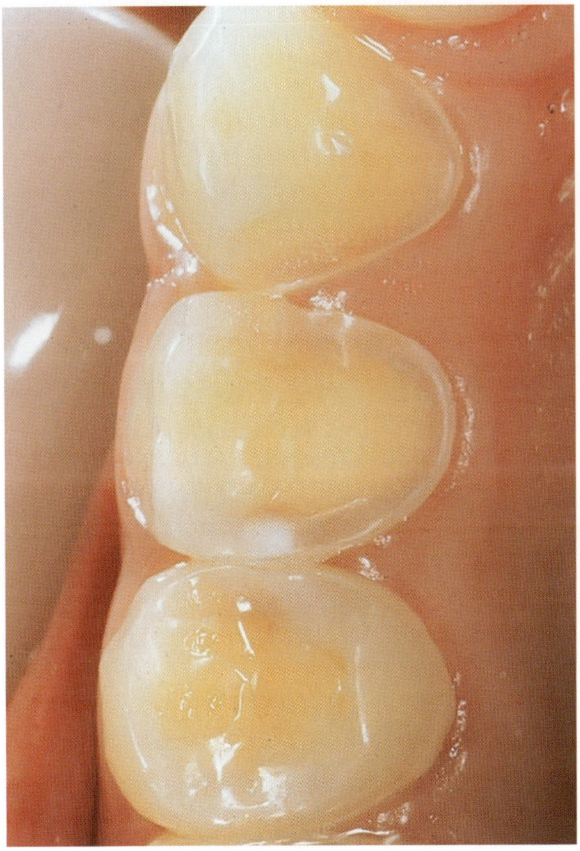

Figure 7-12 Erosions of maxillary premolars.

Initial carious lesions can only be detected after cleaning and drying of the teeth. Such lesions should be examined for surface roughness or actual loss of surface continuity. However, in the case of initial lesions great care should be taken not to expose the subsurface lesions with the probe. Examination of lesions with distinct cavitation should include such signs as the color, size, and depth of the lesion. All previous restorations should be examined for overhang, marginal breakdown and recurrent decay.

Examination for temporomandibular joint problems

The mobility of the temporomandibular joint should be assessed, including the maximum opening. Any restrictions or deviations should be noted (see Chapter 21 for further details).

Examination of occlusion

Finally, the occlusion is examined. Again, a systematic approach is recommended, because the pediatric dentist is the dental professional who is monitoring the occlusal development of the child. Any deviations in dental development, occlusion of the two arches and space conditions are noted.

Records

An accurate record is just as important as a careful examination. Basically, two types of records should be kept:

- recording of findings made during the examination of the child, including the diagnoses
- recording of treatment performed.

Thus, the practice of just recording the treatment needs in the form of fillings needed, for example, is not considered good clinical practice.

No universally adaptable record exists, because the needs will vary according to population, disease pattern, structure of the services, legislation, etc. The importance of the use of uniform recording forms within a dental service should be emphasized, because this allows transfer of information from dentist to dentist. This in turn ensures continuity and improves quality of care.

In Nordic countries, reporting of data to central authorities on, for example, dental caries in children and adolescents is often done on the basis of the data recorded in the child dental service.

Box 7-4 Assessment of dental care can be made

- by members of the dental team
- by the child or its parents.

A method to measure *the dental team's assessment* of the child's reaction to dental care has been described by Rud and Kisling (1):

Acceptance	Criteria
Grade 3	*Cooperative acceptance*: willingness to converse and answer questions, demonstration of interest, relaxed position in the dental chair with arms placed on arm rest, bright, quiet, or alive-and-kicking eyes
Grade 2	*Indifferent acceptance*: hesitating or too quick conversation or answering, cautious or hesitant movements, carelessness. Eye expression indifferent, but still relaxed position in the dental chair
Grade 1	*Reluctant acceptance*: no conversation, no answer, possibly a vague protest, no interest, no relaxed position in the dental chair. Eyes flickering or scowling
Grade 0	*Nonacceptance*: loud verbal protest, physical protest or cry

A complete record of all treatment procedures performed should be made at every visit. The information should be recorded in a standardized way to allow later evaluation of treatment and other interventions.

In pediatric dental care, the reactions of the child and the parents to dental care represent extremely important information for the planning of future dental care. Such information should be recorded in a standardized way, using one of the available scales for reactions to dental care (Box 7-4).

References

1. Rud B, Kisling E. The influence of mental development on children's acceptance of dental treatment. *Scand J Dent Res* 1973; **81**:343–52.
2. Westbom L, Kornfält R. Chronic illness among children in a total population. An epidemiological study in a Swedish primary health care district. *Scand J Soc Med* 1987;**15**: 87–97.

8

Radiographic examination and diagnosis

Hanne Hintze and Ivar Espelid

Radiographic examination in children is essential for diagnosis, treatment planning, and monitoring of a number of changes and pathologies related to teeth and jaws. However, since no exposure to X-rays can be considered completely free of risk, a radiographic examination should be performed only when it is likely that it will benefit the patient; for example, to improve the diagnosis and/or result in a more appropriate treatment considered more beneficial to the patient.

Indications for radiographs in children and adolescents

Before ordering a radiographic examination of a patient the clinician should consider the parameters listed in Box 8-1.

In general, exposure to X-rays must not be undertaken without a previous clinical examination (4). This requirement has been introduced to ensure that radiographs are exposed on the basis of individual prescriptions rather than generalized approaches not taking into consideration individual patient history and clinical findings.

Box 8-1 Parameters to be assessed prior to deciding on radiography, modified from Hintze and Poulsen (7)

Specific parameters
- Patient's symptoms and history.
- Information obtained from clinical examination.

General parameters
- Prevalence in the general population of the disease/anomaly for which the radiographic examination might be required.
- The probability of obtaining additional information from thorough radiographic examination.
- The consequence of an undiagnosed and thereby untreated disease/anomaly.
- The influence of a radiographic finding on the course of the disease or the patient's prognosis.
- Alternative diagnostic methods involving no or lower X-ray exposure.

Principles for interpretation of radiographs

Before image interpretation, the quality of the image should be assessed. Important criteria to be evaluated in this connection are listed in Box 8-2.

Box 8-2 Criteria to be assessed in relation with evaluation of radiographic image quality

- *Region of interest*: is the region imaged sufficiently?
- *Density and contrast*: are these parameters optimal for assessment of the problem?
- *Geometric appearance of the examined structures*: is it good enough for correct interpretation?
- *Sharpness*: is it sufficient?
- *Artefacts*: are such located in areas where they can interfere with image interpretation?

In the case of radiograph being of poor quality, a new radiograph with a higher quality should be exposed before image interpretation can begin. When a radiograph is ready for interpretation it should ideally be observed under proper viewing conditions. For details see Box 8-3.

The best way to start the analysis of a radiograph is to use a systematic viewing procedure including a standard examination sequence ensuring assessment of the different tissues (periapical and alveolar crest bone, number and localization of teeth, each tooth subdivided into crown, root, pulp, etc.) in all parts of the radiograph. The next step is to perform an interpretation including a differentiation between normal and abnormal structures, and a diagnostic decision concerning the latter. The optimal endpoint is a definitive interpretation and a definitive diagnosis.

Box 8-3 Important viewing conditions for radiographic images

Mounting

- Intraoral film radiographs should be mounted and stored in frames.
- Intraoral digital radiographs should be mounted in templates ensuring arrangement in an anatomic identifiable way with a proper orientation (rotation might be necessary).

Displaying

- Film radiographs should be viewed on a lightbox emitting a homogeneous light intensity across the entire surface, and the size of the box should match the size of the radiograph (a large light box can be reduced in size by a sheet of opaque material).
- X-ray viewer with magnification should be used.
- Digital radiographs should be viewed on a high-quality monitor using software with facilities for image enhancement for keeping the radiation dose as low as possible, and for making the image subjectively more appealing in relation to various diagnostic tasks (image enhancement that improves the quality for one specific task might reduce the quality for another task). However, subjectively optimal enhanced images do not necessarily result in improved accuracy of the image interpretation.
- Ambient room light should be turned off or reduced (6).

Radiographic anomalies and pathologies in children and adolescents

Box 8-4 lists the most frequent reasons for radiographic examination in children.

Caries and its sequelae

Using radiographs it is possible to identify approximal enamel and dentine caries lesions and occlusal dentine lesions and to disprove the presence of such lesions. In general, it is recommended to perform a radiographic caries examination when the preceeding clinical examination has not resulted in sufficient information for a final diagnosis or for the planning of treatment. This implies that radiography is considered most useful in surfaces that are not easily accessible with conventional methods such as visual inspection and careful probing.

Box 8-4 The most frequent reasons for radiographic examination of dentomaxillary structures in children and adolescents

- Caries and sequelae.
- Trauma to teeth and supporting tissue.
- Developmental and acquired dental anomalies.
- Systemic diseases and syndromes.
- Treatment planning prior to:
  - orthodontics
  - surgery (most often removal or exposure of impacted teeth).

As caries prevalence decreases in a population there is a continuous need for reassessment of a strategy to take radiographs of individuals where no clinical signs of caries or previous caries experience are present. To do such reassessments, the clinician needs to know the characteristics of the method. Such characteristics are sensitivity and specificity. These parameters are essential in evaluating new methods which are launched to "improve" the caries diagnosis. To determine sensitivity and specificity of a caries diagnostic method a "gold standard" has to be established for every surface included in the study. Often, a histological reference standard is made during sectioning of teeth and thereafter microscopic validation is performed (5,9,29).

Evidence-based reports on caries diagnosis frequently exclude or give a poor-quality rating to studies due to major imperfections in the study design (1,27). In Table 8-1 sensitivity and specificity values from a number of studies judged to fulfill the general principles for good study design are listed. From the table it appears that sensitivity (true-positive ratio) is low in contrast to a relatively high specificity. This means that the radiographic method misses lesions in enamel and even in dentin. On the other hand, relatively few false-positives will occur since the specificity is relatively high. Whether

Table 8-1 Sensitivity and specificity values and ranges in parentheses for radiographic diagnosis of caries based on a systematic review (27)

	Diagnostic accuracy			
	Sensitivity	*N*	Specificity	*N*
Approximal caries in:				
Enamel	0.39 (0.22–0.68)	10	0.87 (0.67–0.97)	10
Dentin	0.45 (0.13–0.61)	9	0.96 (0.89–1.00)	9
Occlusal caries in:				
Dentin	0.58 (0.03–0.96)	17	0.85 (0.71–1.00)	17

Note: in some studies macroscopic methods were used for validation (the gold standard), but microscopic methods were more commonly used. *N* denotes the number of studies which were included after a quality assessment of the literature dealing with the subject.

these values, which are obtained mainly under *in vitro* study circumstances, are also valid in patients is not well researched.

Clinical examination (visual and tactile) is always the prerequisite before any other type of additional examination should be considered. The primary type of supplementary examination should then be the radiographic method. A radiographic image is a good documentation for the dental record and is useful for several purposes including assessment of the caries experience and current activity if undertaken longitudinally. Methods as fiber-optic transillumination, electrical resistance measurements and laser-induced fluorescence (DIAGNOdent) have to be considered as additional techniques that may be used in cases of doubt, but cannot replace the radiographic caries examination so far.

The recommended radiographic technique for caries diagnostics is the bitewing projection. A bitewing radiograph must have a dark density and a good contrast as these factors have a significant influence on the diagnostic outcome (25). A rule of thumb says that good density for caries diagnostics is when image areas representing soft tissue and "air" are intensively black (not dark gray). Usually this will also result in a good contrast. A good contrast ensures optimal differentiation of the various tissues, e.g., that enamel is clearly different from dentin, that demineralized enamel is clearly different from sound enamel, etc. In radiographs with a light density and poor contrast many existing lesions will remain undetected, resulting in false-negative diagnoses. The opposite – that nonexistent lesions are detected – might be the case in radiographs with a very dark density (25). This results in false-positive diagnoses, which may lead to unnecessary treatment (overtreatment).

Deep caries may cause pulp involvement and lead to necrosis of the pulp. Radiographic examination of teeth with pulp involvement may be useful for the detection of internal and external root resorptions and periradicular ostitis. In the primary molars the first sign of necrosis might be a radiolucent zone close to the bifurcation or trifurcation area.

Intervals between bitewing examinations

How often radiographs should be performed for caries detection depends on several factors:

- progression of the disease
- individual caries risk
- value of early diagnosis
- "cost" of dental radiography in terms of radiation, time, and resources.

Caries progression through the approximal enamel will take on average several years, but some surfaces and newly erupted teeth are at a higher risk (18,23). Enamel lesions may arrest, but it is less likely that dentin lesions will, and it is a fact that caries progression in dentin is much faster than in enamel (18).

The combination of strategies based on group levels (e.g., age groups) and individual risk assessment provides a sound basis for deciding intervals between bitewing radiographs. Mejàre (17) has proposed key ages when it is recommended to make radiographs in all individuals. This is largely in line with guidelines for taking radiographs developed by the European Academy for Paediatric Dentistry (EAPD) (3). It is, however, necessary to make a thorough and careful clinical examination to ensure that there are closed, approximal contacts that make the surfaces inaccessible to direct inspection before radiographs are considered. Table 8-2 shows a proposal for an age-based strategy that has to be modified by findings in the individual patient. Mejàre (17) defines the patient at high-risk according to certain age-specific criteria based on a longitudinal study on caries progression of a group of children followed from the age of 11–13 years to young adulthood (19). If the child has no radiographically diagnosed caries at the 5-year control there is low probability that caries will develop over the next 3–4 years. However, radiographic caries experience at the age of 5 years indicates a greater future risk. The information that no caries has been diagnosed also has a value to the child and parents, who will appreciate that their preventive homecare efforts have been successful. Individual caries risk assessment can be based on socioeconomic status, immigrant status, parents' motivation, parental beliefs about oral health, exposure to fluoride, past caries experience, present caries activity, etc. However, risk assessments will never be 100% correct and that is the reason why certain key ages might be helpful for monitoring caries development and progression in low- as well as in high-risk groups. At the age of

Table 8-2 Individual key ages for bitewing radiography and proposed time intervals between radiographic examinations according to Mejàre (17)

Key age (years)	Time interval in years between bitewing examinations	
	In low-risk individuals	In high-risk individuals
5	3–4	1
8–9	3–4	1
12–13	2	0.5
15–16	3	0.5

8–9 years it is reasonable to take radiographs because by then caries may have developed in the first permanent molars and the distal aspect of the second primary molars. At the ages from 12 to 13 years the approximal contacts of premolars and permanent molars have been established for some years and it is reasonable to take bitewings to check caries-prone nonaccessible surfaces. The time before the next bitewing examination should not exceed 2 years. At the age of 15–16 years the teenager still has relatively many newly erupted teeth and runs a considerable risk of caries development.

However, it is important that the proposed intervals should not be misused as an excuse not to see the patient at shorter recalls when reasonable. Clinical examination and caries preventive efforts may be beneficial to the patient at shorter intervals.

When a radiograph is prescribed for caries control, the information should be used to give the best care to the patient. If caries is detected early, treatment without restorations can be performed.

Trauma to teeth and supporting tissue

In children exposed to an acute mechanical trauma of the oral region, radiography is very useful for assessing the extent of possible damage such as displacement of tooth fragments and position of foreign bodies in the soft tissue, root and jaw fractures, tooth displacements, and possible damage to the permanent tooth germs. Patients with moderate to manifest traumas are usually received at an emergency department in a hospital where they will undergo the radiographic examinations specified in the hospital's trauma protocol. Often, such a protocol recommends computed tomography (CT) for severe and multitraumatized patients. Patients exposed to mild traumas that primarily cause damage to teeth and supporting marginal bone only are usually seen in a dental clinic where the radiographic examination should depend on the patient's individual history and clinical appearance.

For correct evaluation of fractures and displacements of teeth, a good radiographic overview (e.g., panoramic examination, occlusal projection, oblique lateral projection) supplemented with periapical radiographs of all involved teeth is recommended. Ideally, each traumatized tooth should be examined from at least two different directions at right angles to one another, but when this is not possible, two projections at two different horizontal or vertical angles might be useful (Fig. 8-1). The angulation of the beam is essential in order to produce an image of the fracture line.

Developmental and acquired dental anomalies

The most frequent dental anomalies in the permanent dentition requiring radiographic examination are:

- tooth agenesis
- unerupted teeth due to: (a) absent eruption space, (b) blocked eruption path caused by an impacted supernumerary tooth, an odontoma or a dentigourous cyst, for example, and (c) ectopic tooth position (mostly upper jaw canines and lower jaw third molars).

Radiographic examination for the assessment of dental anomalies should be undertaken on the basis of individual selection criteria, and the radiographic technique should fit the actual problem in the individual patient. For assessment of a single to few tooth ageneses, periapical radiographs will be the correct choice, whereas for multiple ageneses a panoramic examination might be more relevant to keep the radiation dose to the patient as low as possible (4). For assessment of unerupted teeth the same recommendation is valid. However, a panoramic radiograph will be the most obvious choice if larger pathology or manifest ectopic displacement is suspected clinically. Panoramic radiography will also be the choice when the intraoral image receptor cannot be

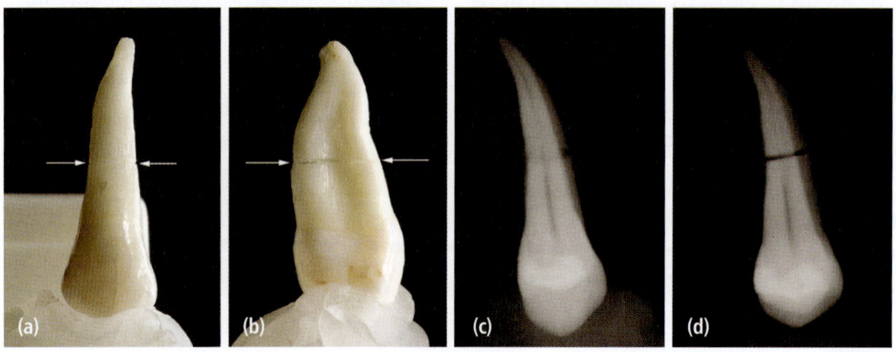

Figure 8-1 A tooth with a root fracture (arrows indicate direction) seen from (a) the facial aspect and (b) an approximal side. On a periapical radiograph this fracture will be shown indistinct or appear (c) as a circle in the case of a steep vertical X-ray beam angulation and as a distinct line in the case of (d) a flat vertical beam angulation.

placed correctly, for example, for the examination of impacted lower third molars.

When the buccal–oral placement of an unerupted tooth is to be assessed, localization radiography conducted by intraoral or extraoral techniques (see below) is indicated.

Systemic diseases and syndromes

Systemic diseases and syndromes causing developmental changes in the maxillofacial bone and in teeth usually need to be examined and monitored by radiography. Major changes often require CT offering the possibility to view the changes in several anatomical planes.

Treatment planning prior to orthodontics

Radiography prior to orthodontic treatment is essential to establish the diagnosis and treatment plan, and as a reference for follow-up examinations to monitor the results of the procedure. Traditionally, a panoramic radiograph and a lateral cephalometric skull radiograph are the images required. However, the introduction of cone beam CT (CBCT) has been shown to be very valuable for the assessment of growth and development (16,26), and some orthodontists seem to prefer a CBCT examination (see below) to the traditional panoramic and cephalometric radiographs (24).

Treatment planning prior to surgery

Radiography prior to surgery is usually needed to provide the surgeon with information leading to a realistic treatment plan ensuring that no unforeseen problems occur during the operation. In general, this means that the most convenient access to the operative area, the extent in all planes of the surgical object, and its localization in relation to important neighboring structures should appear from the radiographic examination. In children with a mixed dentition, specific focus on the localization of developing permanent tooth germs is often necessary to avoid any damage during operation. These requirements often imply that the radiographic examination had to consist of a combination of intra- and extraoral techniques performed in various anatomical planes. In case of close or uncertain relationship between the surgical object and essential neighboring structures CT will often be preferable.

Intraoral radiographic techniques

Periapical radiographs

Periapical radiographs are indicated when the whole tooth and its supporting tissues are to be examined. For

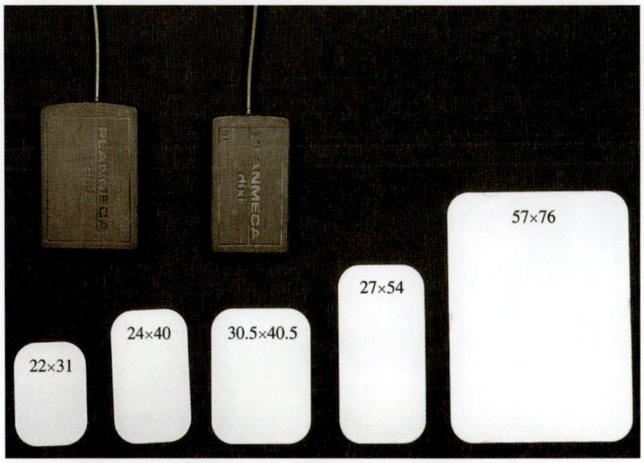

Figure 8-2 Two different sensor sizes and five different phosphor plate sizes. The numbers indicate dimensions in millimeters.

intraoral conventional radiography five film ISO sizes (sizes 0–4) are available on the market. For digital intraoral radiography the same or fewer image receptor sizes are available. Figure 8-2 shows different sizes of digital image receptors. The rule of thumb is that the size of the image receptor should fit the "size of the problem" in the best possible way to minimize the number of exposures. However, in children especially, this rule should be applied with great caution since the discomfort connected with a large receptor usually will have a negative affect on a child's cooperation and acceptance of the radiographic procedure, and in the end result in an inferior radiographic quality.

Periapical radiographs can be performed by a paralleling or a bisecting-angle technique (31). The paralleling technique is preferable because it is easier to perform and gives a more reliable image of the tooth and surrounding alveolar bone (minimal distortion). However, in a young child this technique might be difficult to practice because it requires a film holder, which often will be difficult to place because of the small dimensions of the oral cavity.

In children aged 0–3 years it is in general difficult to obtain periapical radiographs. When necessary due to trauma to the upper front teeth, for example, a dental size 2 image receptor fixed by a needle holder can be placed parallel to the occlusal plane and the X-ray beam angled perpendicularly to the imaginary line bisecting the angle between the surface of the receptor and the long axis of the front teeth in two identical halves (Fig. 8-3). The use of a needle holder makes it easier for a parent to keep the receptor in the correct position during exposure. Another possibility is to place the child backwards on the parent's knee as shown in Fig. 8-4. A needle holder is useful for stabilizing a phosphor plate or a film in the molar region as well, especially in the case

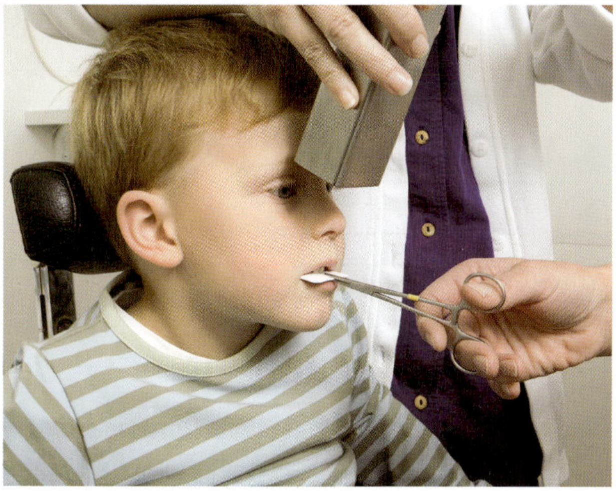

Figure 8-3 Periapical radiography of the upper front teeth. The image receptor is placed in a needle holder parallel to the occlusal plan and the X-ray beam is orientated perpendicular to the line dividing the angle between the surface of the receptor and the long axis of the front teeth in two identical halves.

of a noncooperative child, but cannot be used in combination with a sensor, which is much thicker than phosphor plates and films. If a sensor has to be applied it should to be used in combination with a holder provided with an extraoral beam-aiming device offering the possibility for an accompanying person to hold it in position.

Figure 8-5 shows the "tell–show–do" technique used to introduce a young child to dental radiography. The accompanying parent should be instructed to support the child during exposure to avoid any sudden movement which increases the risk of image blur and subsequently the need of a retake. Box 8-5 gives a number of suggestions to help to obtain good intraoral radiographs in young children.

Bitewing radiographs

The bitewing projection is very useful for determining the presence and extent of caries in approximal and occlusal surfaces. It also gives information about the

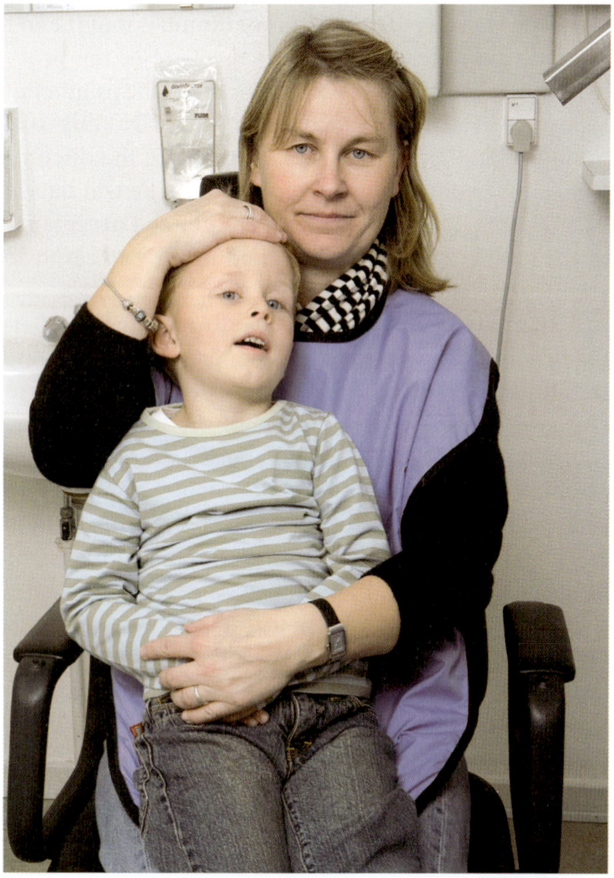

Figure 8-4 A young child placed on the lap of a parent during exposure. To avoid the child moving the parent should hold the child's hands with one hand and support the child's head with the other. The child's head should rest against the parent's shoulder. The legs of very small children can be stabilized between the adult's legs when necessary.

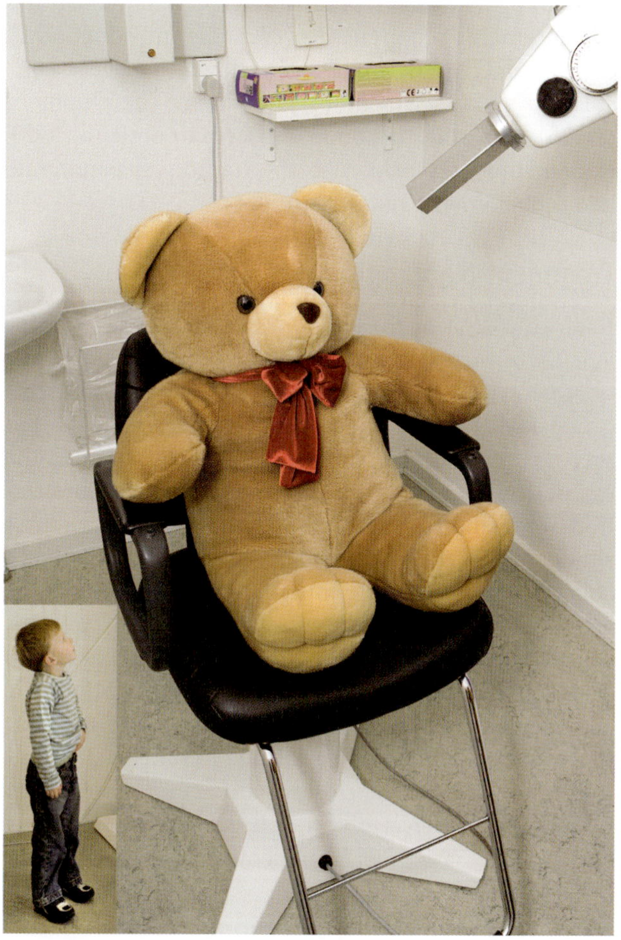

Figure 8-5 "Tell–show–do" technique might be useful to obtain good child cooperation. Before exposure of the child the radiographic procedure can be demonstrated on a teddy bear while the child is watching from a "safe" place.

Box 8-5 Suggestions for obtaining good intraoral radiographs in young children

- Establish good contact with the child.
- Do not separate the child from the accompanying adult except during radiation exposure if the child feels safe. If not, provide the adult with a lead apron and let him or her stay with the child during exposure.
- Explain by using the "tell–show–do" technique what you intend to do. Demonstrate the procedures with the image receptor and the radiographic equipment on the child's doll or teddy-bear or on the accompanying adult using exposure without radiation (Fig. 8-5).
- Be sure that the child is well seated in the radiographic chair. If the child is sitting alone, his or her head should be supported optimally by a headrest. If the child is sitting on the accompanying adult's knee, the child's head should lean against the adult's chest and be fixed by the adult's hand placed on the forehead. This will minimize the risk for patient movement during exposure.
- Before placing the receptor in the holder intraorally, practice with the holder without the receptor. Instruct the child to close the mouth and bite on the bitepiece. When the child manages satisfactorily, mount the receptor in the holder and place them carefully in the mouth without hurting the soft tissue.
- Use a receptor size which can be tolerated by the child. If the receptor cannot be positioned in direct contact or very near the tooth to be radiographed without hurting the child, move the receptor more centrally in the palate or the floor mouth or perform a sharp bend on one of the corners of a film receptor.
- Use a size 0 receptor with a paper loop holder or foam rubber bite block if the child cannot tolerate a common bitewing film holder.
- Involve the child in the procedure, e.g., by breathing through the mouth. Distraction from unpleasant receptor placements can be obtained by counting or letting the child rock one foot calmly.
- Gagging may be caused by dental anxiety, often combined with tactile stimuli to the posterior part of the mouth. Empathy and a relaxed atmosphere combined with a well-organized procedure favor quick exposures and minimize gagging. In cases with extreme gagging, the use of an anesthetic ointment or nitrous oxide sedation can be a valuable adjunct.
- The time with the receptor in the child's mouth can be reduced when two staff members participate in the radiographic procedure.
- If the child does not cooperate, give positive reinforcement and tell the child that you believe it will be easier next time.

status of restorations (overhang, distance to the pulp, secondary caries) and the level of the marginal alveolar bone. The use of a holder device is mandatory in order to place the image receptor correctly in relation to the teeth. A holder with an extraoral beam-aiming device is usually best if it can be tolerated by the patient. If not, a paper loop or a foam rubber bite block glued directly to the front of the image receptor could be used. In that case the X-ray beam should be directed perpendicular to the approximal space between the primary first and second molar in young children and between the second premolar and the first permanent molar in older children. The vertical angulation of the X-ray beam should be +5°–8°. Figure 8-6 shows different image receptor holders for bitewing radiographs.

In general, bitewing radiographs seem to be tolerated even by very young children. In a study of 161 children of 3–5 years, bitewing radiographs of acceptable quality could be obtained in 97% of them (12).

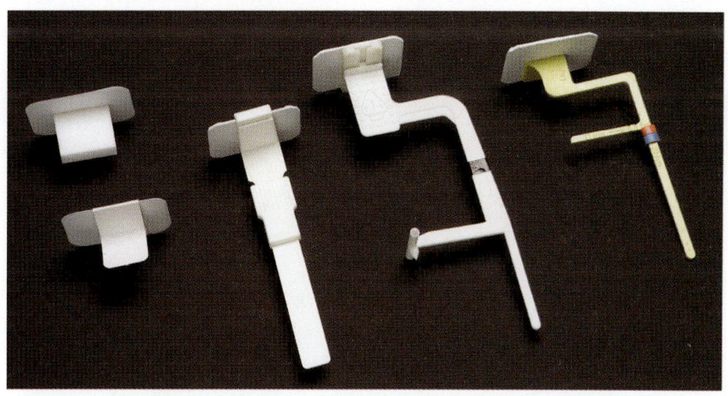

Figure 8-6 Image receptor holders for bitewing radiographs. The three to the right have an extraoral beam-aiming device.

Three-dimensional object localization radiographs

The relative buccal–oral position of two objects can be assessed using parallax movement of the X-ray beam. With a minimum of two intraoral radiographs of the same region taken with different X-ray beam angulations in the same parallel plane (either the horizontal or the vertical) towards the image receptor, the relative depth localization of objects can be visualized. The principle is that the object positioned most orally (nearest the image receptor) will move in the same direction as the X-ray tube while the object positioned most buccally (farthest from the image receptor) will move in the opposite direction to the tube. The localization principle in the horizontal direction is illustrated in Fig. 8-7. Horizontal tube movement is relevant for the depth assessment of impacted teeth in particular (Fig. 8-8),

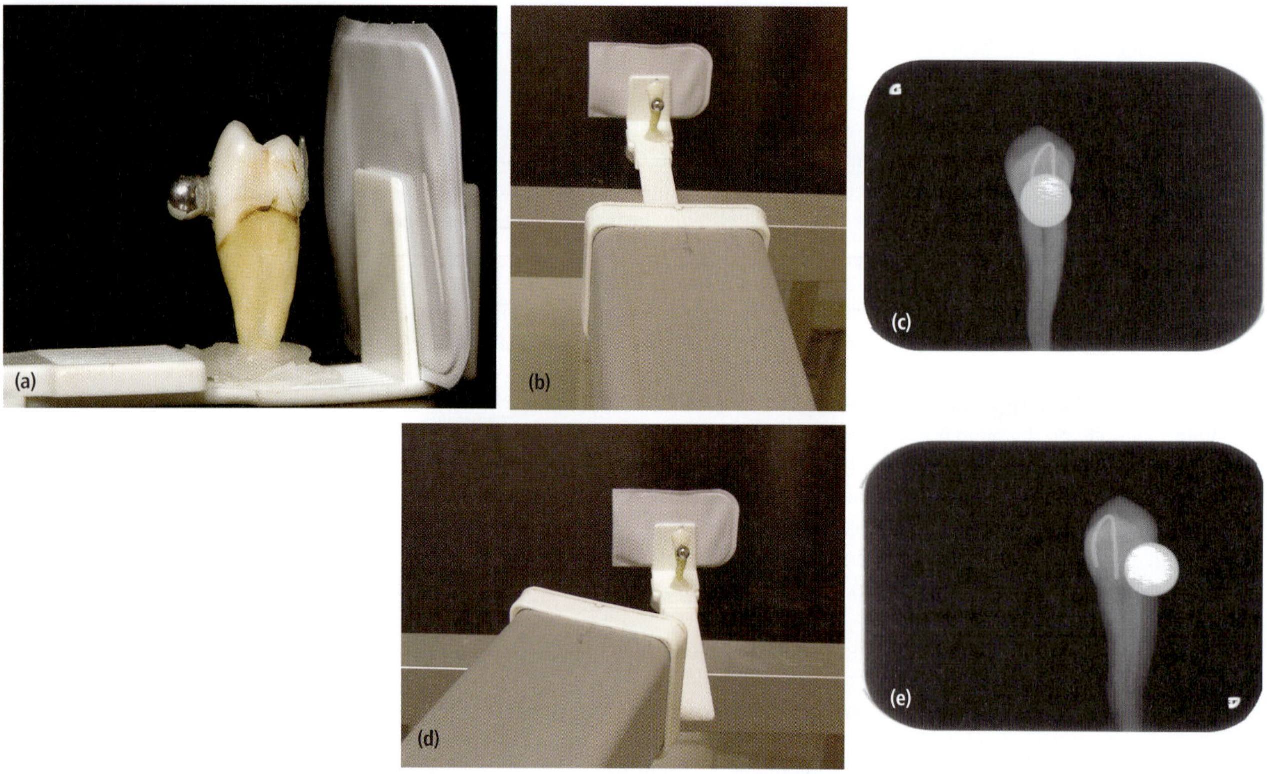

Figure 8-7 Radiographic principle for three-dimensional object localization in the horizontal plan. A metal ball positioned on the facial side of the tooth crown and a metal paper collage positioned on the oral side – nearest the image receptor as shown in (a) will appear as superimposed objects on a radiograph (c) exposed with the X-ray beam orientated perpendicular at the surface of the image receptor (b). On a radiograph exposed with the receptor in the same positioned as in (b) but with the X-ray beam orientated left-sided excentric at the surface of the receptor (d), the metal objects appear separated from each other (e). The paper collage – placed nearest to the receptor – has moved in the same direction as the X-ray beam (to the left) whereas the metal ball – placed nearest to the X-ray focus – has moved in the opposite direction (to the right).

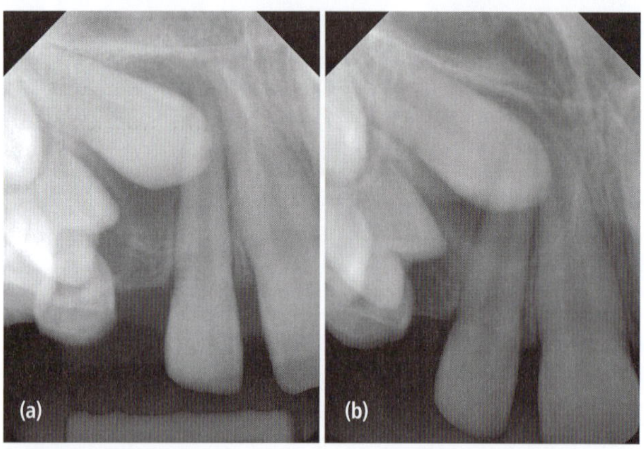

Figure 8-8 Horizontal, three-dimensional object localization of an impacted 13. (a) A periapical radiograph exposed with the X-ray beam orientated perpendicular at the region for 13. (b) A periapical radiograph exposed with the X-ray beam orientated mesio-excentric at the region for 13. Since 13 moves in the same direction as the X-ray beam (mesially) in relation to the root of 12, it is placed nearest the receptor, which means palatally to the root of 12.

radiopaque pathologies, foreign bodies, etc. Vertical tube movement is most relevant for the assessment of the relationship between the mandibular canal and the root of an impacted lower third molar.

From two projections at right angles to each other, the localization of objects in the jaw can also be established. This technique might be useful in connection with the localization of traumatized teeth such as an intruded primary incisor, a supernumerary tooth, or an odontoma. In such cases a combination of an occlusal and a periapical exposure may provide the information needed.

Extraoral radiographic techniques

Panoramic examination

A standard panoramic examination shows the lower part of the patient's face from ear to ear in the horizontal direction and from the inferior point of the chin to the inferior border of the orbit in the vertical direction. Many modern panoramic units are equipped with col-

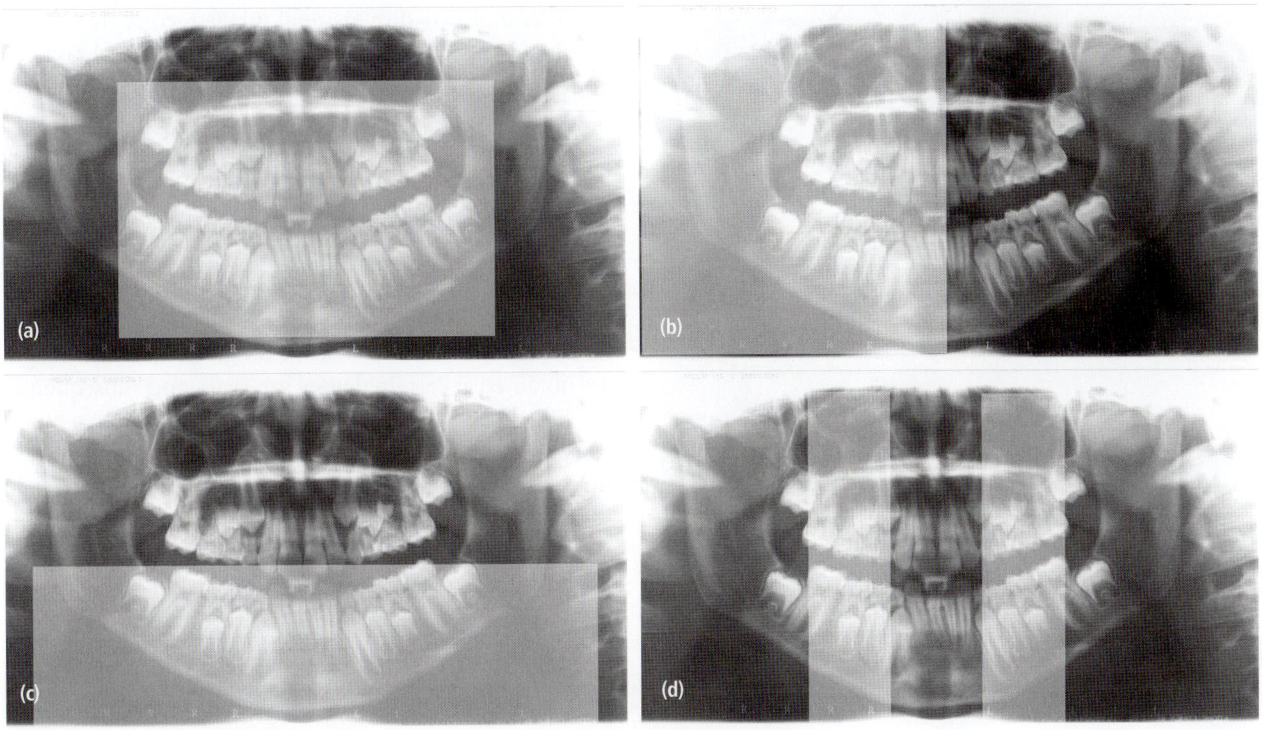

Figure 8-9 Different panoramic segments. (a) A dental panoramic radiograph, (b) a right-sided panoramic radiograph, (c) a lower jaw panoramic radiograph, and (d) a bilateral premolar panoramic radiograph.

limators allowing examination of reduced parts of the area imaged with a standard panoramic examination. Examples of varying panoramic segments can be seen in Fig. 8-9. The clinical problem should be decisive for the selection of panoramic segmentation. A small segment requires a smaller radiation dose than a large segment and should be chosen if possible to optimize the radiation protection of the patient.

Generally, a panoramic examination is comfortable for the patient and can be performed in those patients who are unable to open their mouth due to pain, jaw fixation, unwillingness or inability to cooperate, etc. It requires an effective radiation dose of approximately three to four intraoral radiographs (4) and is rather fast to perform, but it needs the patient to stand still for about 10–20 seconds to avoid moving errors in the image, which makes it unsuitable for diagnostic use. This will often be a problem for children younger than 3–4 years and therefore a very young age might be a contraindication for a panoramic examination. If the radiographer is uncertain of the child's cooperation a test exposure without radiation should be performed.

Scanography

In some modern panoramic units, programs for scanography are available. A scanogram is an image of a restricted area obtained using a narrow collimated radiation beam and a moving image receptor, much the same as applied for the panoramic technique. Due to the technique, scanograms have a higher contrast (important for the perception of small details) than traditional intraoral radiographs.

If scanography is undertaken as a stereo examination at least two scanograms with different X-ray beam angulations towards the same region are obtained (e.g., disto-excentric and ortoradial or ortoradial and mesio-excentric in the horizontal plan). These images can be viewed as stereoscopic pairs in the same way as intraoral radiographs obtained using the principle of parallax. In comparison with the latter, stereo scanograms are easier and faster to perform for the radiographer and more comfortable for the patient (there is no image receptor in the mouth). The dentist gets radiographs of a relatively large size, which leads to a good overview. Stereo scanography is excellent for object localization in the buccal–oral direction. Figure 8-10 shows horizontal stereo scanographic images of an impacted upper second premolar. It is easy to see that the impacted tooth is positioned orally to the root of the first premolar.

Computed tomography

CT can be performed on the basis of the fan beam or cone beam technique (24). With the fan beam technique the patient is exposed to a fan-shaped X-ray beam and the image is produced slice-by-slice in the axial plane. Subsequently, the multiple image slices are stacked

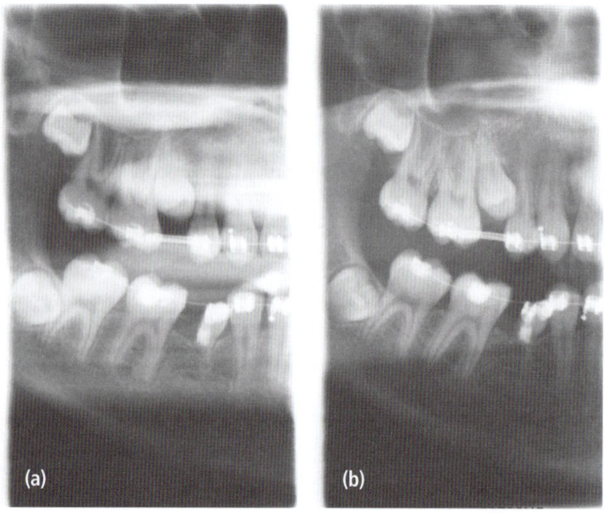

Figure 8-10 Stereo scanogram for depth localization of an impacted 15. The X-ray beam orientation at 15 is "disto-excentric" for the scanogram to the left and "mesio-excentric" for the scanogram to the right. As 15 moves mesially in relation to the root of 14 on the scanogram to the right compared with the scanogram to the left it is located palatally to the root of 14.

together and two-dimensional image reconstructions in all planes (axial, sagittal, coronal, oblique, and curved) and three-dimensional image models can be generated. Fan beam CT scanners are available mainly in hospitals and not commonly used by dentists because of referring restrictions, high costs, and radiation dose being much higher than the doses traditionally used in dental radiography (14,15).

With the CBCT technique the patient is exposed to a cone-shaped X-ray beam rotated around the patient's head during a 180–360° scan. Single projection images are obtained at certain degree intervals, and subsequently the large number of scans is prepared by the machine's software and the images are reconstructed in all planes; three-dimensional image models are available as well. Recently, units for CBCT have been commercially available for dental practice where they have shown to be very useful for the examination of dental and maxillofacial hard tissues (10,20,22). A CBCT two-dimensional examination undertaken for the localization of an impacted supernumerary upper tooth is shown in Fig. 8-11.

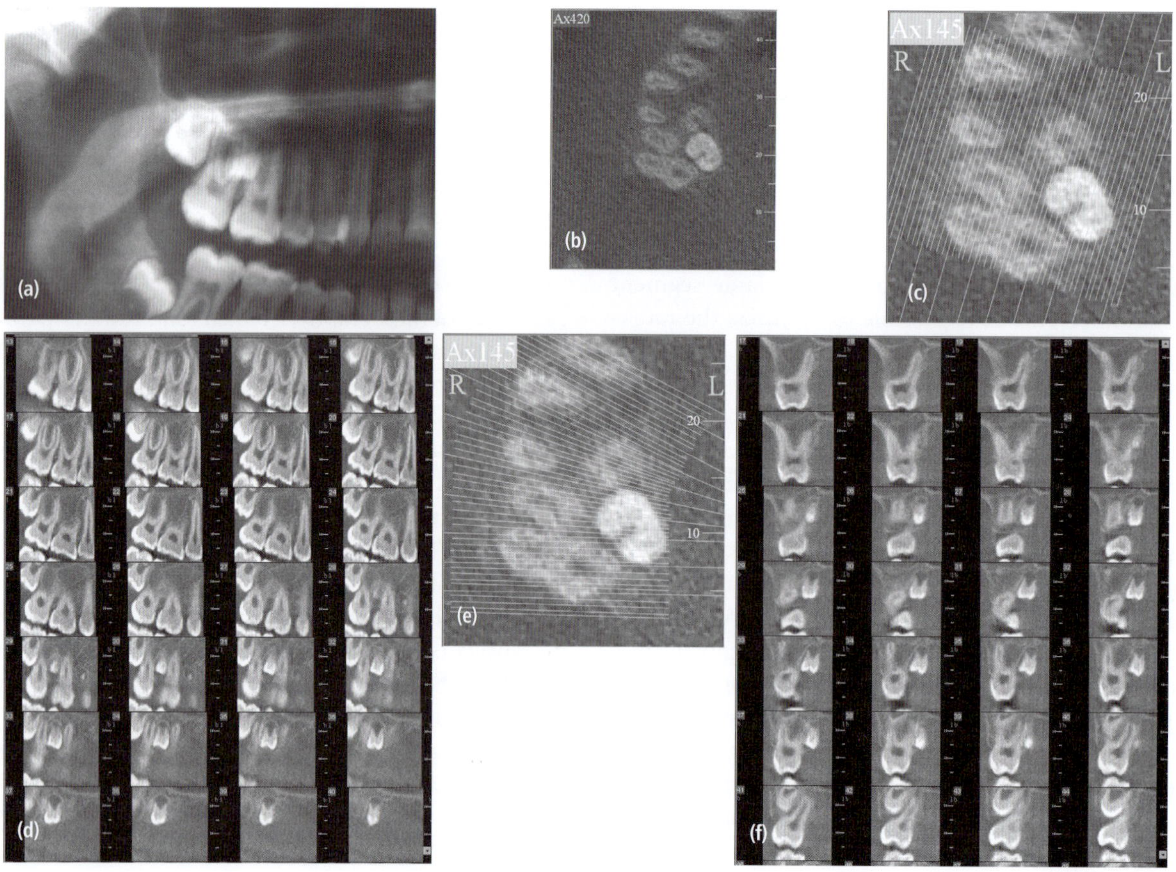

Figure 8-11 (a) Part of a conventional panoramic radiograph showing an upper impacted, supernumerary tooth in region 17 and 16. (b) An axial image from a CBCT examination showing the supernumerary tooth between the palatal root of 16 and the roots of 17. (c) Scout CBCT image showing the orientation of images in the sagittal plan. (d) CBCT sagittal images showing the supernumerary tooth placed palatally to 17 and 16. (e) Scout CBCT image showing the orientation of images in the coronal plan. (f) CBCT coronal images showing the supernumerary tooth placed palatally to 17 and 16.

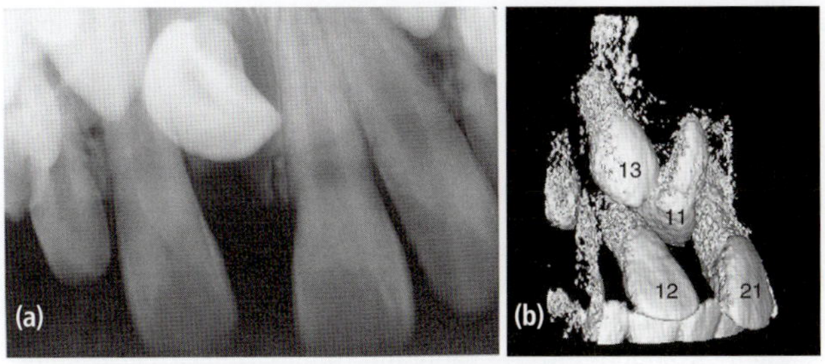

Figure 8-12 (a) Conventional intraoral radiograph showing an impacted, transversally located 11. (b) On a three-dimensional image model from a CBCT examination it is clear that 11 is lacerated and placed with the crown palatally and the root facially to the neighboring teeth.

The three-dimensional image model obtained from CBCT data may facilitate the clinician's perception of the separation level between neighboring structures as illustrated in Fig. 8-12, where the position of an impacted, lacerated upper central incisor in relation to the neighboring teeth appears clearly, often more unequivocally than on the basis of two-dimensional images.

Compared with conventional fan beam CT, CBCT has a number of advantages such as:

- easy to request and to refer to (when fully implemented in dentistry)
- requires a very short scan time
- requires a significant smaller radiation dose [the effective dose for a "full head" CBCT examination performed with a NewTom 3G scanner is equivalent to four to seven single panoramic radiographs compared to a fan beam CT examination which might be equivalent with up to 336 single panoramic radiographs (15)]
- results in fewer relative image artefacts arising from metal objects in the teeth and jaws (fillings, crowns, bridges, implants, bone plate fixtures, etc.)
- study viewers are free or relatively cheap to buy.

Radiation protection

Patient protection in general

Every patient who undergoes an X-ray examination is exposed to millions of photons which can cause cell damage due to ionization. Damage to the DNA in a cell's chromosomes might lead to permanent changes known as mutations. In very rare cases, a mutation may result in the development of a tumor. The risk of a tumor due to a given X-ray dose can be estimated, and dose and risk have been found to be positively correlated. Therefore, it is recommended that patient doses are kept as low as reasonably achievable (4). Since the latent period between X-ray exposure and clinical diagnosis of a resultant tumor is expected to be many years (20–45 years), children are at a higher risk than middle-aged and elderly adults and therefore should be protected most carefully.

Image receptor sensitivity

Dental films are commercially available in ISO speed groups D, E, and F. The F-speed film is the most sensitive (20–25% faster than the E-speed film) and provides a diagnostic quality equal to the other film speed groups and should therefore be used for patient exposures (8,13,21).

Digital image receptors for intraoral radiographs have previously been much more sensitive and thereby require a significantly lower radiation dose than conventional films (8), but for several of the present digital receptors this characteristic is less pronounced when the diagnostic accuracy of the digital image is comparable with that of films (2,28). Problems with smaller digital receptor sizes may lead to more than one exposure to cover the area to be examined, and problems with positioning the digital receptor, in particular bulky sensors, may lead to high rejection rates resulting in retakes (30). These problems might in the end lead to increased patient doses with digital radiography.

For extraoral radiographs, it is unlikely that digital systems will offer any dose reduction when compared to a conventional medium speed film-intensifying screen system.

Beam collimation

For intraoral radiography, a rectangular collimator offers a significant dose reduction to the patient compared with a traditional circular collimator with an opening of maximum size (6–7 cm in diameter) (4). In addition, a rectangular collimator results in higher image contrast owing to lower scattered radiation.

Lead protection

An apron protects against external scattered radiation but seems to have no effect on the gonad dose (11). If the apron is supplemented with a thyroid collar, the dose from both primary and scattered radiation to the thyroid gland might be reduced. However, thyroid shielding is not possible in panoramic radiography, for example. For intraoral radiography, a neck shield as shown in Fig. 8-13 can be used instead of an apron. The neck shield is placed in contact with the inferior part of the mandible and it offers optimal radiation protection to the thyroid gland. However, the shield might interfere with the X-ray tube when exposing periapical radiographs of the lower front teeth, making it impossible to use the paralleling technique in this region.

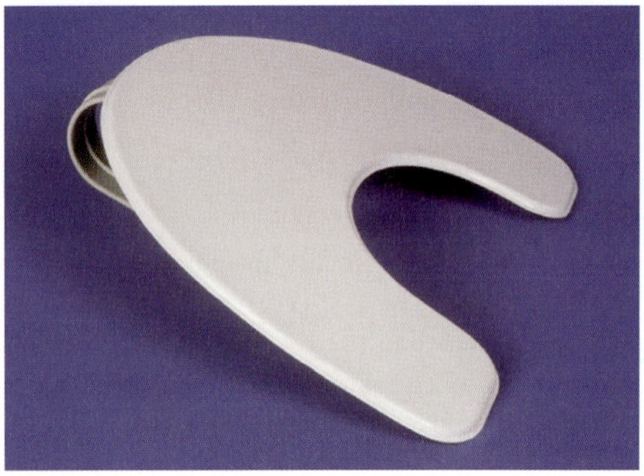

Figure 8-13 A neck shield.

Patient cooperation

Dental radiography may be a frightening experience for a child. With intraoral radiography, the X-ray tube is close to the face and an unpleasant image receptor is placed in the mouth. With extraoral radiography, a young child might find the X-ray unit large and frightening. Techniques to reduce the child's fear should be used, and the technicians should be responsible for ensuring a trustful cooperation with the child, since this is important for an acceptable X-ray examination with a minimum number of retakes.

References

1. Bader JD, Shugars DA, Rozier G, Lohr KN, Bonito AJ, Nelson JP, *et al. Diagnosis and management of dental caries.* Publication No. 01-E056. Rockville, MD: Agency for Healthcare Research and Quality, June 2001.
2. Berkhout WER, Beuger DA, Sanderink GCH, van der Stelt PF. The dynamic range of digital radiographic systems: dose reduction or risk of exposure? *Dentomaxillofac Radiol* 2004;**33**:1–5.
3. Espelid I, Mejàre I, Weerheim K. EAPD guidelines for use of radiographs in children. *Eur J Paediatr Dent* 2003;**4**:40–8.
4. European Commission. *European guidelines on radiation protection in dental radiology.* RP136, Luxembourg, 2004.
5. Grossman ES, Cleaton-Jones PE, Cortes DF, Daya NP, Parak RB, Fatti LP, *et al.* Accurate diagnosis of occlusal carious lesions – a stereo microscope evaluation of clinical diagnosis. *SADJ* 2002;**57**:215–20.
6. Hellén-Halme K, Nilsson M, Petersson A. Digital radiography in general dental practice: a field study. *Dentomaxillofac Radiol* 2007;**36**:249–55.
7. Hintze H, Poulsen S. Pædodontisk radiologi. *Tandlægebladet* 2005;**109**:488–95 (in Danish).
8. Hintze H, Wenzel A. Influence of the validation method on diagnostic accuracy for caries. A comparison of six digital and two conventional radiographic systems. *Dentomaxillofac Radiol* 2002;**31**:44–9.
9. Hintze H, Wenzel A. Diagnostic outcome of methods frequently used for caries validation. A comparison of clinical examination, radiography and histology following hemisectioning and serial tooth sectioning. *Caries Res* 2003;**37**:115–24.
10. Hintze H, Wiese M, Wenzel A. Cone beam CT and conventional tomography for detection of morphological TMJ changes. *Dentomaxillofac Radiol* 2007;**36**:192–7.
11. Horner K. Review article: radiation protection in dental radiology. *Br J Radiol* 1994;**67**:1041–9.
12. Kaakko T, Riedy CA, Nakai Y, Domoto P, Weinstein P, Milgrom P. Taking bitewing radiographs in preschoolers using behaviour management techniques. *ASCD J Dent Child* 1999;**66**:320–4.
13. Ludlow JB, Abreu M Jr, Mol A. Performance of a new F-speed film for caries detection. *Dentomaxillofac Radiol* 2001;**30**:110–13.
14. Ludlow JB, Davies-Ludlow LE, Brooks SL. Dosimetry of two extraoral direct digital imaging devices: NewTom cone beam CT and Orthophos Plus DS panoramic unit. *Dentomaxillofac Radiol* 2003;**32**:229–34.
15. Ludlow JB, Davies-Ludlow LE, Brooks SL, Howerton WB. Dosimetry of 3 CBCT devices for oral and maxillofacial radiology: CB Mercuray, NewTom 3G and i-CAT. *Dentomaxillofac Radiol* 2006;**35**:219–26.
16. Maki K, Inou N, Takanishi A, Miller AJ. Computer-assisted simulations in orthodontic diagnosis and the application of a new cone beam X-ray computed tomography. *Orthod Craniofac Res* 2003;**6**(Suppl 1):95–101.
17. Mejàre I. Bitewing examination to detect caries in children and adolescents – when and how often? *Dent Update* 2005;**32**:588–90, 593–4, 596–7.
18. Mejàre I, Källestål C, Stenlund H. Incidence and progression of approximal caries from 11 to 22 years of age in Sweden: a prospective radiographic study. *Caries Res* 1999;**33**:93–100.
19. Mejàre I, Stenlund H, Zelezny-Holmlund C. Caries incidence and lesion progression from adolescence to young adulthood: a prospective 15-year cohort study in Sweden. *Caries Res* 2004; **38**:130–41.
20. Mengel R, Candir M, Shiratori K, Flores-de-Jacoby L. Digital volume tomography in the diagnosis of periodontal defects: an *in vitro* study on native pig and human mandibles. *J Periodontol* 2005;**76**:665–73.
21. Nair MK, Nair UP. An *in-vitro* evaluation of Kodak Insight and Ektaspeed Plus film with a CMOS detector for natural proximal caries: ROC analysis. *Caries Res* 2001;**35**:354–9.
22. Pawelzik J, Cohnen M, Willers R, Becker J. A comparison of conventional panoramic radiographs with volumetric computed tomography images in the preoperative assessment of impacted mandibular third molars. *J Oral Maxillofac Surg* 2002;**60**:979–84.
23. Reich E, Lussi A, Newbrun E. Caries-risk assessment. *Int Dent J* 1999;**49**:15–26.
24. Scarfe WC, Farman AG, Sukovic P. Clinical applications of cone-beam computed tomography in dental practice. *JADA* 2006;**72**: 75–80.
25. Skodje F, Espelid I, Kvile K, Tveit AB. The influence of radiographic exposure factors on the diagnosis of occlusal caries. *Dentomaxillofac Radiol* 1998;**27**:75–9.
26. Sukovic P. Cone beam computed tomography in craniofacial imaging. *Orthod Craniofac Res* 2003;**6**(Suppl 1):31–6.
27. Swedish Council on Technology Assessment in Health Care. *Caries diagnosis, risk assessment and non-operative treatment of early caries lesions.* SBU Report No. 188, 2007 (in Swedish).
28. van der Stelt PF. Filmless imaging. The uses of digital radiography in dental practice. *J Am Dent Assoc* 2005;**136**:1379–87.
29. Wenzel A, Hintze H. The choice of gold standard for evaluating tests for caries diagnosis. *Dentomaxillofac Radiol* 1999;**28**:132–6.
30. Wenzel A, Møystad A. Experience of Norwegian general practitioners with solid state and storage phosphor detectors. *Dentomaxillofac Radiol* 2001;**30**:203–8.
31. Whaites E. *Essentials of dental radiography and radiology*, 2nd edn. New York: Churchill Livingstone, 1996.

9

Caries prevention

Göran Koch, Sven Poulsen and Svante Twetman

The importance and concepts of caries prevention

Erupting teeth are healthy, and the first carious lesion and its restoration marks the initiation of a series of treatments that during the tooth's lifetime will end up in more and more complicated restorations. Today there is sufficient scientific knowledge about the etiology of caries and about factors that interfere in this process in order for us to develop effective preventive strategies. There is no excuse not to use this knowledge in attempts to control caries. Therefore, caries prevention should be given a high priority by the dental profession as well as by governmental authorities. In this context, the pediatric dentist has a very specific responsibility in meeting the challenge of keeping children and adolescents free from caries. For example, very young children with early signs of caries should be given special attention, as they tend to develop more caries compared to children without early signs of caries (Box 9-1).

Even if the principles of caries prevention are simple, the implementation, management, and evaluation of programs and recommendations can be difficult. For example, it has been shown in clinical trials that professional prophylaxis every second week complemented with strong motivational activities resulted in more or less complete caries control in children (1), whereas a field study with a similar regimen carried out with less enthusiasm or motivation did not give the same results (5).

Different concepts are used to describe preventive activities (Box 9-2). Oral health promotion is an activity which takes place at the community level with the purpose of making it easier for people to live a healthy life. Reducing schoolchildren's access to sweet snacks through school policies is an example of oral health promotion. An important aspect of oral health promotion is that it may also result in the reduction of other health

Box 9-1 Caries development in children 2.5–3.5 years of age

Grindefjord M, Dahllöf G, Modéer T. Caries development in children from 2.5 years of age: a longitudinal study. *Caries Res* 1995;**29**:449–54.

The development of dental caries from the age of 2.5 to 3.5 years was studied longitudinally in 692 children living in the southern suburbs of Stockholm. At baseline examination, 11.3% of the children had caries lesions (initial lesions included). At follow-up, 1 year later, decayed and/or filled surfaces were found in 37% of the subjects. The majority of the new lesions were located on the occlusal surfaces of the second molars. Ninety-two percent of the children with caries lesions at baseline developed new carious lesions during the 1-year follow-up period, compared to 29% of the children who had no caries lesions at baseline ($p < 0.001$). Of the lesions diagnosed at baseline as initial lesions, 64% progressed to manifest lesions during the 1-year period. The study indicates that children with early caries lesions have a high risk of developing new lesions, and that early lesions have a high risk of progression.

Baseline (2.5 years of age)	Follow-up (3.5 years of age)				
	Children with			Mean number of surfaces	
	No caries	New lesions	Restorations	ds	dfs
Children with caries ($n = 78$)	2	72 (92%)	4	6.4	8.2
Caries-free children ($n = 614$)	436	178 (29%)	0	0.9	0.9

Box 9-2 Important concepts in prevention

- *Health promotion*: the process of enabling people to increase control over and improve their health ("making healthy choices").
- *Primary prevention*: disease-specific protection of health.
- *Secondary prevention*: early detection and prompt intervention to control disease and minimize disability.
- *Tertiary prevention*: reducing the impact of impairment, disability, and handicap.

problems such as being overweight, because many health problems have common risk factors. In contrast to health promotion, prevention aims at reducing the risk of a specific disease. Prevention is described at three levels: primary, secondary, and tertiary:

- primary caries prevention is preventing new caries lesions from occurring
- secondary caries prevention is early detection and intervention to arrest early caries lesions
- tertiary caries prevention is restoration of cavitated lesions in order to prevent further destruction, eventually leading to the loss of the tooth.

How does caries develop?

An important basis for prevention is an understanding of causation. In epidemiology, a cause is defined as a factor that influences the risk or disease, and causal factors are often arranged in what epidemiologists know as "webs of causation". This concept has recently been used as a model for understanding dental caries (7), and Box 9-3 illustrates how causes of child dental caries can be identified at several different levels:

- At the tooth surface, where a complex interplay takes place between host factors, diet, and the biofilm.
- In the interaction between members of the family.
- In the living conditions of children and their families.

This understanding has given rise to the concept of "upstream" and "downstream" causal factors. Downstream causal factors are those that are active close to where the caries lesion is observed, i.e., at the tooth surface; while upstream factors are those that affect the living conditions of the family. It is important to underline that it is the responsibility of pediatric dentists to try to reduce causal factors for dental caries at all levels. This means understanding and being interested in health promotion to improve general living conditions and health of children, as well as using all possible methods of prevention to prevent new caries lesions from occurring, and to detect and arrest early initial lesions. The remaining part of this chapter is mainly concerned with prevention, and is based on an understanding of the disease as being multifactorial and caused by the interaction between the biofilm, the substrate available for the biofilm, and host factors. The model developed by Rothman and Greenland (15) for understanding complex diseases and conditions may help in structuring our knowledge (Fig. 9-1). According to this model, disease occurs when a set of *component causes* (in the case of caries: biofilm, sugar, and unfavorable host factors) combine to constitute a *sufficient cause*. Figure 9-2 is a clinical illustration of the development of caries based on the *in vivo* experimental model "caries in man" (18). Even though this experimental model would not obtain ethical approval today, it demonstrates that withdrawal of all mechanical oral hygiene measures and exposure to daily sucrose rinses results in development of initial caries lesions especially in cracks and fissures in the enamel. No initial caries lesions are seen in the mandibular incisors due to the high salivary flow in that region. After a period with oral hygiene, no sugar rinses and topical fluoride applications, the lesions are arrested. The conclusions which can be drawn from this experiment,

Box 9-3 How the causal web can be used to understand causes of caries at many different levels

To the left of the figure below is a common childhood health problem, asthmatic bronchitis, which in itself is caused by a number of factors relating to living conditions, genetic background, etc., as indicated by the arrows to the far left. Children with asthmatic bronchitis often suffer from infections and fever, and may have an increased intake of juice to secure sufficient liquid intake. Parents of asthmatic children may give lower priority to daily toothbrushing. Finally, the medication itself may result in salivary changes increasing the risk of caries. The pie charts to the right indicate which of the component causes are influenced.

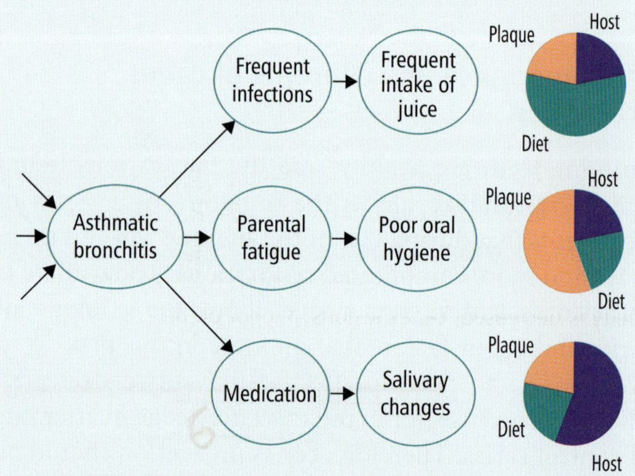

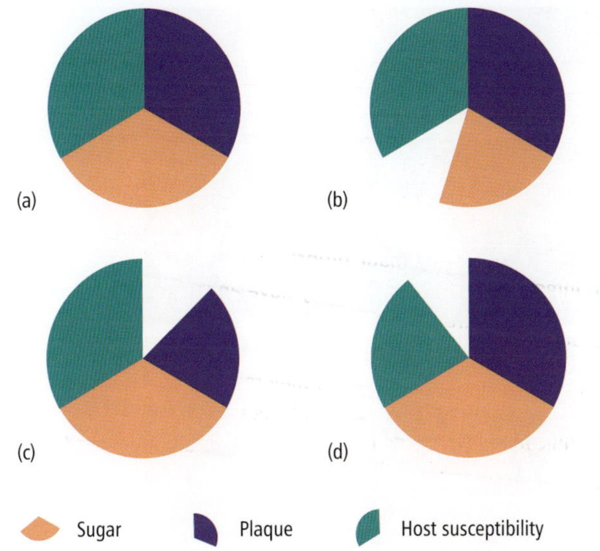

Figure 9-1 A conceptual model, where disease is explained as occurring when a number of component causes (the sections of the circle) act together to form a sufficient cause (the closed circle). (a) High level of plaque, high sugar intake, and high susceptibility to caries will result in a caries lesion. (b) If the sugar intake is reduced, (c) if the plaque level is reduced, or (d) if the susceptibility is decreased, caries lesions will not occur.

projected on the situation for children and adolescents, can be summarized as follows:

- The time needed to develop a clinically detectable carious lesion in the absence of oral hygiene measures and frequent exposure to sucrose-containing preparations is very short. Baby bottle-feeding at night and extensive candy consumption in teenagers, even for short periods of time, are examples of factors that might cause such an effect.
- The retention of bacterial plaque in cracks and fissures increases the risk for caries. This illustrates the need for fissure sealant.
- The presence of saliva is important in order to control the natural ion-exchange balance on the tooth surfaces. This indicates that all children on medication or other treatment affecting salivation have to be given special attention.
- Initial demineralization in the enamel can be arrested with good oral hygiene, reduced sugar consumption, and frequent fluoride applications. Regular oral hygiene measures, sound dietary habits, and topical fluoride applications can keep most children free of caries. Such control of caries is exemplified in Fig. 9-3.

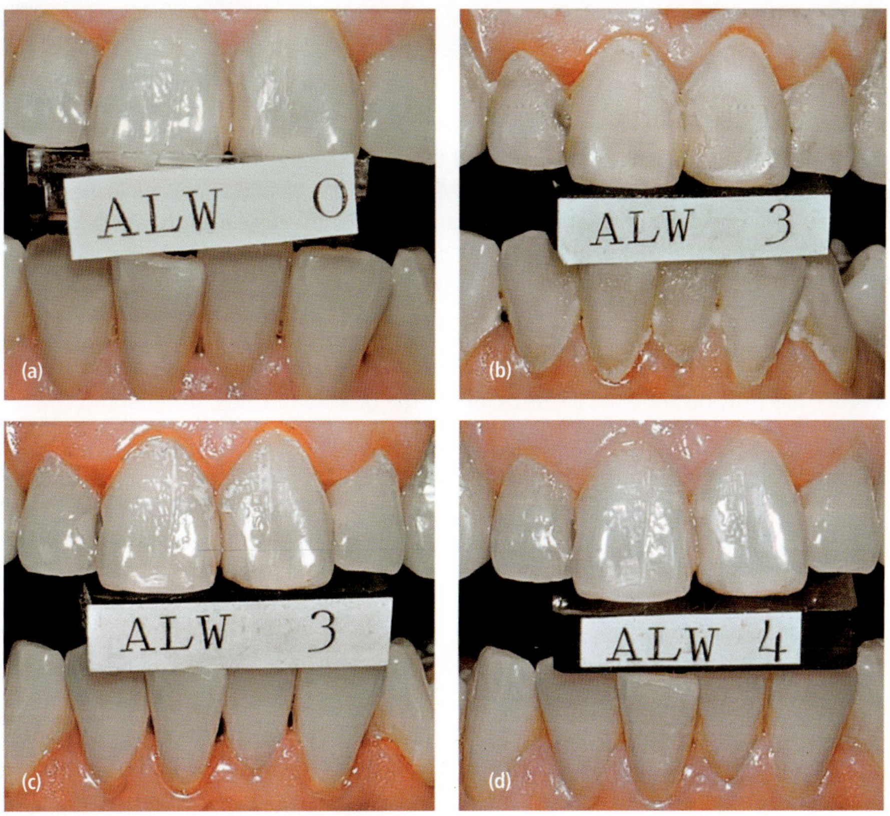

Figure 9-2 Clinical illustrations of the effect of oral hygiene, sugar, and host factors in an experiment. (a) On day 0, all measures of oral hygiene were withdrawn and 10 daily mouthrinses with 60% sucrose solutions were introduced. (b) Three weeks later, plaque was covering the teeth and gingivitis was pronounced. (c) After removal of the plaque, numerous initial carious lesions were observed. (d) One month later. The institution of effective oral hygiene and topical fluorides has reversed the initial carious lesions and the gingivitis.

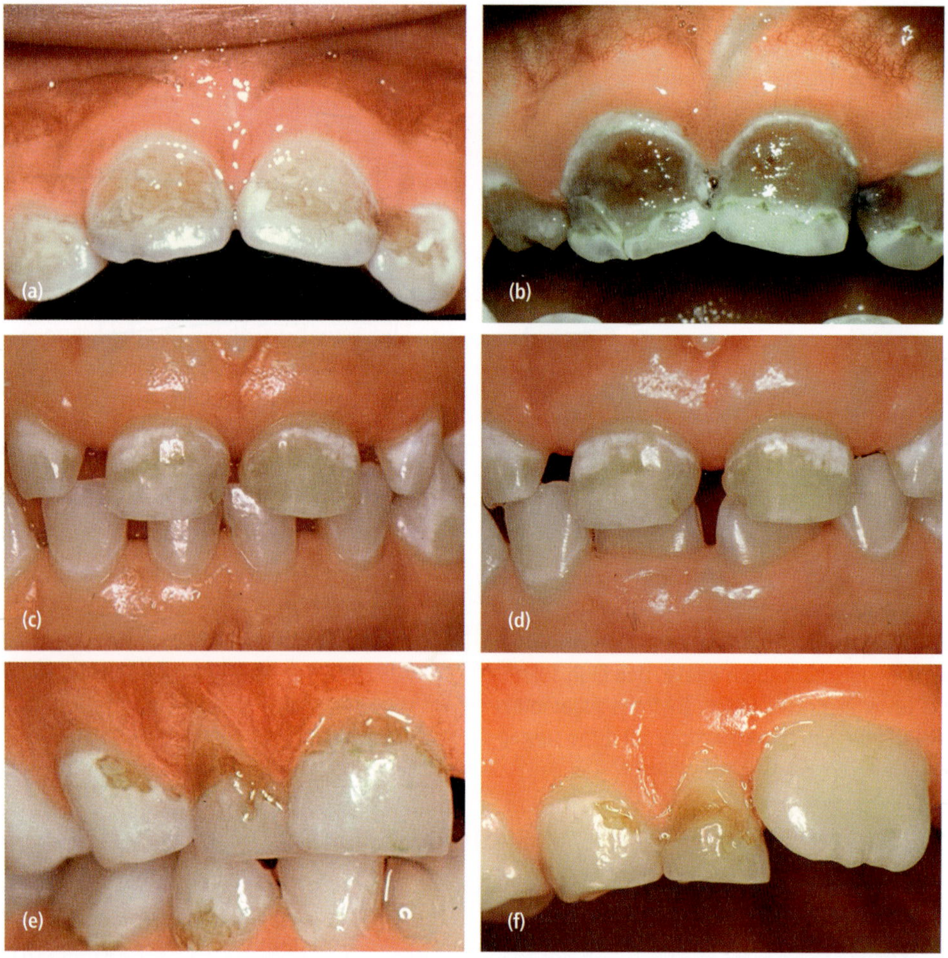

Figure 9-3 Caries progression. (a) An 11-month-old girl exposed to frequent intakes of stewed fruits. The parents could not change the diet. (b) One year later the incisors had to be extracted. (c) A 4-year-old boy with developing initial caries lesions. Good parental cooperation. (d) Status after 1 year shows no progression of the caries lesions. (e) A 6-year-old boy with active caries. Intense prophylaxis. (f) Status 1 year later shows complete control of caries progression.

Evidence-based prevention

Evidence-based practice has now become the focus of all health interventions, including pediatric dentistry, and preventive care for children and adolescents. As pediatric dental care is largely publicly financed, the responsibility of the profession to ensure that all interventions are evidence based is even greater.

The randomized controlled trial

The randomized clinical trial is the most important scientific method in the search for effective preventive methods and has been used for testing a number of caries-preventive agents or procedures over the last few decades. The following section on the use of fluorides is largely based on studies conducted using this design. New preventive methods are, however, continuously being launched. For this reason, the pediatric dentist needs knowledge of the basic characteristics (Box 9-4) of randomized controlled caries trials to be able to assess the quality of trials, understand the results, and skillfully apply them in the development of effective and efficient preventive programs.

The strength of the randomized clinical trial is its ability to eliminate bias through randomization and the use of blinding procedures. The design of a randomized clinical caries trial is shown in Fig. 9-4. It usually runs for 3 years and the outcome is calculated as the difference in new caries lesions between a control group and the experimental group(s). When the first caries-preventive trials of fluoride-containing agents were conducted they comprised one or more experimental groups and a placebo-treated control group (so-called negative controls). Since the caries-preventive effect of fluoride agents is so well established it is no longer considered ethical to include nonfluoride-treated groups in caries-preventive trials.

Box 9-4 Definitions of important characteristics for randomized controlled trials (modified from the Cochrane Handbook, Glossary of Terms, 2005)

- *Randomized controlled trial* (RCT): an experiment in which two or more interventions, possibly including a control or no intervention, are compared by being randomly allocated to participants.
- *Bias*: systematic error in results or interpretation.
- *Confounder*: a factor that is associated both with the intervention and with the outcome of interest.
- *Drop-out*: loss of subjects in the trial due to withdrawal or exclusion.
- *Random allocation*: a method that uses the play of chance to assign participants to comparison groups in a trial, e.g., by using a random numbers table or a computer-generated random sequence.
- A trial is *double-blind* if neither the investigator nor the participants know the type of intervention given to each participant. A trial is single-blind if either the investigator or the participants know the intervention given to each participant.
- A trial is *placebo controlled* when the control individuals receive a placebo that is similar to the active treatment being tested but without the active ingredient (e.g., an inactive pill, a nonfluoride-containing toothpaste, a topical solution without the active ingredient being tested).

Box 9-5 Calculation of measures of effect in randomized controlled clinical caries trials

Absolute difference: $\Delta C - \Delta T$

Prevented fraction (PF): $[(\Delta C - \Delta T)/\Delta C] \times 100\%$

Number needed to treat to save one DMFS (NNT): $1/(\Delta C - \Delta T)$, where ΔC is the mean DMFS increment in the control or comparison group and ΔT is the mean DMFS increment in the treatment group.

The calculation of these three measures is illustrated below.

	Population A	Population B
	DMFS increment	DMFS increment
Control or comparison group	3.09	0.53
Test group	2.32	0.40
Absolute difference	0.77	0.13
PF	25.0%	25.0%
NNT	1.3 ≈ 2	7.7 ≈ 8

The data presented above demonstrate that the same PF (30%) will result in very different absolute differences in populations with high caries increments (as in population A, where 0.93 DMF surfaces are saved) and low caries increments (as in population B, where 0.16 DMF surfaces are saved). In population A two patients would have to be treated in order to save one DMFS compared to eight in population B.

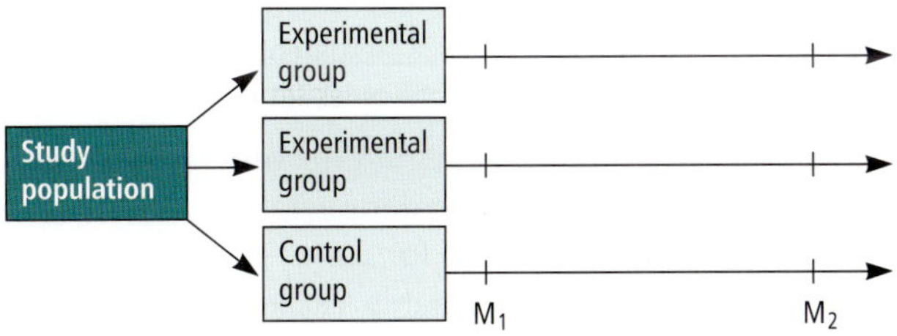

Figure 9-4 The basic design of the randomized controlled caries clinical trial. Study subjects should be assigned randomly to two or more intervention groups, possibly including a control or no intervention one or more group and one (or more) experimental group. The outcome of the trial is measured by comparing caries increment in the group(s) from the beginning to the end of the trial (M_1 to M_2).

An important methodological problem is the size of the trial, which among other things depends on the disease activity in the population. With the relatively high caries level 20–30 years ago, small sample sizes could still give sufficient statistical power. With the decrease in dental caries incidence, sample sizes of 1000 or more subjects per group may be necessary. Some trials may require a sample size so large that they become unrealistic for logistic and other reasons. The statistical power of a trial is important for the interpretation of the results of the trial. A small trial might not have sufficient statistical power to detect an effect, and may erroneously be interpreted as "evidence of no effect", while a correct interpretation is: "no evidence of effect".

The result of trials can be calculated as (Box 9-5):

- absolute difference
- prevented fraction
- number needed to treat.

Absolute differences are dependent on the level of disease in the population, and will have to be recalculated as prevented fractions in order to apply to other populations. Prevented fractions may, however, be misleading when it comes to deciding on implementation in the field, since high percentage reductions in populations with low caries activity may be of little practical importance. In recent years, the number needed to treat (NNT) has been used frequently. NNT has the advantage of giving the clinician an impression of how many individuals have to be treated in order to obtain an effect.

Where to find the evidence

For the pediatric dentist it may be difficult to keep up with the trials published in the literature and to synthe-

Box 9-6 Definition of primary and secondary literature, meta-analysis and systematic reviews

- *Primary literature*: literature that reports results from original studies, e.g., RCTs.
- *Secondary literature*: literature that summarizes results from original studies, e.g., systematic reviews.
- *Systematic review*: a review of a clearly formulated question that uses systematic and explicit methods to identify, select, and critically appraise relevant research, and to collect and analyze data from the studies that are included in the review.
- *Meta-analysis*: the use of statistical techniques in a systematic review to integrate the results of studies.

Box 9-7 List of systematic reviews on the effect of topical fluorides published in the Cochrane Library (2007, Issue 2)

Marinho VCC, Higgins JPT, Logan S, Sheiham A. Fluoride gels for preventing dental caries in children and adolescents, 2002.

Marinho VCC, Higgins JPT, Logan S, Sheiham A. Fluoride varnishes for preventing dental caries in children and adolescents, 2002.

Marinho VCC, Higgins JPT, Logan S, Sheiham A. Topical fluoride (toothpastes, mouthrinses, gels or varnishes) for preventing dental caries in children and adolescents, 2003.

Marinho VCC, Higgins JPT, Sheiham A, Logan S. Combinations of topical fluoride (toothpastes, mouthrinses, gels, varnishes) versus single topical fluoride for preventing dental caries in children and adolescents, 2004.

Marinho VCC, Higgins JPT, Sheiham A, Logan S. One topical fluoride (toothpastes, or mouthrinses, or gels, or varnishes) versus another for preventing dental caries in children and adolescents, 2004.

Benson PE, Parkin N, Millett DT, Dyer FE, Vine S, Shah A. Fluorides for the prevention of white spots on teeth during fixed brace treatment, 2004.

Hiiri A, Ahovuo-Saloranta A, Nordblad A, Mäkelä M. Pit and fissure sealants versus fluoride varnishes for preventing dental decay in children and adolescents, 2006.

Yeung CA, Hitchings JL, Macfarlane TV, Threlfall AG, Tickle M, Glenny AM. Fluoridated milk for preventing dental caries, 2007.

size the information from the many individual trials to decide on what to do for a given patient or community. For instance, a novice search in one of the most commonly used literature databases, PubMed (www.pubmed.gov), in April 2007 yielded more than 3000 hits on the word sequence "topical fluorides". The result included primary literature as well as secondary literature (Box 9-6), and does not automatically include any quality filters with regard to study design. This demonstrates the need for systematic search strategies, critical appraisal, and analysis of the evidence from the literature. A highly formalized review procedure is the so-called systematic review. The most well-known systematic reviews are undertaken by the Cochrane Collaboration (www.cochrane.org) and reviews on a number of caries-preventive methods are now published in the Cochrane Library (2007) (Box 9-7).

Other organizations are, however, also performing systematic reviews of relevance to the pediatric dentist. The Swedish Council on Technology Assessment in Health Care (SBU) has published recent evaluations of caries diagnosis, risk assessment, and caries preventive methods. The full reports as well as short summaries can be downloaded from the SBU website (www.sbu.se).

Basics of caries prevention

There is strong scientific evidence that in order to prevent, reverse, or slow down caries lesions, one or several of the following factors have to be altered or utilized: diet, oral hygiene, fluorides, and fissure sealants. It must, however, be emphasized that the factors should not be looked on as separate entities but as highly interactive. For example, good oral hygiene enhances the effect of topical fluoride applications.

Diet

The relationship between diet and caries has been confirmed in numerous studies. However, diet *per se* can never by itself produce caries. On the other hand, acidic food components can cause demineralization and erosion. To be a potential risk for caries development the food must contain fermentable carbohydrates, which the oral plaque bacteria can use in their glycolytic metabolism to produce acids. Even if sucrose is the fermentable carbohydrate most often implicated in the caries process it has to be remembered that all fermentable carbohydrates can cause acid production. This means that most food products and nearly all snacks, sweets, and soft drinks are potential caries risk factors.

Dietary counseling

Inquiries into the dietary habits of patients are a necessary basis for advice concerning future changes in diet to prevent dental decay. The most valid methods of obtaining exact quantitative data from which to estimate consumption of different dietary items are inventory and weighing procedures. However, these are time consuming and do not lend themselves to practical use. It is more realistic to take a dietary history, which is a semi-quantitative method where the patient or parents record all food consumption during a specific period of time, normally 3–7 consecutive days, on a specially developed form. Without neglecting the general aspects of nutrition, the dentist should concentrate his or her efforts in diet counseling on advice on the consumption of cariogenic products. Thus, dietary counseling concerning improvement of dental health should be aimed at estimating the patient's food habit pattern, the consumption of fermentable carbohydrates, in particular sucrose, and the intake frequency of snacks, sweetened beverages, and adhesive "sticky" food. Bottle feeding with sucrose-containing fluids, especially at night, is an important factor that may cause rampant caries in small children. It should be observed that it is difficult to obtain valid information on consumption. With dietary counseling it is important to develop tools that are understandable and will help the child and family to change their dietary habits. In recent years a more simple "dietary habit evaluation" has been used frequently. This method, based on questionnaires or interviews, concentrates on the number of intakes of well-known cariogenic products, e.g., candy, soft drinks, and cookies. The number of such intakes per day or week is recorded and will form the basis for recommended changes in consumption patterns.

The general guidelines concerning diet and dietary habits to avoid caries are very simple:

- Restrict the frequency of meals and intakes to five or six per day. Usually this means three main meals and three intermediate meals or intakes. Try to avoid sucrose-containing food products and beverages. No "snacking" between meals.
- Restrict candies and sweet snacks to once a week ("Saturday sweets").
- If the intake of sweets and chewing gums cannot be avoided, use products sweetened with sucrose substitutes, e.g., xylitol and sorbitol.
- Advice on infant dietary habits in order to avoid early childhood caries ("baby-bottle caries" or "nursing caries").
- Advice on prevention of erosion, which means reduction of frequent intake of acidic beverages such as soft drinks, fruit juices, and sport drinks.

Sucrose substitutes

Since dental caries forms through a complex interaction over time between acid-producing bacteria and fermentable carbohydrates, it has been an obvious idea to utilize sugar substitutes and artificial sweeteners in order to prevent the disease. Sucrose substitutes can be divided into non-nutritious sweeteners and caloric sweeteners obtained from natural sources. The most widely used sugars in "tooth-friendly" products such as chewing gums, tablets, and candies are the sugar alcohols xylitol, sorbitol, mannitol, maltitol, and lactitol. Although scientifically disputed, it is generally claimed that xylitol is superior for caries prevention. The antibacterial effects are based on metabolic reactions; xylitol is incorporated by oral bacteria with the fructose-specific phosphotransferase system and phosphorylated to xylitol-5-phosphate. This substance hampers further cell metabolism and fewer acids are formed limiting the pH drop in the oral biofilm (see Box 9-8). There are no absolute contraindications for the use of xylitol, but there is a European Union recommendation that the daily intake should be less than 3 g in children under 3 years of age. It is commonly recognized that high

Box 9-8 Combating vertical transmission of mutans streptococci

The strategy to combat early vertical transmission of cariogenic bacteria from parents to their children is often named primary–primary prevention. The preventive intervention is usually directed to mothers of newborn babies with high counts of salivary mutans streptococci and implemented during the eruption of the primary teeth.

A pioneering Swedish study showed that repeated chlorhexidine gel treatments reduced maternal mutans streptococci counts, and had a long-term influence on the caries experience of the child (Isokangas *et al.*, *J Dent Res* 2000;**79**:1885–9).

Two more recent trials with around 150 mother–child pairs studied the effect of xylitol-containing chewing gums on the timing of mutans streptococci detection and subsequent caries development in the children (Köhler *et al.*, *Arch Oral Biol* 1994;**39**:907–11 and Thorild *et al.*, *Eur Arch Paediatr Dent* 2006;**7**:241–5). The rationale was that habitual xylitol consumption would select mutans streptococci strains with less adhesive properties which would subsequently diminish the risk of oral colonization. The protocols were initiated when the children were 6 months old and terminated 1–2 years later. The mothers of the test groups were instructed to consume xylitol-containing chewing gums three times per day for 5–10 minutes. Both trials found results in favor of the xylitol groups when the children were 4–5 years of age with 30–70% fewer caries lesions when compared to the controls.

The studies were, however, conducted in low-caries communities and with parents with good compliance. No health economic analyses of the mother–child concept are yet available and studies in high-caries groups are needed before any public-based recommendations can be formed. Collectively however, these three studies provide some evidence that maternal prevention programs can prevent dental caries in their children by inhibiting the transmission of mutans streptococci from mother to child.

single doses might induce gastrointestinal upsets and soft stools in susceptible individuals.

Xylitol has been extensively studied in controlled trials as well as in field studies. In the pioneering "Turku sugar study" (1975) with almost complete substitution of dietary sucrose with fructose and xylitol, practically no caries lesions developed. Later studies have been conducted in children with a partial sugar substitution and significant reduction of caries lesions has been documented, especially in populations with a high caries prevalence.

Recent clinical trials suggest that the intake of xylitol must exceed 5–6 g/day in fractioned doses to have a clinically significant effect on microbial growth and caries development (Table 9-1). A major obstacle with the use of gums and tablets is the high frequency and large number of pellets that are required to deliver the therapeutic amounts. In addition, the costs for long-term use may be restrictive. Further research is therefore needed before the use of sorbitol- or xylitol-sweetened chewing gums can be considered as a public health measure.

Based on current evidence the following guidelines could be considered:

- products with sugar alcohols could be advocated to children and adolescents at high risk of caries as a supplement to daily fluoride exposure
- xylitol-containing products that actively stimulate saliva secretion, such as chewing gums and sucking tablets, are the first choice
- products should contain as much xylitol per unit as possible and preferable as the only sweetener
- intake should be fractioned at least three times over a day.

Plaque control

Toothbrushing

Proper oral hygiene can be achieved and maintained by mechanical and chemical means at home and at the dental office. There is little scientific evidence that toothbrushing *per se* can prevent dental caries, since normal brushing does not remove plaque from pits, fissures, and other retention sites. Tooth cleaning is, however, of particular importance in the maintenance of a healthy periodontium, and studies (12,21) have demonstrated a relationship between nonbrushing habits and gingivitis and early caries development in infants and toddlers. Toothbrushing skills must therefore be emphasized strongly and taught to children of all ages as well as their parents. It is important that parents are instructed to initiate toothbrushing from the eruption of the very first tooth and that a proper toothbrushing regimen should have been established when the first primary molars erupt. Parents should be shown a technique and be trained on how to use it (Fig. 9-5). Since small children cannot keep up an effective oral hygiene by themselves, parents must perform toothbrushing at least up to the age of 6 years and thereafter regularly supervise the procedure. The special problem associated with the cleaning of the first permanent molar should be underlined. A soft toothbrush of appropriate size and fluoridated toothpaste are the most effective aids for oral hygiene in the primary and mixed dentition. The use of disclosing tablets or liquids should be recommended when necessary. An electric toothbrush has a similar cleaning effect as manual brushing and may be a motivating tool for some children and an excellent help for

Table 9-1 Daily dosage of xylitol, administration form, and main results of some controlled clinical trials published since the mid-1990s

Author (year)	Duration in years, age group	Dose (g/day)	Type	Caries outcome test/control[a]	Reduction (%)	p^b
Kovari (2003)	5, preschool	2.5	Gum	1.2/1.6 ng	25	NS
Machiulskiene (2001)	3, school	3.0	Gum	3.4/4.3 cg	21	NS
Alanen (2000)	3, school	5.0	Gum	1.9/4.4 ng	57	S
Alanen (2000)	3, school	5.0	Candy	1.7/4.4 ng	61	S
Mäkinen (1995)	3.3, school	8.5	Gum	4.6/15.9 ng	71	S
Mäkinen (1996)	2, preschool	10.7	Gum	17.6/50.2 ng	65	S

[a] Values are caries increment expressed as ΔDMF or Δdmf or lesion onset per 1000 surfaces. Key: ng, no chewing gum was used in the control group; cg, control chewing gum without xylitol was used in the control group.

[b] S, statistically significant difference between test and control groups; NS, not statistically different.

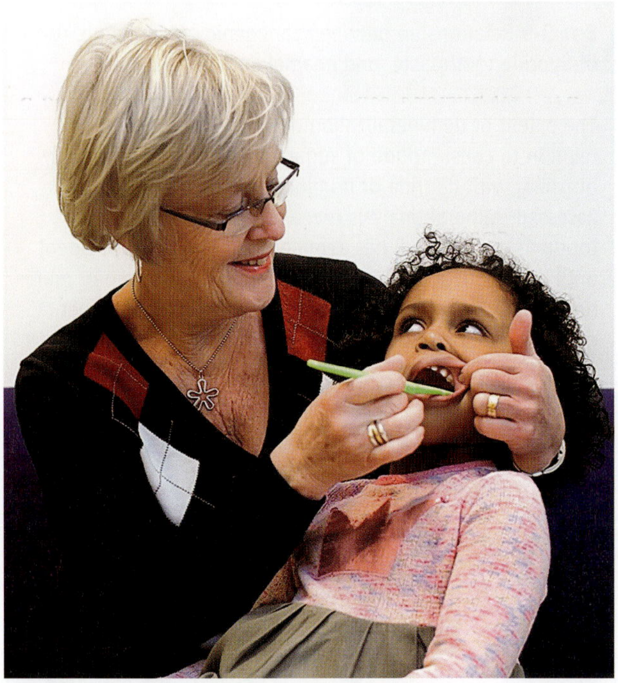

Figure 9-5 How to perform toothbrushing in young children.

disabled patients. Dental floss and toothpicks normally should be considered only for the fully erupted permanent dentition.

Some general recommendations concerning toothbrushing can be given:

- Toothbrushing should be initiated from the eruption of the first tooth and proper regular toothbrushing should have been established when the first primary molar is erupting.
- Brush the teeth twice daily: after breakfast and before bedtime.
- Select a soft brush with a small head and a large handle for the youngest children.
- Use a small amount of fluoridated toothpaste.

Chemotherapeutic agents

Among the antibacterial agents used in the oral cavity, chlorhexidine is considered the gold standard. The drug has a strong affinity to oral structures and interferes with cell wall transportation and metabolic pathways of susceptible bacteria. Chlorhexidine has a general effect on Gram-positive microorganisms; mutans streptococci are particularly sensitive. Within weeks or months after the termination of a chlorhexidine regimen, a regrowth of mutans streptococci normally occurs. A synergistic effect of chlorhexidine and fluoride has been shown in clinical trials (4), extending the time of mutans streptococci suppression compared with chlorhexidine alone. Lactobacilli are less susceptible and many strains are unaffected by chlorhexidine. The drug has a low toxicity and side-effects, except for tooth discoloration, are rare. The somewhat bitter taste may be unpleasant to children.

Chlorhexidine rinses are the treatment of choice for plaque control after oral surgery and for temporary support of oral hygiene in medically compromised and disabled children. After a 0.2% chlorhexidine rinse, the bacterial population in plaque and saliva is reduced by approximately 80%. That does, however, not necessarily imply a reduced risk of caries. Therefore, the evidence for its ability to prevent caries is disputed with studies arguing for and against. The best clinical effect has been achieved when patients highly colonized with mutans streptococci have been treated with gel and when the outcome has been monitored by repeated microbial examinations (4). According to a meta-analysis, the overall caries-inhibiting effect of chlorhexidine gel in the young permanent dentition was 46% (17) but some non-randomized studies with low evidence level were included. A reduction of proximal caries of the same magnitude has been suggested for preschool-aged children.

Chlorhexidine treatments can be carried out professionally in the dental office or at home depending on patient motivation and cooperation. For children at high caries risk and questionable compliance, a professional intensive regimen with a 1% chlorhexidine gel in custom-made soft trays, 3 × 5 min for 2 consecutive days is recommended. For home-care use, a 5-min application once a day for 14 days is preferred. Detergents in toothpaste can inactivate chlorhexidine and toothpaste should therefore not be used within 1–2 hours of the application of chlorhexidine. Topical application of dental varnishes with a sustained release of chlorhexidine may be an alternative professional treatment option that diminishes plaque and gingivitis, but there is limited evidence on its caries-preventive efficacy. Recent research, however, has documented a decreased vertical transmission of cariogenic bacteria from parents to their children after exposure to chlorhexidine and xylitol (Box 9-8).

Fluoride

The introduction of fluoride prophylaxis, starting with water fluoridation in the late 1940s and followed by an extensive utilization of topical fluorides about 20 years later, has resulted in a worldwide reduction in caries, not least among children and adolescents. Although there is no complete scientific agreement on all details of the mechanism of the action of fluoride, there is sufficient evidence showing how to use fluoride for prevention of caries in the most effective way in children.

Mechanism of fluoride in caries prevention

The concept of how fluoride prevents caries has undergone a paradigmatic shift during recent years. Previously, the assumption was that incorporation of fluoride in the enamel apatite lattice during tooth formation and mineralization resulted in a permanent or long-lasting resistance of the enamel to dental caries. The present view on the mechanism of fluoride in caries prevention is that fluoride has to be present in the plaque fluid during the caries challenge, slowing down the dissolution of enamel and supporting the precipitation phase. It has also been found that topical application of fluoride results in the formation of calcium fluoride crystals accumulating on the tooth surface. When pH is lowered during a caries challenge, the crystals are dissolved and provide fluoride that controls the caries attack. Thus, topical applications that form calcium fluoride crystals constitute a pH-controlled fluoride slow-release system ready to act when necessary. This new view on the action of fluoride in caries prevention has to a great extent changed the practical way of utilizing fluoride. In this context it is also important to realize the limitations of the demineralizing controlling effect of topical fluorides in situations with frequent intakes of cariogenic products (Box 9-9).

Box 9-9 Relationship between cariogenic consumption, use of fluoride toothpaste, and enamel demineralization

The extent of demineralization of enamel slabs *in situ* in relation to consumption of sugar-based solutions and daily brushing with fluoride or nonfluoride toothpaste was assessed. Mineral analysis revealed that when fluoride toothpaste was used, net demineralization was not evident until the frequency of sugar consumption was seven or more times a day. When fluoride-free toothpaste was used net demineralization occurred as early as three consumptions a day. (Duggal MS *et al.*, *J Dent Res* 2001;**80**:1721–4.)

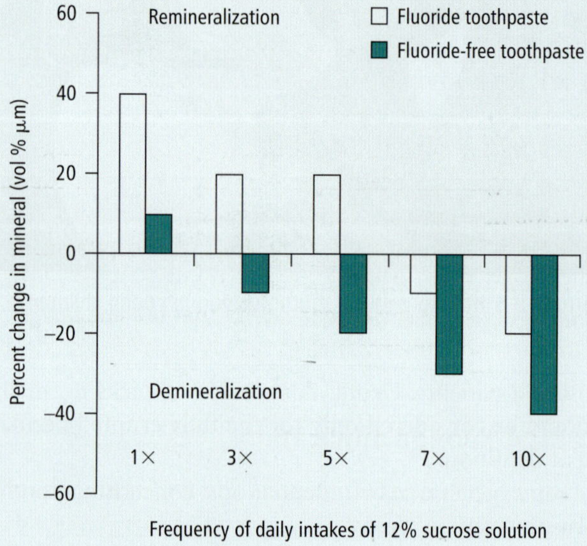

Systemic versus topical application of fluoride

Water fluoridation has been found to be the easiest and cheapest method of systemic administration and caries reductions of 40–50% have been reported. It is recommended by the World Health Organization as an important caries-preventive measure but its use is limited to large communities with water plants of high technical standard. In rural areas with small water plants and less control of the implementation, water fluoridation must be considered unrealistic. Long-term systemic fluoride exposure by water during the period of tooth development and mineralization and thereafter throughout life has a documented caries-reducing effect in both children and adults. However, the caries reduction from community water fluoridation is now considerably less than when the method was introduced, mainly because of the increased exposure to other fluoride sources such as food, beverages, dentifrices, and topical agents. In some areas the addition of fluoride to milk or table salt has been recommended and tested, but the experiences are limited. It has been claimed that the administration of fluoride tablets or other supplements such as fluoride drops may serve as an alternative to fluoridation of drinking water. The administration of fluoride tablets should follow a dosage schedule adjusted to age and fluoride content of drinking water. Even if some well-controlled clinical studies of fluoride tablets have resulted in a statistically significant reduction of caries, the necessity of extremely good parental cooperation for many years and a potential risk of dental fluorosis have caused the use of this regimen to decrease. In addition, there has been an increasing scientific understanding and also acceptance that systemic supplementary administration of fluoride pre-eruptively has little effect in a caries-preventive perspective. Much of the effect of systemic application of fluoride has been explained by the simultaneous topical fluoride exposure posteruptively. So, if fluoride tablets are used they should be sucked or chewed. Pre-eruptive administration of fluoride also always carries a risk for development of dental fluorosis.

Dental fluorosis and toxicity

Dental fluorosis is a qualitative defect of enamel caused by the long-term intake of fluoride during the period of tooth formation. The threshold dose for development of mild fluorosis in permanent teeth has been estimated to 40–100 µg F/kg body weight per day. However, it has been found that for the individual there are no threshold values below which fluorosis cannot occur. In many parts of the world, e.g., North America and Australia, trends towards increasing levels of mild dental fluorosis following fluoride supplements have been reported. The reason might be the increased ingestion of fluoride from water, food, beverages, and dentifrices during the period of tooth formation, in particular the first 2–4 years of life. Control and recommendations of fluoride intake are major obligations of the pediatric dentist. However, it should be emphasized that carefully, professionally applied topical fluorides and the correct use of fluoride toothpaste according to recommendations are not risk factors for dental fluorosis.

Even if the concentrations and amounts of fluoride used in dental practice and in preventive activities outside the clinic are far below toxic thresholds (except for dental fluorosis), it is important to know the levels at which general toxic reactions can be expected.

Acute toxic dose. This situation may occur if 5 mg F/kg body weight has been ingested. The child will rapidly develop nausea and epigastric distress, often followed by vomiting. The child should be referred to hospital immediately for observation and emergency treatment. From reported cases it can be concluded that if a child ingests a fluoride dose in excess of 15 mg/kg body weight, death is likely to occur.

Topical fluoride applications

Topical fluoride application is one of the most effective ways of preventing caries. Numerous clinical studies have been performed over the last few decades. Although the trials differ concerning sample size, age of the children, diagnostic criteria, caries activity, the methods of fluoride application, there is, without doubt, documentation for a considerable caries-reducing effect of topical fluoride application. For detailed information the reader is referred to special textbooks and reviews on the use of fluoride in dentistry, such as the Cochrane Library (Box 9-7). Generally, there is one important basic principle to obtain a good effect: *apply fluoride in such a way that fluoride is present at the plaque/enamel interface where it will control dissolution and reprecipitation of minerals during caries challenges.* This can be achieved by frequent application of low concentrated fluoride solutions or preparations or less frequent application of high fluoride concentration preparations causing fluoride deposits in or on the enamel that will slowly be released to the plaque–enamel interface. As a general rule the fluoride should match the caries activity of the child, that is, the greater the cariogenic challenge, the more intense the fluoride treatment (Box 9-9).

When recommending schedules for topical application of fluoride to children it is important to look at the feasibility, the total fluoride exposure (Box 9-10), and the individual's caries risk.

Box 9-10 Fluoride content in preparations used in caries prevention in children

Preparation	Fluoride concentration (%)	Amount used in a single application	Fluoride dosage in a single application (mg F)
Toothpaste			
1500 ppm F	0.15	0.6 g	0.9
1000 ppm F	0.1	0.6 g	0.6
500 ppm F	0.05	0.4 g	0.2
Mouthrinse solution			
0.2% NaF	0.1	10 ml	10
0.05% NaF	0.02	10 ml	2
Fluoride varnish			
Duraphat®	2.3	0.4 ml	9
Fluoride gel			
High fluoride	1.23	5 ml	62
Low fluoride	0.1	5 ml	5

Fluoride toothpaste is the ideal vehicle to apply fluoride to teeth. Daily use of fluoride toothpaste will result in caries reductions of at least 20–40%. Small children usually swallow about 30% of the amount of toothpaste and for this reason it is important to control the amount of toothpaste that they use. Children can start using a smear layer amount of fluoride toothpaste when the first primary teeth have erupted. From the age of about 2 years the amount of toothpaste should be the size of the child's fingernail (pea size) and from the age of 5–6 years the amount of toothpaste might cover half of the brush head (Fig. 9-6).

Fluoride mouthrinses commonly were used in school-based programs with 0.2% NaF solution weekly or fortnightly during the 1960s–1980s but ceased during later years as most children are using fluoride toothpaste. However, in child populations with high or increasing caries activity, fluoride mouthrinses have been reintroduced with a successful outcome. The effects of the rinsing programs are in the range of 20–40% caries reduction. The best effect is achieved by daily rinsings with 0.05% NaF solution. Mouthrinsing is not recommended for preschool-aged children since they often swallow the rinse solution.

Fluoride-containing varnishes. Fluoride varnishes often contain high concentrations of fluoride and adhere to tooth surfaces for days, thus considerably increasing the fluoride content in the surface and subsurface enamel. The fluoride will then be slowly released to the plaque–enamel interface. A meta-analysis of 12 studies of the effect of Duraphat® fluoride varnish revealed an overall

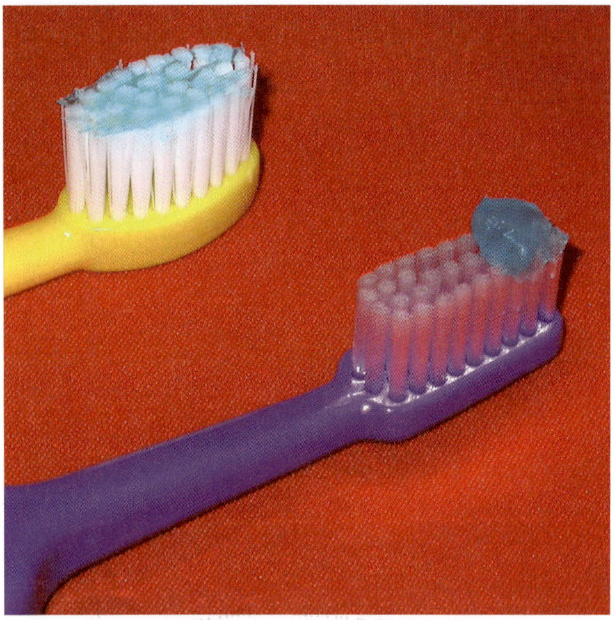

Figure 9-6 Recommended amount of fluoride toothpaste on the toothbrush: smear amount (children 0–2 years of age) and pea-sized amount (children 2–5 years of age) of fluoride toothpaste.

reduction in caries of about 40%. The varnishes are easy to apply and two applications a year will give a good effect.

Fluoride gels are available on the market with different fluoride concentrations and tastes. Most of them are slightly acidic to enhance the fluoride uptake in enamel. They are mostly applied in custom-made trays and are used either in a professional setting or on a daily basis at home. Due to the risk of swallowing, they should not be used in preschool-aged children. The indications are high caries active children and children with reduced salivation.

Fluoride sucking tablets and chewing gum can be a complementary fluoride treatment for children. Fluoride sucking tablets can be used from the age of 3 years and chewing gum from the age of 10 years in children with extreme caries activity.

Some general recommendations for the use of fluorides are as follows:

- Use fluoride-containing toothpaste twice a day from 1–1.5 years of age.
- In areas with a general high caries activity institute school-based fluoride mouthrinsing programs.
- High caries risk patients should have individual fluoride programs based on fluoride varnishes, fluoride gels, or fluoride sucking tablets/chewing gum.

Fissure sealing

Fissure sealing is a method by which a material is placed in the pits and fissures of teeth in order to prevent or arrest the development of dental caries (19). The material is retained on the enamel surface either through an acid-etch technique or the chemical bonding of the material to the enamel surface, as in the case of glass-ionomer-based sealants.

During recent years the distribution of caries in the population and within the dentition has changed dramatically, so much so that it has been stated "caries will be predominantly pit and fissure lesions, with relatively few approximal surfaces affected and virtually no free smooth surfaces affected" (3). It is obvious with this background a method aiming to prevent caries in pits and fissures would be the most relevant (see also Chapter 6).

Since the first resin-based sealants were tested in the late 1960s and the early 1970s, a number of new materials have been introduced on the market. The most commonly used materials are the resin-based sealants, some of which are light cured and some of which are cured chemically. Most of the sealants are clear, but some have a filler material added to improve their resistance against wear. Fluoride-releasing fissure sealants have also been marketed, but there is no convincing evidence that they are more efficacious than nonfluoride-releasing sealants (9).

Many clinical trials have tested the efficacy of sealants. Most of these trials have been conducted using a split-mouth design, where contralateral teeth are assigned randomly to sealing or control/comparison. These trials have evaluated two outcomes: retention of the sealant material and the difference in caries increment in sealed and nonsealed teeth. A Cochrane systematic reviews of clinical trials on fissure sealants has recently been published (Box 9-11). The number of studies on the effect of sealants in primary teeth is limited, but it seems that, with proper moisture control, satisfactory retention can be obtained (13).

Based on the Cochrane review, the effect on caries in permanent molars (most of the studies are conducted on permanent first molars) has been estimated to be between 85% at 12 months and 57% at 48–54 months. The sealing of surfaces with early signs of caries undoubtedly will result in sealing of small caries lesions – even lesions with histologic dentinal lesions. However, studies have shown that counts of bacteria decrease and that progression of dentinal lesions is slower after fissure sealing (11).

Also, when implemented on a population basis, fissure sealants have shown good effect (Fig. 9-7). In the program evaluated by Wendt *et al.* (20), both permanent first and second molars were sealed shortly after eruption, and resealed, if required. After 20 years 65% of sealings in permanent first molars were intact, while

Box 9-11 Excerpt of abstract of a systematic review of fissure sealing published in the Cochrane Library

Ahovuo-Saloranta A, Hiiri A, Nordblad A, Worthington H, Mäkelä M. Pit and fissure sealants for preventing dental decay in the permanent teeth of children and adolescents. *Cochrane Database of Systematic Reviews* 2004, Issue 3. Art. No.: CD001830. DOI: 10.1002/14651858.CD001830.pub2.

Objectives: The primary objective of this review was to evaluate the caries prevention of resin-based pit and fissure sealants and glass ionomer cements or sealants in children and adolescents.
Selection criteria: Randomized or quasi-randomized controlled trials of at least 12 months in duration in which sealants were used for preventing caries in children and adolescents under 20 years of age were included. The primary outcome was the increment in the numbers of carious occlusal surfaces of premolars and molars.
Main results: Based on five split-mouth studies with 5–10-year-old children there were significant differences in favor of the second-generation resin sealant compared with no treatment with pooled relative risk values of 0.14, 0.24, 0.30, and 0.43 at 12, 24, 36, and 48–54 months, respectively. The reductions in caries therefore ranged from 86% at 12 months to 57% at 48–54 months. The 24-month parallel group study comparing second-generation resin sealant with control in 12–13-year-old children found also significantly more caries in the control group children with DFS = 0.65 (95% CI 0.47 to 0.83).
Authors' conclusions: Sealing with resin-based sealants is a recommended procedure to prevent caries of the occlusal surfaces of permanent molars. However, we recommend that the caries prevalence level of both individuals and the population should be taken into account. In practice, the benefit of sealing should be considered locally and specified guidelines for clinicians should be used.

13% had a manifest caries lesion or were filled. For permanent second molars the corresponding figures were 65% intact sealings and 5% manifest caries lesions or fillings.

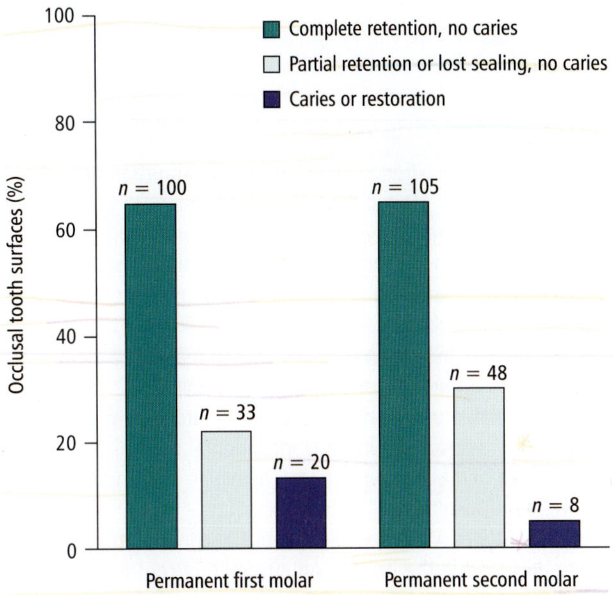

Figure 9-7 Evaluation of a fissure-sealing program after 20 years (20). The majority of the teeth were either completely or partially covered by sealant and caries free.

Preventive strategies

During the era of the high caries level, all Nordic countries implemented preventive programs aiming at reducing the level of disease in the whole population of children and adolescents. This preventive strategy may not be appropriate during a time with a lower level of disease and with a different distribution of disease in the population (see Chapter 6). The word "strategy" is here used in the sense of the art of planning the best way to achieve something or to be successful in a particular field. The present section discusses strategies for implementing the preventive methods, techniques, or technologies described in the previous sections of this chapter.

High-risk and population strategies

Two strategies have been described in preventive medicine: the population strategy and the high-risk strategy. An intermediate strategy is the *high-risk group* strategy. The *population strategy* aims at a general reduction of risk factors for all individuals in a population, whether diseased or not. Examples of population strategies which have been implemented in Nordic countries are fluoride rinses, recommended use of fluoridated toothpaste, and advice to reduce sugar intake. A *high-risk strategy* aims at targeting the program at those *individuals* with the highest risk. The underlying thinking is that scarce resources can be used for those individuals with the highest need. As mentioned above, an intermediate strategy would be a *high-risk group strategy*, where the program aims at known *high-risk groups*, such as certain groups of immigrants in an otherwise low-caries population (Box 9-12). Rose (14) has elaborated the advantages and disadvantages of population strategies as well as population strategies in general preventive medicine, most of which can be recognized from the experience gained with implementing preventive programs in Nordic countries:

- Large-scale preventive programs are difficult to motivate both to the public and the health-care providers involved, because the effort will be directed at all

Box 9-12 An oral health program for preschool children in a multicultural city area in Sweden

Wennhall I *et al.*, *Acta Odontol Scand* 2005;**63**:163–7.

Background and rationale: Rosengård is a suburban district within the city of Malmö, Sweden, where the vast majority of the families are of immigrant origin. An oral health survey showed that 85% of 3-year-old children exhibited signs of dental decay, indicating an urgent need to implement an oral health program targeting preschool children. The challenge was to find an effective way to reach and meet the families at an early age with an attractive and understandable oral health message. The program was planned in association with the local dental public health authorities and based on outreach activities focusing on daily toothbrushing and fluoride exposure.

Project outline: A total of 804 2-year-old children initially were included in the project. An information centre called "The Toothbrush" was established in a popular shopping mall and equipped with comfortable furniture, material for counseling and special facilities for "tell–show–do" training in toothbrushing skills. Color pictures illustrating healthy food and sugar traps were prepared as well as leaflets in foreign languages. The children were recalled four times between 24 and 36 months of age and the program was managed by two specially trained dental assistants. The parents were offered a discounted toothbrush and fluoridated toothpaste (1000 ppm F), provided with free fluoride tablets, and encouraged to give the child one fluoride tablet each day (0.25 mg NaF) in the evening after toothbrushing.

Results: The compliance was higher than expected; 75% of all families showed up as scheduled and 91% used the fluoride tablets regularly. After 1 year, the number of caries-free children had increased significantly. The mean caries experience was 2.0 dmft among the project children compared to 4.4 in a comparable reference group.

Conclusion: This project suggests that a comprehensive outreach program starting early in life can improve oral health in preschool children, suggesting that education and fluoride are key factors, also in poorer socioeconomic areas.

Box 9-13 The effect of a high-risk program based on screening for active initial caries lesions

The graph below illustrates the caries-preventive effect of an intensified preventive program for children with active initial lesions at baseline. Caries at the cavitation level was used as diagnostic criterion at follow-up.

For the entire follow-up period, the preventive fraction was 44.3% (95% CI 30.2, 56.4%).

The conclusion of the authors is, that "a regimen that includes multiple measures for controlling dental caries can significantly reduce dental decay among caries-active children living in an area where the overall level of caries experience is low." (Reproduced from Hausen *et al.*, *Caries Res* 2007;**41**:384–91 with permission from S. Karger, AG, Basel.)

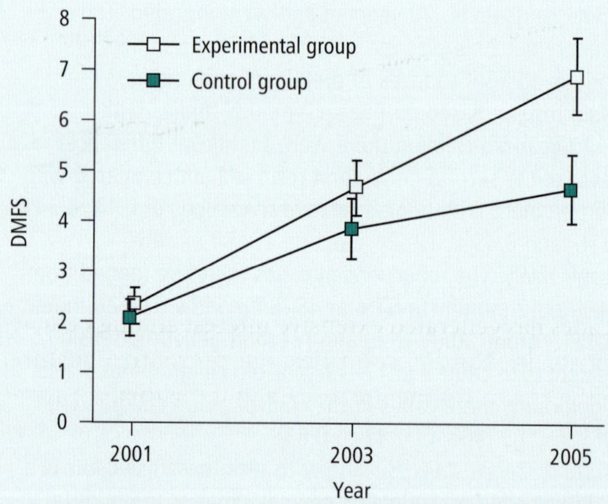

individuals, including those who are at a low risk, and already enjoy excellent dental health and maintain good oral health habits (the "prevention paradox"). This makes it difficult to motivate professionals as well as the population.

- On the other hand, the high-risk strategy suffers from serious disadvantages because it is based on screening for high caries risk (Box 9-13). A number of different screening tests have been developed and tested, but the consensus at the moment is that except for past caries experience, no good screening methods to identify those individuals at a high risk of developing caries are available. Even when past caries experience is used as a screening criterion, the quality of the test is not satisfactory. The consequence is that children at high risk are missed by the test (false negatives) and subsequently not included in the preventive program, while children not at high risk are screened positive (false positives) and unnecessarily included in the program. However, it has recently been shown that screening on the basis of active initial caries lesions, and subsequent preventive action, can be effective (Box 9-14).
- Another important problem relating to the high-risk strategy is that, in spite of the skewness of the distribution of disease in the population, most lesions are still found in individuals with moderate or low DMFS (see Chapter 6). One consequence of this is that the effect of a high-risk strategy aimed at *individuals* will be limited at the *population* level.

Box 9-14 Summary of important issues in screening for high caries risk [for details see review papers by Hausen (6) and Burt (3)]

- Screening is the identification of individuals at high risk of developing a high caries increment. For example, the purpose of a screening test could be to identify the 25% of the children with the highest DMFS increment.
- The best predictor for future caries is past caries, but even for this method, the sensitivity and specificity of the test are not satisfactory. In a literature survey carried out by Hausen (1994) it was concluded, "that the predictive power of even the best screening methods that are currently available is modest".
- With low caries levels, the proportion of children with a given high DMFS decreases. This has consequences for screening:
  - with a decreasing proportion of children in high risk, the predictive value of a positive test decreases, while
  - the predictive value of a negative test increases.

The marked improvement in oral health during recent decades has generated extensive interest among pediatric dentists in Nordic countries on preventive methods aiming at controlling the disease in individuals. A somewhat lower interest has been directed towards reducing the risk factors in the general population. This may be problematic if we want to retain the low general level of disease in the population. Seen from this perspective, population strategies and high-risk strategies should not be considered alternatives but should go hand in hand. Population strategies should aim at reducing the general level of the risk factors in the population, while high-risk strategies should aim at controlling the disease in those individuals with early caries lesions (see Chapter 10). The systematic delivery system for oral health care for children and adolescents developed in Nordic countries makes this strategy very feasible to implement.

Evaluation of caries risk in individuals

The rationale of caries risk assessment is to identify individuals with an increased risk of the disease in order to target the most precise and efficient preventive treatment. Risk is defined as the probability that a harmful or unwanted event will occur and a caries risk assessment is the clinical procedure to predict the probability of future caries development. However, since past caries experience, and especially active initial lesions, is the best single predictor in preschool children as well as in schoolchildren and adolescents, the procedure is also used for the selection of diseased patients in order to control existing lesions with noninvasive treatment (secondary prevention). Each risk assessment is a subjective procedure with an outcome that can be proven to be right or wrong. Based on numerous clinical studies with single predictors, the probability of identifying true high-risk individuals is lower (sensitivity) than the probability of correctly identifing subjects with low caries risk (specificity). However, models that combine several predictors may significantly increase the predictive power (Box 9-12).

Background data and clinical evaluation of caries risk

In Fig. 9-8 some examples of social, behavioral, and biological factors involved in the caries process are illustrated. The oral ecosystem could be regarded as a balance between tooth demineralization and remineralization. For example, in a situation with reduced knowledge, frequent sucrose-containing snacks, and poor oral hygiene, demineralization will dominate due to low pH and bacterial overgrowth, whereas favorable dental habits with regular fluoride exposure will promote remineralization. For an appropriate caries-risk assessment, it is advisable to collect information on the above factors as obtained from: case history, clinical and radiographic examinations, and supplementary tests.

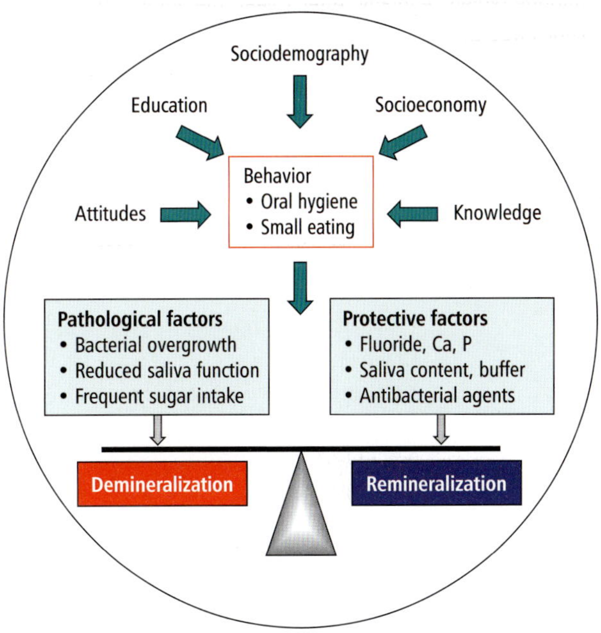

Figure 9-8 The caries balance as influenced by social, behavioral, and biological factors.

Case history

The background factors that may directly or indirectly influence caries risk are:

- general diseases
- medication
- social/family situation
- dietary habits
- oral hygiene routines
- fluoride exposure.

There are few general diseases that directly affect the teeth, although there are several which indirectly influence the carious process. Medication in combination with anxious and sometimes overprotective parents often constitutes a greater caries risk than the disease itself. Several drugs have a high content of fermentable carbohydrates and a low pH. Furthermore, the depressing influence on saliva secretion exerted by various drugs is an established risk. A troubled family or social situation might be reflected by factors such as stress (decreased saliva secretion), lack of interest in hygiene (poor plaque control), and poor economy (cariogenic diet). A dietary history should be obtained as described earlier. Information on present and past fluoride exposure as well as the performance and frequency of the oral hygiene routines should also be collected (Table 9-2).

Clinical and radiographic examination

The clinical examination provides quantitative data on the current caries situation and the prevalence is an indication of host susceptibility. It is important to consider whether or not there are more fillings or extractions than expected for the child's age group. The extension and appearance of lesions, cavities, and fillings should be checked. For example, the presence of white enamel lesions along the gingival margin of newly erupted teeth is a clear sign of ongoing demineralization. In adolescents, proximal enamel lesions visible on bitewing radiographs are markers of increased caries risk. Local aggravating factors such as crowded arches, deep fissures, and enamel morphology should also be taken into consideration. The estimation of the oral hygiene level with a disclosing solution can be recommended, especially in schoolchildren. The presence of gingivitis in preschool

Table 9-2 Risk factors commonly used for caries risk assessment in childhood

Variables	Quantification	Risk value
Social		
Socioeconomic level	Education level	Low
Immigrant background	Parent generation	First generation
Behavioral		
Sucrose intake, small eating	Frequency	Daily
Soft drinks/juice	Frequency	>1 day
Nocturnal meals (toddlers)	Frequency	Present
Toothbrushing	Frequency	Irregular
Fluoride exposure	Frequency	Nondaily
Clinical examination		
Caries prevalence	dmft/DMFT	>1–4
Proximal enamel lesions	Radiographs	>2
Oral hygiene	Visible plaque index	>50%
Gingivitis	Gingival bleeding index	>20%
Saliva tests		
Secretion rate	Sialomethry	<0.5 ml/min (stim)
Buffer capacity	Dentobuff	Yellow (pH 4.0)
Mutans streptococci	Dentocult	Score ≥2
Lactobacilli	Dentocult	≥10^5 cfu/ml

Note: the risk values are suggested indicators of high caries risk but may vary by age and should correspondingly be adjusted.

children could be a marker of insufficient oral hygiene and visible plaque on the labial surfaces of maxillary incisors of a toddler may indicate caries risk.

Supplementary tests

Saliva samples can provide useful information on the component causes of importance for the caries process as discussed earlier in this chapter:

- *bacterial challenge*: levels of mutans streptococci as causative agents
- *diet*: levels of lactobacilli as an indicator of sugar content in diet
- *host susceptibility*: salivary flow rate and buffer capacity as indicators of potential biologic repair.

Samples can be sent to a laboratory or processed with commercial test kits in the dental office. The chair-side methods are generally considered to correspond significantly with conventional techniques. It is important to check whether the child is taking or has recently had antibiotic medication and to avoid sampling immediately after toothbrushing or eating. In addition to the diagnostic value of saliva tests, the didactic properties as a patient-motivating tool in caries prevention are widely acknowledged.

Measurement of saliva flow rate. Since hyposalivation can result in a highly increased caries risk (16), it is important to evaluate whether the secretion is normal or impaired. Decreased flow rate is a common side-effect to radiation therapy and a large number of drugs. In case of hyposalivation, the saliva is often viscous and foamy and follow-up samplings are recommended in order to identify alterations over time. Stimulated whole saliva samples mostly are used for routine work for children over 3 years of age. The stimulation can be done by chewing paraffin or by adding droplets of 3% citric acid on the back of the tongue. The obtained volume of saliva is divided by the collection time and the secretion is expressed as ml/min. In childhood, the stimulated secretion rate is dependent on age and cooperation. For schoolchildren, stimulated values less than 0.5 ml/min should be considered low. Girls generally have a somewhat lower stimulated secretion rate than boys.

Microbial enumeration in saliva. Mutans streptococci are associated with the initiation of dental caries (2) and one chair-side technique, the Dentocult®-SM, utilizes the ability of mutans streptococci to adhere and grow on a nonshedding surface in a selective broth. The kit includes a specially prepared plastic strip for saliva sampling on the tongue. After cultivation, the colony density is evaluated against a chart and scored 0–3, where the highest score corresponds to $>1 \times 10^6$ colony-forming units (cfu)/ml saliva.

Lactobacilli levels are influenced by the intake of carbohydrates and are often found in the deeper parts of a caries lesion (10). The number of salivary lactobacilli can be estimated with the aid of the Dentocult®-LB method, consisting of a dip-slide covered with selective agar. After incubation, the lactobacilli appear as small whitish dots and the number on the agar surface is estimated by comparison with a chart. Values above 1×10^6 cfu/ml saliva are considered high.

In infants and toddlers, bacteria sampling can be carried out with the aid of a wooden cotton pin that is wetted in saliva and streaked along the gingival margin of the upper incisors. The pin is then rolled on the chair-side tests for subsequent cultivation.

Buffering capacity of saliva. The buffering capacity of saliva is important for the maintenance of normal pH levels in the oral cavity. A low secretion might indicate a low buffering effect and an inverse relationship to caries has been described in children (16). Buffer tests, such as the Dentobuff® strip, mainly reflect the bicarbonate buffer system and identify saliva with low (yellow), intermediate (green), and normal (blue) buffer capacity. The yellow color indicates a final pH of 4 or less, meaning that the saliva was unable to raise the pH. Therefore, this result should be regarded as an indication of caries risk.

Some variables used for the assessment of caries in children are shown in Table 9-2. A comprehensive computer-based approach is presented in Box 9-15.

Risk ages

Since the ability to correctly identify patients with increased caries risk is limited, an alternative approach focused on risk ages has emerged. It is well known that all newly erupted teeth are more susceptible to caries than after some years of posteruptive maturation. Moreover, the eruption of a tooth constitutes a risk *per se*, since new surfaces become available for the disease. Thus, all children could be considered at risk at certain ages with population-based preventive measures linked to those periods. The first period in life which merits special attention is 1–3 years during which the majority of the primary teeth are erupting. An early contact with dental health professionals is important to help parents to establish good oral habits. This is of special importance in vulnerable or immigrant groups as exemplified in Box 9-12. The second crucial period in life appears at 5–6 years when the eruption of the first permanent molars constitutes a well-known occlusal risk that could be combated with a structured sealant program. Finally, the early teenage period (12–15 years) offers a high number of molar and premolar surfaces susceptible for decay.

Box 9-15 Caries risk assessment with the "Cariogram" model

The "Cariogram" is an interactive computer-based tool for caries risk assessment in the dental clinic. A caries risk profile for the patient is calculated by entering causal factors of importance for the caries process. The factors are weighted together and the "chance of avoiding caries" in the near future is expressed as a green sector on the screen. The impact of diet, bacteria, susceptibility, and circumstances is presented as dark blue, red, light blue, and yellow sectors, respectively.

The model has been evaluated in a prospective trial in schoolchildren and the program sorted the individuals into risk groups that reflected the actual caries development over a 2-year follow-up period (Hänsel Petersson *et al.*, *Caries Res* 2002;**36**: 327–40). However, the probability was higher of correctly identifing low-risk individuals (specificity) than those with high risk (sensitivity). One advantage of the program is that it may be used as an educational tool facilitating the understanding and discussion with children's patients concerning the multifactorial etiology of caries and its prevention.

The upper figure is an example of a low-risk patient with an 83% chance of avoiding caries (large green sector). The lower example illustrates a child with increased caries risk (24% chance of avoiding caries) due to a sugar-containing diet and frequent snacking (relatively large dark-blue sector).

The program can be downloaded from: www.db.od.mah.se/car/cariogram/cariograminfo.html (accessed August 2008).

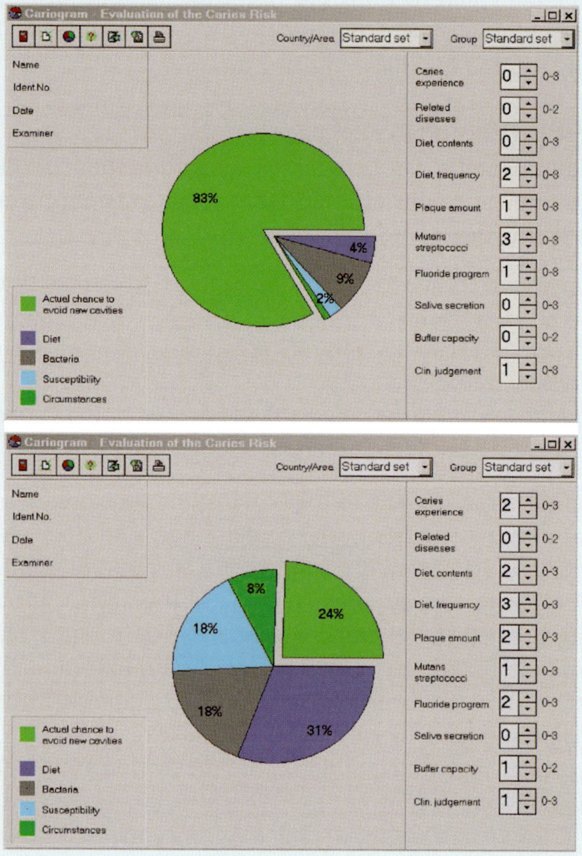

Preventive and operative care: a coordinated approach

The integration of prevention in operative treatment procedures of caries will be dealt with in detail in Chapter 10. However, some comments will be made on the use of the basic concepts of prevention when planning the treatment of children with high caries activity or caries risk. The placement of restorations in children with ongoing high caries activity is not a sound or fair treatment, either ethically or scientifically. The outcome of such treatment will always be poor. Therefore, a strategy has to be found where operative treatment is combined with control of the disease activity.

References

1. Axelsson P. The effect of plaque control procedures on gingivitis, periodontitis and dental caries. Thesis. University of Göteborg, Sweden, 1978.
2. Bratthall D, Carlsson P. Clinical microbiology of saliva. In: Tenovuo J, ed. *Human saliva: clinical chemistry and microbiology*. Boca Raton, FL: CRC Press, 1989; 203–41.
3. Burt BA. Prevention policies in the light of the changed distribution of dental caries. *Acta Odontol Scand* 1998;**56**:179–86.
4. Emilson CG. Potential efficacy of chlorhexidine against mutans streptococci and human dental caries. *J Dent Res* 1994;**73**: 682–91.
5. Hamp S-E, Lindhe J, Fornell J, Johansson L-Å, Karlsson R. Effect of a field program based on systematic plaque control on caries and gingivitis in schoolchildren after 3 years. *Community Dent Oral Epidemiol* 1978;**6**:17–23.
6. Hausen H. Caries prediction – state of the art. *Community Dent Oral Epidemiol* 1997;**25**:87–96.
7. Holst D, Schuller AA, Aleksejuniene J, Eriksen HM. Caries in populations – a theoretical, causal approach. *Eur J Oral Sci* 2001; **109**:143–8.
8. Last JM. *A dictionary of epidemiology*, 4th edn. New York: Oxford University Press, 2001.
9. Lygidakis NA, Oulis KI. A comparison of Fluroshield with Delton fissure sealant: four year results. *Pediatr Dent* 1999;**21**:429–31.
10. Marsh PD. Microbial ecology of dental plaque and its significance in health and disease. *Adv Dent Res* 1994;**8**:263–71.
11. Mertz-Fairhurst EJ, Shuster GS, Williams JE, Fairhurst CW. Clinical progress of sealed and unsealed caries. Part II: Standardized radiographs and clinical observations. *J Prosthet Dent* 1979; **42**:633–8.
12. Needleman IG. Oral hygiene. Today's view. *Int Dent J* 1998; **48**:495–500.
13. Poulsen S, Peltoniemi S. Retention of fissure sealant in primary second molars after 6 months. *Scand J Dent Res* 1979;**87**:328–30.
14. Rose G. Sick individuals and sick populations. *Int J Epidemiol* 1985;**14**:32–8.
15. Rothman KJ, Greenland S. *Modern epidemiology*. Philadelphia, PA: Lippincott-Raven, 1998; 7–16.

16. Tenovuo J. Salivary parameters of relevance for assessing caries activity in individuals and populations. *Community Dent Oral Epidemiol* 1997;**25**:82–6.
17. van Rijkom HM, Truin GJ, van't Hof MA. A meta-analysis of clinical studies on the caries inhibiting effect of chlorhexidine treatment. *J Dent Res* 1996;**75**:790–5.
18. von der Fehr FR, Löe H, Theilade E. Experimental caries in man. *Caries Res* 1970;**4**:131–48.
19. Welbury R, Raadal M, Lygidakis N. Guidelines on the use of pit and fissures sealants in paediatric dentistry. An EAPD policy document. *Eur J Paediatr Dent* 2004;**3**:179–84.
20. Wendt L-K, Koch G, Birkhed D. On the retention and effectiveness of fissure sealant in permanent molars after 15–20 years: a cohort study. *Community Dent Oral Epidemiol* 2001;**29**:302–7.
21. Wendt L-K, Hallonsten A-L, Koch G, Birkhed D. Oral hygiene in relation to caries development and immigrant status in infants and toddlers. *Scand J Dent Res* 1994;**102**:269–73.

10

Diagnosis and management of dental caries

Ingegerd Mejàre, Magne Raadal and Ivar Espelid

The concept of caries diagnosis

The proper management of dental caries in clinical practice requires an accurate diagnosis. Before deciding on a treatment plan, which may include a range of clinical techniques, the characteristics of the manifestations of the caries disease of the individual child must be assessed. This includes the child as a whole, as well as individual teeth and surfaces. In this chapter the concept of caries diagnosis and its diagnostic tools are described. The chapter also describes the concepts of nonoperative and operative treatment and the properties of restorative materials and techniques for their use. Age-specific considerations related to caries diagnosis and treatments are described under separate headings.

Dental caries is the localized destruction of susceptible dental hard tissues by acidic byproducts from bacterial fermentation of dietary carbohydrates (32,61). The disease process is initiated within the bacterial biofilm (dental plaque) that covers the tooth surface. The process is dynamic and numerous episodes of loss and gain of mineral (demineralization and remineralization) take place on the enamel surface. If demineralization prevails over remineralization the result will be permanent and irreversible loss of mineral, cavity formation, and continuous destruction of hard tissues. The signs and symptoms of the disease range from the smallest subsurface loss of minerals to severe destruction of the tooth (Fig. 10-1). In clinical practice, the signs and symptoms of the carious demineralization describe the disease once it is detectable by visual–tactile examination possibly combined with other diagnostic methods such as radiography. In this chapter the term caries is used to describe both the caries process and the caries lesion.

There is some confusion in the literature concerning the terms *caries diagnosis*, *lesion detection*, and *lesion assessment*. Lesion detection merely means that a method is used to determine the absence or presence of caries whereas lesion assessment aims to characterize or monitor a lesion once it has been detected. Caries diagnosis should imply professional, comprehensive assessment of all patient information (82). This means that caries diagnosis involves both the detection of a lesion and the assessment of lesion severity and activity, all of which form the basis for deciding on rational treatment needs.

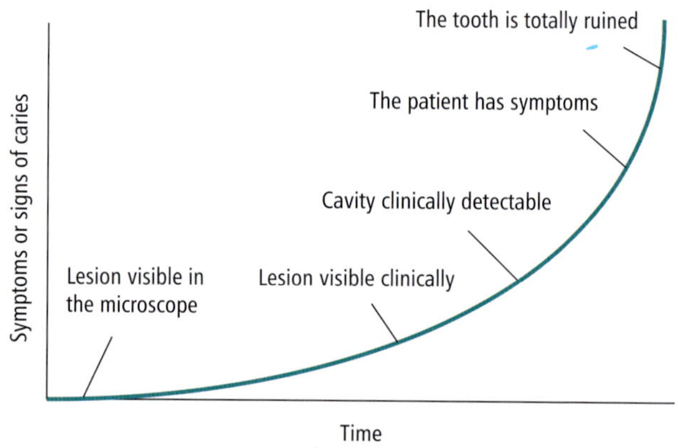

Figure 10-1 How is caries defined? Caries disease is assessed by its signs and symptoms that depend on the severity of the disease. The figure shows the time-dependent development of a lesion from a subclinical level to increasing destruction of dental hard tissues.

Detection and assessment of the caries lesion (caries diagnosis)

Assessment of the presence or absence of a caries lesion is dependent on the cut-off chosen. Traditionally, the presence of a cavity involving the dentin defines a carious (decayed) tooth that needs a filling. Along with changes in caries prevalence, incidence, distribution, severity, and rate of lesion progression, the treatment philosophy has also changed. Thus, there is a growing international trend in clinical practice to move, wherever possible, away from operative intervention towards the nonoperative treatment of caries (83). This has necessitated the need for a more detailed description and assessment of the caries lesion and also methods for monitoring the behavior of a lesion (regression, progression, or no change) (84).

Assessing and grading lesion severity

A valid and reliable system for assessing and grading the severity of the caries lesion has many advantages:

- progression of the disease can be more accurately monitored and the effect of measures to control the disease may be evaluated
- clinicians can calibrate themselves and interobserver and intraobserver reliability can be assessed
- it can facilitate the communication between the clinician, the patient, and the parent
- it can facilitate the communication between clinicians, researchers, and public dental health workers.

The ICDAS (International Caries Detection System) has been introduced for this purpose and great efforts have been made and still continue to make the criteria valid and reliable (82). The ICDAS detection codes range from 1 to 6 depending on the severity of the caries lesion. The basis is essentially the same for all types of surfaces, but varies somewhat depending on surface characteristics (pit and fissures versus free smooth surfaces) and whether or not there are adjacent teeth present (mesial and distal surfaces). The codes and criteria are given in Box 10-1.

Detection and grading the severity of approximal lesions of surfaces contacting neighboring teeth are done from bitewing examination. How radiographic findings should be integrated with the clinical ICDAS criteria is still to be decided. ICDAS-based codes for free smooth surfaces and occlusal surfaces are presented in Fig. 10-2(a). An alternative to the ICDAS criteria, which also includes radiographic scores for approximal surfaces, is given in Fig. 10-2(b).

Box 10-1 Codes and criteria used to assess and grade the severity of a caries lesion according to International Caries Detection System (ICDAS)

0 Sound surface
1 First visual change in enamel (seen only after prolonged air-drying or restricted to within the confines of a pit or fissure)
2 Distinct visual change in enamel
3 Localized enamel breakdown (without clinical visual signs of dentin involvement)
4 Underlying dark shadow from dentin
5 Distinct cavity with visible dentin
6 Extensive distinct cavity with visible dentin

Assessing and grading lesion activity

Assessment of *lesion activity* is as important as lesion detection. This might be done for the single lesion and as an overall assessment based on the caries pattern of the patient. Nyvad *et al.* (81) suggested six grades and criteria, later reduced to four. The criteria were used in a clinical trial where it was observed that active noncavitated lesions had a higher risk of progressing to cavitated lesions than inactive noncavitated lesions (80). A theoretical reasoning for the validity of these criteria was also reported (80). In addition to the visual–tactile appearance, Ekstrand *et al.* (28) added location of the lesion (plaque stagnation areas) to distinguish between active and nonactive lesions. However, the reliability and validity of the proposed criteria in clinical practice are still uncertain and need further evaluation (1). This does not imply that they should not be used. It does, however, call for more clinical research in this field. Criteria for active and inactive caries lesions slightly modified after Nyvad *et al.* (80) and Ekstrand *et al.* (28) are presented in Box 10-2. Figure 10-3 illustrates four lesions corresponding to the criteria.

Diagnostic tools

Visual–tactile and radiographic examination

The two traditional, and still most commonly used diagnostic tools are visual–tactile examination and bitewing radiography. How accurate are these methods? That is, how well do they correspond to the true presence and extension of a lesion? A recent systematic review (1) concluded that visual–tactile examination is a simple, cheap, and reliable method for diagnosing obvious lesions on all tooth surfaces not contacting neighboring tooth surfaces. Also, visual–tactile examination is reliable for detecting early enamel lesions on buccal and lingual surfaces. It is, however, less accurate for detecting enamel and early dentin lesions on occlusal surfaces. For this purpose visual examination of occlusal surfaces should be combined with bitewing radiography. The same applies to enamel and dentin lesions on approximal surfaces in contact with adjacent teeth.

The teeth should be cleaned, dried, and examined in good lighting. A whitish carious spot is detected more easily when the tooth is dry, since the difference in refractive index between carious and sound enamel is higher when the water in the porous carious enamel is removed by drying.

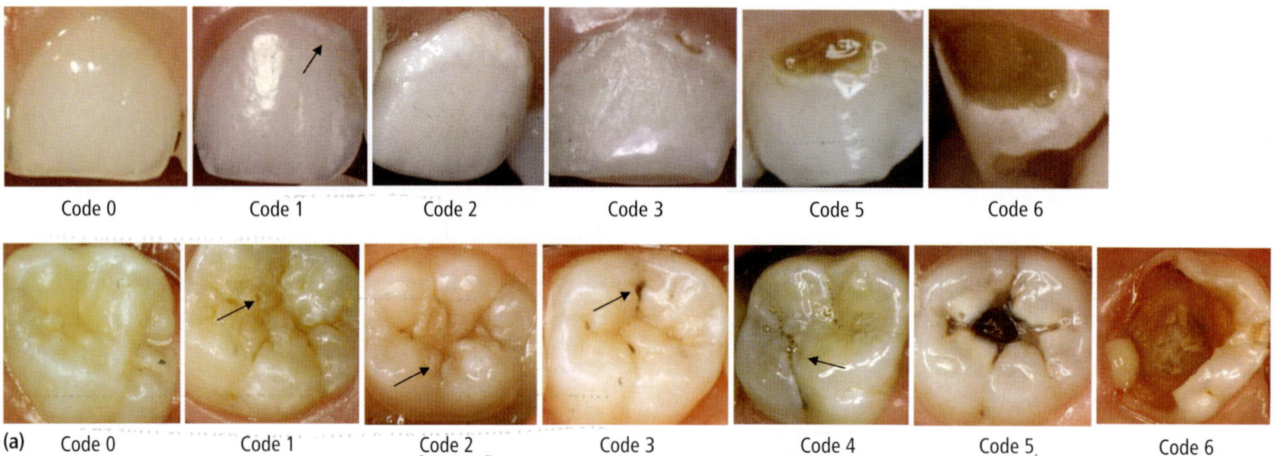

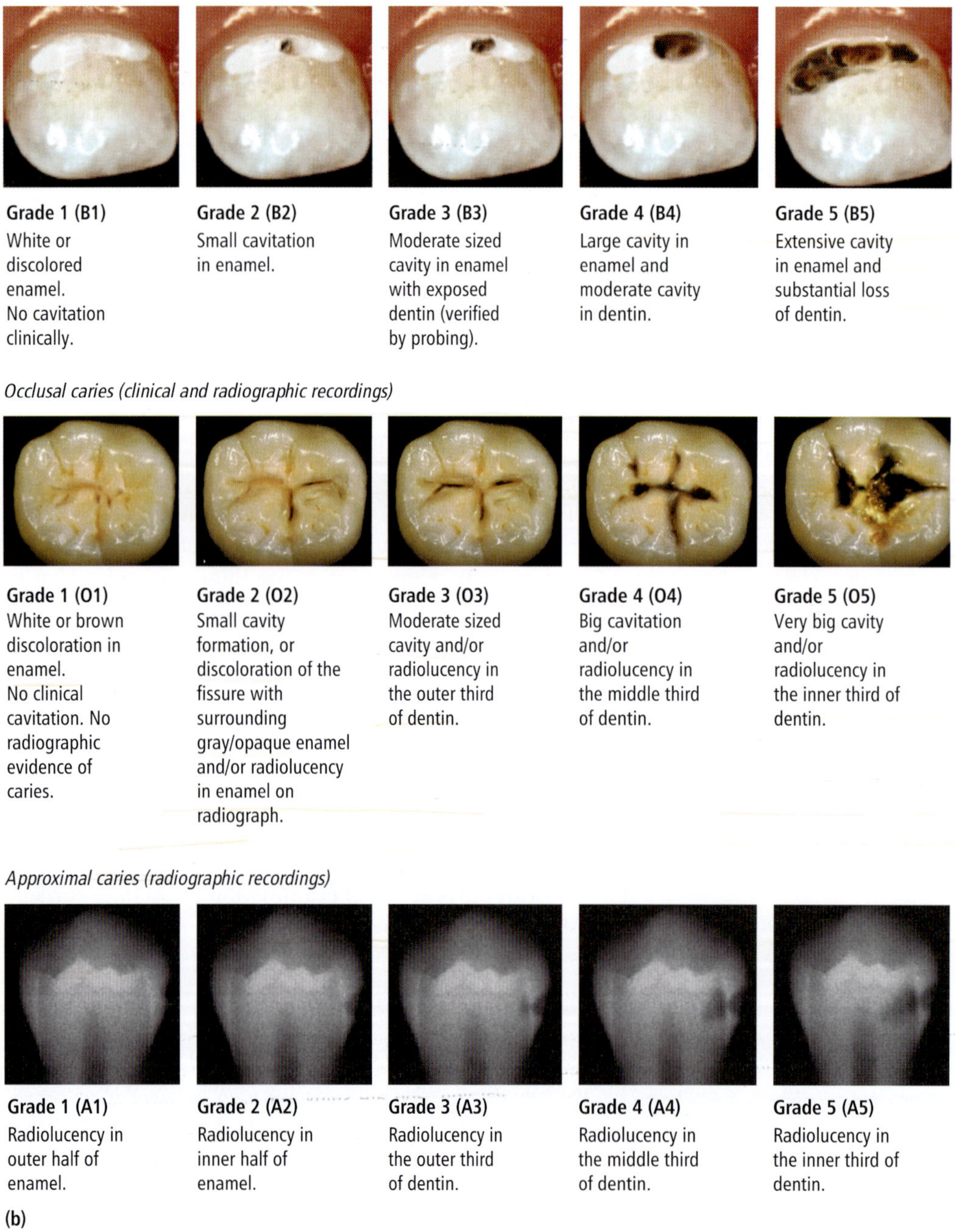

Figure 10-2 (a) ICDAS-based criteria for severity grading of caries on free smooth and occlusal tooth surfaces. (b) Criteria using a five-graded scale for severity grading of caries on free smooth, occlusal and approximal tooth surfaces.

Box 10-2 Clinical characteristics of active and inactive noncavitated and cavitated lesions

	Active caries	Inactive/arrested caries
Noncavitated	Chalky/whitish enamel. Surface is rough on gentle probing. Often covered with plaque and often located close to the gingival line.	Whitish, brownish, or blackish enamel. Shiny, hard surface, smooth on gentle probing. Often located at a distance from the gingival line.
Cavitated	The probe sticks in cavitated areas and the base feels soft or leathery on gentle probing.	The base of the cavity is hard on gentle pressure with probe. Discolored tissue (brown or black). Often open access to cleaning.

Occlusal surfaces (pit and fissures)

Particularly in pits and fissures, the probe should be used carefully in order to avoid irreversible damage (Fig. 10-4). The probe is an important tactile aid and may be necessary to remove plaque. However, solely visual assessment of early (noncavitated) fissure caries lesions is not improved by probing (58). In this context it is also important to recognize that even if the probe "catches", this does not necessarily mean that there is a soft lesion.

Early caries lesions are common during tooth eruption when the occlusal surface of the molar constitutes a plaque stagnation area (16). The reason is that the occlusal surface is located below the occlusal plane and is easily missed by the toothbrush. These early lesions are characterized by whitish opaque areas at the entrance of the fissures. It is easy for them to be overlooked if the surface is not clean and dry and the lighting is not optimal. For the same reasons, small cavitated lesions in these areas may easily be missed.

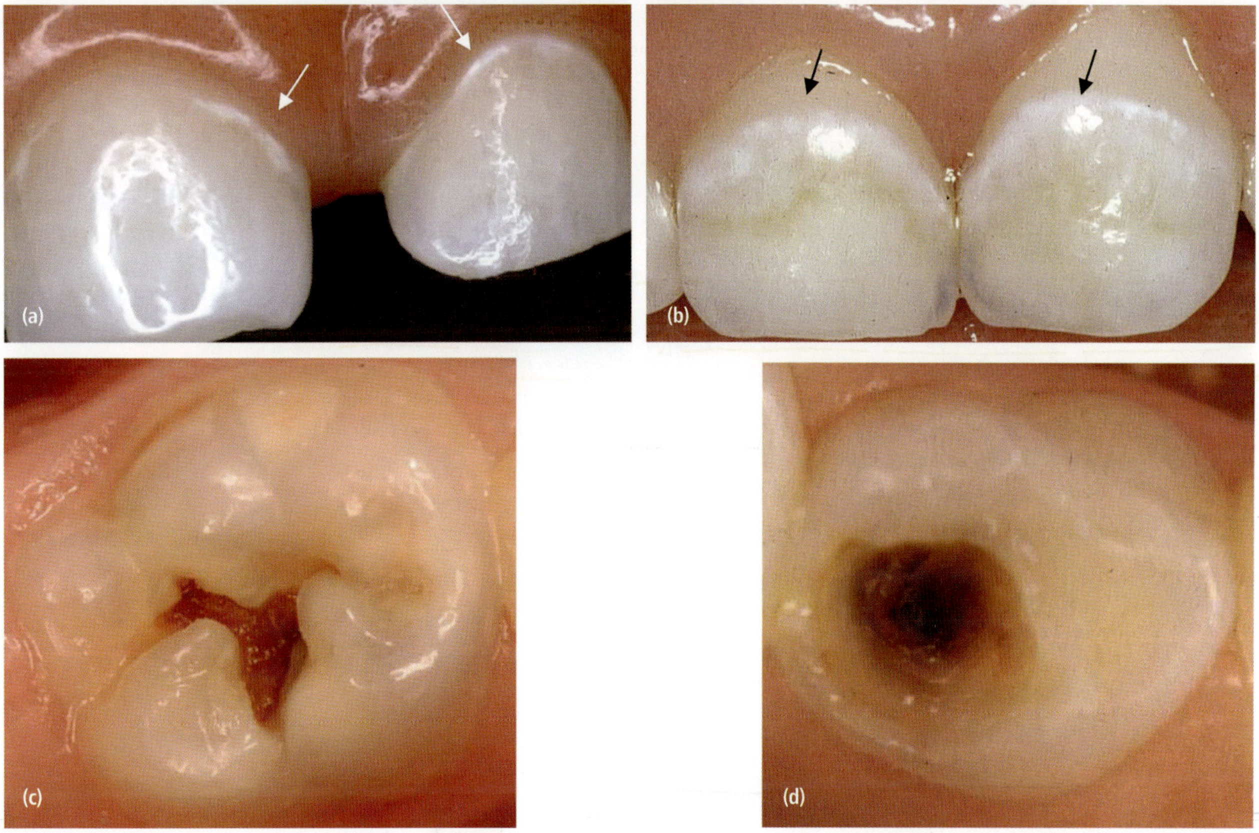

Figure 10-3 Active and inactive/arrested caries lesions. Upper row shows initial (noncavitated lesions) and the lower row shows cavitated lesions. (a) Active noncavitated lesions close to the gingival line on the buccal surfaces of primary upper incisors in a 2 year old. There is loss of luster and the lesions are rough on probing. (b) Arrested noncavitated lesions on the buccal surfaces of primary upper incisors in a 4 year old. The lesions are situated at a distance from the gingival line, and are shiny and hard on probing. (c) Active cavitated lesion in a primary lower second molar in a 5 year old. The dentin is soft on probing and the cavity borders are blunt and irregular. (d) Inactive/arrested cavitated lesion in a primary lower first molar in a 7 year old. The dentin is brownish-black, hard on probing and the cavity borders are sharp and regular.

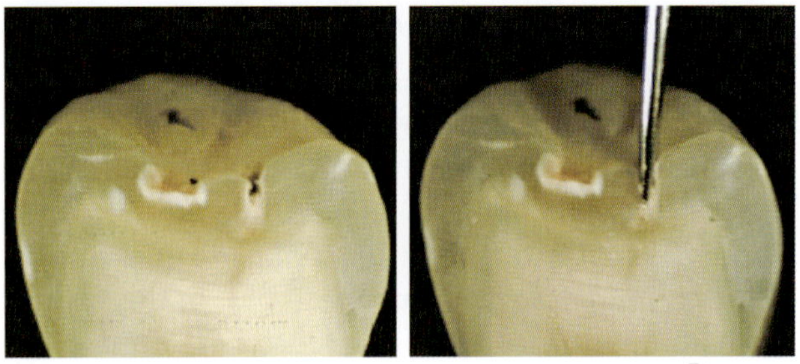

Figure 10-4 Sectioned premolar with an enamel caries lesion in the fissure before probing (left). Intense probing (right) destroys the surface zone of the lesion.

The discolored fissure often poses diagnostic challenges. A discolored fissure does not necessarily indicate an active caries process. To discriminate between active and inactive or arrested lesions, the following characteristics may help:

- *Active lesions* are most frequent seen in erupting and newly erupted teeth in children with other signs of caries activity in the dentition. The discoloration is usually opaque, whitish, or light brownish. Softened enamel at the entrance of the fissure from gentle tactile probing is indicative of an active lesion. When the discoloration also involves obvious loss of continuity of the enamel surface (clinical cavity), bitewing examination frequently reveals a radiolucency in the dentin (Fig. 10-5). Many borderline cases can be difficult to diagnose. For these cases, bitewing radiography is a valuable tool for assessing possible dentin involvement (Fig. 10-6a, b).
- *Inactive lesions* are usually seen in "older" teeth in adolescents with no signs of caries activity. The discoloration is dark brown or black and the surface is hard on probing (Fig. 10-6c). There is usually no dentin involvement.

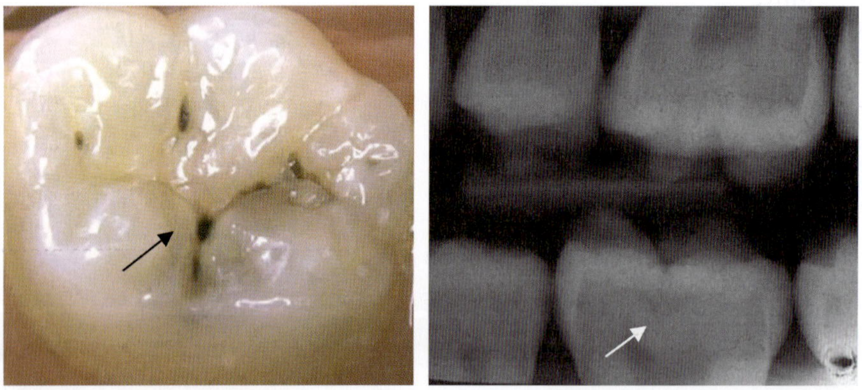

Figure 10-5 A small but obvious occlusal cavity in the central fossa of a permanent first molar (arrow). The borders around the cavity are whitish and rough in texture suggesting an active caries process. There is a shadow from underlying dentin caries. The radiograph reveals a substantial radiolucency in the dentin (arrow).

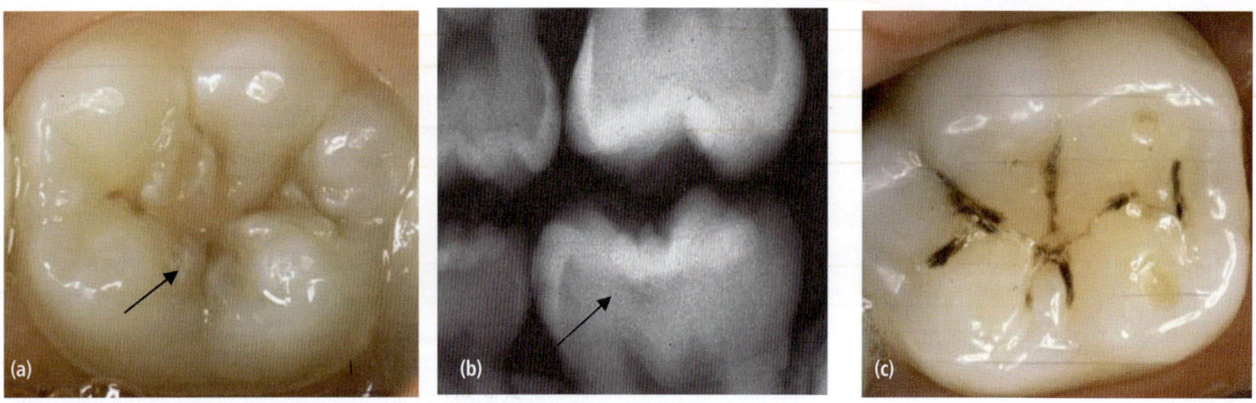

Figure 10-6 (a) Light brown discolored fissures in a permanent first molar of an 8 year old. The enamel around the central fossa is whitish and there is softened enamel at the entrance of the fissure indicating an active lesion (arrow). (b) The radiograph reveals radiolucency in the dentin (arrow). (c) Dark brown/black discolored fissures in a permanent first molar of a 19 year old with a low caries activity. The fissures are hard on probing indicating an arrested (inactive) lesion.

Free smooth surfaces

The buccal and lingual aspects of teeth are easily examined, and it is easier to disclose small changes in surface color and texture of early caries lesions on these surfaces compared to "inaccessible" areas on approximal surfaces or in pits and fissures. The active lesion on free smooth surfaces is usually located near the gingival margin. It is whitish and rough in texture (Fig. 10-3a). In contrast, a typical inactive lesion is seen at a distance from the gingival margin, is hard on probing and may be shiny (Fig. 10-3b).

Approximal surfaces

Radiographic examination is the most commonly used method for detecting and assessing caries lesions on approximal surfaces with adjacent contacting surfaces. The early, noncavitated lesion on these surfaces is, however, not possible to detect in the radiographic image (1) and usually not from direct visual–tactile examination either. It is also important to bear in mind that the proportion of false-positive diagnoses from bitewing radiography is relatively high in low caries prevalence populations. Details on the validity of radiographic caries diagnosis are described in Chapter 8.

For an approximal caries lesion contacting a neighboring tooth, the border between nonoperative and restorative treatment is the presence of an obvious clinical cavity on the tooth surface. This diagnostic decision is therefore crucial. However, on this matter the radiograph does not give straightforward information. An example of this is shown in Fig. 10-7, where only one of two lesions with similar radiographic appearance had a clinical cavity. Studies comparing the radiographic and clinical appearance of approximal lesions in children and young adults report great variation. The percentage of clinical cavities of surfaces with radiolucencies in the outer half of the dentin varies between 41 and 100%, the median (mean) values being 78% (14,23,57,65,67,85,99). The most likely reasons for this variation are different methods used to record the presence of a cavity, different depths of the lesions investigated, and different populations with different caries activity in the various studies. It is obvious, however, that the deeper the lesion, the more likely is cavitation.

Some clues are useful to assess the probability of the presence of a cavity. Cavitation was more frequently found in A2 and A3 lesions (Fig. 10-2) in individuals with high caries activity than in those with lower caries activity (57). Cavitated lesions were found more frequently in surfaces with gingival bleeding (27,93). Tooth separation will allow gentle probing to assess the presence of a cavity. The use of an impression of the approximal surface can also be helpful for diagnosing borderline cases (57,85,93). Admittedly, we lack a simple and valid method for assessing the presence of a cavity on the approximal surface contacting a neighboring surface.

It is likely that the extensive use of fluorides has led to a change in the clinical appearance of pit and fissure caries as well as of approximal caries. The finding of a relatively intact enamel surface hiding a dentin lesion is not uncommon (Fig. 10-8). Continuous fluoride supply seems to delay the progression of the caries process in enamel as well as the breakdown of the enamel surface over the dentinal lesion. This phenomenon is sometimes called occult caries (12). Reported prevalences of hidden occlusal caries in 14 year olds vary (42,110).

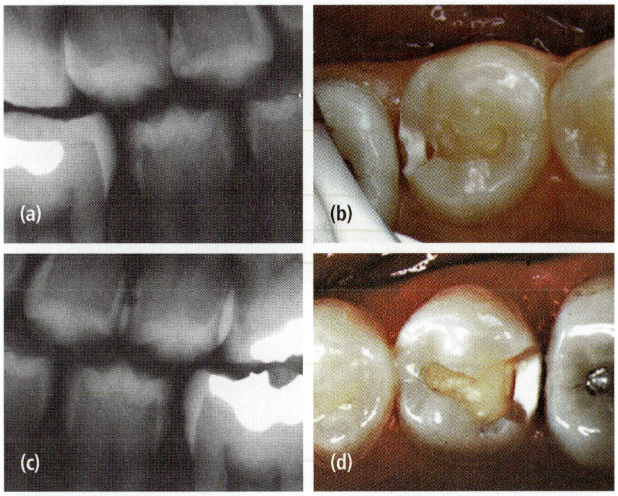

Figure 10-7 Caries lesions on distal surfaces of two mandibular second premolars: both radiographs (a and b, arrows) showed radiolucency in outer dentin, but during cavity preparation, a clinical cavity was observed only in one of them (b).

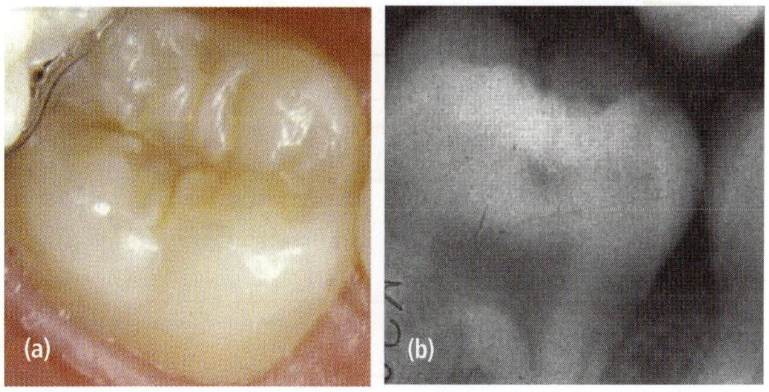

Figure 10-8 Hidden caries under a seemingly sound occlusal surface of a permanent lower second molar in a 14 year old. (a) Visual–tactile examination of the surface did not reveal any clear signs of caries. (b) The bitewing radiograph shows, however, an obvious radiolucency in the dentin. The presence of soft carious dentin was confirmed at drilling.

Alternative/supplementary diagnostic tools

There are a variety of alternative/supplementary diagnostic tools available to the pediatric dentist:

- fiber optic transillumination (FOTI)
- digital fiber optic transillumination (DiFOTI)
- laser fluorescence (DIAGNOdent)
- quantitative light-induced fluorescence (QLF)
- electronic caries measurement (ECM).

The first four are optical methods and the last one is based on electrical impedance. FOTI (DiFOTI) is used as an alternative to bitewing radiography. Holt and Azevedo (43) compared the diagnostic gain from FOTI and radiography and concluded that in terms of accuracy and reliability, the use of FOTI offered no advantage over radiography. In situations when radiography cannot be used, for example children not accepting having radiographs taken, FOTI can serve as an alternative. In a clinical study, DIAGNOdent detected both enamel and dentin lesions with a high sensitivity but at the price of a high proportion of false-positive diagnoses (low specificity) (94). This suggests a considerable risk of overtreatment when relying on this method. QLF can detect small changes in mineral loss with high accuracy but the method is so far little used in clinical practice. ECM was tested in two studies on extracted teeth (29,52). High specificity was found in both but sensitivity varied from low to high in the two studies.

In conclusion, each of these alternatives and supplementary diagnostic tools has shown advantages and drawbacks, but none of them fulfills all of the ideal criteria for assessing treatment needs (79). In addition, a recent systematic review concluded that there is not sufficient evidence to decide on the accuracy of these diagnostic tools (1).

The concept of caries treatment

There has been a strong tradition in dentistry to identify caries treatment with restorative techniques, and to use the term prevention for methods aiming at preventing this kind of treatment. The major drawback with this way of thinking is that it makes dentistry restorative focused. This affects how we make treatment decisions, how we judge the value of restorative treatment, and how resources are allocated. However, since the signs and symptoms of dental caries are the result of a disease process, our treatment should aim at arresting the disease process before repair of destroyed tissue is needed (26). In other words, the primary treatment objective should be to manage the disease by nonoperative measures, while repair of destroyed tissue should come second. It follows that it is very important that resources be allocated accordingly.

Nonoperative treatment aims at reversing, arresting, or postponing progression of the caries lesion and should be the choice of treatment whenever possible. Operative treatment should be used only when progression of the caries lesion cannot be prevented, that is when the lesion is cavitated and adequate plaque control cannot be obtained. From one perspective, nonoperative treatment of noncavitated lesions and operative (restorative) treatment of more advanced lesions both have the same main objective, that is to prevent the disease from further progression leading to further tissue destruction, infection of teeth, and other tissues which may create pain, suffering, and reduced function. The major difference between nonoperative and operative treatment is the long-term benefit of an unrestored tooth.

Nonoperative treatment

The nonoperative treatment techniques are the same as those used to prevent caries, that is, oral health behavior counseling, fissure sealing, and use of fluoride. Nonoperative treatment is used mainly for noncavitated lesions, but there are exceptions such as the management of cavitated lesions in small uncooperative children (see the section "0–3 years" below).

The most commonly used techniques are:

- General intervention (patient): the basic and most important measure is to motivate and teach the patient how to remove dental plaque covering the caries lesion, to keep it clean on a daily basis with the use of fluoride toothpaste. Diet counseling may also be included. In special cases, when the patient and/or the parent is unable to clean the teeth, professional plaque removal may be indicated (106).
- Local intervention (lesion): fissure sealing is used to treat noncavitated caries lesions in pit and fissures. This treatment concept is based on the assumption that a properly placed sealant prevents microleakage from the oral environment. Thereby, supply of nutrients to bacteria in the caries lesion is restrained and the caries process arrested. There is support from the literature that the caries process does not progress as long as the seal is intact, and this applies to both enamel and dentin caries (39,41,72,73). Evidence for the effectiveness of sealing noncavitated caries lesions in pits and fissure in clinical practice is, however, incomplete (2,3). Notably, this does not prove that the technique is not effective; lack of evidence of effect may rather be due to scarcity of well-designed and well-performed clinical studies in contemporary populations.

- Fluoride varnish application is a medical mode of treating noncavitated caries lesions. When topical application of Duraphat® was used in teenagers every third month during a 3-year period, the progression rate of approximal lesions in premolars and molars was reduced significantly (76). This procedure requires resources in terms of professional personnel, time, and equipment but this should be weighed against the benefits. Thus, if successful, this treatment is so much more valuable to the child than a restoration, because it preserves sound tooth tissue. As for fissure sealants, the evidence for the effectiveness of fluoride varnish for treating noncavitated caries lesions is incomplete, implying that there is a need for more studies also in this field (2,3).
- Glass-ionomer cements (GIC) may be used as a temporary sealant in fissures and other lesions, based on their cariostatic and fluoride-releasing properties. This is described later in this chapter.

Operative (restorative) treatment

Irreversible loss of tooth substance and surface continuity has occurred when tooth mineral is lost to the extent that a cavity is formed. This is a critical stage since – unless plaque is effectively removed from the surface of the cavity – destruction of hard tissue will continue. Strictly speaking, the critical border between nonoperative and operative (restorative) treatment is when the patient cannot remove plaque effectively. That border often corresponds to cavity formation (codes 3–6 in Fig. 10-2). This particularly applies to occlusal surfaces and approximal surfaces contacting a neighboring tooth. On buccal and lingual surfaces, even a lesion with an obvious cavity can be arrested without placing a restoration since the surface is accessible to cleaning with the toothbrush.

Most restorative techniques include irreversible loss of sound tooth tissue and therefore permanently weaken the tooth. Furthermore, restorations do not last forever and as a filling is replaced, so the cavity becomes larger and the tooth further weakened. This is true particularly for Class II restorations in primary teeth. Their longevity is further discussed later in this chapter. With Class II restorations there is also an obvious risk of iatrogenic preparation damage to the neighboring approximal surface resulting in an increased risk of lesion progression of the damaged surface (86). It follows that there are several reasons to scrutinize if operative treatment is in the best interest of the patient.

Before deciding to restore, the following factors should be considered:

- *The potential for plaque removal.* The potential for lesion arrest depends on whether or not plaque can be removed from the surface of the cavity. In principle, plaque covering a cavity on a buccal or lingual surface can be removed by the patient with a toothbrush. The critical question is therefore: will the child or the parent be able to clean the cavity effectively? Whether or not this can be done properly has to be decided for the individual patient. Particularly in small children where cooperation for restorative treatment is not good enough, the best option could be to teach the parent to remove plaque from the lesion, that is, to turn an active cavitated lesion into an inactive, arrested lesion. The patient cannot clean an obvious cavity on an approximal surface with a contacting surface effectively – even flossing will only slide over the surface – and the lesion should therefore be restored. The same applies to most cavities on occlusal surfaces. The molar in Fig. 10-5 could serve as an example. The cavity in this permanent first molar cannot be cleaned effectively by the patient since the toothbrush cannot reach the cavity floor because of the undermined enamel. This cavity should therefore be restored.
- *Caries activity – active or arrested lesion.* If there are signs of arrest of a cavitated lesion, restorative treatment may be unnecessary (44). This mostly applies to buccal and lingual lesions. Assessment of caries activity is often difficult for lesions not accessible to visual examination, that is, approximal surfaces in contact with adjacent teeth. Several approximal caries lesions or fillings in an individual often indicate high caries activity with an overall increased risk of relatively fast lesion progression. However, even for the caries-active individual, the rate of progression for a given lesion is difficult to estimate. The only means of deciding whether the lesion is active or arrested is therefore to observe it from repeated radiographic examinations. Here it is important to realize that even with radiographs of good quality, small differences in projection, darkness, and/or contrast can make it difficult to assess whether the lesion has diminished, progressed, or is unchanged. Although it is likely that noncavitated caries lesions visible radiographically can be arrested, the scientific evidence for it is incomplete (1,2). Very few studies are designed to study the efficacy of non-operative caries treatment.
- *Influence of caries prevalence* in the population on the risk of overtreatment. The interpretation of the radiographic image is always associated with risks of making false-negative and false-positive diagnoses (see Chapter 8). The risk of overtreatment mainly concerns approximal lesions. The reason is that the proportion of false-positive radiographic diagnoses is relatively high in low-caries prevalence populations. In other words, the predictive value of a positive diagnosis is

Box 10-3 Main reasons to control caries in the primary dentition

- Prevent pain and discomfort.
- Prevent local infection of jaws and germs of permanent teeth.
- Prevent general infection.
- Prevent negative attitudes and promote interest in keeping good oral health.
- Maintain good masticatory function, aesthetics, and overall well-being.
- Prevent caries in permanent teeth by introducing them to a sound oral environment.
- Prevent malocclusions.

low. This can be compensated for by adopting the philosophy of "when in doubt wait" for borderline cases.

Indications for operative (restorative) treatment of primary teeth

There are several indisputable reasons for maintaining a healthy primary dentition (Box 10-3). However, the benefit and effectiveness of restoring primary teeth are sometimes questioned by practicing dentists as well as by parents of preschool children. The risk of toothache, if not restoring carious primary teeth, was investigated in two studies from England. In one (75), total caries experience in primary molars was the main predictor of pain, while increased levels of restorative care did not lead to either reduced levels of reported pain or to fewer extractions. The authors concluded that if restorative care is not an important factor in predicting dental pain but total decay experience is, then prevention of the disease rather than its repair should form the focus of care for young children. The other study (54) found that 82% of caries lesions extending into the dentin, but left unrestored, exfoliated without symptoms, while 18% had caused pain and were extracted or otherwise treated. The carious teeth most likely to cause symptoms were found in molars that developed cavities with pulpal involvement by the age of 3 years, 34% of which caused pain. Both studies were retrospective and they have several methodological flaws. Bitewing examination was not used and the severity of the lesions at the time of restoration is not stated. In the study by Milsom *et al.* (75) the involved general practitioners were not selected randomly and – perhaps the most serious flaw – the children were not randomly assigned to restoring or not restoring the carious teeth. It is remarkable that restored teeth suffered the same fate as unrestored teeth. This could, however, occur if the lesions were in advanced stages with pulp involvement at the time of restorative treatment. The quality of restorative care may therefore be questioned. Furthermore, the only outcome measure was pain whereas other important parameters were not considered (see Box 10-3). Admittedly, however, there is a need for prospective randomized clinical trials designed to evaluate at what ages and which primary teeth benefit from restorative treatment. Currently accepted best practice for the management of primary molars with dentin lesions not accessible to cleaning involves caries removal with due consideration to the dentin–pulp complex and placement of a restoration.

Treatment planning

Treatment planning for the individual child includes the strategy that one applies after having examined the child and recorded its history. Any treatment action must be adjusted to the child's age, maturity, and ability to cope. This is dealt with in Chapter 4. The treatment is divided into four stages (Box 10-4).

Stage 1: acute treatment

This stage particularly applies to the highly caries-active child. The treatment aims at relieving the child from acute pain and discomfort, or preventing any immediate threat of such suffering. The most commonly used therapies are extraction, pulp treatment, or excavation of deep caries lesions with subsequent application of temporary fillings (Fig. 10-9). Acute treatment in children with coping problems should be carried out under conscious sedation or general anesthesia (see Chapter 5).

Box 10-4 Treatment planning. Background data: case history, clinical and radiographic examinations

Stage 1: acute treatment
- excavation of open cavities – temporary cement
- necessary extractions
- emergency endodontic treatment.

Stage 2: management of the caries disease
- diet history; diet counseling
- salivary tests; bacteriological tests
- oral hygiene instruction; plaque control
- topical fluoride application
- fissure sealing.

Stage 3: restorative (operative) treatment

Stage 4: estimation of risk and establishment of follow-up program

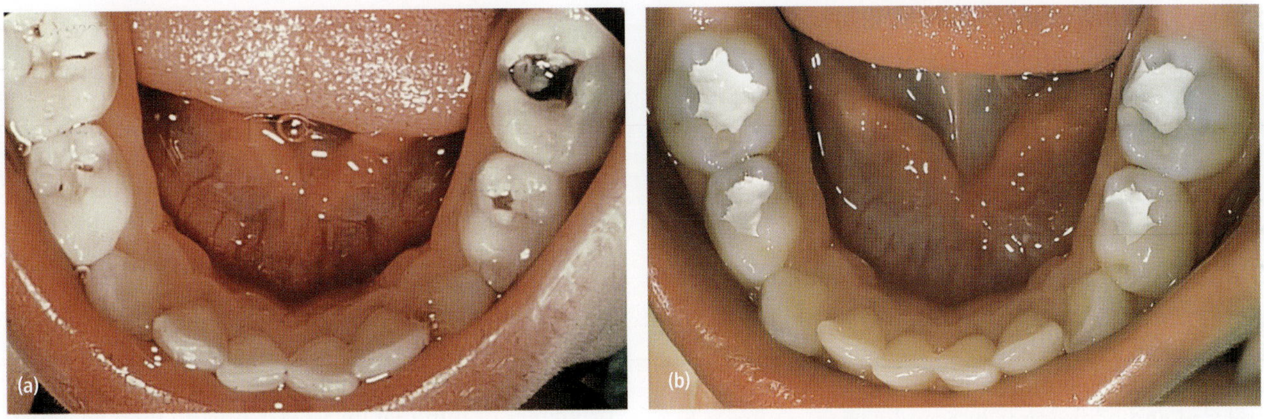

Figure 10-9 (a) A 3-year-old boy with high caries activity due to frequent intake of high sucrose-containing meals. (b) After gross excavation of the caries lesions and application of a temporary zinc oxide–eugenol cement the child is ready for stage 2 which is management of the caries disease.

Stage 2: management of the caries disease; general and local interventions

This stage is based on a general consideration of the caries situation, starting with an estimation of the caries activity. Typical signs of active caries are white spot lesions with rough texture, blunt borders, and location close to the gingival line. The higher the number of active lesions, the higher the activity. In children under regular control and where caries has been recorded over time by the use of a severity grading system, the degree of progression of lesions is also helpful for assessing caries activity. Based on the findings, general and local interventions as described previously in this chapter (nonoperative treatment) should be applied. In individuals with active caries, stage 2 is the most important phase since it involves treatment of the disease itself. In the most difficult cases, it may take months or even years before the disease is brought under sufficient control so that placement of the "final" restorations can be made. The long-term goal should be to reduce the need for restorations and thereby ensure the individual's oral and dental health for a lifetime (Fig. 10-10).

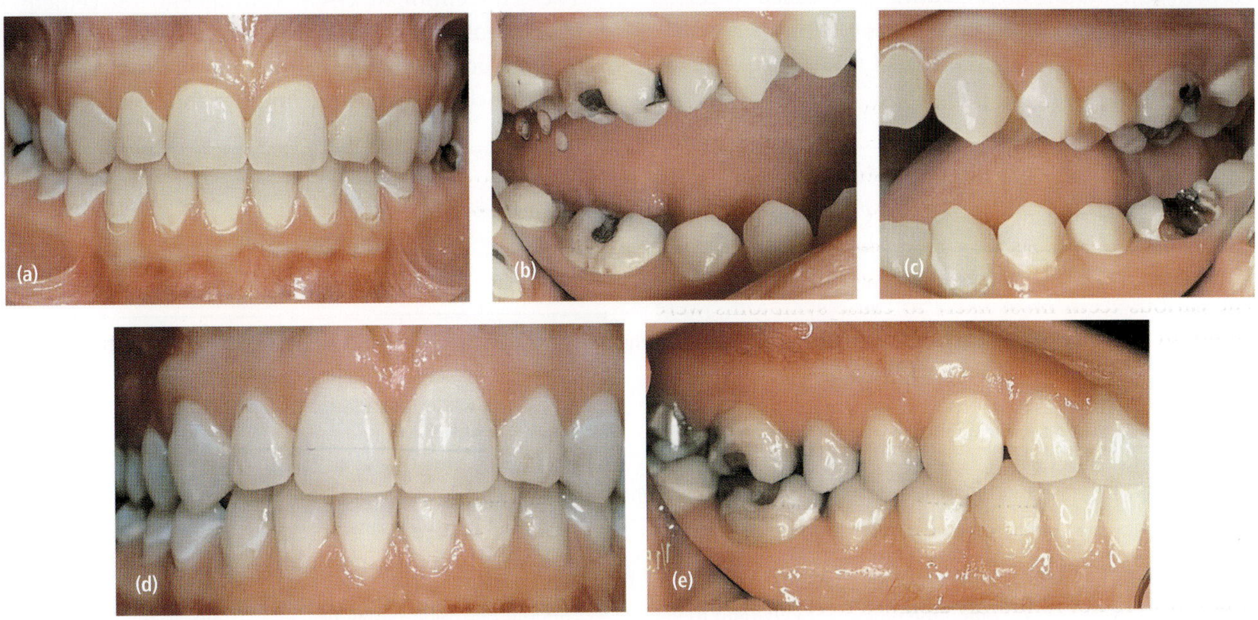

Figure 10-10 (a–c) A 13-year-old girl with active caries and low motivation. Treated by the use of general and local caries-arresting interventions. (d) Five years later: adequate caries control. (e) Another 3 years later: still adequate caries control. Observe the glossy surfaces of the previously active initial caries lesions.

Stage 3: restorative (operative) treatment

The restorative treatment aims at preventing the caries process from further progression as well as restoring the tooth to its original size and form (and color). Indications for this kind of treatment are given in the specific sections for the different age groups later in this chapter.

Stage 4: estimation of risk and recall interval

At the end of the treatment period, an individual risk assessment and a subsequent agreement of recall interval are made. The decreased prevalence of caries among children and adolescents in Scandinavian countries has initiated a discussion of the previously accepted and extensively used 1-year interval (or even shorter) is too short with regard to the cost-efficiency aspect on the use of resources. There are two drawbacks with short recall intervals and frequent check-ups:

- resources that could be allocated to at-risk patients are used for screening healthy individuals, and
- increased risk for overtreatment.

Regarding the first of these drawbacks, we maintain that all dentists, irrespective of type of practice and payment system, should strive for an optimal use of resources allocated to dental services. The second argument is dependent on the dentists' skills and attitudes to dental treatment. Dentists who allocate most of their time and interest to restorative care may constitute a risk group for delivery of overtreatment. In contrast, dentists who focus on preventive and nonoperative techniques for treating caries, and who are sufficiently skilled in caries diagnosis and risk assessment, probably run a very small risk of overtreating. Risk assessment is further discussed in Chapter 8.

Restorative procedures

Restorative materials: basic principles and handling

Due to controversies about possible side-effects of mercury, amalgam is no longer recommended in pediatric dentistry in Nordic countries. Therefore, the materials of first choice are GICs, compomers, and composites. These tooth-colored materials represent a variety of possibilities for improved restorative care in the primary as well as the young permanent teeth due to their ability to adhere to the tooth tissues. In accordance with the principles of minimal invasive dentistry, these materials are appropriate for small cavities with restricted loss of sound tooth substance. The GICs may also have anti-cariogenic properties from fluoride release (15), while compomers and composites have excellent aesthetic properties.

There is a rapid development of new restorative materials following the decreased use of amalgam in dentistry, and it may be difficult for dentists to keep updated in the field when the manufacturers' representatives are boasting all the advantages of their products. The classification of the materials may also seem confusing, for example the resin-modified GICs (RMGIC) and compomers. McLean *et al.* (64) suggest a nomenclature for the classification of adhesive materials and reviews describe the properties and possibilities of these materials (13,19). The general characteristics of GICs, compomers (polyacid-modified resin composite), and composites are summarized in Table 10-1.

The conventional GICs (polyalkenoate cements) adhere to both enamel and dentin and they release fluoride. This occurs mostly during the maturation phase during the first week after application. Still, the low

Table 10-1 General characteristics of GICs, compomers, and composites

Material	Strength and wear	Adhesion	Handling	Fluoride release
GICs; conventional and resin-modified	Low fracture strength. Low wear resistance	Moderate to enamel and dentin	Sensitive to mixture procedure, but capsules are available. Slow setting reaction and low early strength. Not sensitive to moisture	High, possibly caries preventive
Compomers	High fracture strength. High wear resistance	High to enamel and dentin	Easy handling. High early strength. Moisture sensitive	Low, probably not caries preventive
Composites	Very high fracture strength. Very high wear resistance	Very high to enamel (acid etch), high to dentin	Bonding procedure may be complicated. High early strength Moisture sensitive	No

tensile strength and brittleness exclude their use in stress-bearing areas in permanent teeth, other than as a temporary filling material. To improve the physical and aesthetic properties, and to allow a fast set, RMGICs have been developed. The setting mechanism is a combination of light-induced curing and the acid/base reaction. However, they are not considered appropriate for stress-bearing Class II restorations in permanent teeth.

The idea behind the polyacid-modified composites (compomers) is to combine the advantage of fluoride release with improved physical properties. The release of fluoride from compomers is, however, comparatively small and of questionable clinical importance. The advantage of the dual setting mechanism has also been questioned.

The properties of composites have improved continuously during the past decade, and today a number of composites can be used for posterior stress-bearing restorations. The material requires pretreatment of enamel and dentin in order to adhere to these tooth structures. More details about restorative techniques, material properties, and longevity of restorations are given below.

Rubber dam

Acid etching of the enamel and the use of a dentin adhesive are procedures that are extremely sensitive to moisture contamination, and isolation with a rubber dam is therefore preferable. The rubber dam is used for two purposes in restorative dentistry:

- to isolate the operation field from the rest of the oral cavity, and
- for moisture control.

In Scandinavian countries, a rubber dam in restorative dentistry is used mostly for placing composites and other moisture-sensitive filling materials. However, it is acknowledged that the use of a rubber dam facilitates all restorative work in children and increases the quality of the restoration. Thus, the use of a rubber dam during the whole sequence of preparation, filling, and polishing procedures prevents movements of the tongue, cheek, lips, and saliva ejector interfering with the procedures. It also gives a much better control of the operation field. It must be emphasized though that the use of clamps and dental floss to attach the dam to teeth may be associated with pain, and this must be prevented by the use of local anesthesia (injection or topical). Another concern related to use of a rubber dam is the increased prevalence of allergic reactions to latex, which should encourage the use of latex-free rubber dams.

The procedures for applying a rubber dam in two common situations are described in Box 10-5 and illustrated in Figs 10-11 and 10-12. In the first example, the main purpose is to isolate the operation field in the posterior quadrant during the procedures of drilling and filling primary molar teeth (Fig. 10-11). The second example is the upper front region where the main objective is to keep the operation field dry (Fig. 10-12).

Box 10-5 Rubber dams

Rubber dam for isolation of the field before restorative therapy in primary molars

- Suitable clamps are selected, e.g., No.14 or 14A, for the most posterior tooth.
- The dam is applied on the frame and the number of holes necessary punched.
- The clamp is applied in the most posterior hole.
- Clamp with dam and frame is applied in the mouth. The dam is lifted off the ears of the clamp and applied to the teeth to be exposed. (Alternative: the clamp is first applied on the posterior tooth. Then the dam is applied by slipping the posterior hole over the clamp.)
- The dam is attached to the most anterior tooth by the use of dental floss or a wooden wedge if necessary.

Rubber dam for isolation and drying of the field before restorative therapy of maxillary incisors

- Suitable clamps are selected, e.g., #00, for the canines or first premolar bilaterally. (Optional: no clamps, the dam is attached with dental floss only.)
- The dam is applied on the frame and the number of holes necessary punched.
- The dam is applied on the teeth.
- The clamps are applied on the premolars.
- Dental floss is applied around the neck of all teeth to be treated to prevent leakage of gingival fluid.

Specific conditions for different age groups

0–3 years

The current internationally accepted term for caries with early onset is early childhood caries (ECC) (25), which is defined as the occurrence of any sign of caries on any tooth surface during the first 3 years of life (see Chapter 6). ECC is a common condition; in a study from the suburbs of Stockholm in Sweden, 12% of 2.5 year olds had caries (35) and in another Swedish study 28% of 3 year olds had one or more teeth with caries (114). The most common locations are upper incisors and first molars. Caries usually starts as circumferential lesions on the gingival third of the maxillary incisors, while the lower incisors usually remain sound. If the carious process remains active, other teeth are affected as they erupt; most often pits and fissures of primary molars, but also canines and second molars may be affected. Lesion progression can be extremely

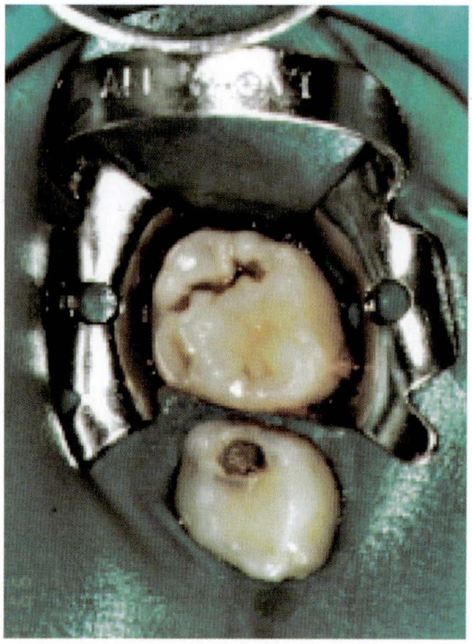

Figure 10-11 Rubber dam for isolating the operation field before restorative therapy of primary molars.

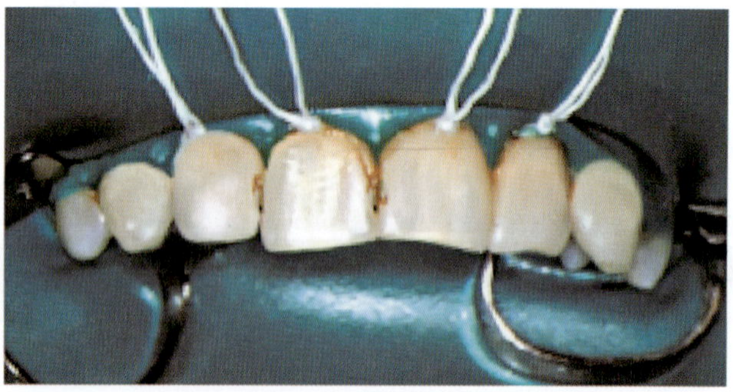

Figure 10-12 Rubber dam for isolating and drying the operation field before restorative therapy of maxillary incisors.

fast and result in pulp involvement if no action is taken (Fig. 10-13). Short episodes of ECC may leave "scars" of previously active caries on areas not prone to caries attacks any more after the tooth has fully erupted (Fig. 10-3b).

Risk factors for ECC

ECC is often associated with *ad libitum* bottle-feeding (74,96). Sugary products in the bottle combined with poor oral hygiene are the main risk factors for the development of ECC. The typical pattern of caries lesions in ECC is due to the nipple blocking the access of saliva to the upper incisors. In contrast, the lower incisors are close to the orifices of the main salivary glands and are protected from the liquid contents of the bottle by the nipple and the tongue. Bottle-feeding with sugary products at night when salivary flow is reduced is particularly devastating (113).

Prolonged breastfeeding (beyond the age of 1 year)

The health benefits of breastfeeding are widely acknowledged and include a reduced risk of gastrointestinal and respiratory infections (50). However, the effects of prolonged breastfeeding on dental caries have been controversial. Some investigators have observed an increased risk and severity of ECC from prolonged breast-feeding (24,38,62,101,111). The relationship is, however, complex and contains several confounding variables such as intake of sugary products in various forms, poor oral hygiene, parental education, and socioeconomic level. Thus, other studies found no association (63,92,111,115). A randomized study provided no evidence of beneficial or harmful effects of prolonged and exclusive breastfeeding on dental caries at early school age (51) and systematic reviews found no conclusive evidence of harmful effects of prolonged breastfeeding (95,107). It therefore seems reasonable to conclude that bad dietary

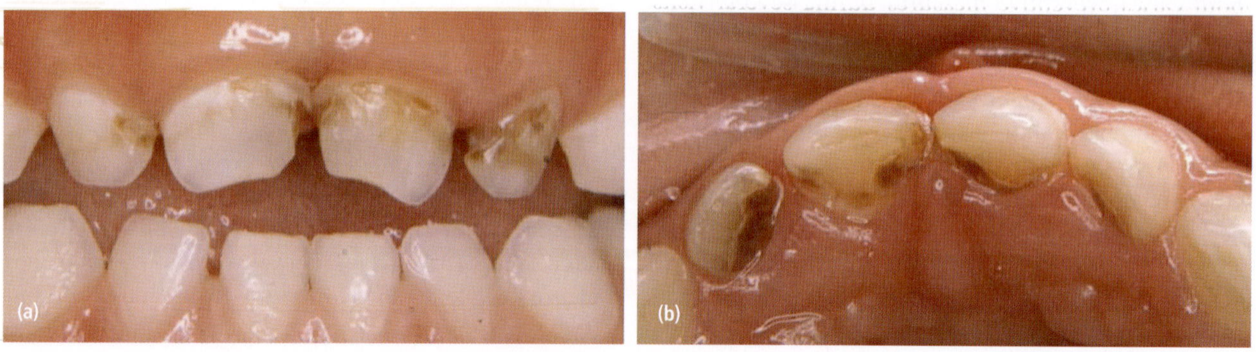

Figure 10-13 Early childhood caries in upper incisors in a 2 year old. The caries process started during the eruption of the teeth due to bottle-feeding with sweetened liquids at night. The severity of the lesions varies depending on the exposure time of the different parts of the teeth: (a) buccal view and (b) palatal view.

habits in general and insufficient exposure to fluoride from poor oral hygiene are the main reasons for ECC in children with prolonged breastfeeding.

Child management and treatment procedures

The major problem related to treatment of children in this age group is their uncooperative behavior due to mental immaturity such as limited perseverance and fear of strangers and stressful situations. Even minimally unpleasant or painful stimuli may generate a fear reaction and subsequent refusal of treatment. This, combined with the fact that these children often have multisurface lesions in the very small and tiny incisors that are extremely difficult to restore, makes restorative care in this age group almost impossible without deep sedation or general anesthesia. However, both deep sedation and general anesthesia are stressful pharmacological encroachments for small children. They require the presence of a specialist in anesthesia, and are very costly. They should therefore be avoided unless absolutely necessary and considered to be the least traumatic treatment mode for the child. General anesthesia is indicated in severe ECC cases with extensive and complicated treatment needs, such as when several teeth have to be extracted or when complicated restorative treatment has to be made. Conscious sedation can be used safely in dental clinics by experienced dentists, and is an alternative for children with less complicated treatment needs (see Chapter 5). Because of what is stated above, a nonoperative treatment approach should be used whenever possible, and all efforts made to turn active lesions into inactive/arrested ones. If successful, restorative treatment becomes superfluous or can be postponed until the child's coping ability allows it.

The nonoperative treatment strategy should utilize all relevant means that can promote the arrest, or at the least a decrease, of the caries activity including both general and local intervention techniques. The general techniques involve information, motivation, and instruction about caries-preventive measures during several visits. When exploring possible etiologic factors by interviewing the parents about food and sleeping habits, one must be extremely careful not to provoke feelings of failure and guilt in the parents. It is well known that many young parents with a variety of difficult problems to handle are struggling with the establishment of normal eating, sleeping, and oral hygiene habits for their children. By showing interest and empathy towards their problem, and by taking the role as a professional helper instead of being a judge, the dentist has better opportunities to obtain compliance, which is an absolute necessity for a positive outcome of the nonoperative treatment approach.

Effective treatment of EEC includes breaking harmful dietary habits and instituting proper daily toothbrushing with fluoride toothpaste. It is extremely important that plaque is removed and the lesions are exposed to fluoride every day. Dietary advice, oral hygiene instruction, and use of fluorides must be adapted individually. If use of a bottle with sweetened liquids at night is the main problem, an abrupt brake may be difficult and create new problems for the family. In such situations, the use of water as the thirst-quencher may be introduced gradually. A schedule for this may help the parent. Regular and frequent (monthly) appointments including professional application of fluoride varnish and encouragement are essential and should continue until arrest of lesions is observed.

Application of a chlorhexidine solution or gel on cotton sticks to the affected teeth may facilitate the cleaning process in cases where brushing is painful due to exposed dentin. Adequate fluoride exposure can be secured by the combined use of tablets (0.25 mg at night) and toothpaste. Since the local effect of fluoride is the most important, children should be encouraged to suck the tablets before swallowing them in order to obtain an increased salivary fluoride concentration.

If the lesions are inaccessible to cleaning, local intervention comprises professional cleaning, careful removal of debris and soft tooth tissue by the use of hand instruments, and the application of fluoride varnish or a thin layer of GIC sealant (e.g., Vitrebond®) on the lesions (Fig. 10-14). This procedure must be repeated frequently, for example once a month, until the caries lesions are arrested. This is seen by the color of the dentin turning from light yellow into dark yellow, brown or black, and the dentin surface becomes hard on probing (Fig. 10-3d). Deep lesions must be excavated stepwise; a procedure that frequently necessitates use of local anesthesia. The Carisolv® technique may be an optional method

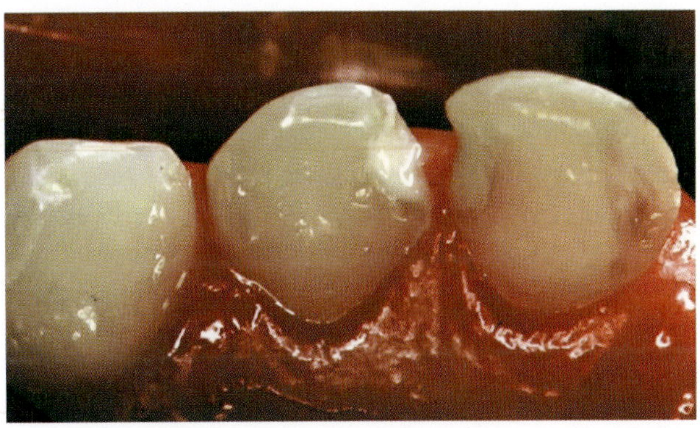

Figure 10-14 Use of a thin layer of GIC for the arrest of approximal dentin caries in primary incisors of a 2-year-old child. A hand instrument was used to remove soft carious tissue before application of the cement.

that is less traumatic to the tooth tissues and less painful for the child than excavators and rotating instruments (33,46,71). GIC is the material of choice for temporary sealing of the cavities, since fluoride release supports the process of arresting (63). It should be noted that there is no evidence-based knowledge on the most effective way to treat ECC apart from the importance of exposure to fluoride (8). The above-mentioned treatment strategies are based on clinical experience mostly from observational studies.

In children with severe ECC, the incisors (and sometimes also the canines and second molars) have multisurface lesions and the first molars large occlusal cavities. Pulpal infection, periapical pathologic changes, and fistula may be present. The second molars are usually less affected due to their later eruption and shorter period of exposure advice and instructions in the mouth. Dependent on the severity, many of these children should preferably be treated under general anesthesia, because it is less stressful for the child as well as for the parents and the dental staff, and probably more cost-efficient, in comparison with a long series of dental appointments. The likelihood of better treatment quality is also higher.

Dental treatment under general anesthesia of small children with extensive and complicated treatment needs usually has to be radical in terms of more extractions and less conservative treatment than under conventional treatment (see Chapter 5). There are two major reasons for this. First, children should be kept under general anesthesia for as short a time as possible, since increased time may be associated with increased risks. The other reason is that only therapies with good prognosis should be selected. Endodontic therapy in primary teeth is associated with a certain risk for postoperative complications. The incisors and first molars should therefore be extracted if there is pulp involvement or extensive cavities, since these teeth are of least value for the continuous development of the dentition. Canines and second molars are more important for the normal development of jaws and for the eruption of the permanent teeth. Therefore, if possible, these teeth should be treated conservatively even if pulp therapy is needed. The restorative treatment may include the use of GIC, composites/compomers, and stainless-steel crowns (see the next section).

3–6 years (primary teeth)

Among 5 year olds, the second molar is the tooth with the highest caries experience. The most frequently affected surfaces in the dentition are the occlusal surfaces of the second molars and the distal surfaces of first molars. More than half of the approximal lesions in the primary molars in 5 year olds are restricted to enamel (7,45), and the proportion of lesions limited to the enamel increases with increasing caries prevalence (45).

Indications for operative treatment

Active lesions in incisors are less common after 3 years of age, but if present, efforts should be made to turn the lesions into inactive stages by nonoperative means. Arrested lesions need no special attention. An active cavitated lesion (usually with dentin involvement) on an occlusal surface should be restored to prevent further lesion progression.

The progression rate of approximal caries lesions in primary molars is relatively fast; the median survival time for a lesion to progress through the enamel was 2.5 years compared to 4 years for young permanent teeth in children and >7 years for young adults (102). Unfortunately, no data are available on the rate of lesion progression in newly erupted primary molars compared to primary teeth with a longer posteruptive age. Another study compared the rate of lesion progression for the distal surface of the primary second molars with the mesial surface of the permanent first molars from the age of 6 to 12 years, and found that the progression rate from enamel to dentin was 1.6 times higher for the primary molar compared with the permanent molar (68).

In conclusion, it is a delicate task to decide on the best time to make a Class II restoration in a primary molar, particularly in the preschool child. Factors such as cooperativeness and caries activity of the child and the expected longevity of the restoration must be weighed against the risk of fast lesion progression. Taken together, the relatively high rate of lesion progression in primary molars in preschool children suggests a more operative-oriented philosophy when compared to permanent molars where lesion progression, in general, is much slower. Another factor supporting this view is that the risk that a Class II restoration in a primary molar will fail increases as the proximity of the cavity to the pulp increases (87). As a general rule, it is suggested that an approximal caries lesion observed at the enamel–dentin border (or deeper) should be restored in the preschool child.

Restorative techniques

The introduction of adhesive techniques has made it less important to focus on cavity design for the retention of the restoration. During preparation for adhesive filling materials such as GIC and composites or compomers, the operator should primarily focus on removal of soft and active carious tissue and secondly finish the margins to remove weak parts of unsupported enamel. The most common cavity preparation techniques used in primary

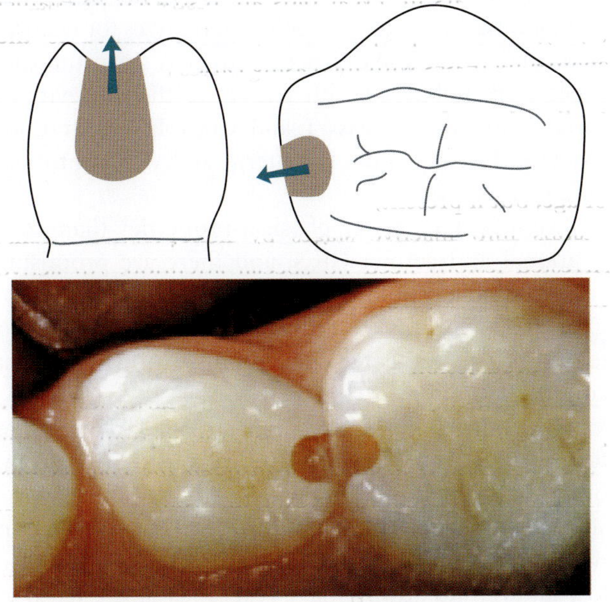

Figure 10-15 Small Class II cavity preparation for GIC in primary molars. Basically, the outline of the cavity is determined by the extent of the caries lesion, but some mechanical retention is advocated in the directions indicated by the arrows.

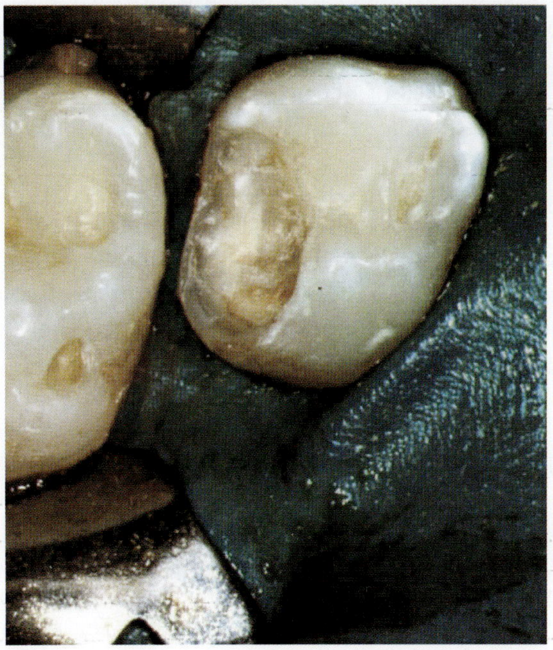

Figure 10-16 Large Class II cavity preparation for compomer or composite materials in a primary molar. Retention of the filling is based on mechanical as well as adhesive techniques.

teeth in patients aged 3–6 years are Class I and Class II cavities in molars and Class III cavities in incisors and canines.

The preparation for Class I cavities in the occlusal surface of primary molars should be guided by the extension of the caries lesion. The opening through the enamel is done with a small round diamond (ISO #014) or steel bur (ISO #009) in a high-speed hand-piece before softened dentin is removed with a slowly rotating round bur of sizes ISO #014 to ISO #021. Sound enamel is removed only to the extent necessary to gain access to remove soft dentin. When filling the cavity, the material (adhesive materials) is extended to cover all parts of the fissure, as in "preventive restorations" (see later).

Resin-modified GICs (RMGIC) are preferred in small Class II preparations where the contact point is maintained partly by sound tooth tissue (Fig. 10-15). The opening through enamel is made close to the marginal crest with a small round diamond (ISO #014) in a high-speed hand-piece. The cavity is widened with a slowly rotating round bur, e.g., sized from ISO #014 to ISO #021 according to the extent of the lesion. GIC is relatively brittle and the cavo-surface angle should ideally be approximately 90°.

Large approximal cavities with total loss of the contact point should preferably be restored with a compomer or composite material since these materials are more resistant to masticatory forces (Fig. 10-16).

Even when adhesive materials are used, some mechanical retention in cavities in primary teeth is recommended, since loss of retention has been reported as a common reason for failure of both compomer restorations (9) and cermet GIC materials (30,48). The manufacturer's instructions should be followed in order to obtain maximum adhesion of the material. Acid etching and bonding procedures both seem to be preferable and safe on enamel as well as dentin when using compomer and composite materials.

Class III preparations in canines and incisors are usually made from the buccal aspect using a slowly rotating round bur for opening and excavation of caries. A high-speed round diamond may also be used to gain access to the caries lesion. The cavity walls are finished and the size and extent of the caries lesion determine the cavity outline.

Material properties in relation to longevity of restorations and possible adverse effects

In the primary dentition, dental restorations should ideally last until natural shedding of the tooth. However, the prognosis for a restoration in primary teeth is poorer than for those in the permanent teeth. It is demanding to make long-lasting restorations in stress-bearing locations in primary teeth. Small tooth dimensions and problems with cooperation are two major problems.

Alm *et al.* (6) found that in the 7–12-year age group about 30% of the restorations in primary teeth were replacements. Wendt *et al.* (116) found that at the age of 8 years, 33% of fillings in primary teeth had failed. The corresponding number for young permanent teeth was 13%.

In a Danish study, the 50% survival times of Class II restorations with RMGIC or compomer were >5 years (87), and the authors concluded that both materials are appropriate for restorations in primary teeth. The median age of the children at restoration was, however, 8 years; that is, the children were rather old at the time of restoration. Presumably, the survival time of Class II restorations in primary molars is shorter in preschool children than in schoolchildren. Furthermore, Qvist *et al.* (88) showed that both RMGICs and compomers are equivalent to amalgam in terms of longevity in everyday practice. The median survival time exceeded 5 years for Class II restorations. Conditioning of dentin improved the success rate of RMGICs. The operator effect was statistically significant for the success rate. In a recent systematic review (49), it was concluded that an approximal Class II amalgam restoration can be expected to survive at least 3.5 years but potentially more than 7 years.

Östlund *et al.* (118) reported a failure rate of 8% after 3 years for Class II amalgam restorations of 16% for composite restorations and of 60% for conventional GICs restorations in primary molars. Other studies confirm that GICs placed in stress-bearing restorations have a lower survival rate than alternative restorations of amalgam or composite (89). A clinical 2-year follow-up study compared the longevity of amalgam and GIC restorations in primary molars. It was concluded that a GIC restoration was "no worse than an amalgam restoration" in primary teeth, but that the GIC restorations underwent greater loss of anatomic form (109). Welbury *et al.* (112) found that after 5 years, the median survival time was 33 months in the GIC group and 41 months in the amalgam group. The amalgams were more durable in terms of anatomic form, marginal integrity, and had fewer overall failures in patients aged 5–11 years. The longevity of dental restorations in children is related to the patient's age at the time of placement, but this seems to be the case only for children below 6 years of age (48,97).

A recent review (18) concluded that conventional GICs should not be used in stress-bearing areas. However, by increasing the powder to liquid ratio and the polyacid concentration or molecular weight, the physical properties are improved (37). The World Health Organization initiated this development for using the material in the atraumatic restorative treatment (ART) technique. These high-viscosity GICs also come with faster setting time and might be useful alternatives for restorations that are not too exposed to stress. A few promising reports are published with respect to the longevity of these materials in Class I and Class II preparations (61,100,117), but more long-term and well-controlled studies are needed.

RMGICs have better physical properties than conventional and cermet GICs, and there are promising results for these materials in Class II cavities (30). One explanation may be fewer problems related to long curing time and vulnerability to early moist contamination.

Compomers are marketed as particularly suitable for restorations in stress-bearing areas in primary teeth, but so far, there are few clinical studies. In a 3-year study by Roeters and colleagues (79,98), the conclusion was that the excellent handling characteristics and the low failure rate during the 3-year study suggested that compomer is a reliable restorative material for primary molars.

It can be concluded that at present there is considerable uncertainty about cavity design, choice of restorative material and adhesive techniques for Class II restorations in primary molars. There is an obvious need for more knowledge, experience, and well-designed clinical studies. Chadwick and Evans summarized in their review (18) that "some operators are better than others" and this expressed the challenge to all clinicians to master the clinical handling of dental materials that is particularly difficult in the case of a restless child.

Atraumatic restorative treatment

ART takes a position between nonoperative and restorative care, since the treatment consists of removing the superficial layer of carious dentin with only hand instruments and using a GIC as a combined restorative and sealing material. The treatment concept is based on the knowledge that the inner carious process is stopped when the lesion is sealed off and microleakage from the oral cavity is avoided. This is a similar treatment concept as in stepwise excavation of deep caries lesions. ART was introduced by Frencken *et al.* (34) as a possible treatment technique in developing countries, demanding minimal technical resources. The ART technique is indicated primarily for treating single-surface cavities in both primary and permanent dentitions. Follow-up studies have revealed that the technique might arrest dentin caries lesions, and that a major factor for success is proper seal of the margins (105). In countries with modern pediatric dental services, the method may be used as temporary caries treatment for small and uncooperative children.

Stainless-steel crowns

Preformed stainless-steel crowns are available for most tooth types, both primary and permanent.

There are two major indications for use of such crowns in pediatric dentistry:

- primary molars with extensive destruction of the crown
- permanent first molars with severe developmental defects.

In the first case, the crowns offer an alternative to extensive, multisurface restorations, which are known to have a poor prognosis and frequent need of repair. When properly made, the steel crowns are known to have a low rate of complications during the lifespan of primary molars (10). In permanent molars where the whole crown is affected by severe tissue damage due to developmental disturbances, the steel crown is used as a temporary restoration until it is decided whether the tooth should be extracted or restored. In the latter case, the steel crown can serve until a permanent cast crown can be made.

The procedure for the adjustment of a stainless-steel crown is given in Box 10-6, and an example is shown in Fig. 10-17. Sufficient local anesthesia of both the pulp and the gingiva is needed. The preparation should be conservative, reducing only enough tooth structure needed for occlusal and approximal adjustment of the crown. Only minor buccal and lingual reduction is needed, since the crowns are elastic to a certain extent and can be pressed over small undercuts, which is important for retention. All soft carious tissue is removed. Large cavities should be restored with GIC before adjusting the crown. The margin of the crown may be adapted to the restoration instead of the cavity margin in cases where the cavity extends deep into the gingival pocket (Fig. 10-18). The crown is cemented with a GIC luting cement, which is favorable for the prevention of secondary caries.

Stainless-steel crowns and orthodontic appliances have been associated with increased risk of nickel sensitivity in children (31). This problem seems to be associated with the old nickel–chromium formulations (72% Ni), and these types of alloys should therefore be omitted.

Box 10-6 Procedure for insertion of stainless-steel crowns

1. Local anesthesia.
2. Excavation of soft carious tissue.
3. Lining of deep dentin areas if needed for pulp protection.
4. Restoration of gross cavities with GIC. The cement is allowed to set (light-cured if resin modified).
5. Occlusal reduction, e.g., with a ball-shaped diamond bur, to allow adjustment of the crown without raising the bite.
6. Slight reduction of buccal and lingual surfaces with a tapered diamond bur. Most of the gingival contour should be kept for mechanical retention of the crown.
7. Removal of approximal contacts, e.g., with a tapered diamond bur, to allow the crown to be adapted between neighboring teeth.
8. A crown is selected based on the mesiodistal space available.
9. The length of the crown is reduced by crown scissors or rotating stone to allow the crown to rest stabilized on the occlusal surface of the tooth with its margins extending into the gingival sulcus.
10. Contouring of the crown with pliers if necessary to obtain a stabilized position with its margins well adapted into the gingival pocket. Pliers may also be used to alter the occlusal surface for adaptation to the bite.
11. Polishing of the gingival margins.
12. Cementing the crown with a GIC luting cement.

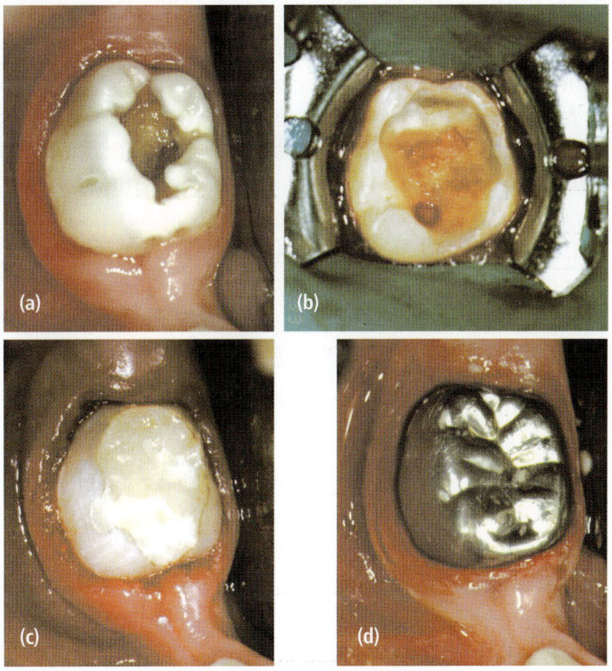

Figure 10-17 (a) Lower right second molar with severe multisurface caries suitable for a stainless-steel crown. (b) Removal of carious tissue reveals pulp exposure. (c) After pulpotomy the cavity is restored with GIC and the crown is prepared for a stainless-steel crown. (d) The tooth is restored with a stainless-steel crown.

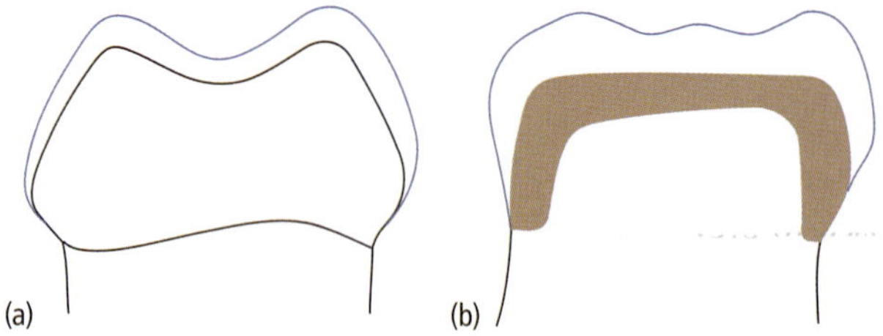

Figure 10-18 (a) Only just enough tooth tissue is removed to adjust the crown to the occluding and neighboring teeth. The gingival contour should be kept intact to retain the crown. (b) Extensive carious defects are initially restored with GIC and the crown is subsequently adapted to the restoration.

6–12 years

Treatment of primary molars in the mixed dentition

Caries increment in primary teeth during this period is predominantly on approximal surfaces of the molars and new lesions may develop, even in children who are caries free at the age of 5 years (103). There may also be substantial caries development in permanent teeth during this period, primarily in permanent first molars. A continuous need for treating the caries disease in primary teeth during this age period, both operatively and nonoperatively, is emphasized, the overall aim being to create the best possible conditions for the permanent dentition. Indications and treatment principles are generally the same as in the previous age period.

As the primary molar approaches exfoliation, a more nonoperative treatment philosophy can be adopted. Simplified procedures such as excavation and a temporary filling may be appropriate. Grinding can also be an option, although the method has not been evaluated. The choice of treatment should be in the best interest of the individual child.

There is a positive association between caries experience in primary teeth and that in newly erupted permanent teeth (103). The ability to predict caries in young permanent teeth from caries experience in primary teeth is, however, limited. According to a recent systematic review the mean sensitivity was 62% and the mean specificity 79% for predicting dentin caries in young permanent teeth from caries experience in primary teeth and other risk factors (1). The results were based on two studies that besides caries experience in primary teeth also used other predictors such as toothbrushing frequency, dietary habits, and sociodemographic factors (104,108). This means that the ability to identify the true nonrisk children is greater than the ability to correctly identify those who will develop dentin caries in permanent teeth. Thus, about four out of five children who do not develop new dentin lesions will be correctly identified, while only about six out of 10 children who do develop new dentin lesions will be correctly identified.

In order to prevent caries on the mesial surface of the permanent first molar, special attention should be given to the distal surface of the primary second molar. The reason is that the risk of caries on the mesial surface of the permanent first molar increases substantially if the distal surface of the primary second molar develops caries (68). Early detection, mainly based on radiographic information, and appropriate treatment of caries on the distal surface of the second primary molar are therefore of utmost importance. If operative treatment is required, GIC should be used because of its potential caries-preventive effect on the contacting surface of the permanent first molar.

Treatment of pits and fissures in permanent first molars

Pits and fissures in the permanent first molars are the most frequent locations for caries lesions in this age group. This is ascribed to the favorable conditions for plaque accumulation in these sites (16). Preventing and treating caries here is therefore of major importance in modern pediatric dentistry (Fig. 10-19).

Fissure sealing is a method where the fissure systems or pits are sealed with a material that is retained on the enamel surface either by the acid-etch technique (resin sealants) or through chemical bonding (GIC sealants). Since the technique was introduced in the late 1960s, based on resins and the acid-etch technique, a variety of methods for the prevention, nonoperative treatment of noncavitated lesions, and restoration of pit and fissure caries have been developed in its wake (20). In this textbook, the term *fissure sealing* applies to techniques for

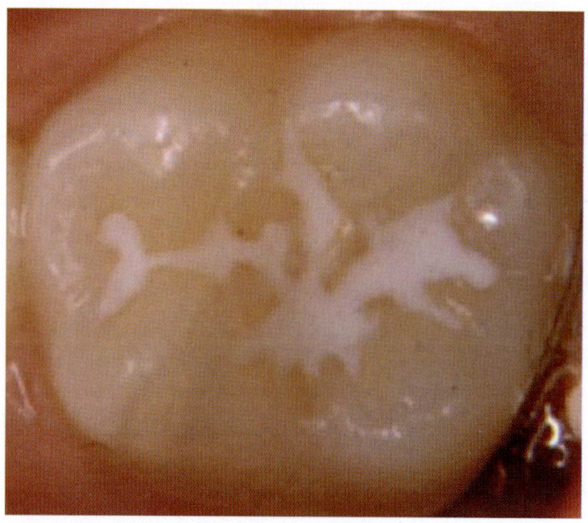

Figure 10-19 Fissure sealing covering all parts of the fissure without overfilling and overextension.

pits and fissures that are either caries free or only have initial caries lesions without cavity formation, and where the removal of soft carious tissue is not advocated. *Preventive restoration* is the term used for a combined restorative and sealing procedure.

Fissure sealing. Two types of materials are presently used: resins and GIC. They have different properties (47). While the caries-preventive effects of resins are based solely on their ability to prevent microleakage of nutrients from the oral cavity to the microflora in the fissure (40), the GICs also inhibit caries by releasing fluoride. Resins are favorable with respect to long-term retention and resistance to abrasive wear, but their ability to prevent caries is dependent on optimal moisture control. The GIC sealants have low strength and short retention rate compared with resins (91), but their major advantage is that they can be applied to teeth which are difficult to isolate with no increased risk of caries. The GIC sealant may therefore be considered as a temporary sealant and a fluoride vehicle. The procedures for resin and GIC fissure sealing are presented in Boxes 10-7 and 10-8. The procedures may differ between different brands, and the manufacturer's instructions should be followed. There are only a few GICs specially designed for fissure sealing on the market. A resin-reinforced light-polymerized GIC liner (Vitrebond®) has been tested by Raadal *et al.* (91) and was found to be easy to handle.

Box 10-7 Fissure sealing with resin

1. Plaque and pellicle must be carefully removed by pumice or air-polishing instruments in order to obtain an optimal acid etch pattern of the enamel surface.
2. Acid etch for at least 20 s, rinse thoroughly with water.
3. Dam is optimal, but should not be used in partly erupted teeth due to pain and damage to the gingiva.
4. Apply the sealant to cover the fissure completely without overfilling and overextending it (Fig. 10-22). Polymerization may be induced by light or by mixing with initiator before the application.
5. Check that the resin is set, retained, and covers the whole fissure.

Box 10-8 Fissure sealing with a resin reinforced light polymerized GIC cement (Vitrebond®)

1. Plaque and debris are carefully removed from the fissure by the use of pumice and rubber cup to allow an optimal bond.
2. The tooth surface is dried, but not desiccated (the GIC cement bonds optimally to slightly humid enamel surfaces).
3. Apply the sealant and cure with light for 30 s.
4. Check for retention and full coverage.

Indications for fissure sealing. Fissure sealing can be used to prevent caries as well as to arrest caries lesions. Several studies have shown that resins are able to stop lesion progression even in the dentin, provided that the quality of the seal is effective in preventing leakage of nutrients to the bacteria in the dentin (40). The crucial points are sufficient removal of soft debris and optimal dryness of the fissure before application of the resin. Many dentists are, however, reluctant to leave carious dentin underneath a sealing, and it is recommended that obvious softened tooth tissue be removed before sealing (preventive fillings, see next section). This means that, generally, noncavitated enamel lesions (codes 1 and 2, Fig. 10-2) can be sealed without the preparation of a cavity, while cavitated lesions (codes 3 and higher) should be restored.

Should all pits and fissures be sealed? First of all, the question is a matter of use of resources and in this respect the caries prevalence level of both individuals and the population should be taken into account (5). Even if a qualified application of sealants to sound fissures does not harm the tooth, it has a cost since each application takes considerable time for highly qualified personnel (dentists, dental hygienists, dental assistants). A "sealing-all-teeth" policy also increases the risk of negative effects, i.e., the treatment initiates caries in sound fissures due to poor moisture control, as has been shown to be an inevitable result of most such programs. The primary indication for the use of sealants should therefore be pits and fissures with initial caries lesions without cavity formation (active enamel lesions) (47). Children with high caries prevalence in primary teeth constitute a risk group for developing occlusal caries in permanent first molars and they should therefore be candidates for fissure sealing (90).

The use of resin sealants is usually contraindicated in erupting teeth due to the difficulties in maintaining good moisture control. Since GIC is suitable as a temporary sealant and fluoride vehicle in cases where moisture control is difficult, it is the material of choice for non-operative caries treatment of initial caries in newly erupted teeth. The eruption period is usually a high-risk period for caries in molars. Even if many lesions are arrested without treatment when the teeth reach occlusion and are subjected to the masticatory forces (16), the GIC sealant is a quick and nonrisky method for fissures with initial caries.

Preventive resin/GIC restorations. A variety of terms are used for the procedure that combines restoring and sealing techniques with resins or GICs (21). The

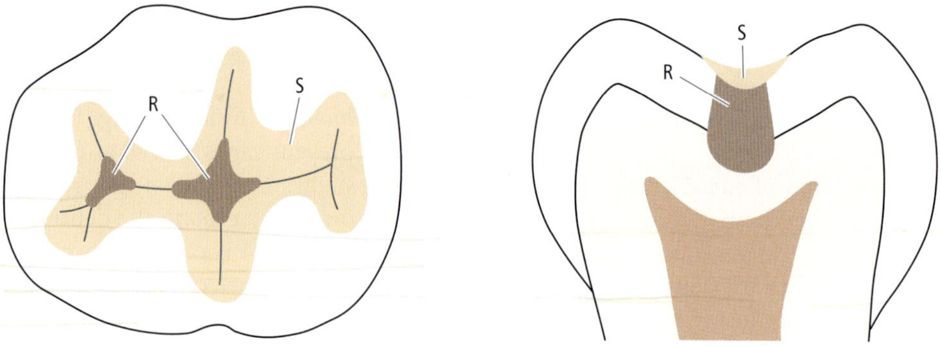

Figure 10-20 Preventive resin/GIC restoration; R = restorative material (resin or GIC), S = sealant.

procedure includes removal of soft carious tissue in parts of the fissure followed by the application of a restorative/sealant material covering all parts of the fissure (Fig. 10-20). The main idea is minimal loss of sound tissue combined with the prevention or arrest of caries in other parts of the fissures.

The removal of soft tissue must be made by using slowly rotating burs to avoid the removal of sound enamel and dentin. The whole fissure must be carefully cleaned for plaque and debris as part of the fissure sealing procedure. The filling material may be GIC, compomer, or composite, depending on the case. For newly erupted teeth or other situations where moisture control is difficult to obtain, GICs should be preferred ("preventive GIC restoration"). The material is applied with a syringe, thereafter covered with a plastic foil and adjusted with a burnisher. After the initial cure, excess material is removed with a rotating bur under water spray and finally the surface is covered with a film to protect the cement during its further maturation process.

Since the GICs are more susceptible to loss of retention and abrasive wear, the longer lasting resin sealants should be preferred in cases where moisture control is not a problem. The cavity is filled with a composite resin or a compomer, and after having trimmed away excess material, the whole fissure is acid etched and covered with resin sealant ("preventive resin restoration").

The combination of modern restorative and sealing techniques allows a variety of preventive, nonoperative, and restorative approaches for fissure caries. The general principles based on the individual caries status and possibilities for moisture control are suggested in Box 10-9. It should, however, be emphasized that the basic methods for caries prevention based on plaque removal and fluoride application can be effective also for preventing fissure caries. This has been shown in studies from Nexø in Denmark (17), where the program was based on intensive patient education combined with individualized professional tooth cleaning during the eruption of permanent first molars.

The mesial surface of permanent first molars

The mesial surface of the permanent first molar is most often the first approximal surface to be restored in the permanent dentition. At the age of 12 years, this surface accounted for more than 90% of all restored approximal surfaces in permanent teeth (70).

If a cavitated lesion is directly accessible after exfoliation of the second primary molar and before eruption of the second premolar, or after preparing the adjacent approximal surface, a modified one-surface restoration can be made. Presupposing that the lesion is limited and does not undermine the marginal ridge, the material of choice would be a composite resin or compomer where the retention is based on the adhesive techniques (acid etching and dentin bonding). After polishing the filling, acid etching of the enamel surface and a layer of resin should be placed to make the surface as smooth as possible. In extremely caries-active individuals, GIC should be placed, although this material probably will degrade with time and therefore needs to be replaced.

Box 10-9 Indications for fissure sealing/preventive resin restorations

Fissure caries status	Individual caries risk (child/tooth)	Possibility for moisture control	Treatment decision
	Low risk	Good or poor	No
Sound Code 0	High risk	Good	Resin sealant
		Poor	GIC sealant
Caries Code (grade) 1–2	Low or high	Good	Resin sealant
		Poor	GIC sealant
Caries Code (grade) 2–3	Low or high	Good	Preventive resin restoration
		Poor	Preventive GIC restoration

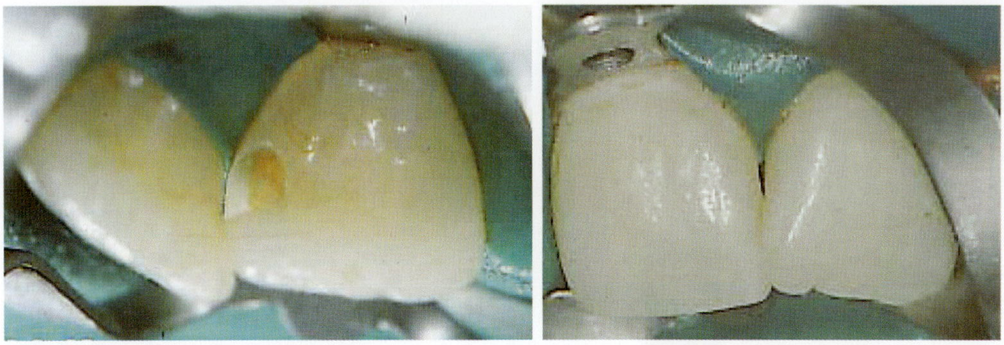

Figure 10-21 Class III cavity in maxillary incisor.

If access to the lesion has to be made from the occlusal surface, two options are available: the conventional Class II preparation or the saucer-shaped cavity form. These are described later in this chapter.

Approximal surfaces of young permanent incisors

Access to approximal caries is obtained from the buccal or lingual aspect, where the least loss of sound tooth substance can be achieved (Fig. 10-21). The size of the cavity is determined by the extent of the lesion. A slight beveling of the cavo-surface margin, giving an increased area for acid etching, is recommended if a composite resin is used. Before the acid etching and bonding a liner should be used to cover the deepest part of the cavity if the lesion is deep and judged to be close to the pulp. In extremely caries-active individuals, GIC or RMGIC may be preferable although its longevity is limited.

12–19 years

Between 6 and 13 years of age, occlusal caries in permanent molars dominates over approximal caries; at the age of 13 years, more than 80% of all decayed dentinal lesions or filled surfaces involve occlusal surfaces (70). During adolescence and young adulthood, the proportion of affected approximal surfaces continues to increase in relation to affected occlusal caries (56,70). At 27 years, almost half of the decayed and filled surfaces involve approximal surfaces as illustrated in Fig. 10-22. This clearly shows that approximal surfaces deserve special attention during adolescence.

Rate of lesion progression: caries rates and survival times in permanent teeth

Occlusal surfaces. The occlusal surface of permanent first molars is still considered the most caries-susceptible surface in children and adolescents. It has been shown, however, that the first year after eruption constitutes the highest risk period (4,59) and after the age of 13 years there is a significant drop in the incidence of dentinal

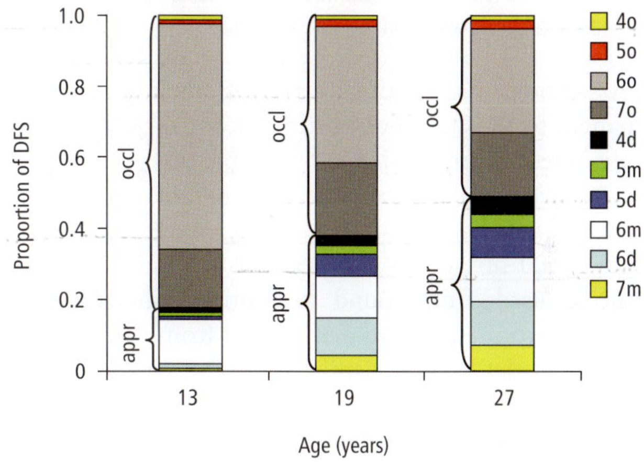

Figure 10-22 The relative percentage distribution of approximal (appr) and occlusal (occl) DFS (decayed and filled surfaces) at ages of 13, 19, and 27 years evaluated from radiographic examinations. For approximal surfaces D equals a radiolucency at the enamel–dentin border or deeper and for occlusal surfaces D equals an obvious radiolucency in dentin. The same individuals ($n = 250$) are followed from 13 to 27 years of age. From Mejàre *et al.* (100).

caries (70). The permanent second molar experiences its highest risk period within the first 3 years after eruption (4,11,70). Therefore, preventive and nonoperative measures directed towards occlusal surfaces of permanent molars should focus on the first year(s) after their eruption. Compared with molars, the occlusal surfaces of premolars run a small risk of developing dentin caries (69). This is illustrated in Fig. 10-26 where it can be seen that more than 90% of occlusal surfaces of premolars remained healthy ("survived") until the age of 27 years without developing radiographically visible dentin caries.

Approximal surfaces of premolars and molars. Figure 10-22 shows that the mesial and distal surfaces of the permanent first molar and the distal surface of the second premolar are the most caries-susceptible surfaces during adolescence and young adulthood. In a population with a generally low caries prevalence, the rate of

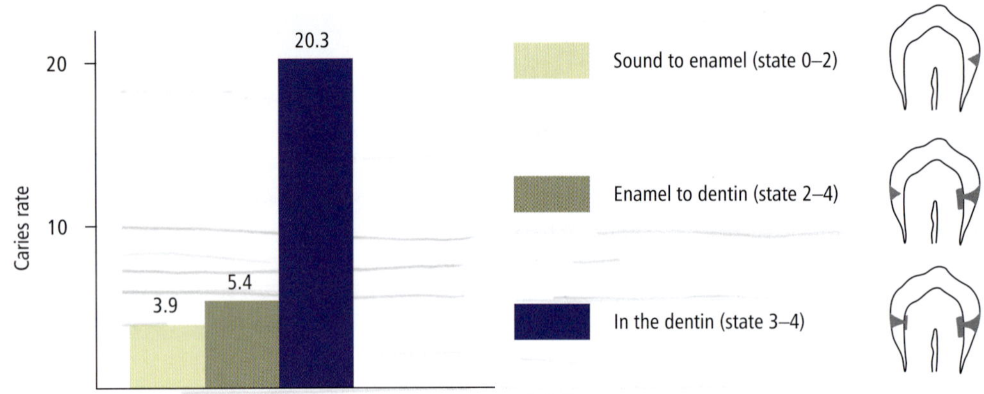

Figure 10-23 Caries rates (number of new lesions/100 tooth surface-years) of approximal surfaces from 11 to 22 years of age. Median values of all surfaces. From Mejàre *et al.* (105).

progression of approximal caries lesions in young permanent teeth is, however, usually slow (53,66,102). The rate of lesion progression can be expressed as incidence rate (*caries rate*). For example, a caries rate of 3.9 means that 3.9 new caries lesions can be expected to develop out of 100 surfaces at risk per year. Several transitions can be used: from sound to dentin, from sound to enamel, from enamel to dentin, and from the enamel–dentin border to outer dentin. From Fig. 10-23 it can be seen that the annual caries rate was 3.9 new enamel lesions during an 11-year period (from age 11 to 22 years). The caries rate was higher from enamel to dentin (5.4), and after the lesion had reached the dentin, the rate was almost four times higher (20.3). These are median values, and there were considerable differences between individuals.

The rate of lesion progression can also be expressed as the *survival time*, i.e., the period of time a lesion remains in a particular caries state until it progresses to the next state. In low-caries prevalence populations the median survival time for a lesion at the enamel–dentin border until it has progressed into the outer half of the dentin is about 3 years. This implies that about half of these lesions progressed into the dentin during this time, while the other half did not. Some lesions progressed faster than 3 years. The survival time seems to be about the same in nonfluoridated and fluoridated areas (56,66). Figure 10-24 shows the ninetieth percentiles for three transitions; sound to enamel, enamel to dentin, and in dentin. Ninety percent of lesions that were confined to the inner part of the enamel survived 31 months before progressing to a dentin lesion. This means that 10% of them progressed into the dentin during this period. Likewise, 10% of enamel–dentin border lesions progressed within 8–9 months.

Factors influencing caries development and lesion progression. Can lesions with a high risk of progression be identified? In the individual case we can never be sure.

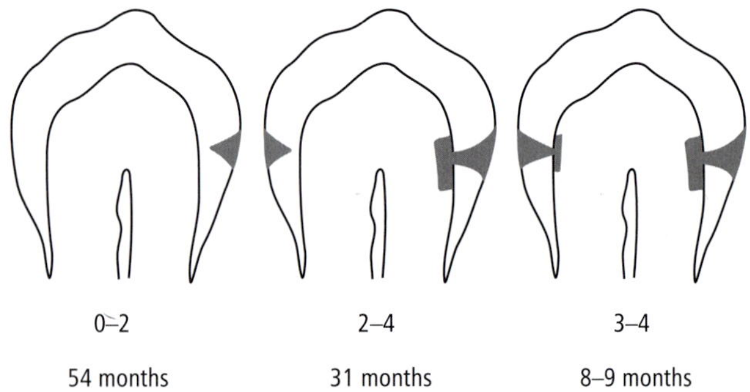

Figure 10-24 Survival times of approximal caries lesions from 11 to 22 years of age. The ninetieth percentiles of three progression states: from 0 to 2, from 2 to 4, and from 3 to 4. From Mejàre *et al.* (100).

As mentioned earlier, cavitation is the crucial turning point for the rate of lesion progression. Some additional factors influence lesion progression:

- *Type of tooth surface.* Considerable differences in survival time of lesions were observed for different surfaces (66). For lesion progression in the dentin, lesions in the distal surface of the maxillary second premolar had the shortest survival time of 2.1 years (Fig. 10-25). Lesions in the distal surface of the mandibular first molar and the mesial surface of the mandibular second molar were also at risk of relatively fast progression with a survival time of 2.8 years, which is lower than the median value of 3.1 years.
- *Posteruptive age of the tooth.* Few studies have investigated the rate of progression as a function of posteruptive age. In a study including both Swedish and US children and young adults, Shwartz *et al.* (102) reported that the median survival time of enamel lesions was about 4 years in 10–11-year-old children and more than 7 years for those aged 17–22 years (the ages at the end of the study). In another study (68), the caries rate for the mesial surface of the permanent

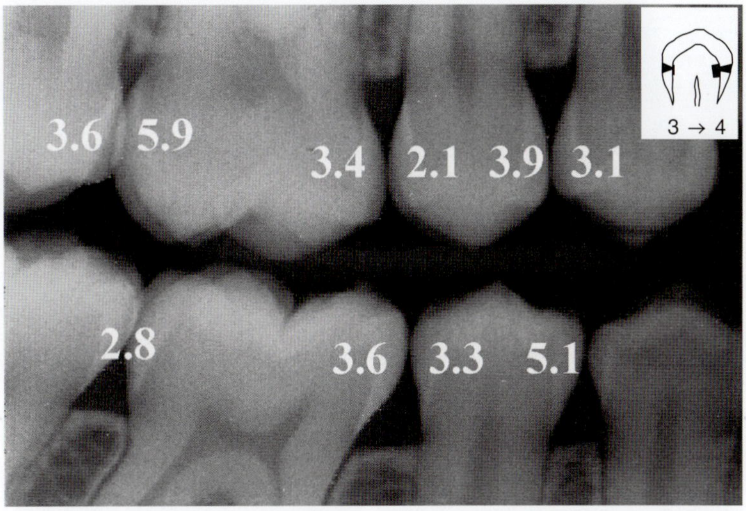

Figure 10-25 Median values of survival times (years) from caries state 3 to state 4 (progression within dentin) at different approximal surfaces. From Mejàre *et al*. (105).

first molars was compared in two age groups, 6–11 and 12–22 years, in the same individuals. While the rate of progression from sound to the inner half of the enamel was not significantly higher in the younger age group, the rate from the inner half of the enamel to the outer half of the dentin was almost four times faster in the younger age group. Thus, progression through the enamel is comparatively fast in newly erupted young permanent teeth, particularly for the mesial surface of the permanent first molar, while it is slower in older adolescents and young adults.

In a longitudinal 15-year study, the rates of lesion progression were compared for three age groups: 12–15, 16–19, and 20–27 years (Fig. 10-27). It can be seen that the survival time of both sound surfaces and progression of enamel and dentin lesions depend on age:

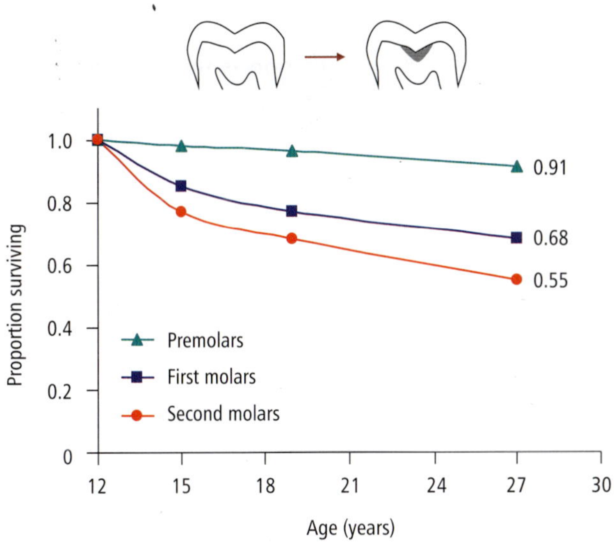

Figure 10-26 Cumulative survival curves of occlusal surfaces (premolars, first and second molars) from radiographically sound to obvious radiolucency in dentin. The slopes of the curves of molars show that most new dentin lesions occurred between 12 and 15 years of age and particularly concerned the second molar. It should be noted that, for the first molar, the data show only those who were radiographically sound at age 12 years. From Mejàre *et al*. (100).

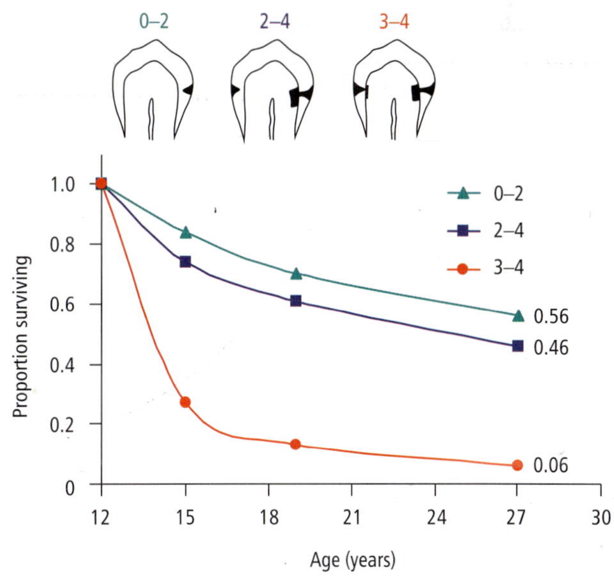

Figure 10-27 Cumulative survival curves of approximal surfaces from radiographically sound to inner enamel caries, from inner enamel caries to caries in outer dentin and from caries at the enamel–dentin border to caries in outer dentin from 12 to 27 years of age. From Mejàre *et al*. (100).

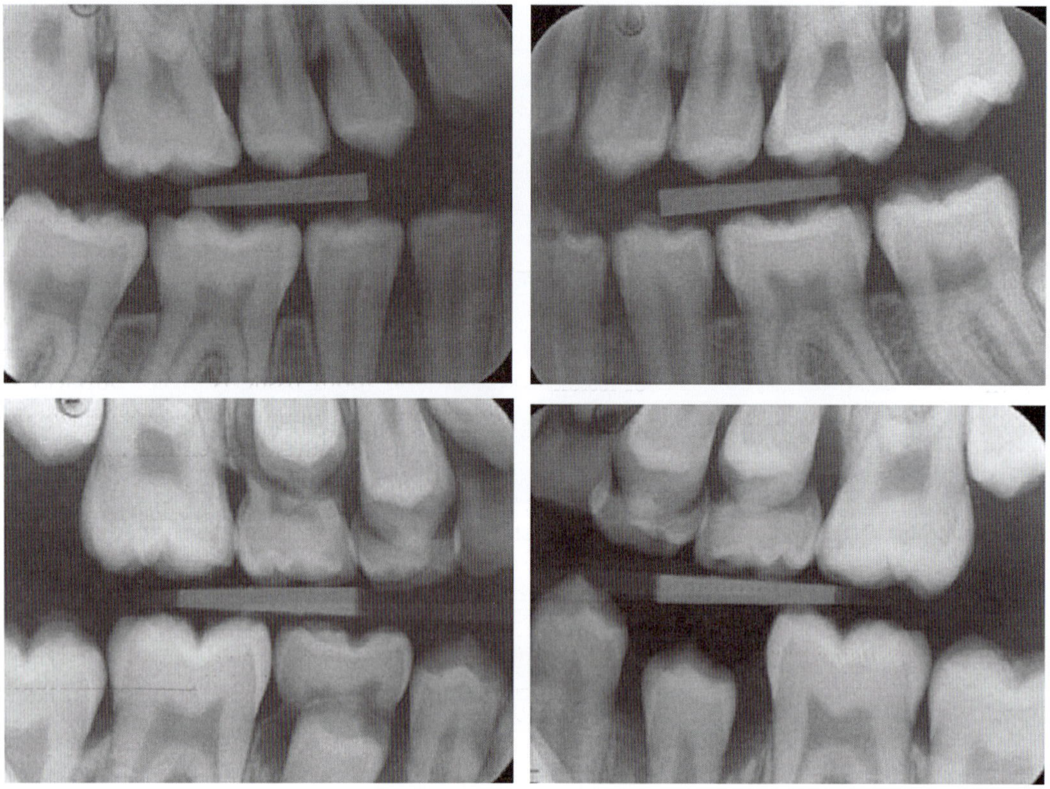

Figure 10-28. Two 12 year olds; one has almost fully erupted premolars and second molars while the other still is in the process of shedding primary molars.

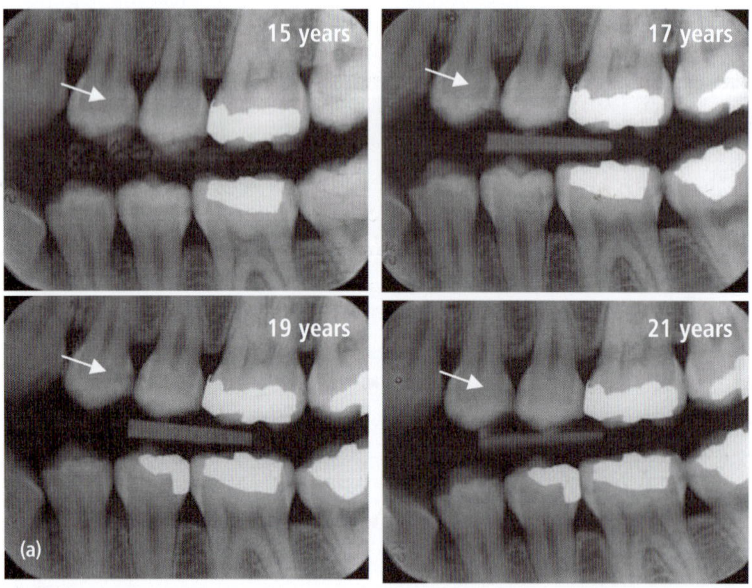

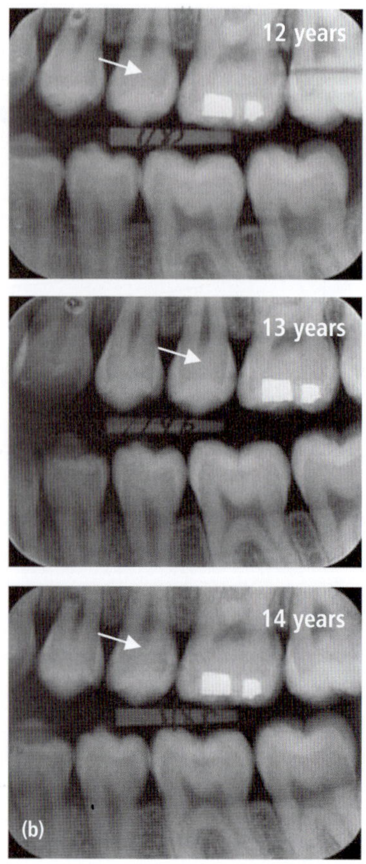

Figure 10-29 (a) Bitewing radiographs from the same individual from 15 to 21 years of age showing slow progression of lesions on the distal surface of upper left first premolar and mesial surface of the second premolar. The enamel lesions on these surfaces have not progressed into the dentin during these 6 years. (b) Bitewing radiographs from age 12 to 14 years showing relatively fast progression of a lesion on the distal surface of the upper left second premolar. The enamel lesion present at age 12 years has progressed into the dentin within 2 years.

the older the individual, the longer the survival times. It is obvious that the first 2–3 years after eruption constitute a risk period for new approximal caries lesions as well as for progression of established lesions. For the younger age group (12–15 years), it is important to be aware of the variation in age at tooth eruption between children. This is illustrated in Fig. 10-28. The survival time for enamel–dentin border lesions (from state 3 to 4) suggests that for lesions at the enamel–dentin border we can use the "wait-and-see" philosophy more safely in young adults than in young teenagers where a substantially higher risk of lesions progression can be expected. An example of the difference in approximal lesion progression is given in Fig. 10-29.

- *Neighboring tooth surface.* Limited data exist on the effect on lesion development of caries on neighboring approximal tooth surfaces. A Swedish study of 6–12 year olds showed that the mesial surface of the permanent first molar had a negligible risk for developing caries when adjacent to a sound approximal surface of a primary second molar. If the primary molar had a caries lesion, the rate was almost 15 times higher (69).
- *Caries experience.* Several studies show that children with approximal dentin lesions at the age of 12–13 years run a higher risk of developing new approximal lesions, as well as progression of existing lesions, than those with none or few such lesions (36,55,66). For example, children showing enamel lesions in premolars and second molars at the age of 12 years are at high risk of developing several lesions in need of operative treatment (22). The number of lesions also plays a role. Thus, the more lesions, the higher the risk of relatively fast progression of at least one lesion.
- *Iatrogenic damage on neighboring surfaces.* During the preparation of a Class II cavity the surface enamel of the neighboring approximal surface was damaged in about 70% of the cases in a Danish study (86). The authors also observed a faster caries progression on damaged surfaces compared with nondamaged. The reasons for this are probably that the bur had removed the outer well-mineralized and relatively caries-resistant layer of the enamel, and that the surface became rough and more susceptible to plaque accumulation. The use of a protecting device during approximal cavity preparation is therefore mandatory.

These factors can aid in assessing the risk of new caries as well as the risk of lesion progression in individuals and in individual teeth and tooth surfaces. They can also be of help in deciding the appropriate time for restoring and the proper length of recall intervals.

Indications for operative treatment

Incisors. Active cavitated caries lesions in incisors are relatively uncommon in low-caries populations. If present on approximal surfaces, operative treatment is usually necessary not least for aesthetic reasons. The same may apply to buccal surfaces.

Occlusal surfaces. The indication for operative treatment is the same as for primary molars, that is, an active cavitated lesion (usually with dentin involvement) should be restored to prevent further lesion progression. In this way, the cavity preparation becomes relatively small and tooth tissue is saved. Surfaces with dentin involvement as observed radiographically only (hidden caries) also require intervention in terms of operative treatment or fissure sealing. Any cavity preparation should be conservative (preventive resin/glass-ionomer cement restoration). Arrested lesions need no special attention.

Approximal surfaces of premolars and molars. A Class II restoration in a young permanent premolar or molar involves the removal of the marginal ridge. The contours of the tooth are restored, but no restorative material has so far been able to match the ingenious construction of the tooth tissues forming the marginal ridge and its ability to withstand high loads during function. Furthermore, there will always be a vulnerable border between the restoration and the tooth. It follows that it is important to use nonoperative alternatives instead of drilling and filling unnecessarily. On the other hand, postponing restoration until severe destruction of hard tissue, including undermining of cusps, which seriously weakens the tooth crown, is of no benefit to the patient either. The risk of pulp involvement also has to be considered. It is therefore a challenge to select the right treatment option and choose the proper time for restoring. A number of factors have to be considered; some of them have been mentioned earlier in this chapter.

Two factors dominate: one is the estimated rate of lesion progression if the decision is to use non-operative treatment and monitor instead of restoring, and the other is the expected survival time of a placed restoration. In general, the rate of lesion progression is slower in permanent premolars and molars, and the survival time of Class II restorations is longer compared to primary molars (see also earlier).

The critical border between a fairly slow and fast lesion progression is the formation of an obvious cavity and, as mentioned before in this chapter, cavitation is often difficult to determine. We therefore have to rely on bitewing radiography and the behavior of the lesion as judged from repeated radiographic examinations. The imperfection of the radiographic assessments (see

Chapter 8) also must be taken into account and be part of the treatment decision. The rate of lesion progression varies depending on the caries activity of the individual. Different tooth surfaces show different rates of lesion progression, and the number of lesions present in an individual and the post-eruptive age of the tooth also play a role. These factors were described previously in this chapter.

There may also be practical circumstances to consider. Postponing restorative treatment involves monitoring and sometimes rather close recall intervals. The question "can I trust that the patient will attend at the proposed recall interval?" may therefore also be a factor to take into account and could be decisive for the treatment decision. It is a challenging task to decide on the proper time for restoring an individual lesion and it is equally challenging to express clear and unambiguously. The following general rule should be interpreted and used with the above-mentioned arguments in mind:

The presence of a clinical cavity or a radiolucency that has progressed into the dentin strongly indicates the need to restore a contacting approximal caries lesion. An important finding supporting this rule is that, irrespective of cavitation or not, lesions in the outer half of the dentin were all infected, although the level of infection was significantly lower in noncavitated lesions (93) (Fig. 10-7).

Cavity designs

In accordance with principles of minimally invasive dentistry, the Class II preparation has changed towards a more conservative design. The reasons for this change are several: a lower caries activity, more effective preventive regimens, development of adhesive techniques, and concern about saving tooth substance, and aesthetic considerations.

The saucer-shaped cavity. Along with improvement of the physical properties of composites, the saucer-shaped cavity design (Fig. 10-30) has more and more replaced the conventional Class II preparation and become the first choice for small primary approximal lesions. The saucer-shaped cavity preparation is a conservative procedure that saves sound tooth tissues and preserves dentin supporting the enamel cusps (Fig. 10-31). The outline of the cavity should aim at preserving natural

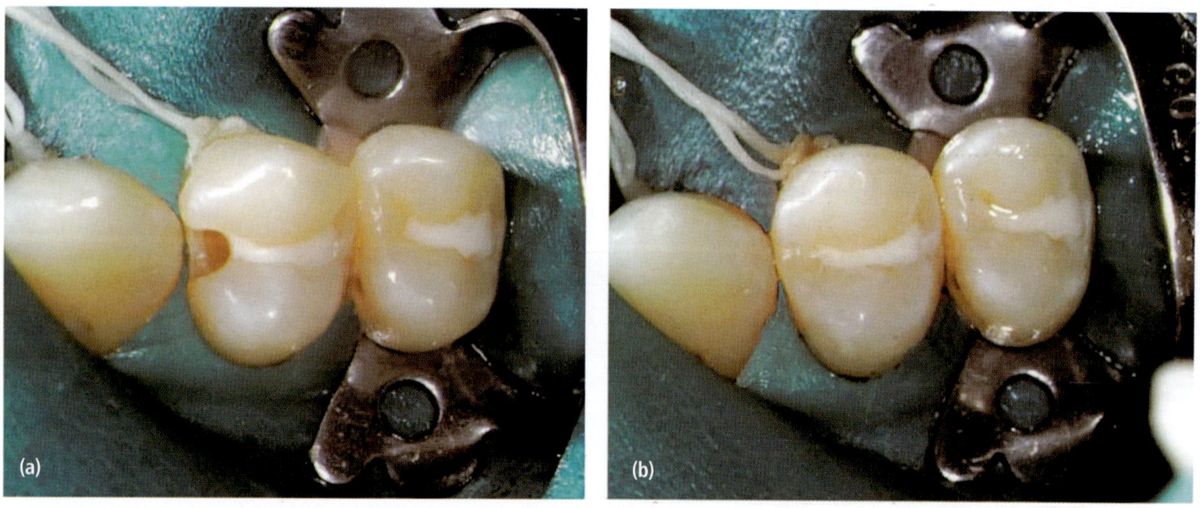

Figure 10-30 The saucer-shaped cavity design: (a) before filling and (b) after filling with a composite resin.

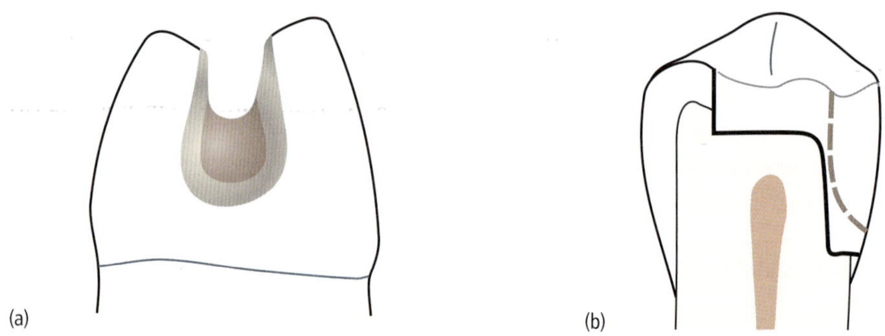

Figure 10-31 (a) The design of the saucer-shaped cavity is based on adhesion of composite resins to enamel and dentin. (b) The saucer-shaped cavity design (dotted line) saves more tooth tissue than the traditional Class II preparation.

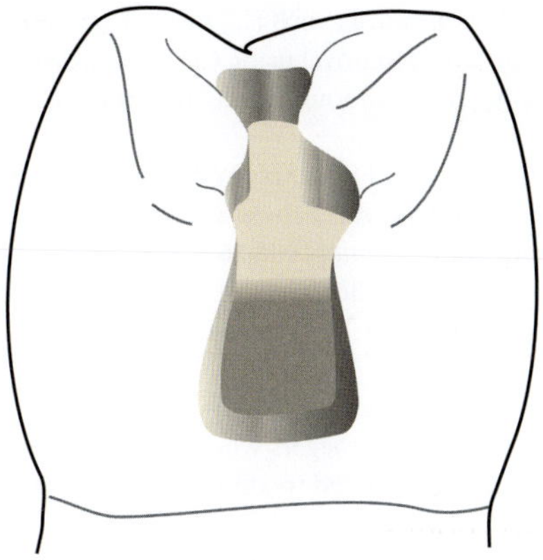

Figure 10-32 Conventional Class II amalgam preparation with minimal buccal–lingual extension.

tissue contacting the neighboring tooth in order to prevent mesial migration resulting from proximal wear.

Important factors for obtaining a successful result are adequate bonding of the composite resin to enamel and dentin, enamel present along the whole preparation outline, and incremental placement of the material in order to avoid adverse shrinkage patterns of the composite. Effective polymerization of every part of the restoration is mandatory and only thin layers should be polymerized at a time. This conservative preparation technique disregards the old principle of "extension for prevention" and relies on adequate oral hygiene and fluoride preventive regimens.

Long-term clinical studies on the success rate of saucer-shaped approximal restorations are relatively scarce. Nordbø *et al.* (77,78) found that 82% of the restorations in young permanent teeth were assessed as successful after 3 years while 70% were acceptable after 7.2 years. The most common cause of failure was recurrent caries and poor marginal adaptation. These authors concluded that the saucer-shaped Class II resin composite restoration should be considered a routine operative treatment for small approximal lesions in posterior teeth.

Important factors that determine the longevity of restorations are given in Box 10-10.

The conventional Class II cavity. The conventional Class II cavity is justified for large cavities where both occlusal and approximal lesions are involved (Fig. 10-32). The cavity design may be used for composites and amalgam. When using amalgam, isthmus fractures are a common cause of failure, most often due to either sharp angles or too small bulk of material. The cavity should be at least 1.5 mm deep in the isthmus area. Beveling the axial–pulpal line angle as well as rounded cavo-surface angles are other important measures to prevent fractures. When composites are used based on adhesive techniques, the occlusal preparation should be conservative in line with the principles of preventive resin restorations (see previous), while the approximal outline is in accordance with the saucer-shaped cavity.

Box 10-10 Important factors determining longevity of approximal restorations

Operator
- Knowledge, skill, and attitude.
- Material properties and handling.

Patient
- Caries activity and quality of oral hygiene.
- Adverse habits such as bruxism and special food preferences.

References

1. Caries Diagnosis, Risk Assessment and Non-operative Treatment of Early Caries Lesions. The Swedish Council on Technology Assessment in Health Care. SBU report No. 188, 2007 (in Swedish).
2. Diagnosis and Management of Dental Caries. In: Evidence report/Technology Assessment. No. 36: AHRQ Publications No. 01-E056; 2001.
3. Prevention of Dental Caries. A Systematic review. The Swedish Council on Technology Assessment in Health Care. SBU report No. 161, 2002 (in Swedish).
4. Abernathy JR, Graves RC, Greenberg BG, Bohannan HM, Disney JA. Application of life table methodology in determining dental caries rates. *Community Dent Oral Epidemiol* 1986;**14**: 261–4.
5. Ahovuo-Saloranta A, Hiiri A, Nordblad A, Worthington H, Makela M. Pit and fissure sealants for preventing dental decay in the permanent teeth of children and adolescents. *Cochrane Database Syst Rev* 2004:CD001830.
6. Alm A, Wendt LK, Koch G. Dental treatment in the primary dentition of 7–12 year-old Swedish schoolchildren. *Swed Dent J* 2003;**27**:77–82.
7. Amarante E, Raadal M, Espelid I. Impact of diagnostic criteria on the prevalence of dental caries in Norwegian children aged 5, 12 and 18 years. *Community Dent Oral Epidemiol* 1998;**26**: 87–94.
8. Ammari JB, Baqain ZH, Ashley PF. Effects of programs for prevention of early childhood caries. A systematic review. *Med Princ Pract* 2007;**16**:437–42.
9. Andersson-Wenckert IE, Folkesson UH, van Dijken JW. Durability of a polyacid-modified composite resin (compomer) in primary molars. A multicenter study. *Acta Odontol Scand* 1997; **55**:255–60.
10. Attari N, Roberts JF. Restoration of primary teeth with crowns: a systematic review of the literature. *Eur Arch Paediatr Dent* 2006;**7**:58–62; discussion 63.
11. Baelum V, Machiulskiene V, Nyvad B, Richards A, Vaeth M. Application of survival analysis to carious lesion transitions in intervention trials. *Community Dent Oral Epidemiol* 2003;**31**: 252–60.

12. Ball IA. The 'fluoride syndrome': occult caries? *Br Dent J* 1986;**160**:75–6.
13. Berg JH. The continuum of restorative materials in pediatric dentistry – a review for the clinician. *Pediatr Dent* 1998;**20**:93–100.
14. Bille J, Thylstrup A. Radiographic diagnosis and clinical tissue changes in relation to treatment of approximal carious lesions. *Caries Res* 1982;**16**:1–6.
15. Burke FM, Ray NJ, McConnell RJ. Fluoride-containing restorative materials. *Int Dent J* 2006;**56**:33–43.
16. Carvalho JC, Ekstrand KR, Thylstrup A. Dental plaque and caries on occlusal surfaces of first permanent molars in relation to stage of eruption. *J Dent Res* 1989;**68**:773–9.
17. Carvalho JC, Thylstrup A, Ekstrand KR. Results after 3 years of non-operative occlusal caries treatment of erupting permanent first molars. *Community Dent Oral Epidemiol* 1992;**20**:187–92.
18. Chadwick BL, Evans DJ. Restoration of class II cavities in primary molar teeth with conventional and resin modified glass ionomer cements: a systematic review of the literature. *Eur Arch Paediatr Dent* 2007;**8**:14–21.
19. Croll TP. Alternatives to silver amalgam and resin composite in pediatric dentistry. *Quintessence Int* 1998;**29**:697–703.
20. Croll TP. Repair of Class I resin-composite restoration. *ASDC J Dent Child* 1997;**64**:22–7.
21. Croll TP, Cavanaugh RR. Direct bonded Class I restorations and sealants: six options. *Quintessence Int* 1997;**28**:157–68.
22. David J, Raadal M, Wang NJ, Strand GV. Caries increment and prediction from 12 to 18 years of age: a follow-up study. *Eur Arch Paediatr Dent* 2006;**7**:31–7.
23. de Araujo FB, de Araujo DR, dos Santos CK, de Souza MA. Diagnosis of approximal caries in primary teeth: radiographic versus clinical examination using tooth separation. *Am J Dent* 1996;**9**:54–6.
24. Dini EL, Holt RD, Bedi R. Caries and its association with infant feeding and oral health-related behaviours in 3–4-year-old Brazilian children. *Community Dent Oral Epidemiol* 2000;**28**:241–8.
25. Drury TF, Horowitz AM, Ismail AI, Maertens MP, Rozier RG, Selwitz RH. Diagnosing and reporting early childhood caries for research purposes. A report of a workshop sponsored by the National Institute of Dental and Craniofacial Research, the Health Resources and Services Administration, and the Health Care Financing Administration. *J Public Health Dent* 1999;**59**:192–7.
26. Edelstein BL. Case planning and management according to caries risk assessment. *Dent Clin North Am* 1995;**39**:721–36.
27. Ekstrand KR, Bruun G, Bruun M. Plaque and gingival status as indicators for caries progression on approximal surfaces. *Caries Res* 1998;**32**:41–5.
28. Ekstrand KR, Martignon S, Ricketts DJ, Qvist V. Detection and activity assessment of primary coronal caries lesions: a methodologic study. *Oper Dent* 2007;**32**:225–35.
29. Ekstrand KR, Ricketts DN, Kidd EA. Reproducibility and accuracy of three methods for assessment of demineralization depth of the occlusal surface: an *in vitro* examination. *Caries Res* 1997;**31**:224–31.
30. Espelid I, Tveit AB, Tornes KH, Alvheim H. Clinical behaviour of glass ionomer restorations in primary teeth. *J Dent* 1999;**27**:437–42.
31. Feasby WH, Ecclestone ER, Grainger RM. Nickel sensitivity in pediatric dental patients. *Pediatr Dent* 1988;**10**:127–9.
32. Fejerskov O, Kidd E. *Dental caries: the disease and its clinical management.* Copenhagen: Blackwell Munksgaard, 2003.
33. Fluckiger L, Waltimo T, Stich H, Lussi A. Comparison of chemomechanical caries removal using Carisolv or conventional hand excavation in deciduous teeth *in vitro*. *J Dent* 2005;**33**:87–90.
34. Frencken JE, Makoni F, Sithole WD. ART restorations and glass ionomer sealants in Zimbabwe: survival after 3 years. *Community Dent Oral Epidemiol* 1998;**26**:372–81.
35. Grindefjord M, Dahllöf G, Ekström G, Höjer B, Modeer T. Caries prevalence in 2.5-year-old children. *Caries Res* 1993;**27**:505–10.
36. Gröndahl HG, Andersson B, Torstensson T. Caries increment and progression in teenagers when using a prevention – rather than restoration-oriented treatment strategy. *Swed Dent J* 1984;**8**:237–42.
37. Guggenberger R, May R, Stefan KP. New trends in GIC chemistry. *Biomaterials* 1998;**19**:479–83.
38. Hallonsten AL, Wendt LK, Mejare I, Birkhed D, Hakansson C, Lindvall AM, *et al.* Dental caries and prolonged breast-feeding in 18-month-old Swedish children. *Int J Paediatr Dent* 1995;**5**:149–55.
39. Handelman SL. Effect of sealant placement on occlusal caries progression. *Clin Prev Dent* 1982;**4**:11–16.
40. Handelman SL. Therapeutic use of sealants for incipient or early carious lesions in children and young adults. *Proc Finn Dent Soc* 1991;**87**:463–75.
41. Handelman SL, Washburn F, Wopperer P. Two-year report of sealant effect on bacteria in dental caries. *J Am Dent Assoc* 1976;**93**:967–70.
42. Hintze H, Wenzel A. Clinically undetected dental caries assessed by bitewing screening in children with little caries experience. *Dentomaxillofac Radiol* 1994;**23**:19–23.
43. Holt RD, Azevedo MR. Fibre optic transillumination and radiographs in diagnosis of approximal caries in primary teeth. *Community Dent Health* 1989;**6**:239–47.
44. Hörsted-Bindslev P, Mjör I. *Modern concepts in operative dentistry.* Copenhagen: Munksgaard, 1988.
45. Hugoson A, Koch G, Hallonsten AL, Norderyd J, Aberg A. Caries prevalence and distribution in 3–20-year-olds in Jonkoping, Sweden, in 1973, 1978, 1983, and 1993. *Community Dent Oral Epidemiol* 2000;**28**:83–9.
46. Kavvadia K, Karagianni V, Polychronopoulou A, Papagiannouli L. Primary teeth caries removal using the Carisolv chemomechanical method: a clinical trial. *Pediatr Dent* 2004;**26**:23–8.
47. Kidd EA, Joyston-Bechal S. Update on fissure sealants. *Dent Update* 1994;**21**:323–6.
48. Kilpatrick NM, Murray JJ, McCabe JF. The use of a reinforced GIC cermet for the restoration of primary molars: a clinical trial. *Br Dent J* 1995;**179**:175–9.
49. Kilpatrick NM, Neumann A. Durability of amalgam in the restoration of class II cavities in primary molars: a systematic review of the literature. *Eur Arch Paediatr Dent* 2007;**8**:5–13.
50. Kramer MS, Kakuma R. Optimal duration of exclusive breastfeeding. *Cochrane Database Syst Rev* 2002:CD003517.
51. Kramer MS, Vanilovich I, Matush L, Bogdanovich N, Zhang X, Shishko G, *et al.* The effect of prolonged and exclusive breastfeeding on dental caries in early school-age children. New evidence from a large randomized trial. *Caries Res* 2007;**41**:484–8.
52. Kuhnisch J, Heinrich-Weltzien R, Tabatabaie M, Stosser L, Huysmans MC. An *in vitro* comparison between two methods of electrical resistance measurement for occlusal caries detection. *Caries Res* 2006;**40**:104–11.

53. Lervik T, Haugejorden O, Aas C. Progression of posterior approximal carious lesions in Norwegian teenagers from 1982 to 1986. *Acta Odontol Scand* 1990;**48**:223–7.
54. Levine RS, Pitts NB, Nugent ZJ. The fate of 1,587 unrestored carious deciduous teeth: a retrospective general dental practice based study from northern England. *Br Dent J* 2002;**193**: 99–103.
55. Lith A, Gröndahl HG. Predicting development of approximal dentin lesions by means of past caries experience. *Community Dent Oral Epidemiol* 1992;**20**:25–9.
56. Lith A, Lindstrand C, Gröndahl HG. Caries development in a young population managed by a restrictive attitude to radiography and operative intervention: II. A study at the surface level. *Dentomaxillofac Radiol* 2002;**31**:232–9.
57. Lunder N, von der Fehr FR. Approximal cavitation related to bite-wing image and caries activity in adolescents. *Caries Res* 1996;**30**:143–7.
58. Lussi A. Comparison of different methods for the diagnosis of fissure caries without cavitation. *Caries Res* 1993;**27**:409–16.
59. Månsson B. Caries progression in the first permanent molars. A longitudinal study. *Swed Dent J* 1977;**1**:185–91.
60. Marks LA, van Amerongen WE, Borgmeijer PJ, Groen HJ, Martens LC. Ketac molar versus Dyract class II restorations in primary molars: twelve month clinical results. *ASDC J Dent Child* 2000;**67**:37–41, 8–9.
61. Marsh P, Martin M. *Oral microbiology*. 4th edn. Oxford: Butterworth-Heinemann; 1999.
62. Matee M, van't Hof M, Maselle S, Mikx F, van Palenstein Helderman W. Nursing caries, linear hypoplasia, and nursing and weaning habits in Tanzanian infants. *Community Dent Oral Epidemiol* 1994;**22**:289–93.
63. Mattos-Graner RO, Zelante F, Line RC, Mayer MP. Association between caries prevalence and clinical, microbiological and dietary variables in 1.0 to 2.5-year-old Brazilian children. *Caries Res* 1998;**32**:319–23.
64. McLean JW, Nicholson JW, Wilson AD. Proposed nomenclature for GIC dental cements and related materials. *Quintessence Int* 1994;**25**:587–9.
65. Mejàre I, Gröndahl HG, Carlstedt K, Grever AC, Ottosson E. Accuracy at radiography and probing for the diagnosis of proximal caries. *Scand J Dent Res* 1985;**93**:178–84.
66. Mejàre I, Källestål C, Stenlund H. Incidence and progression of approximal caries from 11 to 22 years of age in Sweden: a prospective radiographic study. *Caries Res* 1999;**33**:93–100.
67. Mejàre I, Malmgren B. Clinical and radiographic appearance of proximal carious lesions at the time of operative treatment in young permanent teeth. *Scand J Dent Res* 1986;**94**: 19–26.
68. Mejàre I, Stenlund H. Caries rates for the mesial surface of the first permanent molar and the distal surface of the second primary molar from 6 to 12 years of age in Sweden. *Caries Res* 2000;**34**:454–61.
69. Mejàre I, Stenlund H, Julihn A, Larsson I, Permert L. Influence of approximal caries in primary molars on caries rate for the mesial surface of the first permanent molar in Swedish children from 6 to 12 years of age. *Caries Res* 2001;**35**:178–85.
70. Mejàre I, Stenlund H, Zelezny-Holmlund C. Caries incidence and lesion progression from adolescence to young adulthood: a prospective 15-year cohort study in Sweden. *Caries Res* 2004; **38**:130–41.
71. Meller C, Nourallah AW, Heyduck C, Steffen H, Splieth CH. Chemo-mechanical dentine caries removal with Carisolv using a rotating brush. *Eur J Paediatr Dent* 2006;**7**:73–6.
72. Mertz-Fairhurst EJ, Curtis JW, Jr., Ergle JW, Rueggeberg FA, Adair SM. Ultraconservative and cariostatic sealed restorations: results at year 10. *J Am Dent Assoc* 1998;**129**:55–66.
73. Mertz-Fairhurst EJ, Schuster GS, Fairhurst CW. Arresting caries by sealants: results of a clinical study. *J Am Dent Assoc* 1986; **112**:194–7.
74. Milnes AR. Description and epidemiology of nursing caries. *J Public Health Dent* 1996;**56**:38–50.
75. Milsom KM, Tickle M, Blinkhorn AS. Dental pain and dental treatment of young children attending the general dental service. *Br Dent J* 2002;**192**:280–4.
76. Modéer T, Twetman S, Bergstrand F. Three-year study of the effect of fluoride varnish (Duraphat) on proximal caries progression in teenagers. *Scand J Dent Res* 1984;**92**:400–7.
77. Nordbø H, Leirskar J, von der Fehr FR. Saucer-shaped cavity preparation for composite resin restorations in class II carious lesions: three-year results. *J Prosthet Dent* 1993;**9**:155–9.
78. Nordbø H, Leirskar J, von der Fehr FR. Saucer-shaped cavity preparations for posterior approximal resin composite restorations: observations up to 10 years. *Quintessence Int* 1998;**29**: 5–11.
79. Nugent ZJ, Pitts NB. Patterns of change and results overview 1985/6–1995/6 from the British Association for the Study of Community Dentistry (BASCD) coordinated National Health Service surveys of caries prevalence. *Community Dent Health* 1997;**14** Suppl 1:30–54.
80. Nyvad B, Machiulskiene V, Baelum V. Construct and predictive validity of clinical caries diagnostic criteria assessing lesion activity. *J Dent Res* 2003;**82**:117–22.
81. Nyvad B, Machiulskiene V, Baelum V. Reliability of a new caries diagnostic system differentiating between active and inactive caries lesions. *Caries Res* 1999;**33**:252–60.
82. Pitts N. "ICDAS" – an international system for caries detection and assessment being developed to facilitate caries epidemiology, research and appropriate clinical management. *Community Dental Health* 2004;**21**:193–8.
83. Pitts NB. Are we ready to move from operative to non-operative/preventive treatment of dental caries in clinical practice? *Caries Res* 2004;**38**:294–304.
84. Pitts NB. Modern concepts of caries measurement. *J Dent Res* 2004;**83** Spec. No. C:C43–7.
85. Pitts NB, Rimmer PA. An *in vivo* comparison of radiographic and directly assessed clinical caries status of posterior approximal surfaces in primary and permanent teeth. *Caries Res* 1992; **26**:146–52.
86. Qvist V, Johannessen L, Bruun M. Progression of approximal caries in relation to iatrogenic preparation damage. *J Dent Res* 1992;**71**:1370–3.
87. Qvist V, Laurberg L, Poulsen A, Teglers PT. Class II restorations in primary teeth: 7-year study on three resin-modified glass ionomer cements and a compomer. *Eur J Oral* Sci 2004;**112**: 188–96.
88. Qvist V, Laurberg L, Poulsen A, Teglers PT. Eight-year study on conventional glass ionomer and amalgam restorations in primary teeth. *Acta Odontol Scand* 2004;**62**:37–45.
89. Qvist V, Laurberg L, Poulsen A, Teglers PT. Longevity and cariostatic effects of everyday conventional GIC and amalgam restorations in primary teeth: three-year results. *J Dent Res* 1997;**76**:1387–96.
90. Raadal M, Espelid I. Caries prevalence in primary teeth as a predictor of early fissure caries in permanent first molars. *Community Dent Oral Epidemiol* 1992;**20**:30–4.
91. Raadal M, Utkilen AB, Nilsen OL. Fissure sealing with a light-

cured resin-reinforced GIC cement (Vitrebond) compared with a resin sealant. *Int J Paediatr Dent* 1996;**6**:235–9.

92. Ramos-Gomez FJ, Tomar SL, Ellison J, Artiga N, Sintes J, Vicuna G. Assessment of early childhood caries and dietary habits in a population of migrant Hispanic children in Stockton, California. *ASDC J Dent Child* 1999;**66**:395–403, 366.
93. Ratledge DK, Kidd EA, Beighton D. A clinical and microbiological study of approximal carious lesions. Part 1: the relationship between cavitation, radiographic lesion depth, the site-specific gingival index and the level of infection of the dentine. *Caries Res* 2001;**35**:3–7.
94. Reis A, Mendes FM, Angnes V, Angnes G, Grande RH, Loguercio AD. Performance of methods of occlusal caries detection in permanent teeth under clinical and laboratory conditions. *J Dent* 2006;**34**:89–96.
95. Ribeiro M, Ribeiro M. Breastfeeding and early childhood caries: a critical review. *J Pediatric (Rio J)* 2004;**80**:199–210.
96. Ripa LW. Nursing caries: a comprehensive review. *Pediatr Dent* 1988;**10**:268–82.
97. Roberts JF, Sherriff M. The fate and survival of amalgam and preformed crown molar restorations placed in a specialist paediatric dental practice. *Br Dent J* 1990;**169**:237–44.
98. Roeters JJ, Frankenmolen F, Burgersdijk RC, Peters TC. Clinical evaluation of Dyract in primary molars: 3-year results. *Am J Dent* 1998;**11**:143–8.
99. Rugg-Gunn AJ. Approximal carious lesions. A comparison of the radiological and clinical appearances. *Br Dent J* 1972;**133**: 481–4.
100. Rutar J, McAllan L, Tyas MJ. Three-year clinical performance of glass ionomer cement in primary molars. *Int J Paediatr Dent* 2002;**12**:146–7.
101. Sayegh A, Dini EL, Holt RD, Bedi R. Oral health, sociodemographic factors, dietary and oral hygiene practices in Jordanian children. *J Dent* 2005;**33**:379–88.
102. Shwartz M, Gröndahl HG, Pliskin JS, Boffa J. A longitudinal· analysis from bite-wing radiographs of the rate of progression of approximal carious lesions through human dental enamel. *Arch Oral Biol* 1984;**29**:529–36.
103. Skeie MS, Raadal M, Strand GV, Espelid I. The relationship between caries in the primary dentition at 5 years of age and permanent dentition at 10 years of age – a longitudinal study. *Int J Paediatr Dent* 2006;**16**:152–60.
104. Stewart PW, Stamm JW. Classification tree prediction models for dental caries from clinical, microbiological, and interview data. *J Dent Res* 1991;**70**:1239–51.
105. Taifour D, Frencken JE, van't Hof MA, Beiruti N, Truin GJ. Effects of glass ionomer sealants in newly erupted first molars after 5 years: a pilot study. *Community Dent Oral Epidemiol* 2003;**31**:314–19.
106. Thylstrup A, Bruun C, Holmen L. *In vivo* caries models – mechanisms for caries initiation and arrestment. *Adv Dent Res* 1994; **8**:144–57.
107. Valaitis R, Hesch R, Passarelli C, Sheehan D, Sinton J. A systematic review of the relationship between breastfeeding and early childhood caries. *Can J Public Health* 2000;**91**:411–17.
108. Vanobbergen J, Martens L, Lesaffre E, Bogaerts K, Declerck D. The value of a baseline caries risk assessment model in the primary dentition for the prediction of caries incidence in the permanent dentition. *Caries Res* 2001;**35**:442–50.
109. Walls AW, Murray JJ, McCabe JF. The use of glass polyalkenoate (ionomer) cements in the deciduous dentition. *Br Dent J* 1988; **165**:13–17.
110. Weerheijm KL, Groen HJ, Bast AJ, Kieft JA, Eijkman MA, van Amerongen WE. Clinically undetected occlusal dentine caries: a radiographic comparison. *Caries Res* 1992;**26**:305–9.
111. Weerheijm KL, Uyttendaele-Speybrouck BF, Euwe HC, Groen HJ. Prolonged demand breast-feeding and nursing caries. *Caries Res* 1998;**32**:46–50.
112. Welbury RR, Walls AW, Murray JJ, McCabe JF. The 5-year results of a clinical trial comparing a glass polyalkenoate (ionomer) cement restoration with an amalgam restoration. *Br Dent J* 1991;**170**:177–81.
113. Wendt LK, Birkhed D. Dietary habits related to caries development and immigrant status in infants and toddlers living in Sweden. *Acta Odontol Scand* 1995;**53**:339–44.
114. Wendt LK, Hallonsten AL, Koch G. Oral health in preschool children living in Sweden. Part II – A longitudinal study. Findings at three years of age. *Swed Dent J* 1992;**16**:41–9.
115. Wendt LK, Hallonsten AL, Koch G, Birkhed D. Analysis of caries-related factors in infants and toddlers living in Sweden. *Acta Odontol Scand* 1996;**54**:131–7.
116. Wendt LK, Koch G, Birkhed D. Replacements of restorations in the primary and young permanent dentition. *Swed Dent J* 1998;**22**:149–55.
117. Yilmaz Y, Eyuboglu O, Kocogullari ME, Belduz N. A one-year clinical evaluation of a high-viscosity glass ionomer cement in primary molars. *J Contemp Dent Pract* 2006;**7**:71–8.
118. Östlund J, Möller K, Koch G. Amalgam, composite resin and glass ionomer cement in Class II restorations in primary molars – a three year clinical evaluation. *Swed Dent J* 1992;**16**:81–6.

11

Dental erosion

Ann-Katrin Johansson, Göran Koch and Sven Poulsen

Over the past decade the dental community has shown an increasing concern about erosive tooth wear, especially in children and adolescents. This anxiety is based on clinical observations, together with reports from many countries suggesting not only a high prevalence, but also a possible increase of both occurrence and severity of dental erosion. In the young individual the literature points to the global rise in soft-drink consumption as the most significant factor in the development of dental erosion. Other factors such as lifestyle changes, a strong perception of the importance of body image for success, and chronic diseases are other possible reasons for an increasing prevalence of dental erosion. Tooth wear has a multifactoral etiology and is a result of concurrent action of different mechanisms and factors on the teeth in the oral environment. Dental erosion is one of these components and defined as a loss of tooth substance by a chemical process that does not involve bacteria. Besides erosion, dental attrition and abrasion may occur at the same or at different occasions which adds to the complexity of the phenomenon of wear (Box 11-1).

Studies have shown that without presoftening by acid of the dental hard tissue the wearing effect from attrition and abrasion is reduced greatly. Dental erosion is therefore regarded as the most important factor in the development of tooth wear and attrition, with abrasion considered to be of less significance (7).

Box 11-1 Definitions of different types of tooth wear

Erosion	Tooth wear due to a chemical process that does not involve bacteria.
Attrition	Tooth wear due to contact between teeth.
Abrasion	Tooth wear due to foreign objects or substances, e.g., toothbrush, toothpaste or other abrasive components.

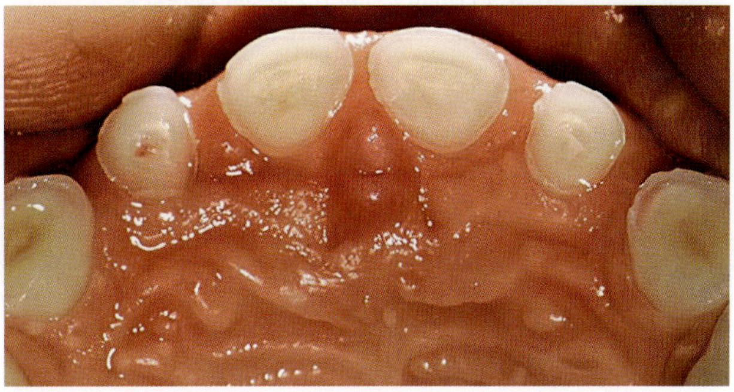

Figure 11-1 Near to pulp exposure on the palatal surfaces of anterior primary teeth.

Microhardness measurements have shown that deciduous enamel is softer than permanent enamel and that the progression of erosion is relatively more rapid than in permanent enamel. In addition, the fact that deciduous teeth are smaller in size further enhances the risk for complications by dental erosion (21) (Fig. 11-1).

Epidemiology

Recent studies claim a high and increasing prevalence of erosions in children and adolescents. Comparison of these studies is often difficult since the diagnostic criteria, scoring systems, and choice of teeth and surfaces to be scored vary. However, there are sufficient studies to give a general idea of the prevalence and distribution of erosion both in the primary and in the young permanent dentition (Table 11-1).

The prevalence of erosion involving dentin in children aged 2–7 years has been reported to vary from 1 to 34%, while erosion limited to the enamel is definitely more frequent. Most reported studies in the young permanent dentition are carried out in children aged 12–14 years and the prevalence of erosion in dentin varies from 2 to 53%. Longitudinal studies indicate an increased number of teeth being affected by erosion and also an increase in severity with increasing age.

Table 11-1 Occurrence of dental erosion in children (primary teeth) and adolescents (permanent teeth) in different countries. Prevalence denotes erosive damage reaching the dentin

Country	Age (years)	No. of individuals	Prevalence (%)	Authors (year)
Children				
UK	4–5	178	30	Millward *et al.* (1994)
UK	5	>1000	24	Downer (1995)
UK	1.5–4.5	1658	8	Moynihan and Holt (1996)
Saudi Arabia	5–6	354	34	Al-Majed *et al.* (2002)
Ireland	5	202	21	Harding *et al.* (2003)
India	5–6	100	30	Deshpande *et al.* (2005)
China	3–5	1949	1	Luo *et al.* (2005)
Germany	2–7	463	13	Wiegand *et al.* (2006)
Adolescents				
UK	14	1035	30	Milosevic *et al.* (1994)
UK	15	>1000	2	Downer (1995)
Saudi Arabia	20	95	16	Johansson *et al.* (1996)
Cuba	12	1010	17	Kunzel *et al.* (2000)
Saudi Arabia	12–14	862	26	Al-Majed *et al.* (2002)
Iceland	15	278	6	Arnadottir *et al.* (2003)
UK	14	1308	13	Dugmore *et al.* (2003)
UK	14	2351	53	Bardsley *et al.* (2004)
Turkey	11	153	28	Caglar *et al.* (2005)
Denmark	15–17	558	1.6	Larsen *et al.* (2005)
Sudan	12–14	157	22	El Karim *et al.* (2007)

The distribution of dental erosion is not uniform within the dental arches. Studies have shown that it is not possible to predict exactly the localization of such lesions depending on their etiology (17). It is, however, clear that erosion will affect some teeth more than others. In children and adolescents, the maxillary anterior teeth (especially the palatal surfaces) and permanent first molars are those most often affected. In severe cases, a shoulder might be present cervically (Fig. 11-2) and occasionally the approximal surfaces may also be affected. Usually the shoulder has a sharp demarcation between the eroded and noneroded surfaces. Cuppings (for explanation see page 146) in the permanent dentition in children and adolescents are most commonly seen on the first mandibular molars, but can be found on all cusp tips or incisal edges. If erosion has been diagnosed on one tooth surface, it is also important to examine other surfaces carefully for signs of tooth surface loss. This could, for example, be the presence of buccal–cervical defects or uprising restorations. Atypical localization of erosion exists and may be the result of lemon sucking for instance (Fig. 11-3).

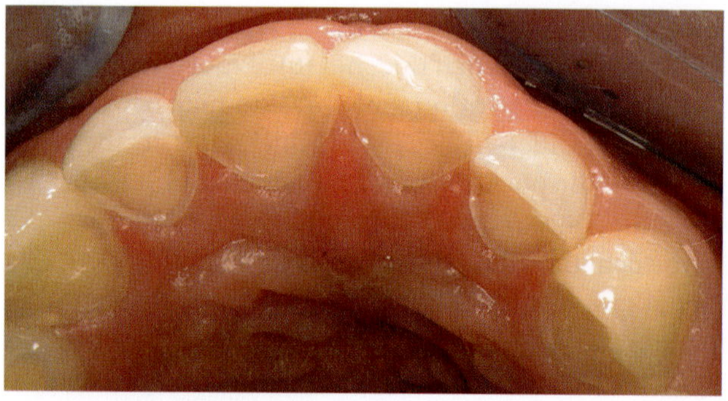

Figure 11-2 On the palatal surface of the upper incisors, the enamel close to the gingival margin is often intact.

Etiology

Traditionally, the etiological factors for dental erosion have been divided into those of extrinsic and intrinsic origin. The term "idiopathic erosion" has been used in cases of unknown etiology, but its clinical application is limited (15) (Box 11-2).

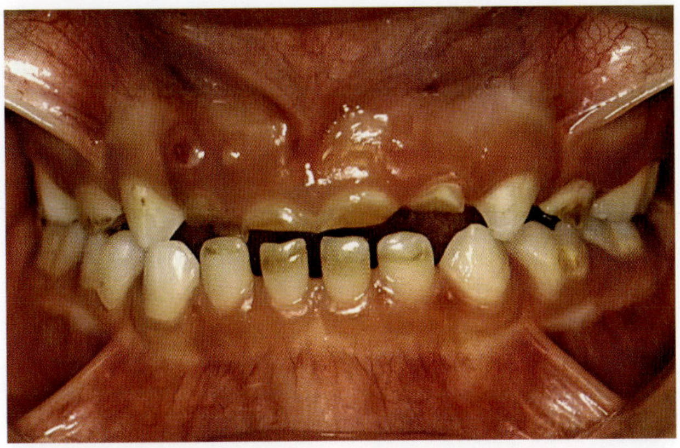

Figure 11-3 Dental erosion as a result of lemon sucking in a 6-year-old child.

Box 11-2 Examples of extrinsic and intrinsic etiological factors as well as modifying factors of importance for the occurrence of dental erosion in children and adolescents, and examples of factors associated with dental erosion

Extrinsic factors (diet and beverages)		• Acidic food, drinks and medications.
Intrinsic factors, general diseases, and syndromes		• Gastrointestinal disturbances. • Eating disorders. • Asthma. • Cerebral palsy. • Down syndrome.
Modifying factors	Pattern of consumption	• Frequency and duration of consumption. • Method of drinking and eating.
	Salivary factors	• Secretion rate. • Buffering capacity. • Composition of saliva.
	Oral hygiene	• Method, intensity, and frequency. • Type of toothbrush, toothpaste, and/or other oral hygiene products.

Examples of factors of extrinsic origins are all acidic drinks, but also acidic foods such as fruits and pickles, acidic medicines (e.g., acetylsalicylic acid and vitamin C tablets), and environmental exposure, such as highly chlorinated swimming pools.

The most common etiological factor for dental erosion in children is the high consumption of soft drinks, including fizzy drinks and fruit juices, which expose the dentition to frequent contacts with citric, phosphoric, or malic acids.

Intrinsic factors include various gastrointestinal and eating disorders, e.g., vomiting, regurgitation, and rumination in which hydrochloric acid from the stomach comes into contact with the teeth.

Several chronic health conditions have been associated with dental erosion, especially those related to gastric acid/stomach disturbances and those affecting salivary secretion.

Gastroesophageal reflux (disease)

Studies have shown that children with gastroesophageal reflux (disease) [GER(D)] have a higher prevalence of dental erosion compared to healthy children albeit it is considered to be a normal physiological condition among infants. In the younger child, the symptoms will be diffuse and frequently described merely as stomach pain or persistent coughing. Symptoms in the older child have a more precise symptomatology: pain from the upper part of the stomach, heartburn, regurgitation, dysphagia, and coughing, especially at nighttime, are examples. In some cases, the patient does not present any typical symptoms at all; this is referred to as "silent reflux". However, this condition may be detected by 24-h pH monitoring, which is the golden standard in GER(D) diagnosis. In rare cases, reflux can be voluntary, which is called "rumination", and most often found in connection with disabilities or eating disorders.

Asthma

Asthmatic problems are common in the child population and many asthmatic children have GER. While some reports have shown an increased prevalence of dental erosion in children with asthma others have not. In an asthmatic patient, broncodilating medication may reduce salivary secretion and relax the lower esophageal sphincter with an increased potential for acidic reflux (34). In addition, the medication itself may be acidic and mouth breathing resulting in dryness of the mouth is common, all of which raises the risk of dental erosion.

Eating disorders

Children and adolescents with eating disorders have an increased risk for erosion. Self-induced vomiting is seen in patients with bulimia nervosa, but also occurs in patients with other types of eating disorders; anorexia nervosa for example. Besides this, a high intake of sugar-free soft drinks and fruits, excessive oral hygiene often combined with gastrointestinal disturbances and salivary impairment are frequent among patients with eating disorders and raise the risk of erosion (31).

A large number of medications cause a dry mouth, e.g., anticholinergic drugs, medicines for GER(D), and psychiatric disorders. Cancer therapy with cytostatics or radiation treatment (often combined with vomiting) frequently compromises the function of the salivary glands and increases the risk for erosion. Diabetes (both types 1 and 2), hypoparathyroidism and hyperparathyroidism, hyperthyroidism, and congenital agenesis of salivary glands, Down syndrome, cerebral palsy, Prader–Willi syndrome or the use of methylenedioxymethamphetamine (ecstasy) are other conditions associated with dental erosion (37).

Other factors associated with dental erosion

Drinking habits

An individual's method of drinking acidic drinks plays an important role in the development of erosive lesions. The erosion damage is likely to be greater in those individuals who retain the drink in their mouth for some time before swallowing, compared to those who do not, as the contact time between the acid and the teeth is increased (20). In one study, 43% of children with dental erosion were found to have a drinking habit such as swishing or holding compared to 3% in caries-free and 15% in caries-active controls (28), and the intraoral pH after drinking soft drinks differed between those with dental erosion and controls (26). Dental erosion has also been associated with the consumption of acidic drinks in a baby's bottle at bedtime or naptime (3). Sucking through a straw might reduce the erosive potential of the drink if the straw is positioned towards the back of the mouth (10) (Box 11-2 and Fig. 11-4).

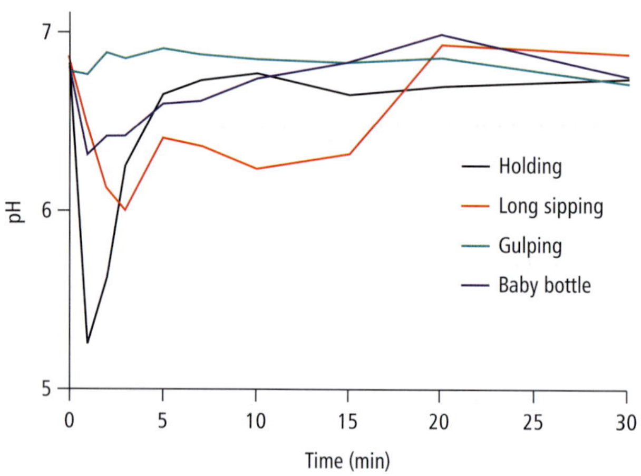

Figure 11-4 pH decrease (mean values) for three methods of drinking and nipping from a baby's bottle using the microtouch method and Cola Light. Holding = holding the drink in the mouth for 2 min. Long sipping = sipping from a glass for 15 min. Gulping = swallowing quickly three times over 5-min intervals. Baby bottle = nipping from a baby's feeding bottle for 15 min. Modified from Johansson *et al.* (20).

Salivary factors

An increased erosive action may be expected if the salivary secretion rate and buffering capacity are reduced. Saliva is important in the prevention of erosions through dilution and clearance of acidic products, and plays an important role in pellicle formation and demineralization and remineralization. The thickness of the pellicle varies between individuals and between different locations in the mouth, and may be reduced by acidic challenges such as soft drinks. A thicker pellicle provides more protection than a thinner one, and it has been suggested that salivary secretion and pellicle thickness strongly influence the location and development of erosion (4,36). When measuring unstimulated and stimulated salivary flow rates, buffering capacity, and number of mutans streptococci in three groups of children, one with extensive erosions, one without caries, and one with high caries prevalence, the following were found: the erosion group showed great similarities concerning caries with the caries-free group and great similarities concerning saliva characteristies with the high caries group (29). Similar results were found in another study where children with erosion showed lower unstimulated and stimulated salivary rates, lower buffering capacity, and lower salivary pH, and a larger maximum pH drop after consumption of soft drinks compared to children without both erosion and caries (Box 11-2).

Oral hygiene practices

Studies have shown that individuals with erosion have better oral hygiene than those without erosion (19). The modern practice of cleaning teeth is certainly more erosion conducive than a more irregular, less methodical, and less vigorous method of oral hygiene, since the erosive lesion develops on surfaces free of plaque. A plaque-free surface could be a result of oral hygiene activities, but also a consequence of natural cleaning from the lips, tongue, and cheeks. Approximal surfaces are seldom free of plaque and this may be the reason why they rarely develop erosive lesions.

Oral hygiene activity, after an acidic challenge on the tooth surface, will result in a greater loss of tooth substance due to its being "presoftened" by acids.

Lifestyle

The view has been expressed that "the lifestyle of today seems to increase the acidic challenge to the dentition and thereby introduces a new risk factor for the dentition" (14). Lifestyle has a large impact on both general and oral health. It varies over time and often reflects social circumstances including dietary habits, physical activity, drug usage, and stress-related factors. One important change in the modern lifestyle is the increase in soft-drink consumption, the decrease in milk consumption, and reduced physical activity in connection to an increasing prevalence of obesity, diabetes, osteoporosis, and being overweight in the child population (5,12).

The fact that most soft drinks are consumed by young children and adolescents (34) especially increases the risk of dental erosion in these groups. Adolescents who frequently consume sport drinks during and after exercise when salivary secretion is lowered (35), as well as the young computer user who stays awake at night with the help of a Coke, will have an increased risk of dental erosion.

A healthy lifestyle may also have an impact on the occurrence and severity of dental erosion, e.g., vegetarianism and dieting practices which are common among vegetarian children and adolescents. Vegetarians and children on a diet often have a high consumption of juices, fruits, and vegetables, perhaps with an added vinegar dressing, and in order to be orally healthy they also perform very thorough tooth hygiene.

The occurrence of dental erosion does not follow any obvious socioeconomic pattern. While some reports show that erosive wear is more common in children and adolescents with low socioeconomic status, other reports demonstrate the reverse. The same applies to gender differences, but in general it seems that boys are more affected than girls, which could be explained by the fact that boys generally drink more soft drinks compared to girls of a similar age.

The consequences of a new lifestyle often become obvious only when it is firmly established and it is difficult to revert to earlier routines. Thus, the oral medical aspects of dental erosion involve not only a proper dietary and medical history, but also knowledge of the person's lifestyle (37) (Fig. 11-5).

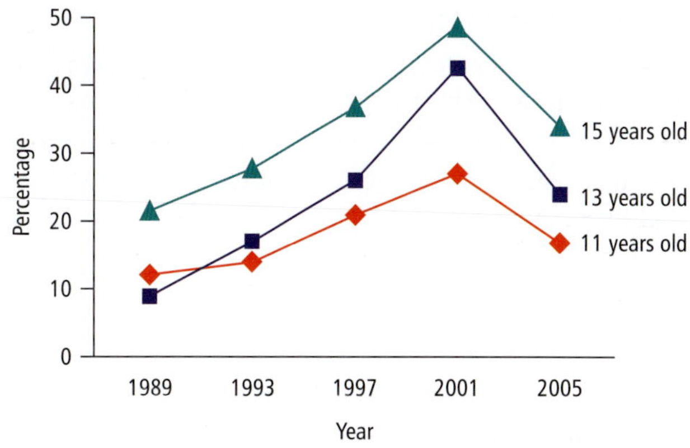

Figure 11-5 Percentage distribution from 1989 to 2005 of Norwegian boys reporting daily intake of soft drinks. (Nordrehaug Åstrøm *et al*., Konsum av sukret mineralvann og søtsaker blant norske skoleelever: sterk økning fra 1989–2001. *Nor Tannlegeforen Tid* 2004;**114**:816–21 and personal communication.)

Case history and clinical examination

Case history

Children and adolescents are exposed to many different erosive challenges which may result in initiation or aggravation of already present dental erosion lesions. Taking a case history in patients with dental erosion is therefore often both extensive and time consuming. Information about general health, e.g., gastric conditions, eating disorders, and asthma, including the type of medication, is relevant. Besides the obvious need for a dietary history, with special reference to acidic intakes including consumption of acidic drinks and fruits, other lifestyle factors also need to be addressed. These include sports activities, computer use, and oral hygiene habits, for example. A dietary history preferably is performed over several days, including one day during the weekend. This can, of course, be difficult especially in younger children, who besides their own family may meet different carers during a day in daycare centers and schools and when being with friends or grandparents. Consideration needs not only to be given to when and what the tooth is exposed to, but also in what way, such as the method of drinking. It is important to remember that an erosive lesion could be caused by earlier periods of acidic challenges such as a period of high consumption of soft drinks. Some practical steps in the clinical assessment of dental erosion are listed in Box 11-3.

Box 11-3 Practical steps in the clinical assessment of cases with dental erosion

Case history including information on:

- medical history and medication
- dietary habits
- oral hygiene habits
- dental problem
- lifestyle factors and earlier challenges.

Clinical examination including:

- visual inspection
- grading of dental erosion
- registrations of other types of dental wear.

Salivary flow and buffering capacity.
Intraoral photographs.
Study casts.

Clinical examination

The first step is a visual inspection of the tooth surface. This should be completed in good operating light and on a clean and dry tooth surface. Since the erosive process might cause endodontic symptoms varying from slight sensitivity to severe pain, any air blow has to be performed carefully. An alternative diagnosis to dental erosion has to be considered, for example, dental caries or endodontic problems. A larger mirror, such as the type of mirror used for occlusal views in intraoral photography, is preferable during the examination of erosion since the enlarged view allows an inspection of several teeth at the same time (22).

The clinical manifestations of erosion are easy to miss in the early stage as there is no discoloration of the lesion, no sticking on probing, and often no or only limited symptoms. In the advanced stages the clinical signs of erosion are more obvious. If the morphology of the tooth surface has changed, not due to mechanical forces or dental caries, dental erosion should be suspected. In cases of severe tooth wear, erosion should always be regarded as a possible underlying factor since the softening of the dental hard tissue by the erosive process may increase the loss of tooth surface. The surface of erosive lesions can have a different appearance. It can be shiny or matte, might be irregular, but is often rounded or flat, as if "melted". The tooth's developmental structures may vanish and in more severe cases the macromorphology is altered. In children, the many macroscopic structures observed in the newly erupted tooth will be lost (Fig. 11-6). Small concavities can sometimes be seen on the buccal surface of the tooth. The pulp might, in severe cases, be visible through the remaining tooth substance: this is most common on the palatal surface of the maxillary central deciduous teeth. There might also be a formation of clinically detectable protective tertiary dentin, or direct pulpal involvement.

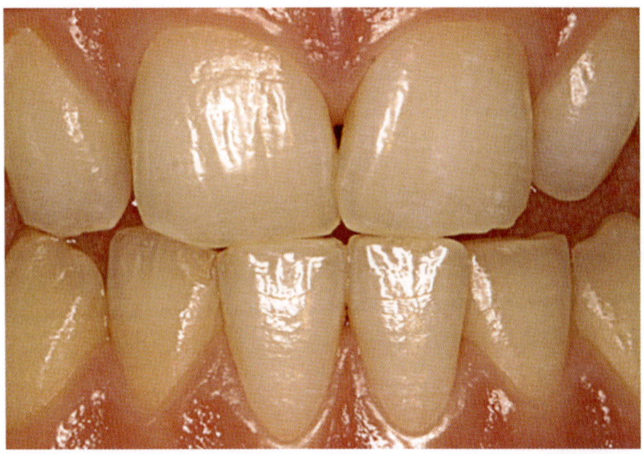

Figure 11-6 Newly erupted permanent teeth showing macroscopic details of the enamel surface.

One common clinical sign of erosion in both permanent and primary dentition is cuppings: a "peephole" in the enamel, most frequently seen on the cusp tips on the first molars. Two or more cuppings may fuse together to form one larger affected area on the occlusal surface (18). Restorations may sometimes be seen rising above the tooth surface as a result of dental erosion. These are not only visible clinically, but may also be detected on radiographs, study casts, and photos.

Besides the more obvious loss of tooth substance resulting in aesthetic and/or functional problems during eating or drinking, the process may also result in malocclusion. The mechanisms behind this are most likely a combination of tooth eruption and compensatory alveolar growth as a result of the erosive loss of vertical crown height. Some clinical characteristics are listed in Box 11-4 and Fig. 11-7.

Study casts are valuable in visualizing the three-dimensional aspects of changes affecting morphological features, but should carefully be prepared to enhance the diagnostic possibilities. The angle at which a cast is viewed will affect the appearance of the lesions. Intraoral photographs are of some value in the clinical assessment, but the two-dimensional image, poorer lightning conditions, and improper angling of the camera strongly limit the information which can be obtained. Salivary secretion rate, of both stimulated and resting saliva, as well as analyses of buffering capacity, should be considered.

Box 11-4 Clinical characteristics of dental erosion. Modified from Johansson *et al.* (18)

- Enamel surface, shiny, matte, irregular, rounded, or flat.
- Developmental structures vanished.
- Macromorphology of the tooth altered.
- Dentinal exposure.
- Cuppings.
- Buccal cervical defects.
- Uprising restorations.

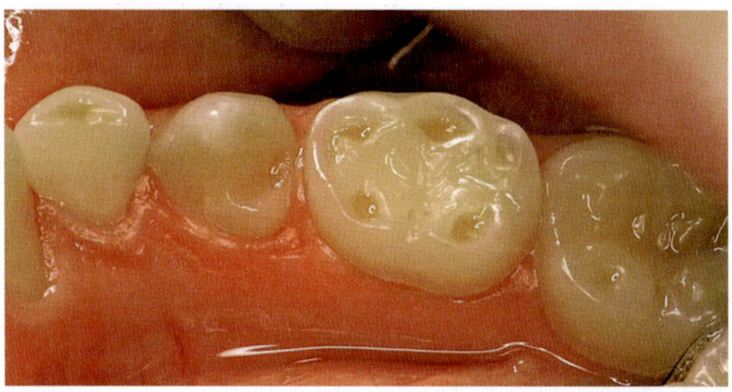

Figure 11-7 Clinical signs of erosion: cuppings on primary molars (teeth 83 and 85) and permanent molar (tooth 46).

Indices for dental erosion

Different index systems for grading dental wear and dental erosion in the clinical situation have been described. Some systems are based on partial recordings of indicator teeth (9,18), while others recommend full mouth scoring (30).

A few indices are designed only for deciduous teeth (30) or only for permanent teeth (24), while others have been used for both deciduous and permanent teeth (9,18). Generally, in most situations, a relatively simple ordinal scale is suitable. A combined approach of grading erosive wear using clinical inspection, examination of study casts and photographs, offers advantages compared to systems which rely on a single or a dual approach. When choosing a scoring system it is important to consider the type of investigation for which the data will be used, e.g., clinical grading for management purposes, population- or laboratory-based research. In the clinical setting, the duration of the examination needs to be kept in mind since some of the systems are very time consuming to use.

Early enamel erosion is found commonly in both children and adolescents. These lesions have to be detected early and if a grading system is to be used it must be able to distinguish between different stages of enamel erosion as well as severe erosion into dentin or close to dentinal exposure. If less refined diagnostic criteria are used, only more severe erosive lesions can be recorded, which increases the risk for overlooking early signs of dental erosion, losing the possibility of early intervention.

Box 11-5 and Fig. 11-8 shows a scale used for grading dental erosion in children and adolescents. Additional registrations should include recording of cuppings on first permanent or deciduous molars and of buccal cervical defects.

Follow-up of patients with erosions

Frequently, the etiological, modifying and/or aggravating factors of dental erosion will persist throughout life. Therefore, a child once diagnosed with dental erosion should be monitored and supervised for a long period. Besides providing the patient and parents with the necessary information about the condition and prophylactic advice, it is possible to use photographs, serial study casts, salivary analysis, and consultations with the patient's family physician (e.g., in cases of gastric problems, eating disorders, or asthmatic problems) as tools to control dental erosion.

The progression of erosion could be assessed by comparing a study cast taken over an appropriate time interval. In some cases radiographs, preferably bitewings,

Box 11-5 Scale used for grading severity of dental erosion on buccal and lingual surfaces of maxillary anterior teeth (13–23 or 53–63), partial recording (18)

Grade	Criteria
0	No visible changes, developmental structures remain, macromorphology intact.
1	Smoothened enamel, developmental structures have totally or partially vanished. Enamel surface is shiny, matte, irregular, "melted", rounded or flat, macromorphology generally intact.
2	Enamel surface as described in grade 1. Macromorphology clearly changed, facetting or concavity formation within the enamel, no dentinal exposure.
3	Enamel surface as described in grades 1 and 2. Macromorphology greatly changed (close to dentinal exposure of large surfaces) or dentin surface exposed by $\leq 1/3$.
4	Enamel surface as described in grades 1, 2, and 3. Dentin surface exposed by $> 1/3$ or pulp visible through the dentin.

Note: approximal erosion and presence of a "shoulder" should be recorded.

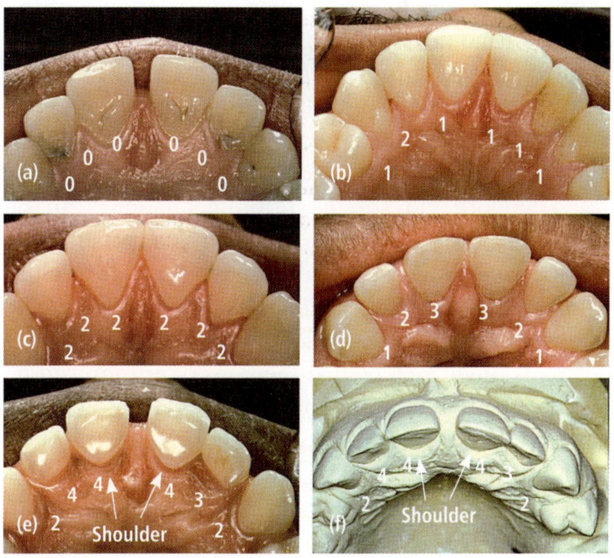

Figure 11-8 Illustrations of different severities of dental erosion graded according to the scale in Box 11-5. (f) is a study model of the patient in (e) illustrating that intraoral photographs could be combined with grading of study models as the two complement each other in assessment of dental erosion (from Johansson AK, Carlsson GE. *Dental erosion: bakgrund och kliniska aspekter.* Förlagshuset Gothia, 2006).

may be of value. Also, it is generally important to predict the longevity for the involved tooth and the impact of this for the patient. One exception to this rule is severely affected deciduous teeth just before exfoliation. Studies have shown that the risk of severe erosion in the permanent dentition increases nearly four times if severe erosion is present in the deciduous dentition (11). The clinical consequence of a diagnosis of dental erosion should be considered on an individual basis since the same severity of erosion may be perfectly acceptable in one patient but not in another. If a child or adolescent is diagnosed with erosion it is more likely that this process is active than if an erosive lesion of the same severity is diagnosed in an adult. As a permanent tooth in a younger individual has a longer life expectancy than in an adult, the same erosive problem may therefore have a higher risk of complications over time in younger compared to older people.

Preventive policies

General aspects

From the preventive point of view, the importance for the dental team to recognize the early stages of erosion and to understand its pathogenesis has been strongly emphasized (22). Equally important are the need and the means to effectively communicate any findings as regards dental erosion to the patient and parents, since the success of preventive measures in most cases will depend strongly on their proper understanding of the condition and their cooperation. If a patient is suspected of suffering from progressive dental erosion it is important to hasten the investigation in order to repress or prevent further tooth surface loss. The defense against erosion varies, as mentioned earlier, between individuals. Therefore, no specific recommendations can be given concerning how much acidic drink a specific child can drink without risk for erosion. However, for a child with diagnosed dental erosion it is clear that the acidic challenges during some period of the life have been too severe. It might well be that the signs of erosion can be linked to earlier habits or conditions and less to present circumstances. Prevention of dental erosion is often complicated, and before any recommendation is decided on it is advisable to evaluate the progression of erosion. Prevention can be primary, secondary, or tertiary, but the prophylactic strategy is in all cases to eliminate or reduce the etiological factors and to strengthen the individually related defense mechanisms.

Elimination of etiological factors

Reduction of all acidic intakes is one method of prevention in cases of erosion due to extrinsic causes, but life-style changes are always difficult to make and especially so for a child or adolescent. Prevention may, therefore, at times involve not only the affected child, but also the whole family. If a proper diagnosis of erosion in the deciduous teeth can be made and the factors involved understood, a preventive strategy for the permanent teeth is possible since the etiological factors will most likely similarly affect the child's permanent dentition (21). Advice and information about erosion at the right time may in some patients totally prevent further damage, while in others the situation may be more difficult. Examples of recommendations in cases of extrinsic dental erosion are given in Box 11-6.

The ultimate goal of prevention is to avoid the initiation of any erosive lesions and to stop progression of existing lesions. In some patients with active erosion the preventive measures may only result in a slowing of the progression. This is especially the case in patients with dental erosion due to intrinsic causes as GER and/or eating disorders, diseases which may be found in both children and adolescents and are difficult to control.

One way to eliminate or reduce intrinsic factors for erosion is to consult the patient's physician. By treating or controlling the general disease, the best possible prevention of dental erosion is obtained. In patient with GER, a proper medical examination, sometimes including 24-h pH measurement of the acidity in the esophagus, and then diagnosis and treatment with medication or surgery is of importance. Within cases of nocturnal reflux, the head of the child's bed could be raised 5–10 cm in order to reduce the risk of the stomach's acidic

Box 11-6 Example of recommendations to children/parents with extrinsic erosion

- Avoid or limit acid-containing drinks, fruits, and other types of foods especially between meals and at nighttime.
- Drink water when you are thirsty especially between meals and at nighttime.
- Be aware of the contact time for acidic intake, e.g., method of drinking.
- Drink milk with meals; finish the meal with cheese or other milk products.
- Eat the whole fruit rather than drinking its juice; do not suck lemons or other fruits.
- Mix acidic foods with less acidic ones to neutralize, e.g., fruit with milk products.
- If you do drink acidic drinks:
  - don't keep the drink in the mouth before swallowing – drink quickly
  - if using a straw, place it far behind the front teeth
  - avoid acidic drinks in a bottle in your bag
  - never put acidic drinks in a baby's bottle.

content reaching the oral cavity. If antacid is used as a medication for gastric reflux this could be kept in the mouth before swallowing in order to neutralize any acid in the mouth (25). Dietary advice should, as always, be given with due consideration to the medical recommendations. If an eating disorder is suspected, contact with parents, school nurse, physician, or psychiatric care is suggested. Dietary advice in patients with eating disorders should be given in collaboration with medical or psychiatric personnel and has to consider not only dental and medical health but also psychiatric health.

Remineralization of newly eroded surfaces can be achieved as long as the affected tooth substance is not completely lost and if sufficient calcium, phosphate, or fluoride is available on the surface. Rinsing the mouth with water when there are acidic challenges will stop the erosive process but does not lead to any remineralization. If the brittle organic network that remains on the tooth surface just after erosive challenges is worn off by abrasion or attrition, the opportunity for remineralization is lost. Therefore, it is recommended that toothbrushing is avoided at least for an hour after an acidic challenge. It is also recommended to avoid abrasive toothpaste just before an acidic challenge. Toothbrushing without toothpaste, after an erosive challenge, has shown deposition of salivary components, inducing remineralization, while brushing with nonfluoridated abrasive toothpaste resulted in abrasion (23). Dental erosion has also been found to be associated with brushing before sleeping and after meals, and also with the type of toothbrush and the brushing technique (1). Salivary secretion rate is very important in order to prevent dental erosion and needs to be increased when insufficient. First, ensure that the intake of liquid is adequate, and second, salivary secretion could be stimulated using fluoride tablets or special sugar-free tablets. Chewing gum can also be recommended even though it should be used with caution since it can increase occlusal wear in some cases. If medication causes reduced salivary secretion or increased reflux, or is acidic itself, elimination or substitution of the medicine should be considered in collaboration with medical expertise. Examples of recommended oral hygiene habits for patients with erosion are given in Box 11-7.

In patients with nocturnal bruxism the use of an occlusal protective splint can be suggested in order to eliminate abrasion or attrition. However, there has been speculation that the splint may act as a reservoir for acid during nocturnal regurgitation, thus increasing the risk of dental erosion.

Fluoride is less important in the prevention of dental erosion than for the prevention of caries. However, fluoride therapy is recommended in patients with erosion even though the effect of the treatment is limited and not fully understood. At the same time it has to be stressed that a change of lifestyle, resulting in a reduction of etiological factors, is much more effective than any other preventive technique.

Box 11-7 Example of recommendation of oral hygiene habits in cases with dental erosion

- Don't brush your teeth just before an acidic challenge and wait at least an hour after the challenge to brush.
- Use a soft toothbrush and if needed warm water.
- Brush your tongue after reflux or vomiting.
- Use a toothpaste with a high fluoride concentration and low abrasives.

Sensitivity due to erosion can be reduced in different ways. The first, and most important, is to eliminate or reduce all acidic challenges. In combination with this, intensive fluoride therapy may be useful, as well as the use of special toothpastes. Other methods could be to block the enlarged dentinal tubules with different types of bonding or desensitizer. This treatment may reduce the sensitivity even though the prognosis depends on the longevity of the blocking agent and its resistance towards further erosive challenges in the mouth. It might, therefore, be necessary to repeat the treatment. In severe cases it can even be necessary to restore the eroded surfaces in order to prevent or eliminate sensitivity and further erosive damage. In some cases fissure sealants may be helpful, e.g., in the prevention and/or restoration of cuppings. Box 11-8 shows examples of clinical preventive measures in cases of erosion.

The child with eroded deciduous teeth presents both a challenge and an opportunity to prevent erosion in the permanent successors.

Population-based prevention

On a population basis it is likely that the most effective prevention of erosion would be to reduce the intake of acidic drinks among children and adolescents both with and without dental erosion. The preventive effect of information about dental erosion is also valuable even though knowledge does not always lead to a change of

Box 11-8 Examples of measures of clinical prevention in cases of diagnosed erosion

- Fluoride varnish or gel, fissure sealants.
- Block dentin tubule, bonding or desensitizer.
- Restoration with adhesive technique.
- Avoid tooth bleaching.

lifestyle. Studies have also shown that the availability of soft drinks in school vending machines is an important factor in the choice of beverage. Campaigns promoting a healthier lifestyle among children and adolescents have mainly targeted being overweight and obesity, but have also been of value for the improvement of oral health and the prevention of dental erosion.

Other appropriate preventive measures are the modification of acidic drinks by the addition of calcium. Such modified products are available in some countries in order to reduce the erosivity of the drink (13).

Restorative treatment

There are a number of indications for restorative interventions in cases of dental erosion. Restorations can be performed to improve aesthetics and function, or to manage sensitivity and pain which does not respond to other preventive actions. In some instances, restorative intervention is needed in order to prevent undesirable orthodontic effects or further loss of tooth substance. However, all reconstructions have a limited longevity, which implies that a future treatment need exists for teeth that have been restored at an early age in children and adolescents. It is equally important to recognize that tooth surface loss does not always need to be restored and that any decision on restorative intervention always should be individually based.

Soft drinks, especially fruit juices, have been proven to reduce the longevity of many dental materials. After a year of immersion *in vitro* in apple and orange juice, conventional glass ionomers have dissolved completely, but were less affected by Coca-Cola. Microhardness was reduced on resin-based glass ionomers and compomers during immersion in Coca-Cola, but was affected less than by fruit juice (2). Studies have shown that even though many dental materials will be affected by acid, resulting in different types of problems, composite materials and ceramics seem to have a good stability (16,27). The effect of soft-drink consumption on the bonding between orthodontic appliance and tooth surface has been investigated in one combined *in vivo* and *in vitro* study. It was shown that children who were exposed to soft drinks several times daily had poorer retention of their brackets than children who were not (32). Another study indicated that the longevity of posterior restorations, with direct and indirect composites, worn by erosion is shorter than control teeth restored due to dental caries. The failure rate after 3 years was 50% in the erosion group and 20% in the control group. Twenty-eight percent of the restorations in the erosion group were completely lost and another 22% were fractured during this period of time (6).

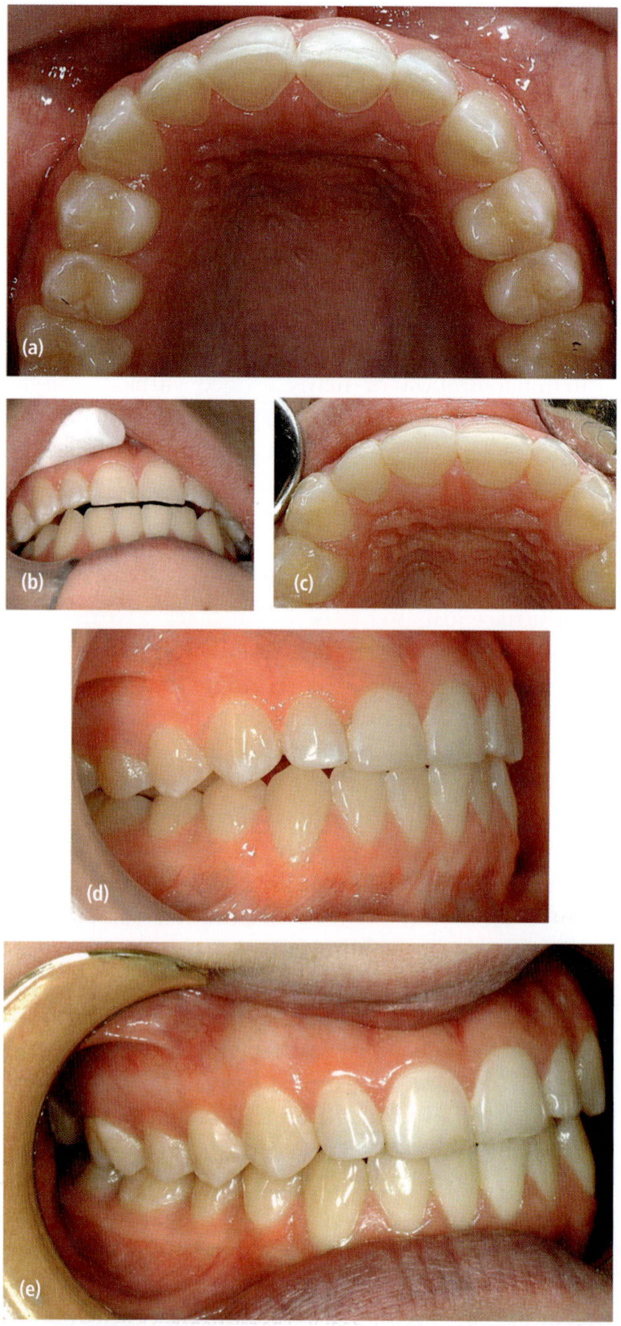

Figure 11-9 (a) Fifteen-year-old girl with palatal erosion and sensitivity on maxillary anterior teeth. (b) Composite restoration took place on tooth 12, establishing a new vertical dimension sufficient for restoring 11, 21, and 22 (c). (d) As a result, posterior disocclusion is present which, however, is normalized after approximately 4 weeks due to (e) compensatory eruption and alveolar growth (from Johansson AK, Carlsson GE. *Dental erosion: bakgrund och kliniska aspekter*. Förlagshuset Gothia, 2006).

In children and adolescents with dental erosion, composites have to be considered as the first choice of restorative treatment even though the long-term performance in cases of dental erosion has not been sufficiently evaluated. In children with erosive wear it is preferable that restorative treatment is performed using a minimally invasive technique. If the retention of the restoration needs to be reinforced, as in the case of restorations of cuppings, it is recommended that a bevel preparation is used. There is an increased risk for progressive wear in a cupping since any acidic challenges may remain inside the cupping thus resulting in a prolonged contact time between the acid and the tooth surface.

In patients with localized worn anterior teeth, the loss of vertical height caused by the erosion might cause a problem with space for the restorative material. Raising the bite using the Dahl technique or a modified Dahl technique can in many cases be a good solution (8). This is performed using an occlusal splint or temporary build-up on the maxillary anterior teeth, which is used night and day for a number of months. At first this technique will create a posterior open bite bilaterally, but with time occlusion will be normalized by a compensatory eruption of posterior teeth and intrusion of anteriors. After removing the anterior splint adequate interocclusal space for permanent restoration has been gained. Often the temporary build-up can be kept as a permanent or semipermanent solution (Fig. 11-9).

Composite restorations can also be used as temporary solutions if prosthetic therapy is indicated in the future. Occasionally, prosthetic therapy is the first choice of treatment even in young individuals.

It has to be remembered that restorative treatment is not causal therapy of the disease. The erosion process can still be active, affecting the dentition, and the patient will be in need of future support and follow-up.

References

1. Al-Dlaigan YH, Shaw L, Smith AJ. Dental erosion in a group of British 14-year-old, school children. Part III: Influence of oral hygiene practises. *Br Dent J* 2002;**192**:526–30.
2. Aliping-McKenzie M, Linden RW, Nicholson JW. Effects of pH on the microhardness of resin-based restorative materials. *Oper Dent* 2005;**30**:661–6.
3. Al-Malik MI, Holt RD, Bedi R. The relationship between erosion, caries and rampant caries and dietary habits in preschool children in Saudi Arabia. *Int J Paediatr Dent* 2001;**11**:430–9.
4. Amaechi BT, Higham SM, Edgar WM, Milosevic A. Thickness of acquired salivary pellicle as a determinant of the sites of dental erosion. *J Dent Res* 1999;**78**:1821–8.
5. American Academy of Pediatrics Committee on School Health. Soft drinks in schools. *Pediatrics* 2004;**113**:152–4.
6. Bartlett D, Sundaram G. An up to 3-year randomized clinical study comparing indirect and direct resin composites used to restore worn posterior teeth. *Int J Prosthodont* 2006;**19**:613–17.
7. Bartlett DW. The role of erosion in tooth wear: aetiology, prevention and management. *Int Dent J* 2005;**55** (Suppl 1):277–84.
8. Dahl BL, Krogstad O, Karlsen K. An alternative treatment in cases with advanced localized attrition. *J Oral Rehabil* 1975;**2**: 209–14.
9. Downer MC. The 1993 national survey of children's dental health. *Br Dent J* 1995;**178**:407–12.
10. Edwards M, Ashwood RA, Littlewood SJ, Brocklebank LM, Fung DE. A videofluoroscopic comparison of straw and cup drinking: the potential influence on dental erosion. *Br Dent J* 1998;**185**:244–9.
11. Ganss C, Klimek J, Giese K. Dental erosion in children and adolescents – a cross-sectional and longitudinal investigation using study models. *Community Dent Oral Epidemiol* 2001;**29**: 264–71.
12. Harnack L, Stang J, Story M. Soft drink consumption among US children and adolescents: nutritional consequences. *J Am Diet Assoc* 1999;**99**:436–41.
13. Hooper S, Hughes J, Parker D, Finke M, Newcombe RG, Addy M, *et al.* A clinical study *in situ* to assess the effect of a food approved polymer on the erosion potential of drinks. *J Dent* 2007;**35**: 541–6.
14. Imfeld T, ten Cate JM. Preface. *Eur J Oral Sci* 1996;**104**:149.
15. Imfeld T. Dental erosion. Definition, classification and links. *Eur J Oral Sci* 1996;**104**:151–5.
16. Jaeggi T, Gruninger A, Lussi A. Restorative therapy of erosion. *Monogr Oral Sci* 2006;**20**:200–14.
17. Järvinen V, Rytomaa I, Meurman JH. Location of dental erosion in a referred population. *Caries Res* 1992;**26**:391–6.
18. Johansson AK, Johansson A, Birkhed D, Omar R, Baghdadi S, Carlsson GE. Dental erosion, soft-drink intake, and oral health in young Saudi men, and the development of a system for assessing erosive anterior tooth wear. *Acta Odontol Scand* 1996;**54**: 369–78.
19. Johansson AK, Lingström P, Birkhed D. Comparison of factors potentially related to the occurrence of dental erosion in high- and low-erosion groups. *Eur J Oral Sci* 2002;**110**:204–11.
20. Johansson AK, Lingstrom P, Imfeld T, Birkhed D. Influence of drinking method on tooth-surface pH in relation to dental erosion. *J Oral Sci* 2004;**112**:484–9.
21. Johansson AK, Sorvari R, Birkhed D, Meurman JH. Dental erosion in deciduous teeth – an *in vivo* and *in vitro* study. *J Dent* 2001;**29**:333–40.
22. Johansson AK. On dental erosion and associated factors. *Swed Dent J* Suppl 2002;(156):1–77.
23. Kuroiwa M, Kodaka T, Kuroiwa M, Abe M. Brushing-induced effects with and without a non-fluoride abrasive dentifrice on remineralization of enamel surfaces etched with phosphoric acid. *Caries Res* 1994;**28**:309–14.
24. Lussi A, Schaffner M, Hotz P, Suter P. Dental erosion in a population of Swiss adults. *Community Dent Oral Epidemiol* 1991; **19**:286–90.
25. Meurman JH, Kuittinen T, Kangas M, Tuisku T. Buffering effect of antacids in the mouth – a new treatment of dental erosion? *Scand J Dent Res* 1988;**96**:412–17.
26. Moazzez R, Smith BG, Bartlett DW. Oral pH and drinking habit during ingestion of a carbonated drink in a group of adolescents with dental erosion. *J Dent* 2000;**28**:395–7.
27. Mohamed-Tahir MA, Tan HY, Woo AA, Yap AU. The effect of Coca-Cola and fruit juices on the surface hardness of glass-ionomers and 'compomers'. *J Oral Rehabil* 2004;**31**:1046–52.
28. O'Sullivan EA, Curzon ME. A comparison of acidic dietary factors in children with and without dental erosion. *ASDC J Dent Child* 2000;**67**:186–92.
29. O'Sullivan EA, Curzon ME. Salivary factors affecting dental erosion in children. *Caries Res* 2000;**34**:82–7.
30. O'Sullivan EA. A new index for the measurement of erosion in children. *Eur J Paediatr Dent* 2000;**1**:69–74.

31. Öhrn R, Enzell K, Angmar-Månsson B. Oral status of 81 subjects with eating disorders. *Eur J Oral Sci* 1999;**107**:157–63.
32. Oncag G, Tuncer AV, Tosun YS. Acidic soft drinks effects on the shear bond strength of orthodontic brackets and a scanning electron microscopy evaluation of the enamel. *Angle Orthod* 2005; **75**:247–53.
33. Rugg-Gunn AJ, Nunn JH. Diet and dental erosion. In: *Nutrition, diet and oral health.* Oxford: Oxford University Press, 1999.
34. Shaw L, Al-Dlaigan YH. Childhood asthma and dental erosion. *ASDC J Dent Child* 2000;**67**:102–6.
35. Sorvari R, Rytömaa I. Drinks and dental health. *Proc Finn Dent Soc* 1991;**87**:621–31.
36. Young WG, Khan F. Sites of dental erosion are saliva-dependent. *J Oral Rehabil* 2002;**29**:35–43.
37. Young WG. The oral medicine of tooth wear. *Aust Dent J* 2001; **46**:236–50.

12

Pedodontic endodontics

Ulla Schröder

Pedodontic endodontics includes pulpal treatment of primary and young, immature permanent teeth. The aim of endodontics with primary teeth is, if possible, to keep the teeth in function until exfoliation, or at least for as long as they are important for occlusal development. This demands thorough knowledge of pulpal conditions and therapies, and also of the value of the individual tooth for the occlusal development. Furthermore, the underlying permanent tooth germ must not be at risk of any developmental disturbance or injury as a consequence of the pulpal and/or periradicular involvement of the primary tooth or the treatment performed.

Endodontic treatment of immature permanent teeth aims to maintain continuing root development and to keep the tooth functional in the dentition. If this is not possible, in cases with poor prognosis, it may sometimes be considered valuable to keep the tooth in the dentition for a certain interval to decide the proper time for its extraction. It may be a question of timing with favorable occlusal conditions for space closure, an implant, or another permanent solution for the dentition and the patient.

Thus, pedodontic endodontics has its own characteristics but must always be seen in the total context of the dentition and the patient. Therapy planning including short- as well as long-term prognosis must be done before any endodontic treatment of primary and immature permanent teeth is performed. Diagnosis and treatment planning for pulp therapy in children should include an appropriate medical and dental history, radiographic evaluation, and clinical tests, such as palpation, percussion, and mobility evaluation. There are clinical challenges when trying to diagnose the pulpal state, depending not only on the condition of the pulp but also on communication problems when treating young patients, especially the preschool child.

Diagnosis of pulp lesions in primary and immature permanent teeth

Diagnostic criteria are in general the same for primary and permanent teeth (Table 12-1). Treatment of primary teeth is usually restricted to vital pulps, which is why the residual pulp that is to be left *in situ* must be normal,

Table 12-1 Diagnostic criteria for pulpal conditions

Diagnostic factors	Diagnostic criteria		
	Partial chronic pulpitis[a]	Total chronic pulpitis	Partial/total pulp necrosis
Increased mobility	No	Yes	Yes
Tenderness on percussion	No	Yes	Yes/?
Sensitivity	Yes	Yes	?/No
X-ray, pathologic changes	No	?/Yes	Yes
Excessive bleeding at the exposure	No	?/Yes	No
Toothache	No/?	?/Yes	?/Yes

[a] Symptomless carious exposure.

since there is no medicament today with healing effect on chronically inflamed or almost necrotic pulp tissue.

A differentiation is therefore essential not only between vital and nonvital pulp, but also between healthy pulp tissue and chronically inflamed pulp tissue, totally or partially involving the pulp (Box 12-1). The pulp of the young permanent tooth copes better with both inflammation and traumatic injury because of a more favorable connection with well-vascularized periapical tissue. The pulp is healthy when exposed by trauma or accidentally during cavity preparation and can be kept healthy if properly treated. Pulp exposed by caries is always chronically inflamed, partially or totally, or may be necrotic.

A correct diagnosis may be particularly difficult to establish in cariously exposed pulps. A diagnostic procedure is therefore necessary to differentiate between the partially and the totally chronically inflamed pulp. An 80% agreement between histologic (Fig. 12-1) and clinical/radiographic criteria has been found for primary teeth with symptomless cariously exposed pulps (partial chronic pulpitis) (17). Teeth with total chronic pulpitis may show clinical as well as radiographic symptoms. In such cases the pulp is not expected to heal.

Partial or total necrosis of the pulp may be the consequence of untreated caries, invagination of enamel or traumatically exposed pulp. Necrosis, a pulpal infarct, may develop following a luxation injury, where the pulpal circulation has been compromised or disrupted apically. X-rays are important diagnostic adjuncts. Radiographic changes such as widened periodontal space with broken cortical bone or apical periodontitis are seen. Lack of narrowing of the pulpal lumen compared with earlier observations and/or discontinued root development are indicative of pulp necrosis.

External root resorption with osteolysis (inflammatory root resorption) may develop in connection with luxation injury with pulp necrosis. The irritation of necrotic pulp tissue through the dentinal tubuli to the injured periodontal membrane may cause the resorption.

Box 12-1 Pulpal conditions of primary and immature permanent teeth

- The pulp is healthy, when exposed by trauma or accidentally during cavity preparation, and can be kept healthy if properly treated.
- The caries-exposed pulp is always chronically inflamed, partially or totally, or may be necrotic.
- Partial or total pulp necrosis may be the consequence of untreated caries, invagination of enamel or traumatically exposed pulp. Necrosis, a pulpal infarct, may develop following a luxation injury, where the pulpal circulation has been compromised or disrupted apically.

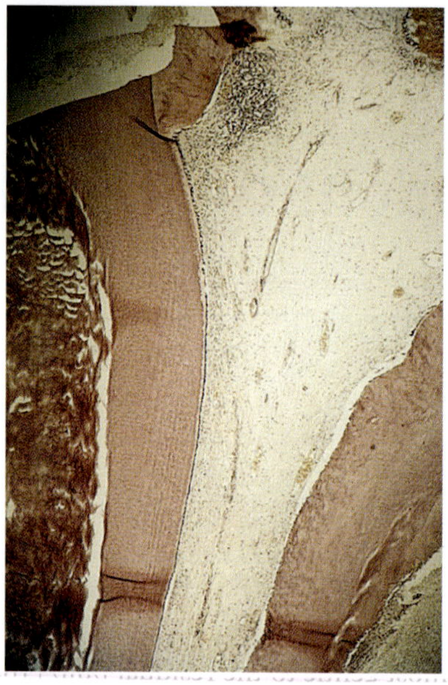

Figure 12-1 Histologic view of partial chronic pulpitis of a primary molar. Note the restricted area of chronic inflammation at the site of carious exposure.

Should endodontic interventions be carried out in the primary dentition?

Important factors other than pulpal diagnosis and occlusal conditions are the patient's ability to cooperate and his or her general and oral health. Can the treatment be performed conventionally or is sedation/general anesthesia needed? Is there any risk of injury/infection of the underlying permanent tooth germ? The choice between endodontic treatment and extraction should also be considered and be based on the value of the tooth for the occlusal development and the child's ability to stand the treatment (Box 12-2). Consequently, pulpal treatment especially is relevant for primary second molars with exposed pulps before or at the time of eruption of the permanent first molar. However, if there is any risk for the underlying permanent tooth germ, e.g., in cases with pulpal necrosis and apical/interradicular periodontitis, extraction should be considered and probably preferred.

Endodontic techniques in primary teeth

The various endodontic techniques are presented in Box 12-3. All endodontic treatment should be performed with due consideration to disinfection. That means that the tooth should be isolated with a rubber dam and the tooth and the operation area disinfected before endodontic therapy.

Since most pulpal treatment of primary teeth involves a vital pulp, it is of utmost importance that the surgical technique is gentle – atraumatic – in order not to decrease the healing capacity of the residual pulp. The recom-

Box 12-2 Important considerations when deciding on extraction or pulpal treatment in the primary dentition

- When the primary dentition is complete, primary incisors are of very limited importance for occlusal development.
- In cases with normal occlusion, loss of primary first molars will result only in temporary loss of space, which will be regained in the mixed dentition (16).
- When the permanent first molars are in occlusion, the primary second molars lose importance for the occlusal development.

mended technique includes use of diamond burs on high-speed equipment and irrigation with water in order not to burn the residual pulp. This procedure has been shown under experimental as well as clinical conditions to be the most gentle to the residual pulp (18,19).

The wound treatment is also important. Calcium hydroxide should be applied in direct contact with the wound surface without any intermediate blood clot. The presence of an extrapulpal blood has been shown to interfere with the healing and cause chronic inflammation and internal dentin resorption (18). The wound surface should therefore be gently irrigated with sterile saline in order to achieve hemostasis before application of calcium hydroxide. If bleeding persists, the addition of calcium hydroxide to the saline may enhance hemostasis. Thereafter it is important to provide a tight seal to the oral cavity to prevent leakage and thereby infection and complications.

Stepwise excavation

In general, a nonexposed pulp has a more favorable healing capacity than an exposed pulp. This is important to consider when treating extensive carious lesions, where an exposure of the pulp may be expected if all carious dentin is removed. The technique includes removal of most of the soft carious dentin, application of calcium hydroxide, and sealing the cavity temporarily with a tight sealing, i.e., resin-reinforced zinc oxide–eugenol cement or glass-ionomer cement. The tooth is left for at least 3–6 months, while secondary dentin formation continues, which means less or no risk of exposing the pulp when re-entering the cavity for final removal of carious dentin and restoration of the tooth (Fig. 12-2). Leaving carious tissue permanently under a restoration, "indirect capping", is not recommended.

Box 12-3 Endodontic techniques

With all techniques it is important to perform a tight seal to the oral environment in order to prevent microleakage!

Therapy	Measures		Indications
Stepwise excavation	Removal of most of the carious dentin. Demineralized dentin covered with calcium hydroxide and left temporarily under an intermediate filling	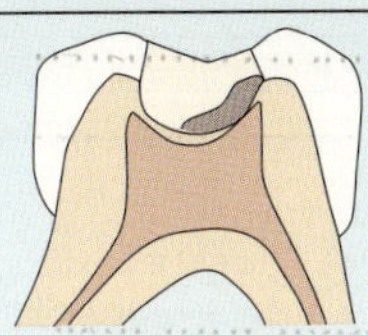	Deep carious lesion, carious softened tissue close to pulp but no exposure. No clinical or slight radiographic signs of pulpitis
Direct pulp capping	No surgical removal of exposed pulp tissue. Pulp covered with calcium hydroxide and the tooth restored	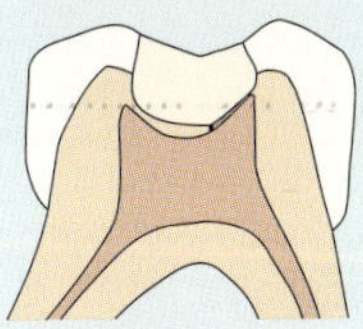	Accidental minimal exposure of healthy pulp during preparation or via trauma. Little or no contamination of the exposed area
Partial pulpotomy	Excision of a superficial part of the pulp. Calcium hydroxide applied in tissue contact with the wound without any extrapulpal blood clot. Tight seal to oral cavity	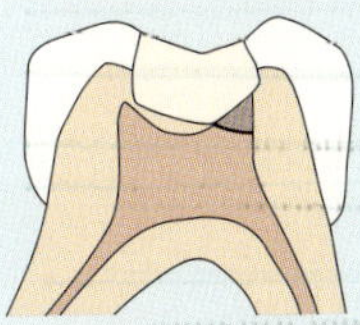	Accidental exposure of healthy pulp; carious exposure – partial chronic pulpitis
Pulpotomy	Removal of the coronal pulp. Wound surfaces placed in the orifices of the root canals	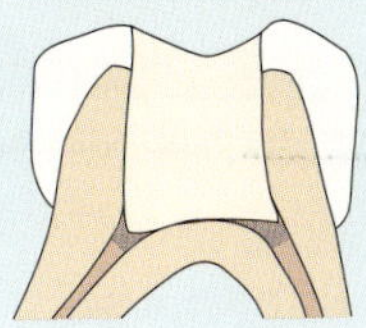	Carious exposure – pulpitis, partial or total chronic pulpitis

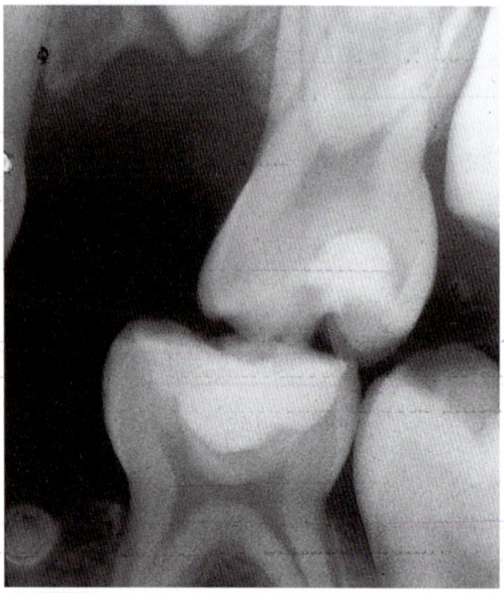

Figure 12-2 Radiograph showing stepwise excavation performed in two primary second molars in order to keep them *in situ* and without subjective symptoms at least until the permanent first molars are in occlusion.

Direct pulp capping

Direct pulp capping means covering the exposed healthy pulp with a medicament, preferably calcium hydroxide, without any surgical intervention. Direct capping has some disadvantages, especially in the primary dentition, due to minimal space for retention of the wound dressing, zinc oxide–eugenol cement, and permanent restoration. Direct pulp capping is rarely used nowadays since partial pulpotomy was introduced and shown to be a more favorable choice of treatment.

Partial pulpotomy

The technique of partial pulpotomy is presented in Box 12-4 and Fig. 12-3. Partial pulpotomy is the treatment of choice for primary molars with healthy pulps or partial chronic pulpitis. The prerequisites of access to the pulp wound, sufficient space for the wound dressing, and establishment of a tight seal against the oral environment, are better met by this technique than by direct pulp capping. The technique includes removal of a small part of the pulp just at the site of exposure using high

Box 12-4 Partial pulpotomy

Prior conditions. Pulpal state: healthy pulp or partial chronic pulpitis/symptomless carious exposure. A more advanced pulpal state might be accepted for the very young permanent tooth: see text.

The tooth has been anesthetized and isolated with a rubber dam. The treatment is performed with due consideration to disinfection.

Procedure	Method	Rationale – comments
Removal of pulp tissue	Starting from the exposure, 1–2 mm of the pulp tissue is removed with a high-speed rotating spherical diamond cooled bur with ample flow of water	As judged by histology, the least trauma to the wound surface is achieved
	The diamond bur should be large enough, if possible, to work in the hard tissue concomitantly with the cutting of the pulp tissue	To gain support for a smooth cut
Control of bleeding	Rinse gently with sterile saline. Dry gently with sterile cotton pellets	A smooth-cut pulp tissue will bleed moderately
	Check that there are no residual tags of pulp tissue	Residual tags may prolong bleeding
	Lime-water [supersaturated solution of $Ca(OH)_2$] may be used for hemostasis	Calcium ions enhance coagulation. Avoid other hemostatics: they either damage tissue or may induce after-bleedings
	If bleeding persists	Remove more pulp tissue or reconsider therapy
Application of calcium hydroxide	Cover the wound with a 0.5–1 mm layer of calcium hydroxide	
	Check carefully that no bleeding has started	A blood clot between the wound and the wound dressing will impair wound healing
Placement of the base	Apply a layer of slow-setting zinc oxide–eugenol cement. Cover with a setting calcium hydroxide base or glass-ionomer cement	Gives the best bacteria-tight seal. The base prevents pressure on the pulpal wound
	Proceed with restorative work	
	Ensure a tight seal against the oral environment	

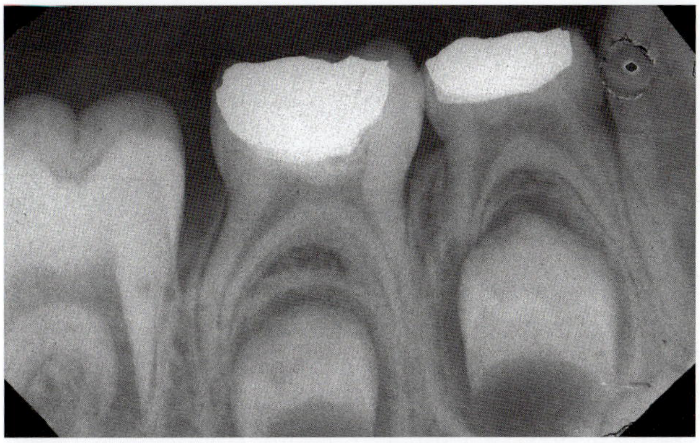

Figure 12-3 Radiograph of primary second molar after partial pulpotomy. The hard tissue barrier indicates wound healing; note absence of periradicular pathology.

speed and a diamond bur during irrigation with water in order not to traumatize the pulp. The wound treatment is as described before, i.e., application of calcium hydroxide in tissue contact without any intermediate blood clot. Slow-setting zinc oxide–eugenol is applied and covered by a cement. The tooth is restored.

Pulpotomy

Pulpotomy, or vital amputation of the coronal pulp, includes removal of all the coronal pulp. The surgical technique and the treatment of the wound are the same as described for partial pulpotomy, but the wound surface is placed at the orifices of the root canals.

Before partial pulpotomy was introduced, pulpotomy was the traditional treatment for pulpally involved primary teeth.

Pulpectomy and root canal therapy

The modern (up-to-date) approach is to avoid pulpectomy and root canal therapy in the primary dentition and to choose extraction. As mentioned before (Box 12-2) the risk for occlusal complications is rare and should be seen in relation to the risk for the underlying permanent tooth germ if perforating the roots and/or pushing infected material through the apical foramen.

In cases when the second premolar is missing, conventional pulpectomy or root canal treatment with guttapercha as root-filling material may be performed.

Wound dressings and tissue reactions

A proper wound dressing for use in pedodontic endodontics should not induce any persistent pathologic changes of the residual pulp or the periapical tissues. In the case of primary teeth the wound dressing should not carry any risk to the underlying tooth germ. Two main groups of wound dressings have for a long time been at choice, calcium hydroxide and formocresol. For some years two other medicaments have been in use, mineral trioxide aggregate (MTA) and ferric sulfate (Box 12.5).

Calcium hydroxide preparations are used because of their biological effect, i.e., stimulation of a hard tissue barrier, which allows healing in an organ such as the pulp, which lacks epithelium. MTA is a new wound dressing material with very promising results.

The use of formocresol has been questioned for several years. Since the International Agency for Research on Cancer (6) classified formaldehyde as carcinogenic to humans, efforts have been reinforced to prevent formocresol being used in endodontic treatment. The present trend is away from devitalizing medicaments and towards searching for medicaments able to keep primary teeth with total chronic pulpitis or partial necrosis in the dentition without causing any periapical pathologic changes. Ferric sulfate belongs to this category and has so far showed similar success rates as formocresol. In this context, the possibility of extraction of primary teeth with more advanced pathologic pulpal changes should be seriously considered.

Calcium hydroxide and MTA

Calcium hydroxide is strongly alkaline with a pH about 12 and initially causes a chemical injury to the vital pulp with a zone of firm necrosis adjacent to vital pulp tissue.

Box 12-5 Wound dressings

Calcium hydroxide
- Biological effect.
- Contributes to wound healing in healthy pulp tissue and apical closure of nonvital teeth.
- Contributes to dissolution of nonvital pulp remnants when used in relation to root canal treatment of immature permanent teeth.
- Can be used in both primary and permanent teeth.

MTA
- A cement – biological effect.
- The same as for calcium hydroxide except no ability to dissolve nonvital pulp tissue remnants.

Formocresol
- Devitalizing effect – nonbiological.
- Causes chronic inflammation and necrosis.
- Has systemic negative effects.
- Has no pulp healing effect.
- To be used very restrictively *if ever* and only in primary teeth.

Ferric sulfate
- Nonbiological.
- Produces hemostasis and forms a ferric ion complex.
- To be used in primary teeth.

The response of the residual pulp tissue is characteristic of wounded connective tissue. It begins with a vascular and inflammatory reaction to control and eliminate the irritating agent. Thereafter, the repair process starts, including proliferation of cells and formation of new collagen. When the pulp is protected from irritation, new odontoblasts differentiate and the newly formed tissue assumes a dentin-like appearance, which indicates that pulp function has been restored. Mineralization of the newly formed collagen starts with dystrophic calcification of the zone with firm necrosis leading to deposition of mineral in the newly formed collagen as well (18).

MTA induces similar tissue reactions when applied to pulp tissue. MTA, when mixed with water, forms crystals of calcium oxide in amorphous structure of 33% Ca^{2+}, 49% PO_4^{3-}, 2% C, 3% Cl^-, and 6% Si^{2+}. MTA was developed as an apex filling material, but has also been proven successful in vital pulp therapy procedures (12). It is a powder that sets in the presence of moisture and has a pH of 12.5, similar to calcium hydroxide. It has an ability to actively promote hard tissue formation.

The hard tissue barrier is a criterion of wound healing and must be considered favorable because it facilitates the clinical handling of the tooth. The hard tissue barrier does not mean a tight seal against the oral cavity. It is therefore of utmost importance that the restoration of the tooth provides a tight seal to prevent infection through microleakage.

Calcium hydroxide and MTA contribute to wound healing but, as with any other pulpal medicament, they have no healing effect on chronically inflamed pulp tissue. Consequently, these two medicaments are more delicate to work with, regarding the diagnosis of the residual pulp, the surgical technique, and the wound treatment.

The two medicaments must be restricted to teeth with healthy pulps or with partial chronic pulpitis in order to achieve a favorable outcome. However, in young, immature permanent teeth with a more favorable ability to heal, they may be used in cases with more advanced pulpal conditions as well.

In root canal therapy of immature permanent teeth calcium hydroxide induces an apical seal, a hard tissue barrier, and dissolves necrotic tissue remnants left in the root canal; all beneficial effects (1,4). MTA contributes to a rather immediate apical seal, since it is a cement and also induces hard tissue formation, but has no dissolving effect on remnants of pulpal tissue.

Formocresol

The use of formocresol as pulp medicament should be avoided because of its negative systemic properties. Formaldehyde has a known carcinogenic, immunogenic, toxic, and mutagenic potential which makes it questionable and unsuitable for use in pedodontic endodontics (6,8). Formaldehyde is the devitalizing ingredient in formocresol. Formaldehyde, the aqueous solution of the gas formaldehyde, is used for fixation of tissue in histologic studies. The same process is considered to occur *in vivo*. The clinical procedure includes a pulpotomy, followed by application of cotton pellets moistened with formocresol *to* the root pulps at the canal openings for 5 minutes. The treated root pulps and the furcation area are then covered with slow-setting zinc oxide–eugenol cement in order to get a bacteria-tight seal and the tooth is restored.

The rationale for use of this type of wound dressing is to create a chemically altered zone at the medicament interface that will be stable over time and leave the deeper untreated pulp tissue vital and uninflamed. Studies show, however, that the degree of penetration of formaldehyde is time and dose dependent (11). Furthermore, clinical–histologic investigations have shown that chronic inflammation or even partial necrosis of the residual pulp often results (15).

In conclusion, formocresol does not induce healing of the pulp but does cause pathologic changes in the residual pulp. Formocresol very seldom gives rise to clinical complications but should be used very restrictively because of its systemic risks.

Instead of using formocresol, ferric sulfate may be used or the tooth extracted.

Ferric sulfate

Ferric sulfate (15.5%) has been used as pulpotomy agent as a substitute for formocresol for 15–20 years. Ferric sulfate (Fe_2SO_4) in contact with blood forms a ferric ion–protein complex, which seals the cut blood vessels mechanically, producing hemostasis (3). The effect of ferric sulfate is hemostatic but not bactericidal or fixative. After application of ferric sulfate for 15 seconds, the pulp is covered with zinc oxide–eugenol and the cavity sealed. Research has shown similar results both regarding clinical, radiographic, and histologic results as formocresol. Healing has not been achieved, but the teeth could be retained in the dentition for shorter or longer intervals. There are no known systemic risks of using ferric sulfate in pulpal treatment.

Regarding endodontic treatment of primary teeth with more advanced pulpal involvement than partial pulpitis, extraction of the tooth should be considered as first choice of treatment. Extraction of a primary molar often has no or only a slight influence on the occlusal development. In very rare cases space maintenance is needed. Extraction is especially important to consider in seriously carious primary dentitions in order to avoid overtreatment and therapies with uncertain prognosis. The capacity of the family to meet necessary preventive demands is also to be evaluated in order to spare the child from unnecessary treatment or treatment with uncertain prognosis.

Complications (primary teeth)

Internal dentin resorption is a common complication irrespective of medicament used, but is often reported to be caused by calcium hydroxide. However, investigations have shown that the reasons for resorption are most probably chronic inflammation of the residual pulp and/or the presence of an extrapulpal blood clot on the wound surface before capping with calcium hydroxide (18). There is no support for the statement that calcium hydroxide *per se* causes chronic inflammation and resorption.

MTA has not been used in the primary dentition for a long enough time to allow estimation of complications with any certainty.

Formocresol fixates parts of the underlying pulp, and the outcome is consequently not dependent on the pulpal state or healing. Most studies report various degrees of chronic inflammation and/or necrosis of the residual pulp, which in time might cause clinical and radiographic complications, though very seldom within 2–3 years following treatment (15). Negative effects on the underlying permanent tooth germ have been reported in some but not all studies.

Using ferric sulfate gives similar pulpal reactions to formocresol.

Follow-up and long-term prognosis (primary dentition)

Long-term prognosis might be an inappropriate term considering primary teeth. It is, however, reasonable to consider the necessity for and outcome of the treatment planned. It is not ethically justifiable to let a child undergo treatment, perhaps experienced as both difficult and stressful, if the outcome is uncertain or poor.

Stepwise excavation is a treatment that is easily accepted by the child and usually includes a seriously carious tooth of a very young child or a tooth with a short-term importance for the occlusal development. The clinical experience of this therapy is favorable.

Partial pulpotomy is the therapy of choice in cases with partial chronic pulpitis (the symptomless cariously exposed pulp). Partial pulpotomy does include some strain on the young patient, but the treatment is usually short, since the surgical intervention is minimal, and the control of the bleeding is easy because no major vessels are cut. Compared to direct capping, the possibility to seal the cavity efficiently is better and consequently the risk of future bacterial contamination and failure is less. According to the literature, the prognosis for partial pulpotomy of primary molars is about 80% after 1 year (19) and 75% after 2 years, which is more favorable than that reported for traditional pulpotomy.

Pulpotomy (coronal pulpotomy), using calcium hydroxide, became a more favorable therapy when a gentle surgical technique was introduced, where no blood clot was left on the wound surface and calcium hydroxide was applied in tissue contact with the pulp. The rate of success, however, seldom exceeded 60% after 2 years. There are still clinical problems in controlling the bleeding because the technique includes cutting the greater vessels of the pulp.

Pulpotomy, using formocresol or ferric sulfate as wound dressing, has shown favorable clinical and radiographic success rates (5,10).

Pulp therapy in immature permanent teeth

The wound dressing most used is calcium hydroxide. The techniques are described in Box 12-3. However, MTA has been introduced as a wound dressing for partial pulpotomy, pulpotomy, as apex filling at pulpectomy, and root canal treatment in very young and immature permanent teeth.

Stepwise excavation

This therapy is very successful in young permanent teeth with extensive carious lesions with obvious risk of pulp exposure. It alleviates subjective symptoms and, according to literature (7,14), the risk of pulp exposure at the final treatment is dramatically decreased compared to removal of all caries at the first treatment session. Furthermore, when treating a young dentition with extensive carious lesions, stepwise excavation provides time for a more considered evaluation of the long-term prognosis for the dentition as well as for the patient (Fig. 12-4).

Partial pulpotomy

Partial pulpotomy has been shown to be the treatment of choice in traumatically as well as cariously exposed pulps of young permanent teeth (Box 12-4). The partial pulpotomy makes physiologic narrowing of the coronal pulp lumen possible, which means a mechanically stronger tooth less prone to future fracture (Fig. 12-5), compared to a tooth subjected to coronal pulpotomy. Partial pulpotomy is also to be preferred to pulp capping, since there is a much better possibility to control the wound surface, avoid any extrapulpal blood clot, to

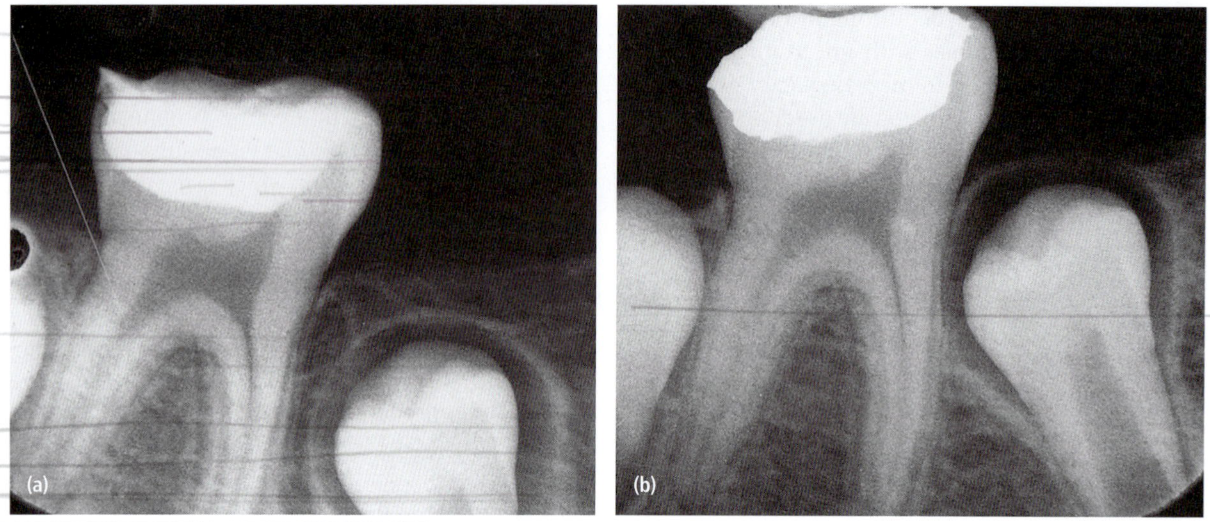

Figure 12-4 Stepwise excavation of a permanent molar, (a) at the time of treatment and (b) 9 months later. The formation of dentin between the temporary filling and the pulp has proceeded and the risk of pulp exposure at the time of final restoration of the tooth is minimal.

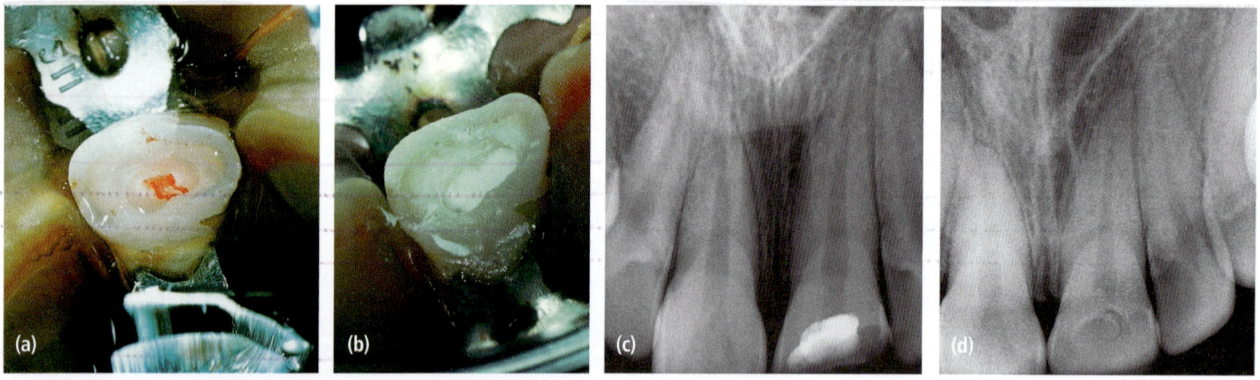

Figure 12-5 Partial pulpotomy of a permanent incisor with complicated crown fracture. (a) At the time of treatment; (b) application of calcium hydroxide; (c) radiograph at the time of treatment; and (d) several years later.

get sufficient retention for wound dressing and a tight seal, and thereby prevent bacterial infection. Partial pulpotomy of traumatized incisors has a success rate of 95% following an observation period of 3–15 years (2).

Partial pulpotomy is also the therapy for young permanent teeth with carious exposure of the pulp (Fig. 12-6). The outcome is favorable. Studies show a 89–91% success rate with a follow-up of about 3–4.5 years, irrespective of root development at the time of treatment (12). A recent study using MTA as wound dressing showed high success rate, 93% after about 3 years (13).

Partial pulpotomy is a permanent treatment and should only be followed by a pulpectomy if there is a need for a post in the root canal in the future.

Pulpotomy

Since partial pulpotomy was introduced, pulpotomy has become a rare therapy. It was most often looked on as a temporary measure, especially in molars, until root development was complete and a pulpectomy and permanent root filling with guttapercha could be done. Calcium hydroxide or MTA are the wound dressings to be used.

Pulpectomy

This type of endodontic treatment should be avoided in immature permanent teeth because continuing root development is compromised. In permanent teeth with complete or almost complete root development this therapy does not differ from that given in adult teeth. The reader is referred to textbooks on endodontics for further information.

Root canal treatment

Nonvital pulp of an immature permanent tooth includes, for incisors, a great risk of future fracture of the tooth

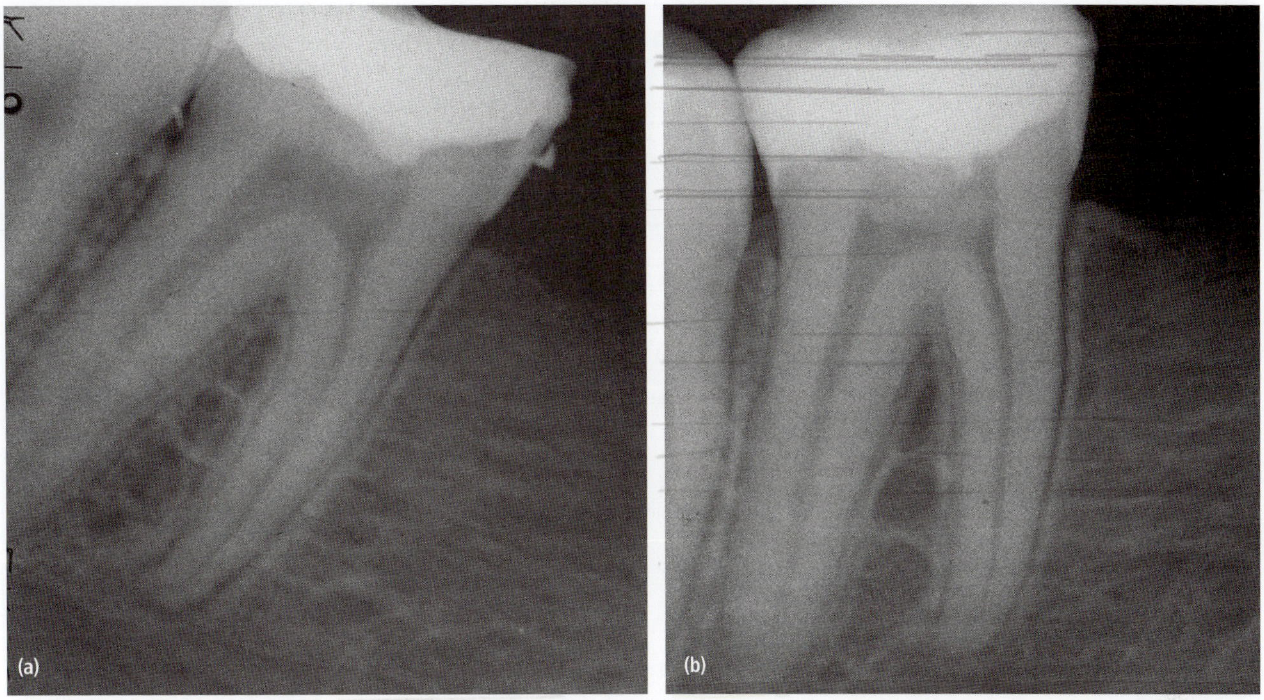

Figure 12-6 Partial pulpotomy of permanent molar. (a) Radiograph taken at the time of treatment and (b) 2 years after treatment.

because of a wide pulpal lumen and short roots with thin walls. The more immature the root, the greater the risk of tooth fracture. This usually does not contraindicate root canal treatment of immature traumatized permanent incisors, which mostly should be kept to maintain the space until favorable conditions for space closure, orthodontic treatment, or inserting an implant are attained.

The technique when treating a nonvital immature permanent incisor might be somewhat different because of the difficulty of removing all necrotic pulp tissue (Box 12-6). It is essential to fill the canal with calcium hydroxide for two reasons: first, to get calcium hydroxide in contact with periapical tissue to promote the hard tissue barrier formation and second to enable the calcium hydroxide to dissolve necrotic pulp tissue that has unintentionally been left (4). The level of calcium hydroxide, which has a radiopacity similar to that of dentin, is checked radiographically every 3–6 months. The treatment is repeated when the level of calcium hydroxide is coronal to the apical third of the canal. Usually two or three changes are necessary until a hard tissue barrier has formed apically and any apical periodontitis has healed. Thereafter, a permanent root filling is made. The frequency of success of this sequence of endodontic interventions has been reported to be very high, about 95%, 4 years after the permanent root filling with guttapercha (1).

MTA will most probably be a better alternative than calcium hydroxide. When applied apically in the root canal, a prompt apical seal is obtained, which also induces hard tissue formation against the vital periapical tissue. The treatment has to be combined with an interval of calcium hydroxide filling of the canal in order to dissolve unintentionally left necrotic tissue. The permanent root filling with guttapercha can be done shortly afterwards. Extraction or resorption of a tooth with an apical seal of MTA cement might pose a problem, since the cement might be difficult to remove and it might complicate the insertion of any implant.

Bleaching of nonvital discolored permanent teeth

The clinical procedure for bleaching with sodium perborate is presented in Box 12-7.

Bleaching of teeth may be complicated by cervical external root resorption and the treatment should therefore be carefully performed and followed up. Leakage of the bleaching agent through the rubber dam may cause periodontal damage and the periodontium may be injured by the bleaching agent leaking via the dentinal tubules. If carefully performed, bleaching of discolored nonvital incisors has a favorable outcome (9) and the frequency of cervical resorption can be expected to be low.

Box 12-6 Root canal treatment of immature permanent incisors

Prior conditions (use of calcium hydroxide):

- The pulp is necrotic.
- The tooth is isolated with a rubber dam. The treatment is performed with due consideration to disinfection.
- A radiograph of the tooth is available.

Procedure	Method	Rationale – comments
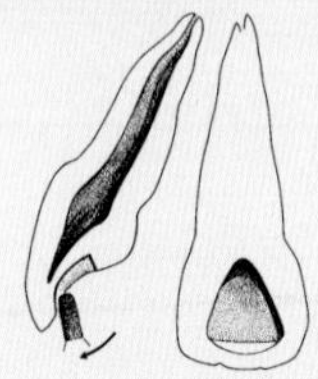	Use a cylindrical/spherical bur on high-speed drill and make a triangular cavity into dentin	The shape of the cavity corresponds to the outlines of the pulp chamber
	Raise the bur more vertically and slope the wall at the base of the triangle outwards	To accommodate a direct-line access into the pulp chamber and root canal in the long axes of the tooth
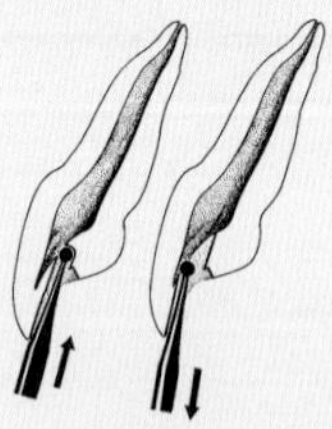	Perforate the pulp with a round bur at low speed. Then move the bur incisally, from inside the pulp chamber and outwards down to the tip of the pulpal horn	Perforation in apical direction omits compromising the labial wall. Working from inside restricts removal of dentin to the roof of the chamber
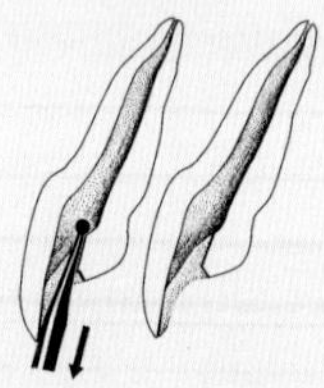	Shift to a round bur with a long shank. Place the bur apical to the lingual ledge of dentin and move the bur out to the cavo-surface	The groove in the ledge should be just wide enough to allow passage into the canal of properly sized root canal instruments
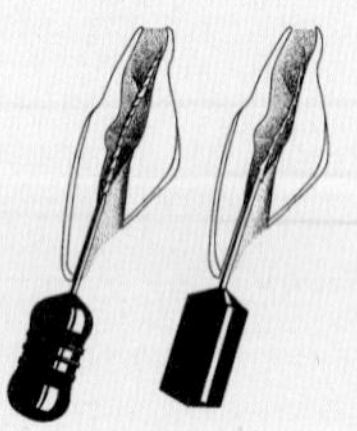	Clean the access cavity. Use barbed broaches around the periphery of the root canal	To reach the irregularities of the root canal walls
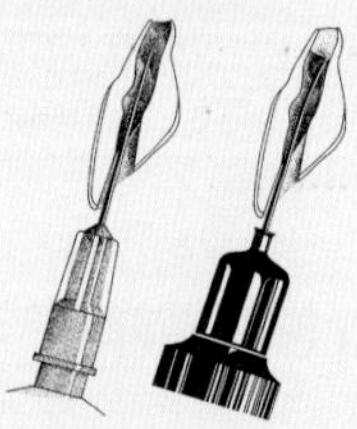	Irrigate with 0.5% sodium hypochlorite or sterile saline. Dry the canal with coarse paper points	For mechanical and chemical debridement
Calcium hydroxide as medicament		
	Fill the canal stepwise with calcium hydroxide paste using a cartridge syringe	For disinfectant and activity and to promote apical closure. Also to dissolve pulp tissue remnants
	Be sure of contact with vital tissue apically	Necessary in order to achieve a hard tissue formation
	Pack the paste stepwise with the blunt end of a thick paper point. Seal the cleaned opening with IRM-cement	To blot excess moisture. The radiopacity of a well-packed canal is similar to that of dentin
MTA		
	First appointment: place the MTA cement at the apical foramen. Apply calcium hydroxide in the root canal to make sure there is a humid environment. Further appointments: the canal is filled with guttapercha and the tooth restored	In order to set the cement and dissolve pulp tissue remnants

Box 12-7 Bleaching of nonvital discolored teeth

Prior conditions:

- The tooth has an adequate guttapercha root filling, and has been carefully isolated with a rubber dam following careful cleaning with an aqueous slurry of pumice.
- A radiograph should be available.

Procedure	Method	Comments
Gaining access to pulp chamber	Remove all restorative material and as much discolored dentin as possible without weakening the tooth unnecessarily	Permits easier penetration of the bleaching agent
Removal of root filling	Remove guttapercha 1–2 mm below the level of the dentinogingival junction. Apply a 1–2 mm layer of zinc oxide–eugenol cement	To prevent seepage into the root canal/or into the periodontium via dentinal tubules
Pretreatment of the cavity	Carefully etch the dentin. Clean with chloroform or acetone. Blow the pulp chamber dry	To dissolve any fatty material
Bleaching		
Preparation of the bleaching paste	Mix sodium perborate with 3% H_2O_2 or water to a thick paste	H_2O_2 might be omitted because of its possible resorption-inducing ability
Application of the paste	Fill the pulp chamber with the paste	Leave enough space for sufficient sealing. Carefully remove any bleaching paste from enamel margins
Sealing of the cavity	Seal with zinc oxide–eugenol cement and phosphate cement between appointments. If necessary, repeat the procedure one to three times at 1-week intervals	
Rinsing of the gingival crevice	Rinse carefully with water	To avoid chemical injury to the soft tissue and thereby the risk of cervical external root resorption
Final sealing	Remove all bleaching agents. Flush the cavity carefully with water and finally with chloroform. Acid etch the cavity, use dentin bonding, and restore the tooth with the lightest composite available	To enhance the result of the bleaching

Handling the emergency child patient

In this chapter, discussion of emergency treatment will be restricted to the preschool child with toothache due to extensive carious lesions. For treatment of acute trauma and the use of sedation and pain control the reader is referred to Chapters 5 and 18.

Symptoms may vary depending on the extent of the carious lesion and the involvement of the pulp. The aim of the emergency treatment is to provide pain control and to eliminate the cause of pain. The pain control usually includes local analgesia and may also include sedation and oral analgesics. History taking should focus on the general health of the child and how and when the pain is occurring, followed by the examination of the mouth and the teeth.

After the diagnosis has been made, a decision is made for conservative treatment or extraction. Should the final treatment be performed immediately or should temporary measures be taken? Is sedation necessary? Are antibiotics necessary? Finally, the parents must be given thorough information before treatment.

Pain at food intake

The tooth is painful when the child is eating, especially sour, hot, or sweet food. In such a case the tooth usually has an extensive carious lesion with retentive capacity. This is why the pain appears when ingredients of the food irritate the pulp when stuck in the cavity. The radiograph shows a deep carious cavity, not necessarily with pulp lesion.

The emergency treatment involves stepwise excavation avoiding exposure of the pulp, application of calcium hydroxide and a temporary filling. The family of the child should be provided with some analgesics and information about caries-preventive measures; later the tooth is restored with a more permanent filling material.

Toothache at night

This type of pain is usually not related to food intake but appears spontaneously, especially at night, and the child wakes up. Symptoms commonly have been apparent for a period of time and the child has been avoiding drinking and eating on the painful side of the mouth and might therefore be tired and difficult to handle. The tooth is mostly grossly carious, has some distinct clinical symptoms such as tenderness on percussion and/or pressure and increased mobility, indicating involvement of the periodontal membrane. Spontaneous pain that is not relieved by analgesics is usually an indication of advanced pulp pathology. Although X-rays may not show pathologic changes, widening of the periodontal space is usually seen, indicating more advanced pathologic changes. The treatment may include some temporary measures but the final treatment is extraction of the primary tooth. When there are definite radiographic signs of periradicular and/or interradicular periodontitis, the tooth is extracted with due consideration to sedation and pain control (see case description in Box 12-8).

Box 12-8 The emergency child patient – description of a case

History

A physically healthy 5-year-old boy is seeking your help because of:

- toothache for 3 weeks
- no sleep for the last 3 nights due to increasing pain and discomfort
- fever and pain which have during the last 2 days been treated by analgesics with varying effect.

Status

The boy is tired and difficult to handle:

- extraorally
  - a slight nonpainful swelling along left mandible
  - regional lymph nodes are involved
- intraorally:
  - several molars show large carious lesions and heavy plaque accumulation especially in the left mandible
  - 75, only remnants of the crown are left and there is a buccal fistula; radiograph shows apical periodontitis
  - 74 is also carious and shows increased mobility as well as tenderness on percussion; radiograph shows interradicular periodontitis and widening of the periodontal space apically

Therapy

There are two alternatives, both of which have to be followed up in order to re-create good oral health for the boy:

- prescription of antibiotics and adequate pain control; extractions done a few days later under antibiotic cover
- immediate extraction with due consideration to pain control including local analgesia as well as oral analgesics.

Most probably the patient needs some sedation as well, for instance rectal/oral sedation with midazolam or nitrous oxide/oxygen sedation.

The emergency patient with toothache may also show general symptoms such as fever and tiredness. The oral symptoms are often more pronounced, with involvement of the regional lymph nodes and swelling of the oral tissues surrounding the tooth. Evaluation of the nature of the swelling includes the size and extent of the swelling, and the location, intraoral and/or extraoral. Is the swelling increasing? There are distinct pathologic radiographic signs and purulence might be present. The child may be in need of antibiotics. A few days later, the tooth is extracted under antibiotic cover. Temporary measures may include opening the tooth, exposing the pulp and draining the pus. The tooth should not be left open to the oral environment, risking further infection, but should be sealed temporarily.

The rationale for being radical in the emergency situation is based on the value of the tooth and the consideration that the child should not suffer more strain than necessary. If an extraction is done with adequate sedation, preferably with amnesic effect, and analgesia, the emergency treatment is adequate and the child will soon recover. There is very seldom any need for several treatment sessions of pulp treatment with doubtful outcome as these usually end up with extraction anyway. Concern about the child's future attitude to dental care is more important than the child losing a painful tooth.

Use of antibiotics

Antibiotics should always be used restrictively, which is also the case in children's dentistry. There are medical conditions that demand antibiotic cover even for ordinary dental treatment and the reader is referred to Chapters 22 and 23 regarding medically compromised children. With emergency treatment, however, there are situations where antibiotics may be indicated, most often when the child's general state or a tooth is seriously infected with a risk of spread to neighboring tissues, teeth, tooth germs, and ultimately a risk of a general spreading to more vital organs.

In general, penicillin V (phenoxymethylpenicillin) is the drug of choice, but with anerobic microorganisms, which is often the case in oral infection, metronidazole may be used. Metronidazole is to be preferred when there is an infected pulp, for instance following a luxation injury. Although the treatment with calcium hydroxide may be bacteriostatic, there is a risk of persistent infection of periradicular tissues.

Erythromycin is the third alternative with dental infections in children. It is used in cases where there is an allergy to penicillin V.

Dosage may vary between different countries. However, the regimen for penicillin V is usually 12.5 mg/kg body weight two to three times a day for 10 days, for metronidazole 7.5 mg/kg body weight every 8 hours for 5–6 days, and for erythromycin 15 mg/kg body weight every 24 hours for 10 days. For very small children, there are special dosages. For other dosages, see local reference guides.

References

1. Cvek M. Prognosis of luxated non-vital maxillary incisors treated with calcium hydroxide and filled with gutta-percha. A retrospective clinical study. *Endod Dent Traumatol* 1992;**8**:45–55.
2. Cvek M. Partial pulpotomy in crown-fractured incisors – results 3 to 15 years after treatment. *Acta Stomatol Croatia* 1993;**27**: 167–73.
3. Fischer DE. Tissue management. A new solution to an old problem. *Gen Dent* 1987;**35**:178–82.
4. Hasselgren G, Olsson B, Cvek M. Effects of calcium hydroxide and sodium hypochlorite on the dissolution of necrotic porcine muscle tissue. *J Endod* 1988;**14**:125–7.
5. Ibricevic H, Al-Jame Q. Ferric sulphate and formocresol in pulpotomy of primary molars: long term follow-up study. *Eur J Paediatr Dent* 2003;**1**:28–32.
6. International Agency for Research on Cancer, WHO, 2004; Press Release No. 153, June 15.
7. Leksell E, Ridell K, Cvek M, Mejàre I. Pulp exposure after stepwise versus direct complete excavation of deep carious lesions in young posterior permanent teeth. *Endod Dent Traumatol* 1996; **12**:192–6.
8. Lewis B. Formaldehyde in dentistry: a review for the millennium. *J Clin Pediatr Dent* 1998;**22**:167–77.
9. Marin PD, Heithersay GS, Bridges TE. A quantitative comparison of traditional and non-peroxide bleaching agents. *Endod Dent Traumatol* 1998;**14**:64–7.
10. Markovic D, Zivojinovic V, Vucetic M. Evaluation of three pulpotomy medicaments in primary teeth. *Eur J Paediatr Dent* 2005; **6**:133–8.
11. Mejàre I, Hasselgren G, Hammarström LE. Effect of formaldehyde-containing drugs on human dental pulp evaluated by enzyme histochemical technique. *Scand J Dent Res* 1976;**84**: 29–36.
12. Mejàre I, Cvek M. Partial pulpotomy in young permanent teeth with deep carious lesions. *Endod Dent Traumatol* 1993;**9**: 238–42.
13. Qudeimat MA, Barrieshi-Nusair KM, Owais AI. Calcium hydroxide vs. mineral trioxide aggregates for partial pulpotomy of permanent molars with deep caries. *Eur Arch Paediatr Dent* 2007;**8**:99–104.
14. Ricketts DN, Kidd EA, Innes N, Clarkson J. Complete or ultra-conservative removal of decayed tissue in unfilled teeth. *Cochrane Database Syst Rev* 2006 29,3.CD003808.
15. Rölling I, Thylstrup A. A 3-year clinical follow-up study of pulpotomized primary molars treated with the formocresol technique. *Scand J Dent Res* 1975;**83**:47–57.
16. Rönnerman A, Thilander B. A longitudinal study on the effect of unilateral extraction of primary molars. *Scand J Dent Res* 1977; **85**:362–72.
17. Schröder U. Agreement between clinical and histologic findings in chronic coronal pulpitis in primary teeth. *Scand J Dent Res* 1977;**85**:583–7.
18. Schröder U. Effects of calcium hydroxide-containing pulp-capping agents on pulp cell migration, proliferation and differentiation. *J Dent Res* 1985;**64**(Spec Iss):541–8.
19. Schröder U, Szpringer-Nodzak M, Janicha J, Wacinska M, Budny J, Mlosek K. A one-year follow-up of partial pulpotomy and calcium hydroxide capping in primary molars. *Endod Dent Traumatol* 1987;**3**:304–6.

13

Periodontal conditions

Bengt Sjödin and Lars Matsson

Inflammatory reactions in the periodontal tissues are common in children and adolescents. In most instances the inflammation is restricted to the gingival tissues. Gingivitis is characterized by the presence of gingival inflammation without detectable loss of bone or connective tissue attachment. Periodontitis in children and adolescents may, as in adults, have varying manifestations, and the present nomenclature distinguishes between *aggressive* (i.e., severe) and *chronic* (i.e., moderate) forms of the disease.

As in adults, gingivitis and periodontitis in children and adolescents are primarily caused by accumulation of bacterial plaque on the teeth, and especially in the case of gingivitis, the state of the gingiva thus mirrors the oral hygiene level of the individual. However, severe forms of inflammation may also signal the presence of a general disorder, especially if the gingival inflammatory reaction is out of proportion to the amount of bacterial plaque present (1).

Early treatment of periodontal diseases is usually very effective and early recognition increases the chances of preventing loss of tooth support or limiting the progression of the disease. Thus, there are good reasons to pay attention to inflammatory reactions in the periodontal tissues of young individuals (9). In addition, there are other conditions, such as gingival recessions and gingival enlargements, which need the pediatric dentist's attention.

Normal periodontal conditions

Primary dentition

The marginal edge of the primary tooth gingiva has a bulky and rounded appearance (Fig. 13-1). The typical stippling in healthy gingiva develops slowly from the age of 2 or 3 years. In areas with diastema between primary teeth, the interdental tissues are comparable to saddle areas. When the molars have established proximal contacts the interproximal area is completely filled by an interdental papilla, with a marginal concavity, a col, corresponding to the contact area (22).

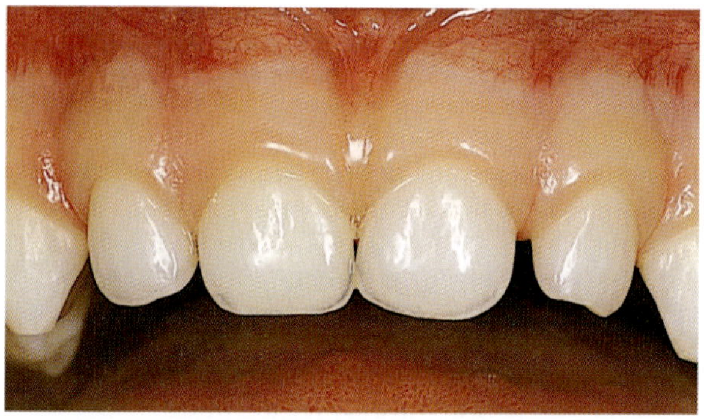

Figure 13-1 Clinically healthy primary tooth gingiva.

The connective tissue has a similar composition to that around young permanent teeth. However, compared to permanent teeth the primary teeth are associated with a thicker junctional epithelium, which may influence the permeability of the epithelial structures by bacterial toxins. The junctional epithelium of the primary dentition would be less permeable and thus more resistant to inflammation.

On radiographs, the alveolar bone surrounding the primary teeth has a distinct, but thin, lamina dura and a comparatively wide periodontal membrane. There are few trabeculae and large marrow spaces with rich vascularization. The root cementum is also thin and mainly cellular.

Permanent dentition

The exfoliation of primary teeth and the eruption of permanent teeth entail considerable morphological and histological changes, as described in Chapter 15.

Compared to the primary tooth gingiva, the healthy marginal gingiva around permanent teeth is thin and is characterized by a pink color (Fig. 13-2). After the tooth

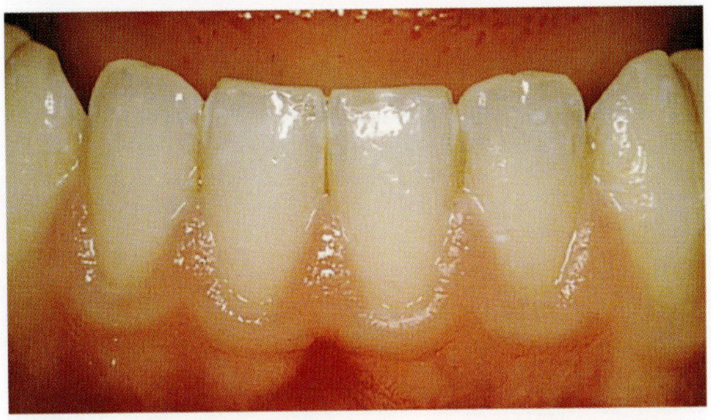

Figure 13-2 Clinically healthy permanent tooth gingiva.

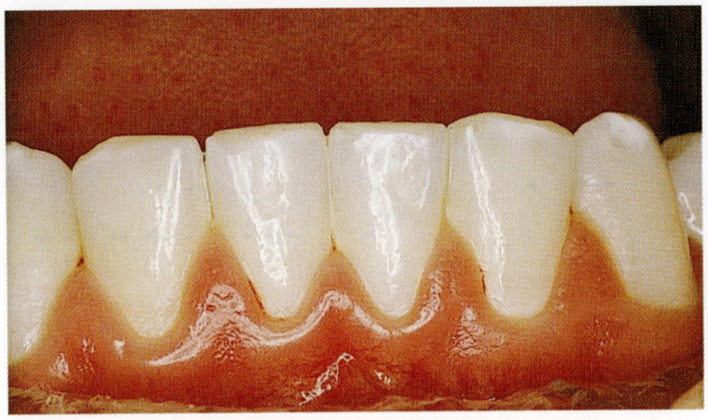

Figure 13-3 Chronic gingivitis.

is fully erupted, the gingival margin is located on the enamel surface approximately 0.5–2 mm coronal to the cemento-enamel junction. During the period of passive eruption, i.e., the period of slow withdrawal of the marginal soft tissue, the length of the junctional epithelium is considerable in children. Although a periodontal probe is easily inserted deep along the tooth surface, there is no justification for unnecessary explorations interfering with the junctional epithelium.

Bacteria-induced inflammatory periodontal diseases

One of the major problems in understanding the pathogenesis of periodontal diseases is the difficulty in distinguishing clearly between normal and pathological conditions. When the gingival tissue is kept free from plaque, leukocytes will still be found migrating through the junctional epithelium towards the gingival sulcus. A few inflammatory cells may also be present in the connective tissue.

The balance between irritation, and the individual phagocytic capacity and immunological competence, will be decisive for the severity of the disease. If plaque accumulation is minimal and the defense mechanisms operate normally, there will be no clinical symptoms. More pronounced plaque accumulations or defects in the defense reactions result in clinical symptoms (20).

Gingivitis

Clinical picture

The inflammatory reaction includes a vascular response and an accumulation of inflammatory cells. When the vascular response has reached a certain level, clinically noticeable signs of inflammation will occur. The marginal gingiva becomes reddish, with a swollen appearance and papillae protruding from the interproximal spaces (Fig. 13-3). The volume is increased and the surface is shiny. Crevicular exudation is clinically obvious, especially when light pressure is applied to the free gingiva. There is also an increased tendency towards gingival bleeding on probing.

The vascular and cellular reactions in the marginal gingiva should primarily be regarded as a natural defense against microorganisms. Since the causative factor is plaque accumulation, an efficient oral hygiene regimen will eliminate the clinical symptoms rapidly. However, a new period of poor oral hygiene will result in a recurrence. Subclinical reactions and episodes of clinical gingivitis may alternate over long periods.

The diagnosis of gingivitis is based on the clinical symptoms visible to the eye, such as redness, swelling, and bleeding tendency. The tendency today is to simplify the diagnostic criteria using gingival bleeding tendency as a measure of the gingival inflammatory condition. The gingival bleeding index (GBI) is based on one simple criterion: whether or not the marginal gingiva bleeds on gentle probing. The index is calculated as the percentage of bleeding gingival units of the total number of units examined (20).

In healthy children, gingival affections usually remain superficial, and when a child shows severe generalized long-standing gingivitis, the dentist should consider having the child's general health investigated.

Age-related differences

Epidemiological as well as experimental studies have revealed an age-dependent difference in the tendency to develop gingivitis during childhood. Thus, preschool children tend to be less susceptible to gingivitis than adolescents and adults (22). The reasons for this difference are not fully understood. It has been shown that spirochetes and black-pigmented *Bacteroides*, although frequently found in adults, are not regularly present in the microbial plaque of children with normal gingiva. In addition, the microbial plaque of children with gingivitis has lower proportions of *Fusobacterium*, *Eubacterium*, and *Lactobacillus* species (8). The increased cell proliferation and turnover of collagen, compared with adults, may also be significant. The cellular infiltrate of established gingival lesions in children is dominated by T-lymphocytes and the adult lesion by B-lymphocytes, indicating age-related differences in immunologic response. The thicker junctional epithelium in the primary tooth gingiva, a factor that could influence the permeability of the epithelial structures, may also be important for the age-related differences in developing gingivitis.

Etiology

There is unanimous agreement that gingivitis is caused by microbial plaque. A large number of bacteria exist as a part of the normal ecology of the mouth. Many of these have virulence potential but the gingivitis infection is characterized as nonspecific in terms of predominance of any particular pathogen. Most studies of the role of microorganisms in the pathogenesis of gingivitis have concluded that the quantity of bacteria and bacterial products that accumulates locally is of prime importance in the pathogenesis of gingival inflammation. Nevertheless, gingivitis must be regarded as a multifactoral disease and a number of intrinsic as well as extrinsic factors influence the severity of its manifestation (23).

Factors influencing plaque formation

Calculus is formed by mineralization of microbial plaque. Supragingival calculus is predominantly found adjacent to the ducts of the major salivary glands (Fig. 13-4). Subgingival calculus is found in areas of periodontal pockets (Figs 13-5 and 13-6). The surface of the calcified deposits is rough and further enhances bacterial colonization, and calculus is therefore deleterious to periodontal health (4).

Disturbances in enamel mineralization may cause a rough surface, which accumulates plaque. The early stages of eruption of hypoplastic teeth may be accompanied by pronounced gingivitis, which disappears later if the cervical part of the tooth has unaffected enamel.

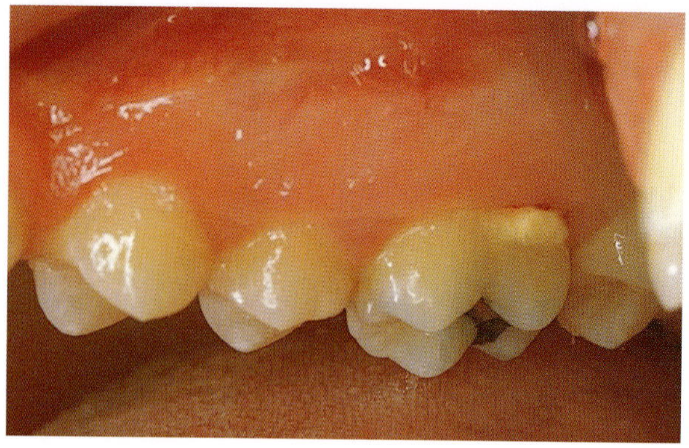

Figure 13-4 Supragingival calculus.

Manifest carious lesions increase plaque accumulation and gradually impair oral hygiene. Cervical carious lesions are almost without exception accompanied by a local, chronic gingivitis.

Restorations with defective margins, rough surfaces, or faulty contacts will all cause chronic gingivitis due to increased plaque accumulation. The dentist who inserts the first proximal or cervical restoration has a great responsibility for the patient's future periodontal health.

Malocclusions do not play a dominant role in the etiology of periodontal disease, but crowding of teeth may render oral hygiene measures difficult.

Fixed orthodontic appliances may impair oral hygiene procedures; bands and brackets accumulate plaque (Fig. 13-7), and removable plates can cause denture stomatitis. Any possible harm to the supporting tissues caused by the appliances must be adequately treated and controlled.

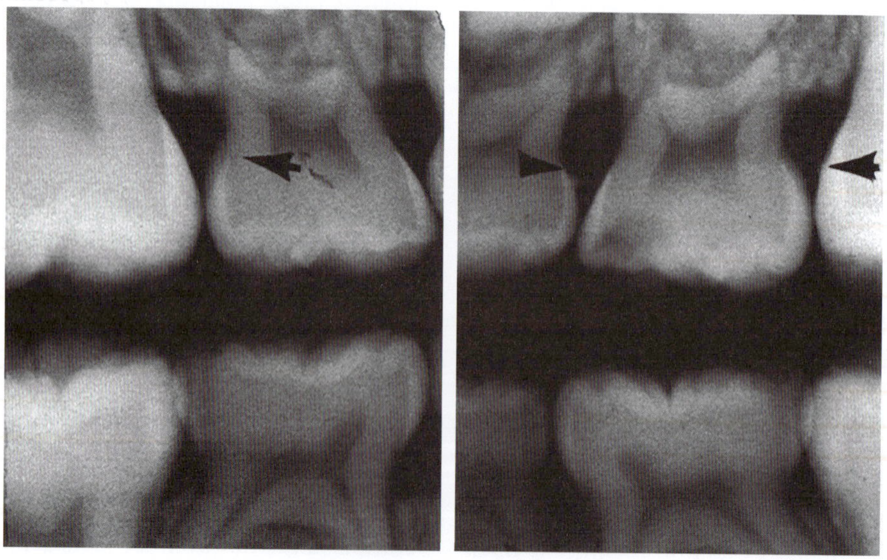

Figure 13-5 Bitewing radiographs showing proximal calculus on primary teeth.

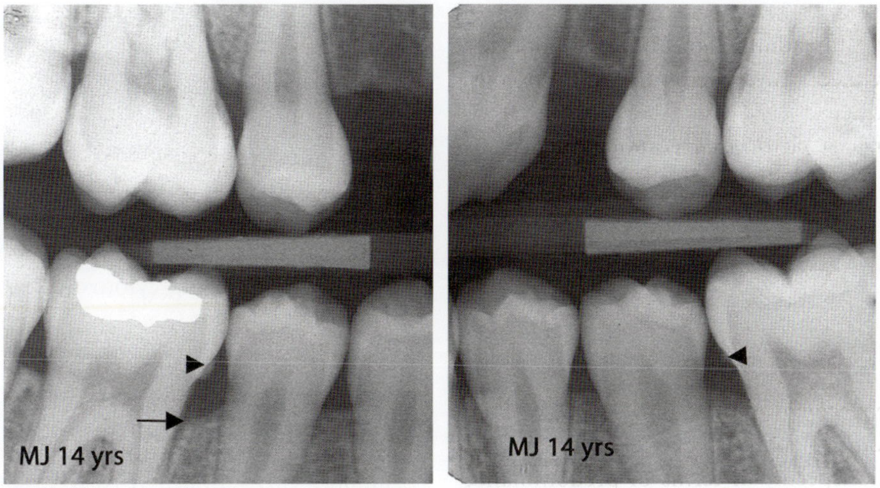

Figure 13-6 Radiographs of a 14-year-old boy showing proximal subgingival calculus and minor bone loss at mandibular permanent first molars. Arrow indicates bone loss and arrowheads indicate subgingival calculus.

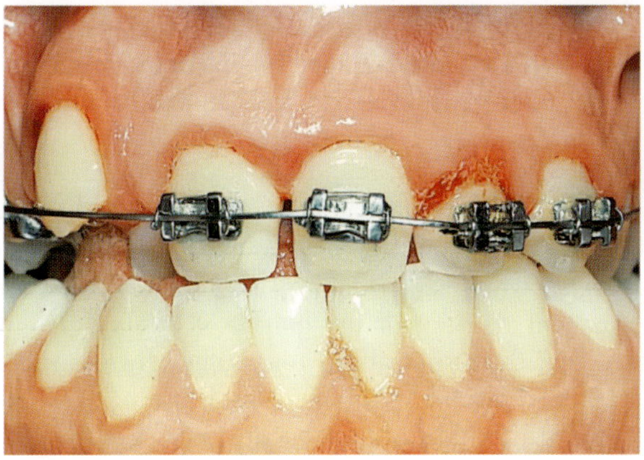

Figure 13-7 Poor oral hygiene and gingivitis in a patient undergoing orthodontic treatment.

Factors modifying the defense system

- *Mouth breathing.* Clinical observations and epidemiological studies indicate an association between mouth breathing or deficient lip closure and chronic gingivitis (Figs 13-8a, b) (31). Mouth breathing may cause frequent drying out of the gingiva in anterior areas. It has been suggested that this may result in vasoconstriction and decreased host resistance.
- *Hormonal changes.* It is an established fact that hormonal changes contribute to the increased susceptibility to gingival affections during pregnancy. Correspondingly, a specific "puberty gingivitis" has been described, with pronounced edema in the marginal gingiva (Fig. 13-9). Epidemiological studies have shown that the incidence of gingivitis reaches a peak 2 or 3 years earlier in girls than in boys, approximately coinciding with puberty. Findings of a correlation between the degree of gingivitis and parameters describing pubertal

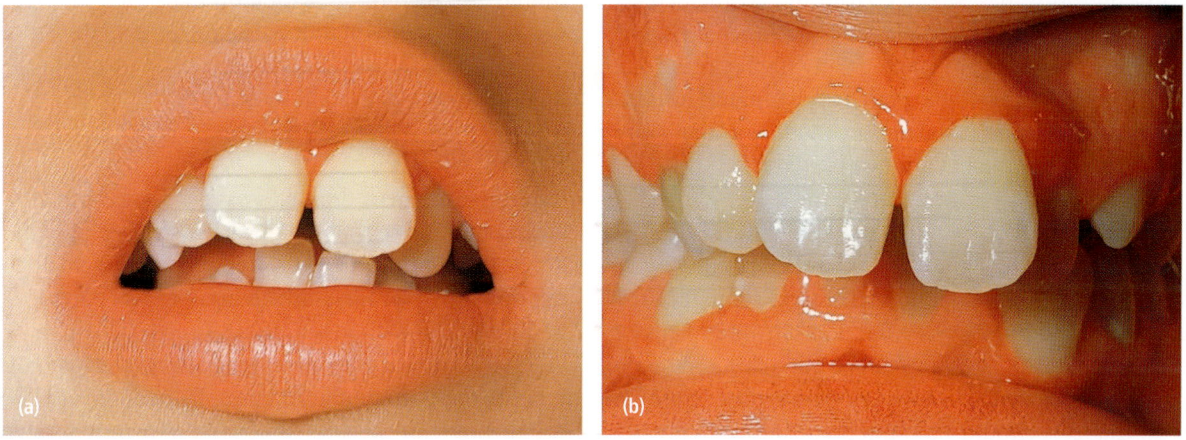

Figure 13-8 Chronic gingivitis associated with mouth breathing.

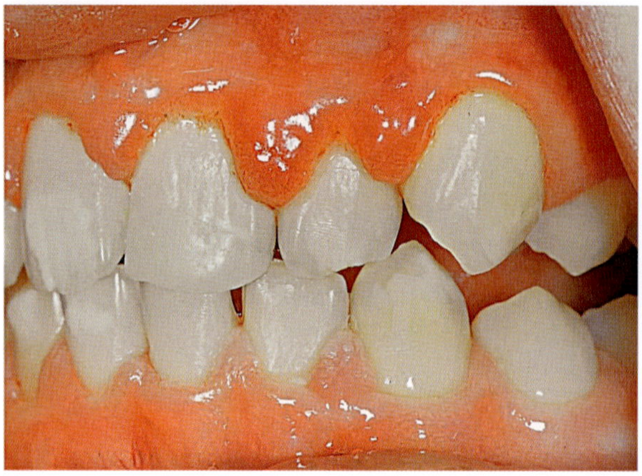

Figure 13-9 Edematous gingival inflammatory reaction during puberty.

maturation further strengthen the theory of an influence of sex hormones on gingival status during puberty (23).

- *Eruption gingivitis.* This term is used to describe more intense forms of gingival inflammatory reactions around erupting permanent teeth. In areas of shedding primary teeth and erupting permanent teeth there is a great risk of plaque accumulation, as tooth cleaning may be difficult or even unpleasant to perform, leading to an inflammatory reaction. Furthermore, a gingival response is sometimes seen that is out of proportion to the degree of bacterial irritation, indicating that other factors modify the inflammatory response. It has been shown that during the phase of eruption, the epithelium displays degenerative changes at the site of fusion between dental and oral epithelia. This indicates a weak point in the epithelial barrier, and an enhanced permeability of the newly formed junctional epithelium may make the area especially vulnerable to bacterial accumulation. Another factor of importance is that once gingival inflammation has been established, the long dental epithelium of the erupting tooth may separate from the enamel, creating a niche for pathogenic bacteria and a risk of deeper tissue involvement. Such an establishment of a subgingival plaque may explain why a gingival inflammatory reaction at an erupting tooth is often more difficult to cure than at a fully erupted tooth (22).

Systemic diseases and syndromes

- *Diabetes mellitus.* Children with diabetes are more susceptible to periodontal diseases than healthy children. The tendency to develop chronic forms of gingivitis is most pronounced in children with poorly controlled diabetes. Consequently, children with diabetes should be trained and motivated early to maintain efficient plaque control (25).
- *Leukemia.* The most common form during childhood, acute lymphoblastic leukemia, is often accompanied by severe oral symptoms at the time of hospitalization and during the period of cytotoxic treatment. The low resistance of the tissues to infection is explained by drug interference with the replication of epithelial cells, in addition to a low number of circulating leukocytes. Therefore, plaque control is essential both before commencing cytotoxic treatment and during medical treatment (25,32).
- *Agranulocytosis.* This malignant type of neutropenia is rare in children, but as in cyclic neutropenia and chronic neutropenia, oral ulceration and periodontal manifestations are common. In chronic cases the gingiva will become hyperplastic, with granulomatous changes (25).
- *Heart conditions.* The severity of oral manifestations is directly proportional to the general cyanosis. The gingiva has a bluish-red hue. As the lowered tissue respiration impairs the defense against microorganisms, children with peripheral cyanosis exhibit a high gingivitis prevalence. Indications for antibiotic prophylaxis are given in Chapter 22.

Treatment

Gingivitis involving marginal and papillary tissues is reversible with plaque control and heals without any permanent damage of the gingiva. However, parents must bear the responsibility for plaque control in their preschool children. A simplified Bass brushing technique using a soft toothbrush is adequate in cases of marginal gingivitis.

In cases of more severe forms of gingivitis, professional tooth cleaning is usually necessary in order to secure the removal of subgingival plaque and calculus. This often needs to be performed under local anesthesia. The treatment may be supported by chemical plaque control during the initial phase. Treatment of gingivitis should also include education on the etiology of the disease as well as instruction in the use of dental floss (11).

Periodontitis

Clinical picture

Inflammatory periodontal disease includes both gingivitis and periodontitis. Not all patients with gingivitis will develop periodontitis. The latter term implies an ongoing inflammatory process involving deeper parts of the periodontium with loss of tooth support.

Periodontitis differs from gingivitis in the histological appearance of the inflammation. In periodontitis larger proportions of plasma cells and B-lymphocytes are found compared to what is found in gingivitis.

Periodontitis is accompanied by few if any subjective symptoms, and the patient therefore has to rely on early diagnosis by professionals. The diagnosis primarily is based on recording of probing depth, attachment loss and/or loss of marginal bone assessed on radiographs. These methods, however, do not discriminate between current disease, previous episodes of disease, and loss of periodontal support due to other reasons, and therefore have to be supplemented with an evaluation of the inflammatory status. Signs indicative of ongoing disease are excessive bleeding on probing, suppuration, and presence of subgingival calculus. However, owing to the specific morphology of the gingiva at erupting or newly erupted permanent teeth, insertion of a probe into the crevice should be avoided. In general, there is no point in carrying out systematic measurements of pocket depth or probing attachment level until the age of 13–14 years.

Classification and epidemiology

Classification

The first reports on periodontitis in children and adolescents described medically compromised individuals. Since the late 1970s cases of otherwise healthy children and adolescents with periodontitis have been reported. On account of the early onset, the seemingly rapid progression, a specific microflora, and frequently localized lesions, it has been suggested that periodontitis in children and adolescents represents unique forms of disease entities differing from periodontal disease in adults.

The terms *prepubertal periodontitis, juvenile periodontitis, early onset periodontitis, early periodontitis,* and *incidental attachment loss* have been used and are still used in the literature. According to the results of recent research, there has gradually been a change in the perspective and today there is a common understanding that the diagnosis based mainly on the age of onset cannot distinguish periodontal disease entities. In the classification today the expressions *aggressive periodontitis* and *chronic periodontitis* replace the previously used terminology (Box 13-1). Both forms of disease have been subgrouped according to severity and distribution within the dentition as a *localized* or a *generalized* form (1). There are still questions about using the number of sites involved as a criterion. Do localized and generalized form of periodontitis truly reflect diverse forms of periodontal diseases with distinct etiological factors and pathogenesis, or does the clinical picture reflect different stages of the same disease (3,21)?

Box 13-1 Classification of bacteria-induced inflammatory periodontal diseases

Gingivitis
- Inflammatory reaction involving the gingiva. Clinical diagnosis based on redness, swelling, and bleeding tendency.

Chronic periodontitis
- Moderate signs of inflammation except at areas of periodontal destruction.
- In children and adolescents often solitary lesion.
- Affects apparently healthy individuals.

Aggressive periodontitis

Localized
- Moderate signs of inflammation, except at areas of periodontal destruction.
- Two or more teeth involved, usually permanent first molars and incisors.

Generalized
- Permanent dentition:
  - severe signs of inflammation
  - periodontal destruction at first molars and incisors and at least three other teeth.
- Primary dentition:
  - usually severe signs of inflammation
  - several teeth involved
  - often associated with a systemic condition.

Epidemiology

Whereas epidemiologic studies in young children are few, a large number of studies including teenagers have been performed. A wide variation of prevalence has been reported. The variation may, of course, represent true differences between populations, but there is no doubt that disparate findings most likely are also due to the use of different modes of examination procedures, different criteria and methods of population sampling.

While early epidemiological studies used probing clinical attachment loss (CAL) as diagnostic criteria, recent studies have used radiographic criteria. Usually the distance between the cemento-enamel junction and the marginal bone level is measured. According to methodological studies, distances >2 mm should be regarded as a deviation from normality both in the primary and in the permanent dentition. In developed countries, the reported prevalence of radiographic bone loss is 2–13% both in children and in adolescents (18,28,33).

Most epidemiological studies do not distinguish between individuals with minor loss of periodontal attachment (chronic periodontitis) and individuals with severe loss (aggressive periodontitis), but most cases found in epidemiologic studies are probably individuals with minor lesions. However, longitudinal studies of adolescents have shown that individuals with minor or few lesions more frequently develop attachment at additional sites or more severe attachment loss at the original site (aggressive periodontitis) compared to adolescents with no signs of attachment loss (2,10).

Chronic periodontitis

Chronic periodontitis is most prevalent in adults but may also occur in young individuals. This form of periodontitis is characterized by minor loss of periodontal support and a slow progression rate (Fig. 13-6). The patients often show considerable plaque accumulation, and subgingival calculus is a frequent finding.

In young children the loss of periodontal support usually manifests as single lesions at primary molars. The pocket deepening at affected primary teeth is limited. Scandinavian studies report that 2–4% of 7–9-year-old children display solitary sites of radiographic bone loss in the primary dentition (28). Most of these sites could be characterized as incidental attachment loss, associated with various types of local trauma or with factors related to the development of the dentition. This type of defect may also represent an earlier inflammatory process, which has healed. However, more importantly, it may represent an initial stage of progressive periodontal disease. Patients with clinical or radiographic attachment loss should be regarded as being at risk of developing early periodontitis.

In developed countries, most epidemiologic studies on loss of periodontal support in adolescents report frequencies of less than 5%. As in younger children, most affected individuals show solitary sites. However, the number of sites per individual as well as the amount of attachment loss seems to increase with age. Usually, the first permanent molars are affected. Subgingival calculus is a frequent finding in these patients (Fig. 13-6) (4,26).

Aggressive periodontitis

No strict definition of the level of attachment loss and number of teeth involved has been proposed. The few epidemiologic studies performed, focusing on aggressive periodontitis, indicate prevalence rates of less than 0.5%, but some populations show a considerably higher prevalence (3). A great majority of the reported cases show localized lesions. The patients, in general, display moderate signs of gingival inflammation except at diseased areas.

In young children, the generalized form is often associated with systemic diseases, although otherwise healthy cases are reported (Fig. 13-10). The periodontal destruction often start early after eruption and is usually characterized by severe gingival inflammation and may lead to premature loss of teeth. Patients should be referred to a pediatrician for medical examination (3).

Localized aggressive periodontitis in adolescents is a rapidly progressing disease with onset in the early permanent dentition. It usually involves permanent first molars and incisors (Fig. 13-11a, b). The inflammatory signs are often restricted to the areas of attachment loss. Radiographs disclose a vertical or arch-shaped pattern of bone loss.

The diagnosis generalized aggressive periodontitis is used when the patients exhibit widespread bone loss including at least three teeth that are not first molars and incisors. This form of disease is accompanied by severe inflammation. In both types of disease the periodontal pockets often harbor subgingival calculus.

Studies indicate that aggressive periodontitis in the permanent dentition is often preceded by bone loss in the primary dentition (Fig. 13-12) (12,26,27). In addition, it has been shown in longitudinal studies of adolescents that those who have experienced loss of periodontal

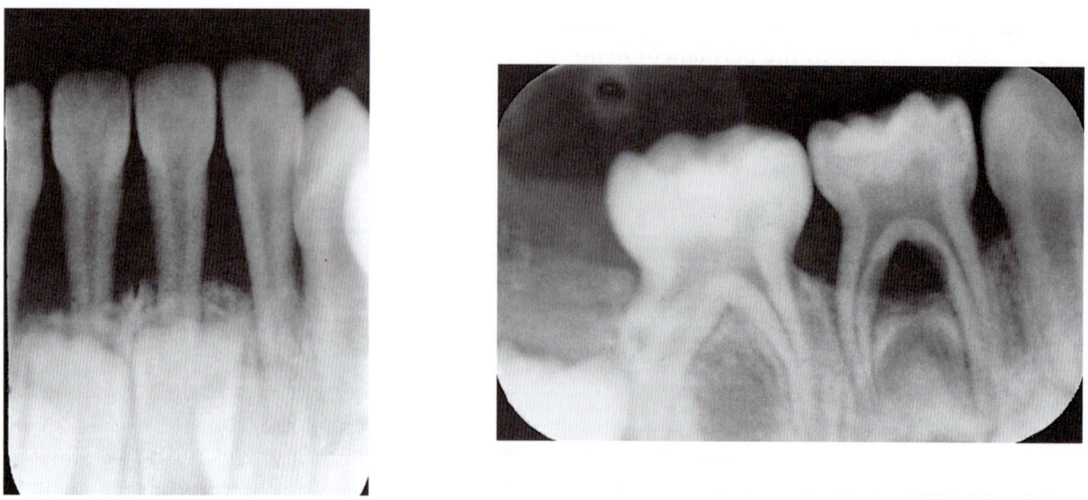

Figure 13-10 A 3-year-old boy with a generalized form of aggressive periodontitis. The primary teeth in all quadrants are involved.

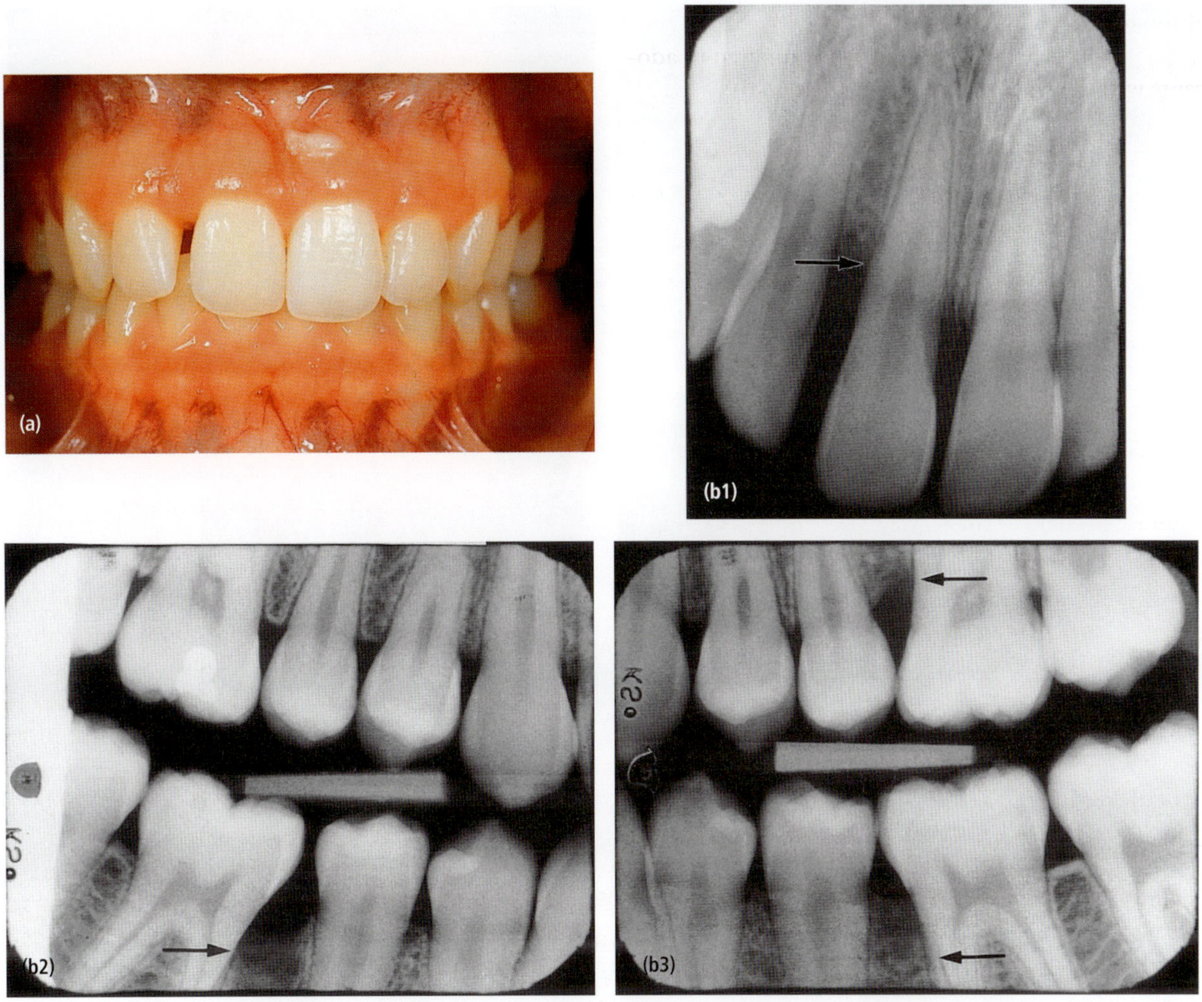

Figure 13-11 (a) A 13-year-old girl with a localized form of aggressive periodontitis, clinically identified with a diastema between maxillary incisors. (b) The radiographs show bone destruction in the same area as well as in the molar regions (arrows).

support (even minor damage) are at higher risk of developing further attachment loss later in life. Thus, by a systematic use of available bitewing radiographs, taken for caries diagnosis, patients at risk of developing destructive periodontal disease in the permanent dentition may be identified and subjected to early treatment (Fig. 13-13).

Etiology and risk factors

General factors

Periodontal disease is a chronic infectious disease of the supporting tissues. If the gingival tissues are exposed to microbial plaque over a long period of time, deeper parts of the periodontium may be involved and slowly destroyed by the action of the inflammatory process. If untreated the teeth may lose their ligamentous support. Most children and adolescents show varying degrees of gingivitis. Why some individuals do and others do not develop destructive periodontitis is not fully understood.

Although bacterial exposure is a prerequisite for the occurrence of gingivitis and periodontitis, its presence alone explains only a limited proportion of the variance in disease expression. The wide variation in the expression of the destructive forms regarding progression rate, number of teeth involved, and clinical appearance implies a multifactoral disease.

Most studies on possible etiological factors in young individuals have focused on cases with aggressive periodontitis. The research has mainly concerned specific infections, variation in host response, and possible impact of genetic factors.

Microbiology

A large number of different microorganisms are found in the oral cavity. An increasing body of evidence suggests that only a subgroup of these microbes might be

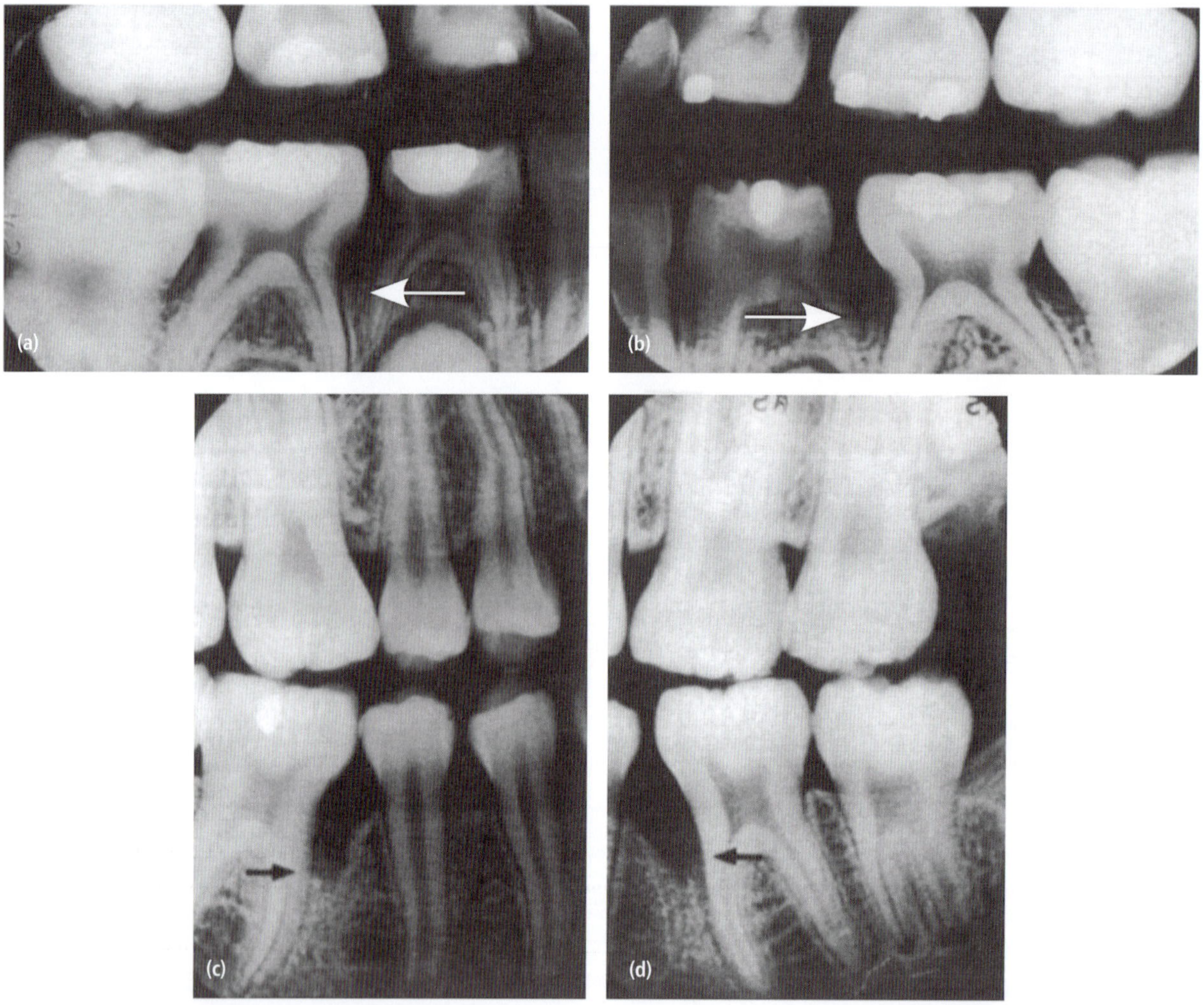

Figure 13-12 A 14-year-old boy with localized aggressive periodontitis (c, d). Previously obtained and filed radiographs from the age of 8 years show loss of bone support (a, b) (arrows).

responsible for the tissue destruction. Particular attention has been paid to the role of *Aggregatibacter* (*Actinobacillus*) *actinomycetemcomitans* in the pathogenesis of aggressive periodontitis. This bacterium is a nonmotile, short facultative anerobic rod, which possesses several virulence factors. Of specific interest is the capacity to produce a leukotoxin with the ability to harm and kill human leukocytes. Other virulence factors include cytolethal-distending toxin which reduces the content of collagen in the tissues. It seems as if *A. actinomycetemcomitans* also has the capacity to invade the periodontal tissue. A majority of young individuals with aggressive periodontitis harbor this species, but the mere presence of this microorganism does not necessarily indicate ongoing disease since many healthy individuals also carry this microorganism. There seems to be variation of virulence between different clones. A recent study indicates a specific clone (JP2) to be more strongly associated with development of aggressive periodontitis (16).

While *A. actinomycetemcomitans* has been associated with localized aggressive periodontitis, generalized aggressive periodontitis has been associated with both *A. actinomycetemcomitans* and periopathogens such as *Porphyrmonas gingivalis*, *Prevotella intermedia*, and a number of other microorganisms. It seems reasonable today to assume that periodontal disease is a result of a polyinfection by different microorganisms and the interaction of this infection with the varying efficiency of the host response (8,14).

Host-defense factors

The host-defense system comprises a great number of cells and molecules whose role is to protect the body against infection. The function of the polymorphonuclear neutrophil cell (PMN cell) is an important part of the innate host-defense system against bacterial infection. The PMN cell has the ability to migrate to extravascular sites, adhere, produce phagocytes, and kill

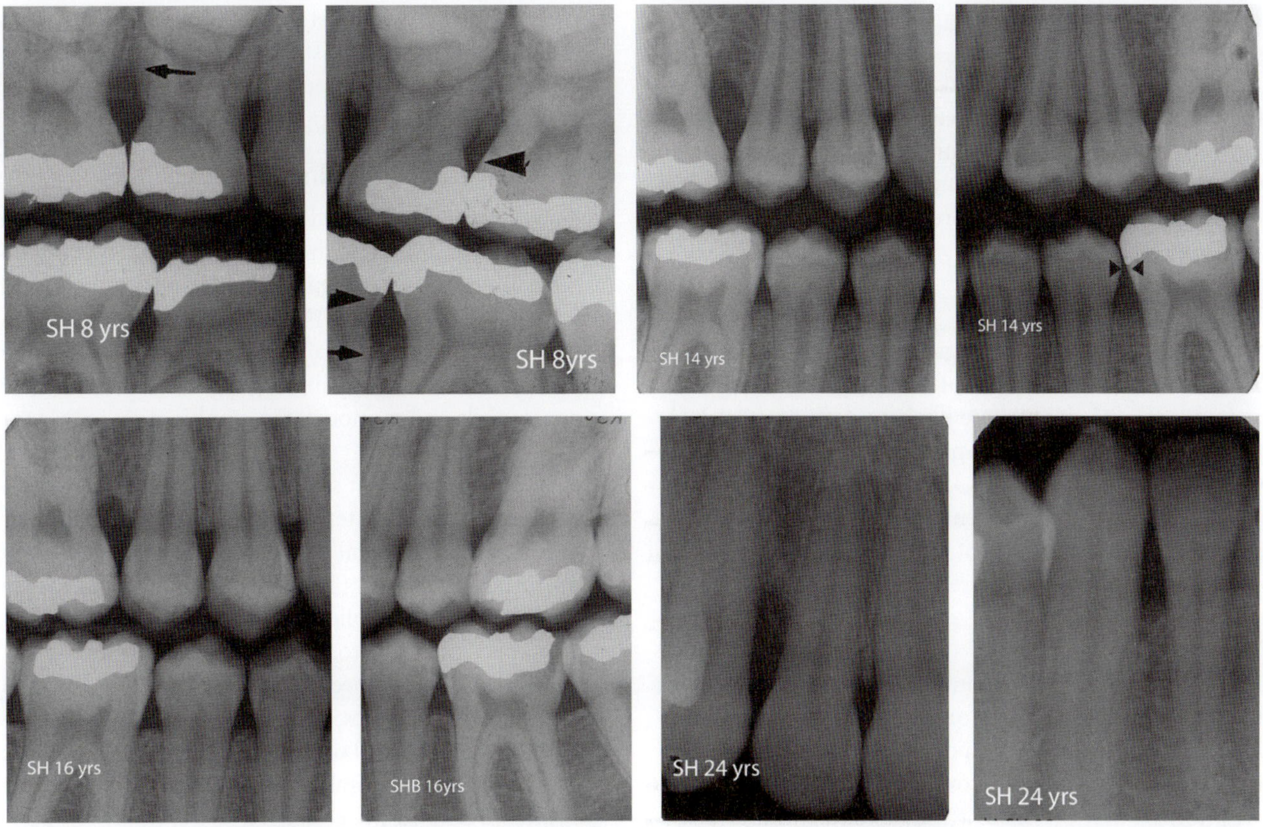

Figure 13-13 Radiographs of an 8-year-old girl showing calculus and alveolar bone loss at primary molars. At the age of 14 years deep pockets and bone loss were found mesially of the maxillary right and left molars and distally of the mandibulary left molar. Scaling and root planing resulted in clinical healing and some bone fill. No detoriation occurred during the 5-year maintenance program. At the age of 24 years the patient was referred to the clinic. New periodontal lesions at the maxillary right canine and the mandibulary left canine were found.

microorganisms. The first findings of reduced host defense in young patients with periodontal disease were the discovery of neutrophil dysfunction of peripheral PMN cells of adolescents with aggressive periodontitis. These findings include abnormalities of adherence, chemotaxis, phagocytosis, and bactericidal activity. Chemotactic dysfunction has particularly been found in high percentages of patients with aggressive periodontitis. Whether this is due to intrinsic defects in PMN cells or due to extrinsic factors is not fully known. The defect chemotaxis has mainly been found in patients of African-American origin. However, studies including European and Japanese populations have not confirmed these results.

The roles of the specific immune response in the pathogenesis of aggressive periodontitis have been studied extensively over the past decade. A major finding has been a significant elevation in serum immunoglobulin G levels particularly to *A. actinomycetemcomitans* but also to other periopathogens. The relationship between antibody level and periodontal disease is, however, complex. It has been suggested that a deterioration of the periodontal status from a localized to a generalized expression might be explained by a weak antibody response in patients developing generalized aggressive periodontitis (20).

Genetic factors

In some families there is a marked aggregation of severe periodontitis. This finding together with results from epidemiological studies indicates that hereditary factors are important for the development of aggressive periodontitis. Segregation studies of affected families have revealed different modes of inheritance. Both autosomal dominant and recessive as well as X-linked transmission have been suggested.

The familial clustering of aggressive periodontitis might be an expression of enhanced susceptibility to microbial infections, in part determined by the host's genotype. Studies including a substantial numbers of probands have shown a wide variation: 8–63% of near relatives have been reported to have severe periodontitis (15,17). It is obvious that the different results can be attributed not only to variations in the populations included, but also to diagnostic criteria and the number of relatives examined.

Even if there have been conflicting suggestions as to the modes of inheritance, it seems established that inheritance is a risk factor to be considered. For the clinician this emphasizes the importance of clinical examination of children, siblings, and parents of patients identified with aggressive periodontitis.

Ethnicity

Comprehensive epidemiologic surveys in the United States have demonstrated that black or Hispanic adolescents were 5–15 times more likely to develop aggressive periodontitis or chronic periodontitis compared to Caucasian adolescents (3,33). In addition, Swedish studies have revealed an enhanced risk of developing periodontitis in immigrant children of Asian origin compared to Swedish children (24).

Modifying factors

In areas of defective restorations or manifest carious lesions, localized inflammatory reactions may progress to involve deeper parts of the periodontium. In a dentition under development, eruption disorders such as ectopic eruption of first permanent molars and infraocclusion of primary molars may favor plaque accumulation, leading to chronic gingivitis and possibly the development of destructive periodontal disease.

Early reports often state that adolescents with localized aggressive periodontitis generally demonstrate little dental plaque and subgingival calculus. In contrast, more recent investigations have reported levels of plaque and calculus similar to cases with chronic periodontitis. Proximal subgingival calculus is often seen in areas of marginal bone loss in the primary dentition and the young permanent dentition, and is always connected with signs of chronic inflammation (Figs 13-5 and 13-13). Calculus is found more often in individuals with bone loss than in individuals without any sign of loss of periodontal support (4,26). The exact role of calculus in the initiation and progression of the periodontal lesion is however unclear, and the finding of an association between subgingival calculus and periodontal disease does not automatically imply that calculus is of primary etiologic importance for the development of the disease. However, the rough calcified deposits facilitate bacterial colonization and should be removed.

Smoking is considered to be among the most significant risk factors for periodontitis in adults and should be regarded as a factor of importance for the initiation of the disease in adolescents as well (20). The reasons for the enhanced risk of developing periodontitis in smokers are not fully known, but smoking-related substances are known to act as vasoconstrictors, possibly resulting in tissue ischemia. These substances may also exert a negative effect on fibroblasts and inflammatory cells, thereby affecting the wound-healing capacity.

Systemic diseases and syndromes

- *Down syndrome.* Periodontal disease is a common finding in children with Down syndrome. Marginal bone loss is more severe in the anterior segments, and especially in the mandible. The reasons for the high susceptibility to periodontal disease in these children are probably an impaired phagocytic function of neutrophils and monocytes in combination with poor oral hygiene (6).
- *Type 1 diabetes.* Most studies of adolescents with diabetes demonstrate a tendency to higher susceptibility to loss of periodontal support compared to healthy controls (Fig. 13-14) (19). Whether or not this is also valid for well-controlled patients is uncertain. However, it is reasonable to consider these individuals as at risk and address special prophylactic programs to children with diabetes. Impaired function of the polymorphonuclear leukocytes and vascular changes, coupled with poor oral hygiene, have been suggested as factors behind the enhanced susceptibility to periodontal disease in patients with diabetes.
- *Hypophosphatasia.* This hereditary metabolic syndrome results in low serum alkaline phosphatase activity, ricket-like skeletal changes, and loss of alveolar bone, usually limited to the area of anterior primary teeth (Fig. 13-15). The result is a precocious exfoliation of these teeth. Microscopically, teeth from affected areas exhibit aplasia and hypoplasia of root cementum, large pulp chambers, and interglobular dentin formation. Findings indicate that permanent teeth can also be affected, which puts children with

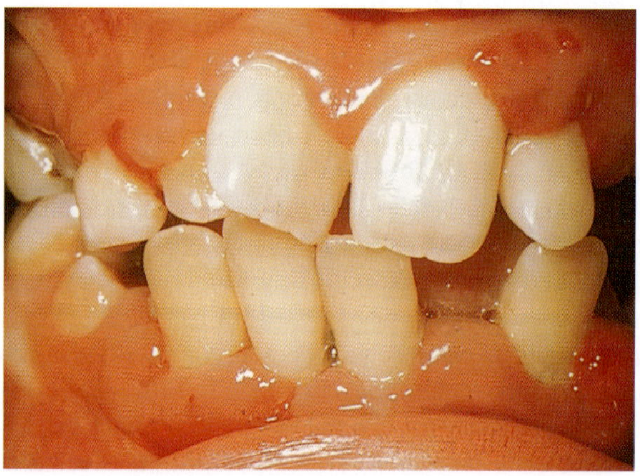

Figure 13-14 Severe periodontal involvement in a young child suffering from diabetes mellitus.

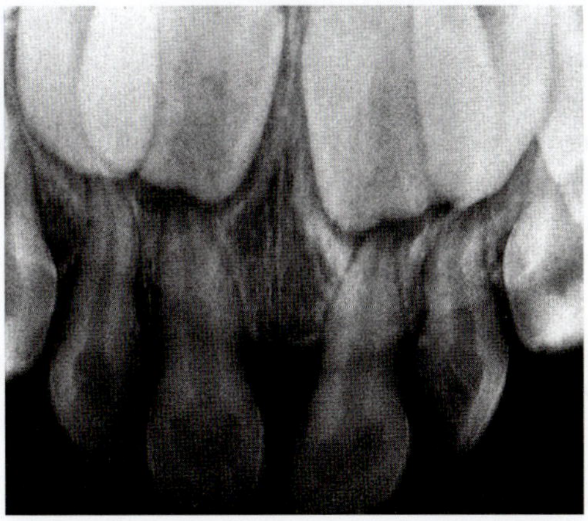

Figure 13-15 Alveolar bone loss in a child with hypophosphatasia.

hypophosphatasia at risk of developing periodontal complications during adolescence and adult life (29).

- *Histiocytosis-X (reticuloendotheliosis).* This condition may cause alveolar bone destruction in connection with lesions in the jaws. Eosinophilic granuloma (histiocytosis in bone) is more frequent in the mandible than in the maxilla. Hand–Schüller–Christian disease (chronic disseminated histiocytosis) may lead to gross bone destruction extending around the roots and causing exfoliation. The treatment of the disease (corticosteroids, irradiation, and cytostatics) may produce secondary negative effects in the periodontium (29).
- *Papillon–Lefèvre syndrome.* This is a rare genetic disease affecting the hands and feet (keratosis palmaris et plantaris) and leading to fulminant types of periodontitis with rapid bone destruction. The oral symptoms start immediately after eruption of the primary teeth and cease after the premature loss of the first dentition only to start again after eruption of the permanent teeth (30).

Screening and treatment

Screening

Evidence is available that a proportion of young individuals with early clinical or radiographic signs of attachment loss are at risk for disease progression. There are also data suggesting that young patients enrolled in organized dental health care have better prerequisites to stabilize or improve their periodontal conditions (2). Although the prevalence of attachment loss is low in most populations, it should be considered to include periodontal assessment in the regular oral examination of children and adolescents (Box 13-2).

The necessity to do a full mouth periodontal probing in all children and young teenagers can however be questioned since only a small fraction of the population will develop the disease. A partial periodontal probing including proximal sites of the first molars is an alternative. The evaluation of periodontal status in children and young teenagers can also be based on radiographic analysis of the marginal bone level.

Box 13-2 Screening and treatment schedule

Primary dentition
- alveolar bone loss >2 mm

Permanent dentition
- alveolar bone loss >2 mm
- probing attachment loss >2 mm

Clinical examination
- plaque
- gingival bleeding
- probing pocket depth
- calculus
- pus

→ **No signs of periodontal disease**
- ordinary regular examinations

↓

Periodontal disease
- oral hygiene training
- scaling and root planing

→ **Healing**
- regular controls
- maintenance care

↓

Nonhealing
- microbiological sampling
- antibiotic medication
- surgery
- extraction (primary teeth)

→
- regular controls
- maintenance care

The clinical examination of individuals in risk groups (earlier disease, near relatives with aggressive periodontitis, systemic disease) should include a more thorough examination.

Clinical or radiographic signs of bone loss should always lead to a supplementary clinical examination. Presence of pathologic pockets, excessive bleeding, suppuration, or subgingival calculus calls for treatment. An early diagnosis of periodontitis is a must for an easy and effective treatment with predictable results.

Treatment

The initial therapy includes training of the patient in plaque control, and professional scaling and root planing. As in all periodontal treatment, optimal oral hygiene is a prerequisite for a successful treatment outcome (7,8). It has been shown in cases with chronic as well as aggressive periodontitis that disease progression is related significantly to the dental plaque load of the patient. Thus, treatment is always combined with a preventive program to reduce plaque accumulation.

Scaling and root planing are effective methods to remove subgingival plaque and calculus, reduce the gingival inflammation, and promote healing. Thoroughly performed, this technique substantially reduces the bacterial load and results in reduction of pocket depths or pocket elimination. Scaling and root planing are generally performed under local anesthesia.

Most chronic cases will be managed by this standard treatment. For young patients with aggressive periodontitis many authors recommend the use of systemically administrated antibiotics since the elimination of putative pathogens is considered hard to achieve with debridement only. However, a number of studies report a successful outcome without including antibiotics in the therapeutic regime of patients with localized aggressive periodontitis (Fig. 13-16).

A careful evaluation of the effectiveness of the treatment should be performed 4–6 weeks after scaling and root planing. The purpose is to check whether the healing process is continuing or if further therapy is needed. The absence of healing calls for further treatment, improved effectiveness of self-performed plaque control, and repeated scaling. Surgical pocket elimination is considered for permanent teeth. The goal is pocket elimination and hopefully the bone fill of vertical bone defects.

After successful clinical treatment, the patient should be subjected to a regular maintenance program. At recalls, a re-examination of oral hygiene, gingival conditions, probing depth, and attachment level is performed. If deterioration is seen, scaling is repeated. Subgingival sampling to test for the presence of potential pathogenic bacteria is considered, including antibiotic susceptibility testing. In severe forms of aggressive periodontitis, systemic antibiotics may be useful in combination with mechanical treatment. In cases of aggressive periodontitis in young children, extraction of severely affected primary teeth may be the treatment of choice. In adolescents, surgery is often indicated to accomplish proper debridement in deeper periodontal pockets.

Prevention of bacteria-induced inflammatory periodontal diseases

Mechanical plaque control

Toothbrushing. Mechanical removal of plaque by oral hygiene leads to remission of gingivitis. Plaque control is thus critical for the maintenance of gingival health. It has been shown that parents have to brush their children's teeth at least until school age to ensure optimal oral hygiene (11). Parents will also appreciate a simple, straightforward method, especially for use in small children. The simplified Bass technique, involving a horizontal movement of the toothbrush along the outside and the inside of the dental arches, is effective for both children and parents.

A convenient method for a parent to brush a child's teeth is illustrated in Fig. 9-5. Systematic brushing of all tooth surfaces is important. The toothbrush recommended for children should be small, soft, and have a large handle which is easy to hold. The quality of the oral hygiene is more important than the frequency. Hastily performed and haphazard toothbrushing adds little to oral hygiene. It is vital to train parents and children in toothbrushing, and to monitor the procedure with disclosing agents at regular intervals. Toothbrushing should

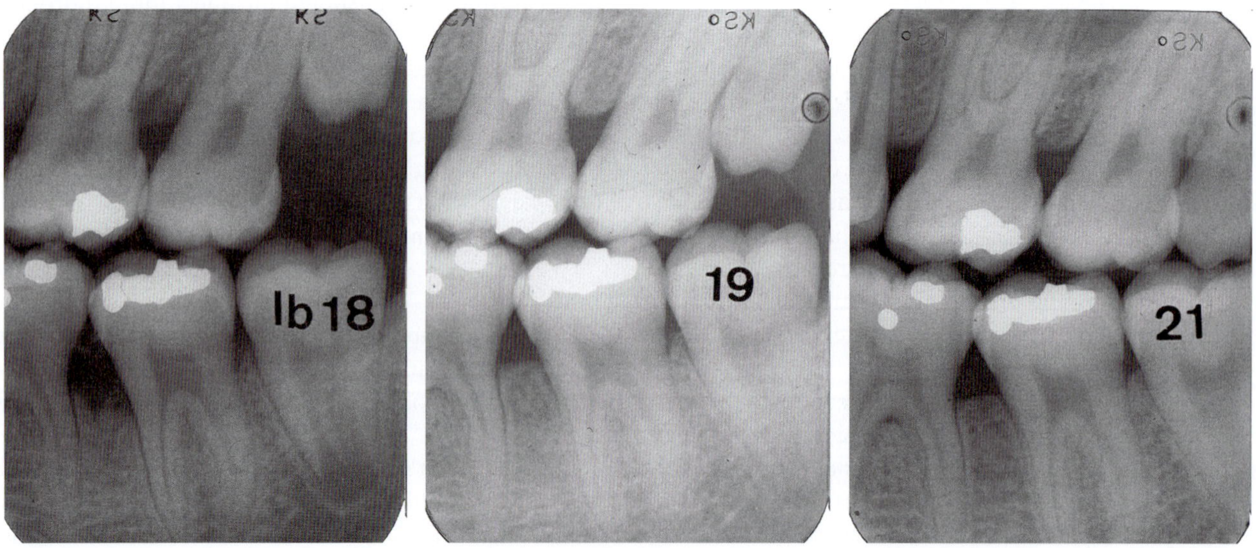

Figure 13-16 Aggressive periodontitis at molars of an 18 year old. Thorough scaling and root planing was performed. Radiographs taken 1 and 3 years later show substantial healing of the bone defects.

be performed twice a day, in the morning and in the evening before bed.

Toothpicks. The use of toothpicks in children is recommended only in very specific cases and after careful instruction by a dentist or a dental hygienist. As the gingival tissues in children fill the interproximal spaces almost completely, the use of toothpicks will result in gingival retraction and unnecessary exposure of the proximal surfaces.

Flossing. Interproximal areas are the least accessible to toothbrushing, and dental floss is advocated as an aid to cleaning these regions. Studies have shown that flossing does not result in further improvement when oral hygiene and gingival health are already reasonably good. However, it can benefit individuals whose gingival health is poor.

Chemical plaque control

Much attention has focused on the use of chemical agents which exhibit an effect on dental plaque either as an inhibitor of biofilm formation, or as an inhibitor of microbial metabolism. Both have the potential for the prevention or reduction of periodontal diseases. The most thoroughly investigated substance is chlorhexidine. Preparations are available as mouthrinse, dental gel, and varnish in many countries. Regular or intermittent long-term use of chlorhexidine seems justified to control the gingival situation in high-risk patients, where no other effective means of oral hygiene are applicable. In addition, chlorhexidine is sometimes appropriate as a supplement to mechanical oral hygiene in relation to oral surgery or trauma to teeth and surrounding tissues.

Gingival recession

Localized gingival recession is found in approximately 10–15% of teenagers (Fig. 13-17). In young children the lesion frequently occurs on the labial surfaces of the mandibular incisors while in teenagers the buccal surfaces of upper molars and premolars are the most affected areas. In young individuals, recession is often seen in association with labial and irregular position of teeth, trauma from toothbrushing, history of orthodontic therapy, or poor plaque control (5). A predisposing factor to gingival recession in the mandibular incisor area is high attachment of a frenum (5).

The first step in the treatment of a localized gingival recession is to identify the etiology and predisposing factors. In most cases instruction of the patient in adequate toothbrushing technique, resulting in good plaque control, can arrest recession. For this, a soft toothbrush is mandatory. In cases of labially or irregularly positioned mandibular incisor, alignment due to spontaneous space creation by increased intercanine width favors normalization. If the gingival recession is associated with a high frenulum attachment, which retracts the marginal gingiva when the lip is stretched, frenectomy is recommended. In rare cases a successful treatment may require surgical intervention such as free gingival grafts.

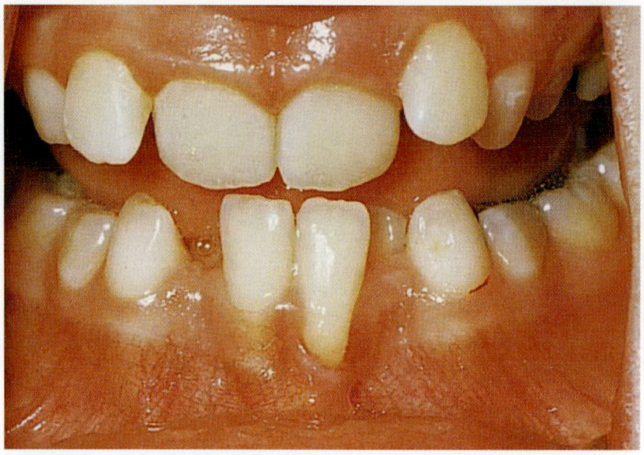

Figure 13-17 Gingival recession at permanent lower central incisor.

Gingival enlargements

Chronic marginal gingivitis in children is usually characterized by marked vascular reactions and tissue edema. In uncomplicated marginal gingivitis the edema is limited to the free marginal gingiva. Gingival enlargement dominated by edema is sometimes seen during puberty and in children with peripheral cyanosis. Enlargement of the gingival margin is also seen in cases of mouth breathing.

Drug-induced gingival overgrowth

Drugs such as calcium channel blockers (nifedipine), immunosuppressives (cyclosporin A), and anticonvulsants (phenytoin) can induce gingival overgrowth (Fig. 13-18). It has also been reported that the use of the antiepileptic agent sodium valproate can result in development of gingival overgrowth (13).

Phenytoin is used in children with grand mal but also in patients with psychomotor seizures. Connective tissue reactions are a common result of this antiepileptic treatment. Phenytoin-induced gingival overgrowth occurs more frequently in children than in adults. The front regions are usually more severely affected than other areas of the dentition. It starts as a lobulate enlargement of the interdental papillae. By introducing a plaque control program before or at the start of phenytoin therapy, gingival overgrowth can be minimized but not totally prevented. In outpatients, the thickness of the marginal gingiva is increased bucco-lingually, especially in the

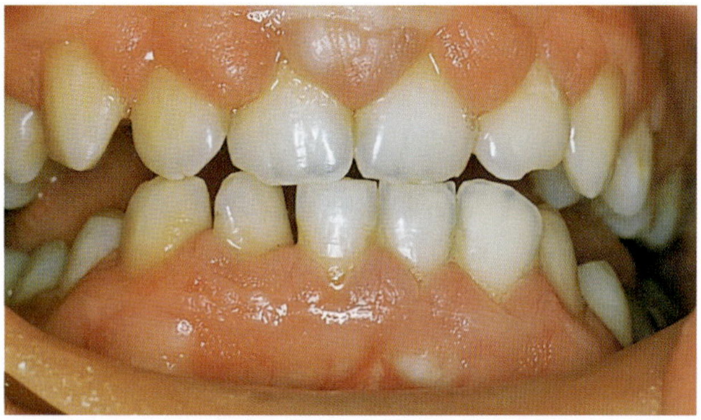

Figure 13-18 Phenytoin-induced gingival overgrowth.

anterior region. Approximately 50% of children, where oral hygiene is not controlled, develop gingival overgrowth in the form of pseudopockets (probing depth >4 mm). A few patients develop a severe form of gingival overgrowth where gingival tissue covers a substantial part of the anatomical crowns. In such cases surgical intervention is indicated, and an intensive preventive program must be established to minimize the risk of recurrence of tissue enlargement.

Gingival overgrowth represents tissue with an altered composition compared with normal gingiva, and contains an increased noncollagenous matrix with increased amounts of glycosaminoglycans.

Gingival fibromatosis

Gingival fibromatosis is a special type of diffuse, non-inflammatory gingival enlargement (Fig. 13-19a, b). It is often autsomally inherited. The fibrosis of the gingival tissue, generalized or localized in the molar areas, is usually symmetrical, and affects the entire gingiva up to the muco-gingival junction. The extent can be so great that it changes the facial contour of the patient. Onset is early and the disease is often diagnosed in connection with retarded eruption. The enlargement is very firm and pale in color, and may be treated with gingivectomy or, when extensive, with a replaced flap procedure.

Necrotizing periodontal diseases

Necrotizing gingivitis (NG), also named acute necrotizing ulcerative gingivitis, is a disease with rapid onset characterized by painful necrotic ulcerative gingival lesions and affected interdental papillae. Occasionally, the necrotic ulcerative lesions may extend into the attached gingiva and oral mucosa, and are covered by grayish-white pseudomembranes. Often NG is accompanied with *foetor ex ore*. In severe cases the infection may involve deeper parts of the periodontium and is termed necrotizing periodontitis.

NG is mostly seen in child populations suffering from malnutrition, but is rare in developed countries today. The microorganisms *Treponema* spp., *Selenomonas* spp., *Fusobacterium* spp., and *Prevotella intermedia* are often demonstrated in NG lesions, together with an unspecified, variable flora. The pathogenic role of the microorganisms is, however, not fully understood. Changes in the leukocyte function and the immune system have also been reported.

In children, professional plaque removal is indicated, combined with mouthrinsing with 0.5% hydrogen peroxide or with 0.1% chlorhexidine. Antibiotics are administered in cases of the patient's nonresponse to debridement, risk of spread of the infection, or affected general health.

Traumatic ulcerative gingival lesions

These types of lesions start in the marginal gingiva and are caused by bacterial superinfection of traumatized gingival tissue. The trauma is predominantly the result of excessive use of the toothbrush or poor brushing technique. The bacterial infection is caused by the normal mixed flora of the oral cavity. Usually the ulcers

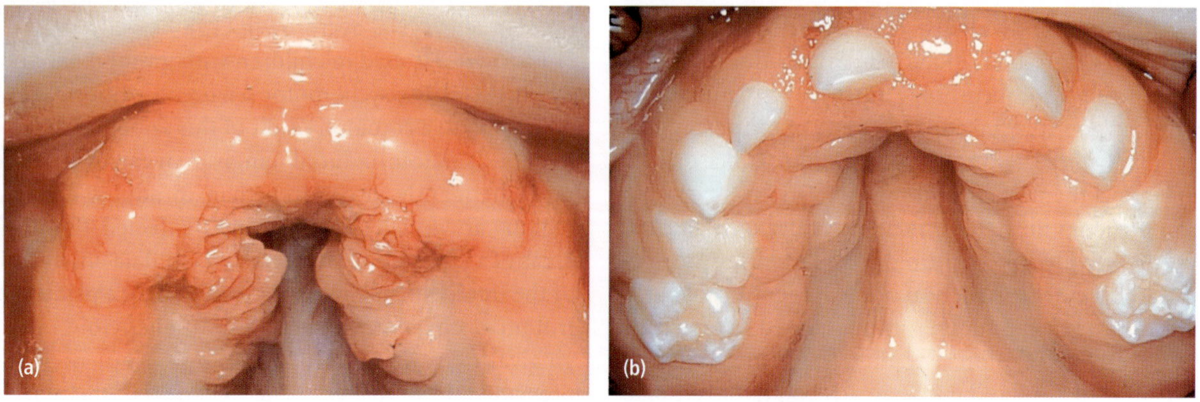

Figure 13-19 Gingival fibromatosis (a) in a newborn child and (b) at 5 years of age after surgical correction.

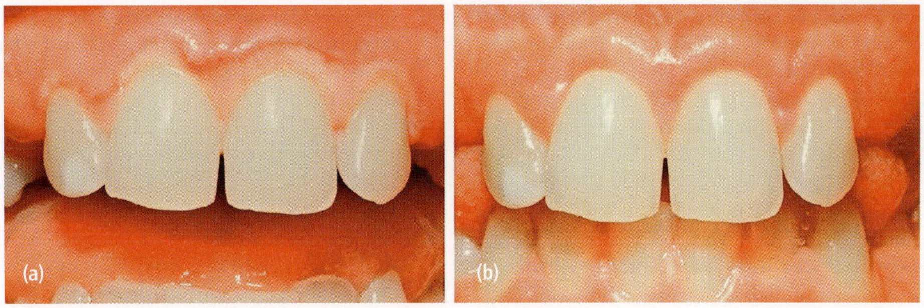

Figure 13-20 (a) Traumatic ulcerative gingival lesion and (b) after treatment.

are covered with a thin, yellowish or grayish exudate and the patients often complain of pain in the affected area. The lesions are located in the buccal gingiva and there is no necrosis of the interdental papillae as in NG, or vesicles as in herpes simplex virus infections (Fig. 13-20a). Initial professional cleaning of the teeth followed by cessation of toothbrushing for 7–10 days is recommended. During this period the child should rinse twice daily with a 0.1% chlorhexidine solution. Instruction in adequate toothbrushing technique should also be given (Fig. 13-20b).

Streptococcal gingivitis

In rare cases of streptococcal tonsillitis, the infection may spread to involve the gingival tissues. The gingiva is painful, appears red and swollen, and tends to bleed spontaneously. Treatment includes improved oral hygiene and antibiotics. Prescription of antibiotics should be preceded by microbiological diagnosis.

References

1. Academy Report. Position paper. Periodontal diseases of children and adolescents. *J Periodontol* 2003;**74**:1696–704.
2. Albandar J, Baghdady VS, Ghose LJ. Periodontal disease progression in teenagers with no preventive dental care provision. *J Clin Periodontol* 1991;**18**:300–4.
3. Albandar J, Rams T. Global epidemiology of periodontal diseases in children and young persons. *Periodontology 2000* 2002;**29**: 153–76.
4. Albandar JM, Brown LJ, Brunelle JA, Löe H. Gingival state and dental calculus in early-onset periodontitis. *J Periodontol* 1996; **67**:953–9.
5. Andlin-Sobocki A. Gingival recession, keratinized and attached gingiva in anterior teeth of children. Thesis. Umeå, 1993.
6. Barr-Agholme M. Periodontal disease in adolescents with Down syndrome. Thesis. Stockholm, 1999.
7. Bimstein E. Periodontal considerations in the child dental patient. *Acta Odontolol Pediatr* 1987;**8**:13–19.
8. Bimstein E, Ram D, Irshied J, Naor R, Sela MN. Periodontal diseases, caries, and microbial composition of the subgingival plaque in children: a longitudinal study. *J Dent Child* 2002;**69**: 133–7.
9. Bimstein E. Seven-year follow-up of ten children with periodontitis. *Pediatr Dent* 2003;**25**:389–96.
10. Brown LJ, Albandar JM, Brunelle JA, Löe H. Early-onset periodontitis: progression of attachment loss during 6 years. *J Periodontol* 1996;**67**:968–75.
11. Clerehugh V, Tugnait A. Diagnosis and management of periodontal diseases in children and adolescents. *Periodontology 2000* 2001;**26**:146–68.
12. Cogen RB, Wright JT, Tate AL. Destructive periodontal disease in healthy children. *J Periodontol* 1992;**63**:761–5.
13. Dahllöf G. Phenytoin-induced gingival overgrowth in epileptic children. A clinical, histological and biochemical study. Thesis. Stockholm, 1986.
14. Darby I, Curtis M. Microbiology of periodontal disease in children and young adults. *Periodontology 2000* 2001;**26**:33–53.
15. Diehl SR, Wu T, Michalowicz BS, Brooks CN, Califano JV, Burmeister JA, Schenkein HA. Quantitative measures of aggressive periodontitis show substantial heritability and consistency with traditional diagnoses. *J Periodontol* 2005;**76**:279–88.
16. Haubek D, Ennibi O-E, Poulsen K, Væth M, Poulsen S, Kilian M. Risk of aggressive periodontitis in adolescent carriers of the JP2 clone of *Aggregatibacter* (*Actinobacillus*) *actinomycetemcomitans* in Morocco: a prospective longitudinal cohort study. *Lancet* 2008;**371**:237–42.
17. Hodge P, Michalowicz B. Genetic predisoposition to periodontitis in children and young adults. *Periodontology 2000* 2001;**26**: 113–34.
18. Källestål C. Periodontal conditions in Swedish adolescents. Thesis. Umeå, 1991.
19. Lalla E, Cheng B, Tucker S, Greenberg E, Goland R, Lamster IB. Periodontal changes in children and adolescents with diabetes: a case-control study. *Diabetes Care* 2006;**29**:295–9.
20. Lindhe L, Karring T, Lang NP eds. *Clinical periodontology and implant dentistry*, 4th edn. Copenhagen: Munksgaard Blackwell, 2003.
21. Lopez R, Baelum V. Classifying periodontitis among adolescents: implication for epidemiological research. *Community Dent Oral Epidemiol* 2003;**31**:136–43.
22. Matsson L. Development of experimental gingivitis in pre-school children and young adults. A comparative experimental study. *J Clin Periodontol* 1978;**5**:24–34.
23. Matsson L. Factors influencing the susceptibility to gingivitis during childhood – a review. *Int J Paediatr Dent* 1993;**3**:119–27.
24. Matsson L, Sjödin B, Blomquist HK. Periodontal health in adopted children of Asian origin living in Sweden. *Swed Dent J* 1997; **21**:177–84.
25. Meyle J, Gonzáles R. Influences of systematic diseases on periodontitis in children and adolescents. *Periodontology 2000* 2001; **26**:92–112.

26. Sjödin B, Matsson L, Unell L, Egelberg J. Marginal bone loss in the primary dentition of patients with juvenile periodontitis. *J Clin Periodontol* 1993;**20**:32–6.
27. Sjödin B, Matsson L. Marginal bone loss in the primary dentition. A survey of 7–9-year-old children in Sweden. *J Clin Periodontol* 1994;**21**:313–19.
28. Sjödin B. Loss of periodontal support in children with primary teeth. Thesis. Umeå, 1994.
29. Sollecito TP, Sullivan KE, Pinto A, Stewart J, Korostoff J. Systemic conditions associated with periodontitis in childhood and adolescence. A review of diagnostic possibilities. *Med Oral Patol Oral Cir Bucal* 2005;**10**:142–50.
30. Ullbro C. Studies on clinical expression, genotype, and gingival crevicular fluid characteristics in young patients with Papillon-Lefèvre. Thesis. Umeå, 2004.
31. van Gastel J, Quirynin M, Teughels W, Carels C. The relationships between malocclusion, fixed orthodontic appliances and periodontal disease. A review of the literature. *Aust Orthod J* 2007;**23**:121–9.
32. Wahlin Y-B. Changes in the oral microbiota, mucosal lesions and salivary secretion in patients with acute leukemia. Thesis. Umeå, 1990.
33. William M, Jenkins M, Papapanou P. Epidemiology of periodontal disease in children and adolescents. *Periodontology 2000* 2001;**26**:16–32.

14

Tooth development and disturbances in number and shape of teeth

Göran Koch, Irma Thesleff and Sven Kreiborg

Mechanisms of normal and abnormal tooth development

Teeth develop as epithelial appendages from the ectoderm covering the oral cavity. The morphological aspects of tooth development at the microscopic level have been described in great detail long ago, and more recent research has started to uncover the molecular details underlying the morphogenesis of teeth, dental cell differentiation and extracellular matrix formation, and mineralization. The genetic regulation of normal tooth development has been elucidated by experimental studies mainly using mouse teeth as models, and studies in human molecular genetics have led to the identification of gene defects causing dental aberrations.

Principles of tooth development

Tooth development starts from thickenings of the oral epithelium which bud to the underlying neural crest-derived mesenchyme. This is accompanied by condensation of mesenchymal cells around the bud and subsequent folding of the epithelium starting at the tip of the bud. Rapid growth of the tooth germ leads to the cap stage of development, and the shape of the tooth crown becomes established during the bell stage when the locations and heights of tooth cusps are set by additional foldings and growth of the epithelium. The odontoblasts and ameloblasts differentiate during the bell stage, and deposit the extracellular matrices of dentin and enamel, respectively. Differentiation, matrix deposition, and mineralization start from the tips of the cusps and proceed cervically, and after they reach the future cementoenamel junction, root development starts (Box 14-1).

Permanent teeth develop from the epithelium of the primary (deciduous) tooth germs, and their budding starts during the bell stage of primary tooth development. Bone formation is initiated in the maxilla and mandible only after the initiation and budding of primary teeth, but the subsequent development of alveolar bone from the mesenchyme surrounding the tooth germs is tightly coordinated with tooth morphogenesis. At the time of eruption, the teeth are surrounded by bone, and their eruption depends on precisely regulated bone remodeling, i.e., bone resorption between crown and the oral cavity and bone apposition at the base of the roots.

The most important mechanism regulating tooth development is the interaction between the epithelial and mesenchymal cells. During the initiation of tooth development, the epithelium has an instructive role and determines the type of the tooth to be formed as well as the odontogenic fate of the mesenchymal cells. The capacity to regulate tooth development shifts to the mesenchyme during budding and, subsequently, mesenchymal signals regulate the morphogenesis of the epithelium and the shape of the tooth. The differentiation of the odontoblasts, ameloblasts, and cementoblasts, as well as their matrix deposition, is also regulated by interactions between the different tissues. Hence, tooth development is controlled by a series of reciprocal tissue interactions. It is noteworthy that similar sequential and reciprocal cell interactions govern the development of all organs in the embryo.

Molecules regulating tooth development

The most important molecules regulating tooth development are those that participate in the signaling networks mediating epithelial–mesenchymal interactions. The actual signals are hormone-like small peptides which are secreted by one cell and exert their influence on nearby cells through binding to specific receptors (Fig. 14-1). This leads to changes in gene expression in the responding cell and subsequent changes in cell behavior. Extensive studies on the signaling molecules in teeth and other organs and in different animals have shown that they have been conserved to an astonishing extent during evolution. It is now known that the same

Box 14-1 Stages of tooth development

Initiation

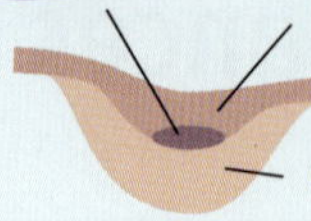

- Oral epithelium thickens and induces mesenchymal cells to odontogenic lineage.
- The dental placode forms.
- The sites and types of teeth are determined.

Bud stage

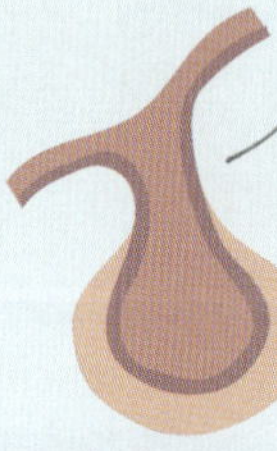

- Dental mesenchyme has condensed and induces growth and folding of epithelium.

Cap stage

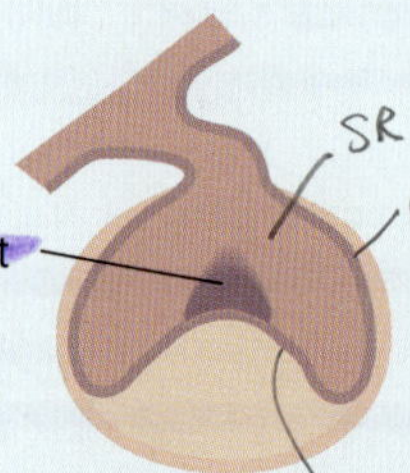

- Onset of shape development.
- Signaling center forms in the enamel knot.

Bell stage

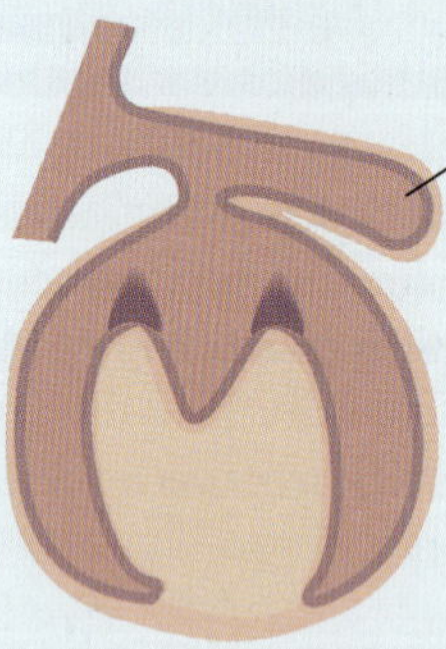

- Crown shape is determined by secondary enamel knots.
- Odontoblasts and ameloblasts differentiate.
- Dentin and enamel formation and mineralization start.
- Development of permanent tooth has started.

Maturation stage

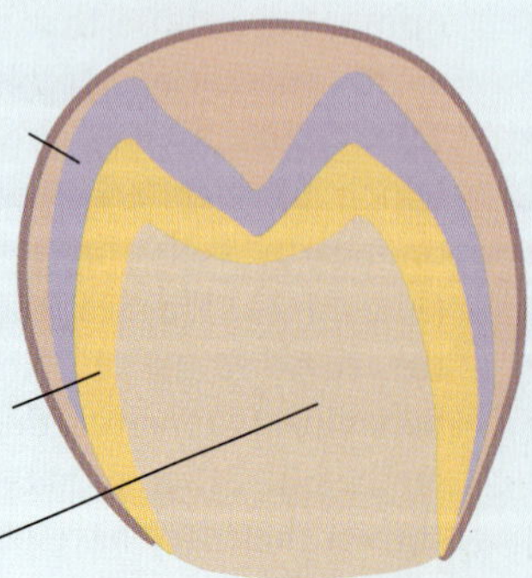

- Crown development is completed.
- Root development has started.
- Eruption begins.

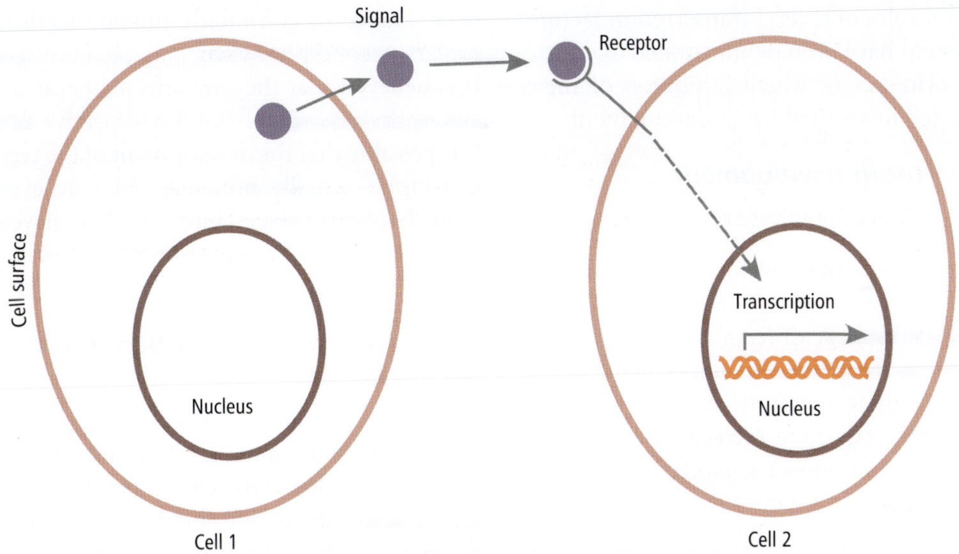

Figure 14-1 Cells communicate via soluble signals regulating gene expression (transcription).

signals regulate the development of practically all organs in the embryos of all species, but depending on the organ and stage of development, the signals elicit different responses.

The actual signals belong to a few families, of which four have been mostly studied and they also, importantly, regulate tooth development. These are the hedgehog, FGF (fibroblast growth factor), BMP (bone morphogenetic protein) and Wnt families. These signals are expressed in the very early dental epithelium and regulate the initiation of tooth development. They also signal back from mesenchyme to epithelium and initiate epithelial folding and thereby shape development. During advancing development several signals are locally expressed in the dental epithelium in small clusters of cells, the dental placodes and the enamel knots, which are signaling centers regulating tooth initiation and crown shape. The placodes form at sites where the dental epithelium buds to mesenchyme. The primary enamel knot forms at the tip of the bud and induces the folding of the epithelium and onset of cap formation. In molars, secondary enamel knots appear at the sites of new cusps and produce FGF signals, which stimulate the growth of the cusps (Fig. 14-2). The signals regulate a great number of different transcription factors which determine the ways in which the cells respond to the

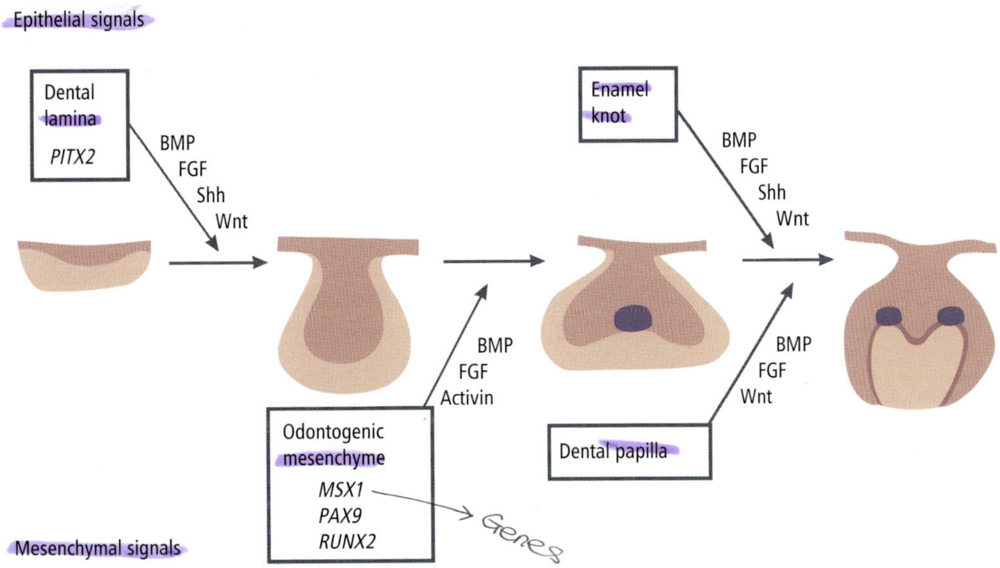

Figure 14-2 Reciprocal interactions between the epithelial and mesenchymal tissues are mediated by conserved signaling molecules (BMP = bone morphogenetic protein; FGF = fibroblast growth factor; Shh = sonic hedgehog, Wnt). Numerous transcription factors are associated with signaling, and only those in which mutations cause dental abnormalities are indicated in the boxes (PITX2, MSX1, PAX9, RUNX2).

signals. The central roles of several transcription factors in tooth development have been demonstrated by transgenic mouse experiments in which inhibition of their function has resulted in arrested tooth development.

Disturbances in tooth development

Disturbances in tooth development are seen as:

- numerical variations (missing or supernumerary teeth)
- variations in size and shape of teeth
- defects in the mineralized tissues, enamel, dentin, and cementum, which may result from defects in the composition of the respective extracellular matrices and/or their mineralization (see Chapter 17)
- problems in eruption (see Chapter 15).

It is obvious that tooth development may be disturbed at different stages of morphogenesis, and that the end result depends on the timing and the type of insult. Variations in the number, shape, and size of teeth are commonly linked. In particular, hypodontia together with small and peg-shaped teeth are often seen in the same patient. In these cases it is apparent that there is an inhibition of the early morphogenesis, and that it leads either to a complete arrest of development or to small teeth depending on the tooth type and extent of disruption. The most commonly missing teeth are the third molars, second premolars, and maxillary lateral incisors. It is believed that they are affected because they are the last teeth to develop from the respective dental placode. It is possible that the development of the teeth ultimately missing is actually initiated and may even have proceeded to early stages but that their development has been arrested because the tooth germs did not reach threshold size.

Genetic causes of disturbed tooth development

Tooth development is under strict genetic control and apart from some mineralization disturbances which are commonly caused by environmental factors, disturbances in tooth development result from gene mutations. It has been known for a long time that dental abnormalities run in families, and the inheritance patterns of numerous isolated, as well as syndromic, dental defects have been examined in detail. Many gene mutations have been identified that cause abnormal tooth development.

It is noteworthy that most mutations that have so far been identified as causing abnormalities in tooth number and/or shape, affect molecules of the signaling networks regulating early tooth morphogenesis (Box 14-2). In

Box 14-2 Gene mutations causing aberrations in number and shape of teeth

Syndrome	Phenotype	Causative gene	Type of molecule
Oligodontia	Severe hypodontia	PAX9	Transcription factor
Oligodontia	Severe hypodontia Cleft palate (occasionally)	MSX1	Transcription factor
Oligodontia–colorectal cancer syndrome	Hypodontia of permanent teeth Colorectal cancer	AXIN2	Signal inhibitor
Rieger syndrome	Oligodontia Eye and umbilical defects	PITX2	Transcription factor
Hypohidrotic Ectodermal dysplasia	Oligodontia Small peg-shaped teeth Hypoplasia of hair and glands	EDA/Ectodys Plasin EDAR EDARADD	Signal molecule Signal receptor Signal mediator
EEC syndrome	Ectodermal dysplasia Ectrodactyly Cleft palate	P63	Transcription factor
CLPED	Ectodermal dysplasia Cleft lip/palate	PVRL1	Cell adhesion molecule (Nectin-1)
Cleidocranial dysplasia	Supernumerary teeth Impaired eruption Deficient bone formation	RUNX2	Transcription factor
Tricho-dento-osseous syndrome (TDO)	Taurodontism Enamel hypoplasia Hair and bone defects	DLX3	Transcription factor

contrast, most of the currently known mutations that cause inherited defects in dentin and enamel are in genes encoding major components of their respective extracellular matrices and include, e.g., type I collagen and amelogenin.

Hypodontia and abnormal tooth shape

The gene defect(s) causing the most common form of hypodontia, affecting one or a few incisors and/or premolars, have not yet been identified, but mutations causing rare and syndromic forms of hypodontia have been found in several genes. Autosomal dominant hypodontia has been shown to be caused by mutations in the transcription factors MSX1 and PAX9. The patients with PAX9 mutations have no other congenital defects whereas patients with MSX1 mutations may be affected by cleft palate. MSX1 and PAX9 have central functions in the early dental mesenchyme where they mediate epithelial–mesenchymal signaling. Mutations in AXIN2, an inhibitor of Wnt signaling, cause a rare form of oligodontia (lack of more than six teeth) affecting only permanent teeth. These patients develop colorectal cancer later in life.

Most of the hypodontia genes that have been identified are associated with syndromes affecting several other organs besides the teeth. That the development of different organs is disturbed by mutations in one gene is not surprising, taking into account the fact that similar mechanisms and the same genes regulate the development of all organs. The causative gene in Rieger syndrome is PITX2, a transcription factor expressed very early in dental epithelium. The most common form of ectodermal dysplasia (syndromes affecting several ectodermal organs including teeth, hair, glands, and nails) is hypohidrotic ectodermal dysplasia in which oligodontia is severe (sometimes all teeth are missing) and the rest of the teeth are small and peg-shaped. This syndrome is usually caused by the loss of function of the signal molecule, ectodysplasin (EDA) belonging to the tumor necrosis factor family, or other molecules participating in the mediation of EDA signaling, e.g., its receptor EDAR. Ectodermal dysplasia may be associated with cleft lip and palate and mutations in the transcription factor P63 and the cell adhesion molecule Nectin-1 have been identified as causes of such syndromes (Box 14-2).

Hyperdontia

Compared to hypodontia, hyperdontia, or the formation of supernumerary teeth, is quite rare, and the genetic background has been clarified in only two conditions. Cleidocranial dysplasia is an autosomal dominant syndrome mainly affecting bone development (hypoplastic clavicles, open fontanelles, short stature). The patients have multiple extra teeth, which develop successively from the secondary teeth and form a partial third dentition. The eruption of teeth is impaired most likely because of defective bone remodeling. The causative gene is RUNX2, a transcription factor that is a master regulator of osteoblasts, the bone-forming cells. Experiments in mouse embryos have shown that in addition to bone, the gene is intensely expressed in dental mesenchyme during the bud and bell stages of tooth development, and that it is critically involved in signaling interactions between the epithelium and mesenchyme. Supernumerary teeth together with odontomas and impacted teeth occur in 10–20% of patients with familial adenomatosis coli (FAP). The causative gene is APC, which is a modulator of Wnt signaling. Interestingly, the stimulation of Wnt signaling in dental epithelium of transgenic mice results in massive production of supernumerary teeth which form successively from previously forming teeth. Hence, the Wnt signal pathway likely is a key regulator of tooth initiation and replacement (3).

Clinical aspects

Chronology of dental development

Data on the chronology of tooth development are usually given as mean values from series of observations. Even if the chronology in tooth development has a documented stability, deviations may occur. The timing of onset to completion of mineralization/development of the primary and permanent dentition is presented in Box 14-3 and Figs 14-3 and 14-4. The mineralization of the primary teeth starts during 14–18 weeks *in utero*. The root formation of the primary teeth is completed between 1.5 and 3 years. The crowns are halfway mineralized at birth and become fully formed during the first year of life (Fig. 14-3). Mineralization of the permanent teeth starts at birth with the first molars. The incisors

Box 14-3 Initiation of mineralization of primary teeth (mean ages)

Central incisors
- 4 weeks *in utero*.

First molars
- 15.5 weeks *in utero*.

Lateral incisors
- 16 weeks *in utero*.

Canines
- 17 weeks *in utero*.

Second molars
- 18 weeks *in utero*.

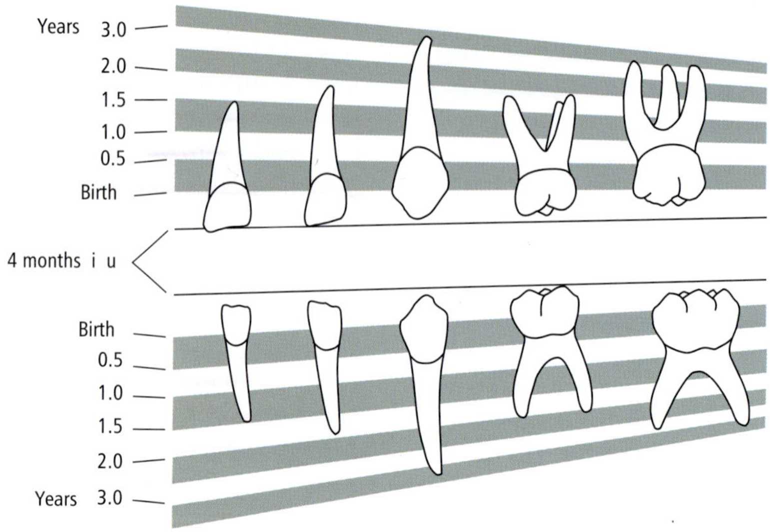

Figure 14-3 The chronology of mineralization of primary teeth.

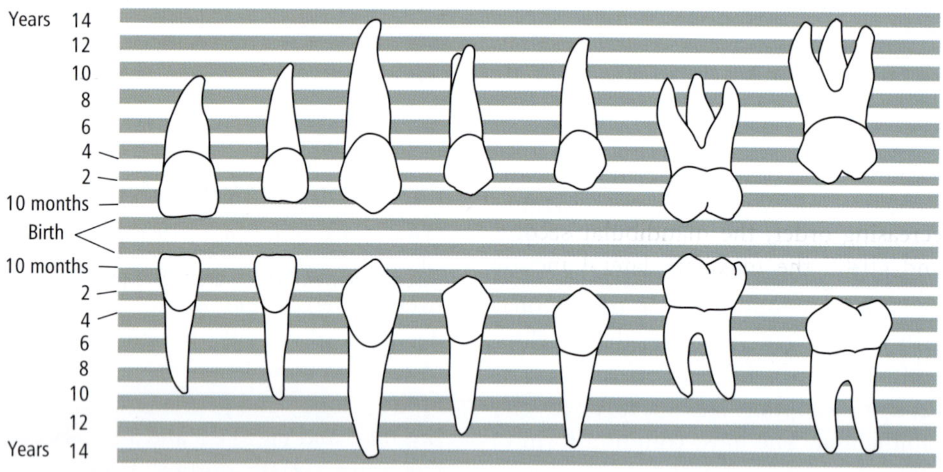

Figure 14-4 The chronology of mineralization of permanent teeth.

and canines start their mineralization during the first year of life, the premolars and second molars between the second and third years of life, and the third molar between the eighth and eleventh years of life. However, the normal range is wide. The crowns of the permanent teeth (except third molars) are generally completed between 5 and 7 years of age. Root development takes about 6–7 years. In general, the mandibular teeth develop earlier than the maxillary teeth (Fig. 14-4). A marked sex difference has been observed in tooth formation, girls being on average half a year ahead of boys.

Dental age estimation

The reasonable stability of the chronology of tooth development has been helpful in the evaluation of general growth and developmental disturbances and also in estimation of the chronological age of children with unknown birth date. Dental age may be evaluated from assessments of pre-eruptive tooth formation as judged from orthopantograms. Several systems have been developed (see Chapter 2) where various stages of tooth development are given numerical values (scores).

Terminology and definitions

The terminology used to describe congenitally missing teeth has been confusing, as terms such as agenesis, anodontia, aplasia, hypodontia, and oligodontia have been used interchangeably. Recently, Schalk van der Weide (6) proposed definitions to overcome this (Box 14-4).

Numerical variations in the primary dentition

Epidemiological investigations report a prevalence of hypodontia between 0.1 and 0.7%. The mandibular central incisors are almost exclusively affected and then mainly the laterals. Oligodontia or anodontia is rare but

> **Box 14-4** Terminology of congenitally missing teeth (6)
>
> **Hypodontia**
> - Fewer than six teeth, excluding the third molar, congenitally missing.
>
> **Oligodontia**
> - Six or more teeth, excluding the third molar, congenitally missing.
>
> **Anodontia**
> - All primary and/or permanent teeth congenitally missing.

may be found in connection with ectodermal dysplasia. There is a rather strong correlation between hypodontia in the primary and permanent dentition. The prevalence of supernumerary teeth varies between 0.3 and 0.6%. Ninety percent of all supernumerary teeth are located in the maxillary anterior region.

Numerical variations in the permanent dentition

Hypodontia is more frequent in the permanent than in the primary dentition, with a prevalence reported between 6 and 10% excluding the third molar. The most affected teeth are, in decreasing order, the mandibular second premolar (around 40%), the maxillary lateral incisor (around 20%), the maxillary second premolar (around 20%), and the mandibular central incisor (around 4%). Hypodontia in the permanent dentition usually affects two or more teeth in 50% of the cases (Fig. 14-5). Oligodontia and anodontia are rare (5). Symmetrical hypodontia often occurs for maxillary lateral incisors and second premolars. There is a particular relation between hypodontia and microdontia in the maxillary laterals and strong evidence that this form of hypodontia is inherited as an autosomal dominant trait.

Hyperdontia, or supernumerary teeth, are found with a frequency of 0.1–3.6%. The most frequent supernumerary tooth is the mesiodens in the midline of the maxilla (Fig. 14-6) or a supernumerary lateral in the maxilla. Supernumerary teeth are common in children with clefts and in cleidocranial dysplasia.

Syndromes involving congenitally missing teeth

There are a great number of syndromes with reported congenitally missing teeth. When any of the recently developed computer-aided syndrome diagnosis systems, e.g., OMIM (Online Mendelian Inheritance in Man), POSSUM (Pictures of Standardized Syndromes and Undiagnosed Malformations), or LDDB (London Dysmorphology Database), are consulted more than 100

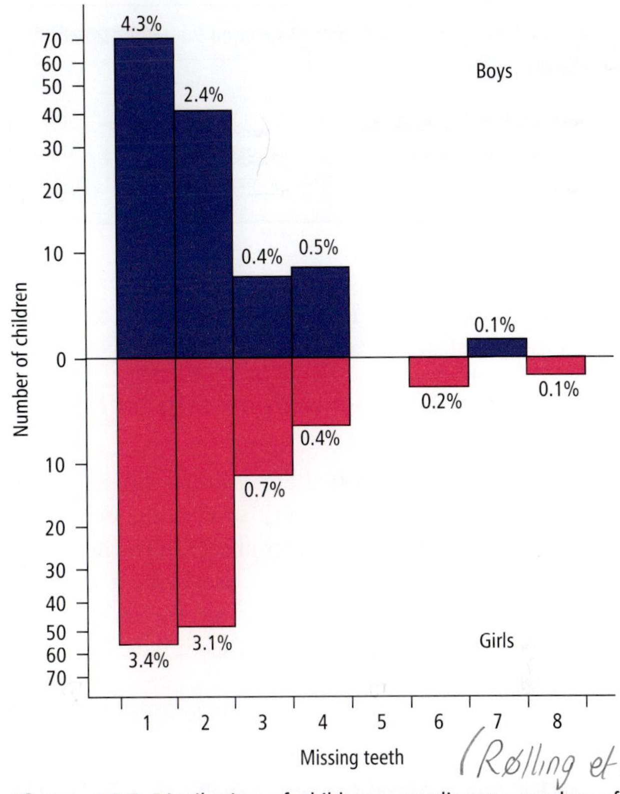

Figure 14-5 Distribution of children according to number of missing teeth. The horizontal axis shows the number of missing teeth per child. The vertical axis is logarithmic and shows the absolute number of children. The proportion of children is given above each column (5).

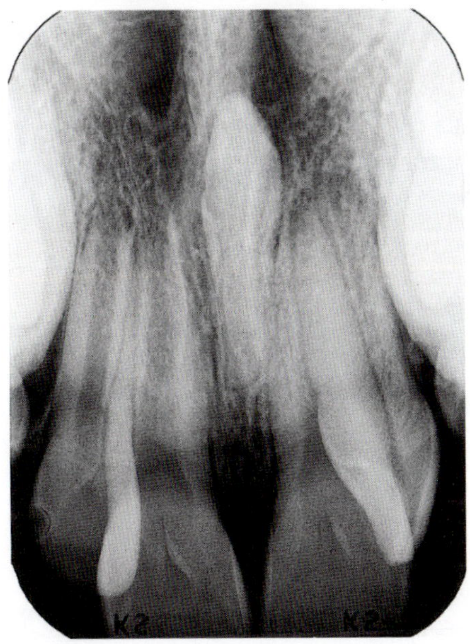

Figure 14-6 Mesiodens in an inverted position in the midline of the maxilla.

Box 14-5 Frequent syndromes associated with congenitally missing teeth

- Ectodermal dysplasias.
- Incontinentia pigmenti.
- Clefts of all types.
- Down syndrome.
- Rieger syndrome.
- EEC syndrome.

syndromes with missing teeth as a trait are presented. The most common syndromes with missing teeth are listed in Box 14-5.

Treatment of children with missing teeth or hyperdontia

In the primary dentition there is often no need for treatment unless there is a very severe oligodontia or anodontia. In such cases, uncomplicated prostheses are prepared to facilitate speech and also to be a psychological support. Such treatment can also be necessary in situations where a large number of teeth have been lost due to trauma or caries.

Congenitally missing teeth in the permanent dentition need thorough treatment planning and a serious consideration of different therapies in order to save tooth substance and to optimize the outcome in a lifelong perspective. In the premolar region, the treatment is mostly aimed at spontaneous closure of the space supported by timing of extraction of primary molars. In the frontal region, orthodontic treatment should always be considered before prosthodontic therapy. The hypodontia often concerns the laterals in the maxilla. The morphology of the canines is important if they are expected to erupt in the place of a missing lateral incisor. However, slight grinding and morphologic rebuild with composites can achieve good aesthetics. Composite-retained onlay bridges are also used to replace missing laterals (Fig. 14-7a, b). Hypodontia of permanent mandibular incisors may result in a frontal collapse with a deep overbite (Fig. 14-8). Early prosthetic treatment in the mandible is therefore indicated, e.g., an onlay bridge. In cases with extensive lack of teeth a multidisciplinary team approach is strongly recommended (2). In this

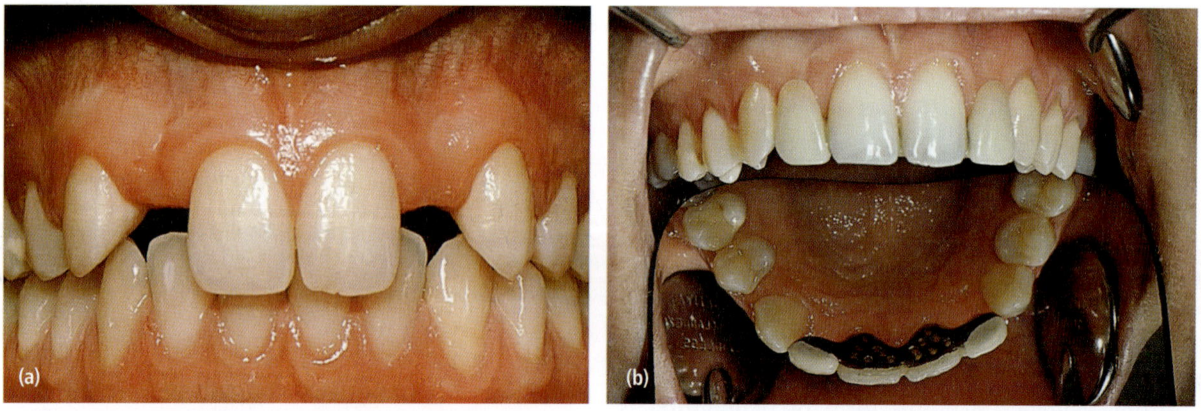

Figure 14-7 (a) Hypodontia of the permanent maxillary lateral incisors in a 15-year-old boy. (b) The same boy with the laterals replaced with a composite-retained onlay bridge. The material in the Rochette-bridge is stainless steel and fused porcelain.

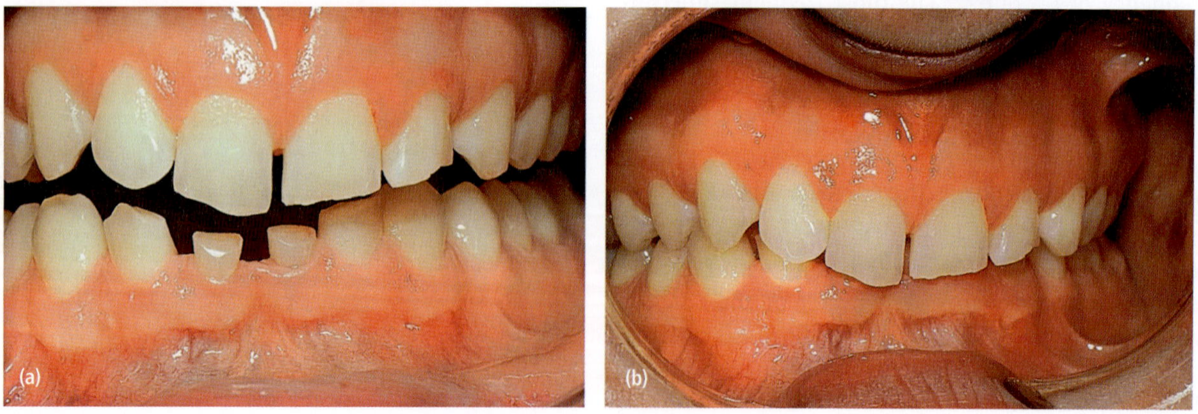

Figure 14-8 Hypodontia of permanent mandibular incisors in an 18-year-old boy resulting in elongation of the maxillary central incisors and a deep bite.

team, specialists in pediatric dentistry, orthodontics, oral surgery, prosthodontics, radiology, and a consulting psychologist should be represented. The treatment will often cover a 10–20-year period and may involve orthodontics, tooth transplantations (auto), implants, and fixed and removable prosthodontics. This team should follow the child from the time when the diagnosis of oligodontia or anodontia has been settled and continuously plan and supervise the treatment to adulthood (1–3). In Fig. 14-9, the treatment of a boy with ectodermal dysplasia is presented, following a team-approach model.

The treatment of hyperdontia is usually extraction or surgical removal of the supernumerary tooth, especially if there is a disturbance of the eruption of surrounding teeth.

Morphologic abnormalities

A variety of tooth morphology abnormalities can occur. As discussed above in this chapter, tooth morphology is predominantly determined by genetic factors. Consequently, many aberrations are better understood in an anthropological context. However, there are also a number of external influencing factors, e.g., effect of cytotoxic medication, trauma, radiation, or pulpal complications to the teeth during their development (4).

Variation in tooth size

Generally men have larger teeth than women. Racial differences have also been seen. Tooth size is defined as abnormal when dimensions deviate two standard deviations from average. The deviation may be general or local and may involve the whole tooth or only parts of it.

Microdontia is defined as teeth smaller than normal. General microdontia is a rare condition occurring in connection with congenital hypopituitarism, ectodermal dysplasia, and Down syndrome. *Local microdontia*, involving single teeth, is more common and often associated with hypodontia. Microdontia mostly concerns maxillary laterals and third molars. The frequency of microdontia in maxillary laterals is slightly less than 1%. Radiation to the jaws during tooth development may cause microdontia in the area involved. *Macrodontia* is defined as teeth larger than normal. General macrodontia is extremely rare but can be seen in cases with gigantism. Double formations might sometimes be misinterpreted as macrodontia (Fig. 14-10). In congenital hemifacial hypertrophy, macrodontia may be seen unilaterally in the affected side in combination with a difference in developmental stage (Fig. 14-11).

Rhizomicry means that the length of the root is shorter than the height of the crown. This is seen in osteoporosis and in dentinal dysplasia.

Local rhizomicry may be acquired as a result of trauma, pulpal infections, and radiation during root development and later due to root resorption. A familiar pattern of rhizomicry has been reported, predominantly affecting maxillary incisors and premolars. In cases of established heredity this aberration is designated SR-anomaly (short root). Abnormally large roots, *rhizomegaly*, are an unusual anomaly mainly affecting maxillary canines.

Variation in tooth morphology

The maxillary lateral incisor frequently exhibits variation in the form of the crowns. Conical peg-shaped form and accentuated cingulum often connected to the incisal edge are the most common aberrations. The "cusp-shaped" cingulum of maxillary anterior teeth, Talon cusp, can interfere with normal occlusion (Fig. 14-12). The same abnormality may also be seen in premolars or molars and is called evagination. The two conditions usually contain an extension of the pulp. The treatment is therefore careful, successive grindings to avoid pulp involvement or, if this is not possible, to perform a partial pulpotomy (see Chapters 12, 17, and 18).

The permanent maxillary first molar and also the primary maxillary second molar may appear with an extra tuberculum, Carabelli's cusp, which is located on the palatinal side of the mesiopalatal cusp. The third molar exhibits the greatest variation of size and morphology of all teeth. The shovel-shaped incisor is seen more frequently among Eskimos, Mongolians, and American Indians.

Dens invaginatus (Fig. 14-13) is a common malformation due to an invagination of enamel epithelium resulting in a channel or lumen surrounded by hard tissues within the tooth. The anomaly occurs most frequently in the palatinal surface of maxillary laterals but can be found in other teeth. A frequency of 3% has been reported in a Swedish population. The defect varies in severity and a classification into three types has been described (Box 14-6).

Invagination can be suspected at clinical examination if the tooth has a marked cingulum or palatal cusp. The entrance to the invagination can be extremely narrow, thus X-ray examination is necessary.

Taurodontism (Latin *taurus* = bull) is a rare anomaly found in multirooted teeth in both dentitions and is characterized by elongated root-stem with the furcation more apical than normally. The anomaly is genetically determined (see Box 14-2) and the degree of taurodontism increases from the first to the third molar.

Double formation of teeth

In contrast to other dental anomalies, double formations appear more frequently in the primary dentition

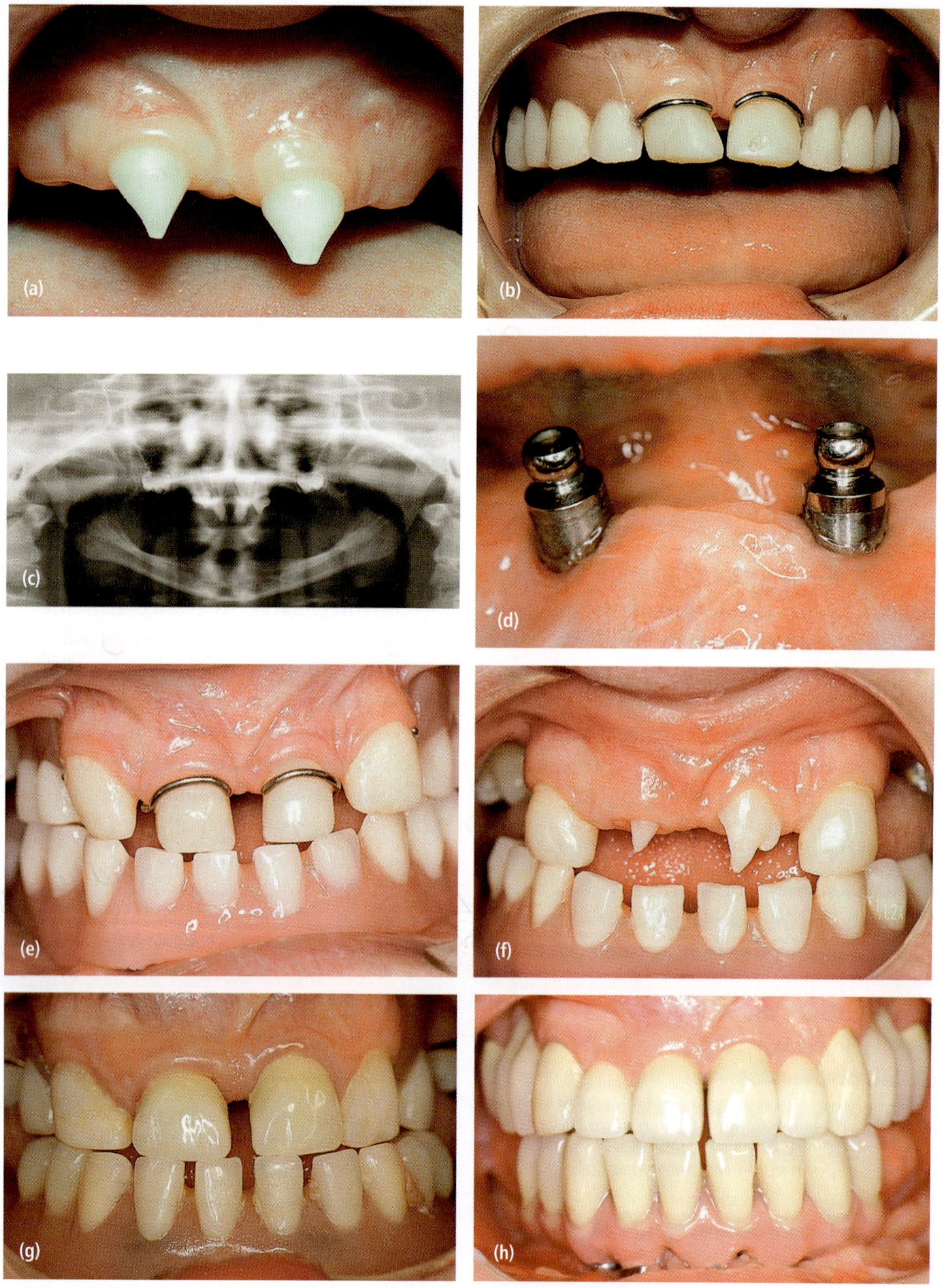

Figure 14-9 A boy with ectodermal dysplasia. (a) Intraoral view at the age of 2 years. Conically shaped primary incisors 51 and 61. (b) Teeth 51 and 61 rebuilt with composite resin and a removable partial denture in the maxilla at the age of 3 years. (c) Radiographic examination at the age of 4 years. No teeth in the mandible. In the maxilla 16, 11, 21, 26 and 53, 51, 61, 63 are present. (d) Two fixtures installed in the mandible at the age of 6 years. (e) Removable partial denture in the maxilla and implant retained over denture in the mandible at the age of 7 years. Note small, "primary" acrylic teeth. (f) Eruption of malformed permanent maxillary central incisors at the age of 8 years. (g) Temporary crowns 11 and 21 and rebuilt maxillary and mandibular denture at 18 years of age. (h) At 20 years of age, two fixed bridges were placed in the maxilla (53 and 63 were used in the bridges as they were stable and showed no root-resorption) and two more implants were placed in the mandible, enabling the construction of a bridge in the mandible as well (1).

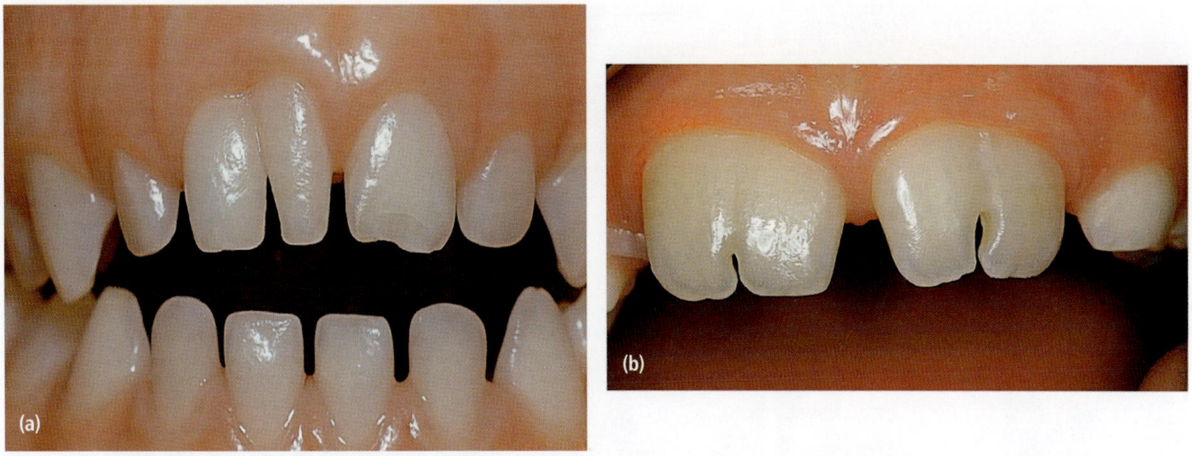

Figure 14-10 Double formation in (a) primary and (b) permanent teeth in the maxillary frontal region.

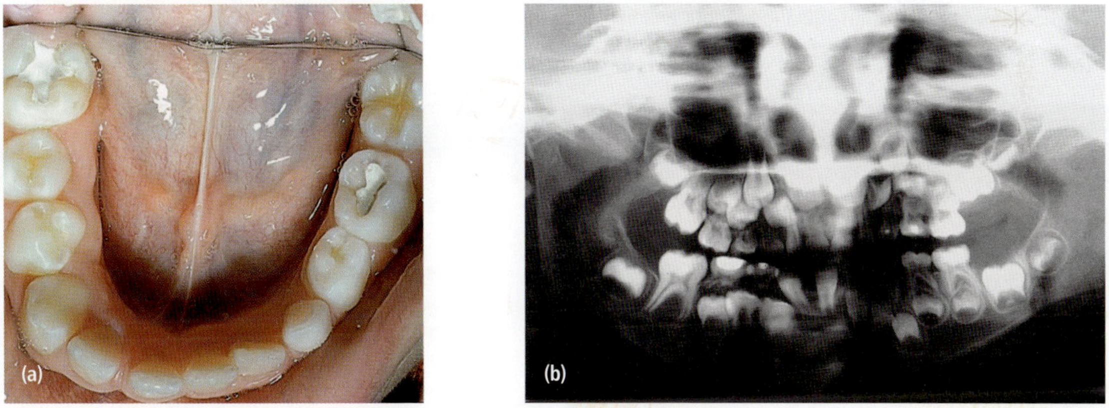

Figure 14-11 (a) A 4-year-old girl with hemifacial hypertrophy on the right side. Observe the difference in size and developmental stage between the left and the right sides. (b) Orthopantomogram of the same girl. Compare the developmental differences between the permanent first molars in the left and right sides.

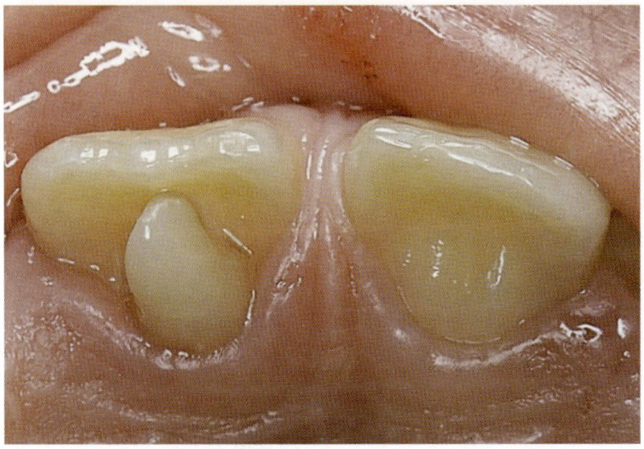

Figure 14-12 "Cusp-shaped" cingulum of permanent central incisor interfering with occlusion.

Box 14-6 Types of invagination according to severity

Type I
- Enamel-lined cavity confined to the tooth crown.

Type II
- Enamel-lined cavity extending into the root.

Type III
- Enamel-lined cavity perforating the root apically or laterally.

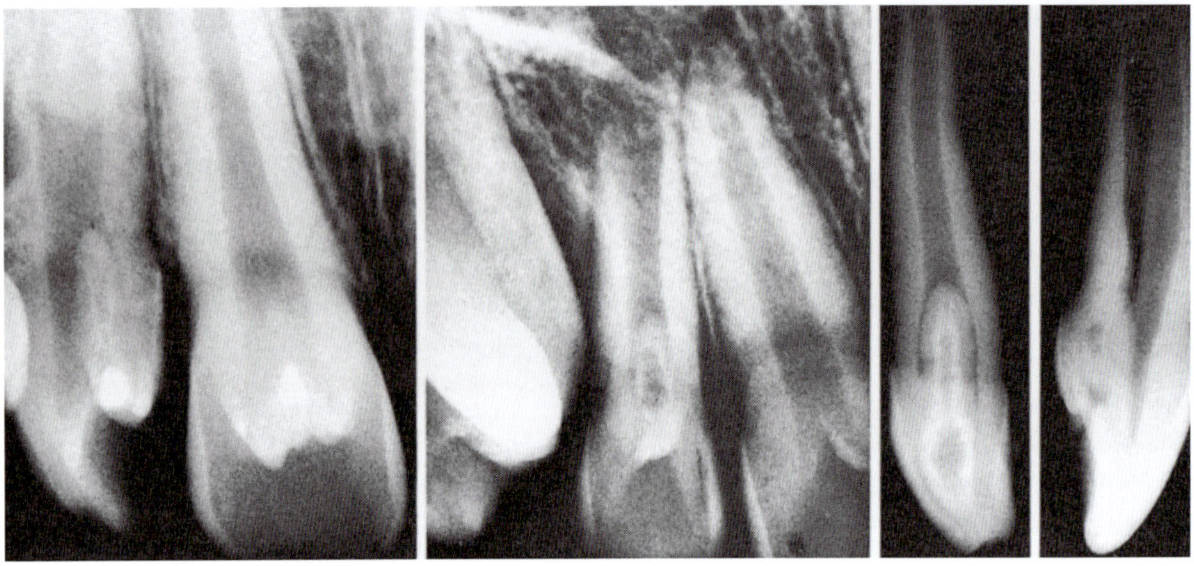

Figure 14-13 Some examples of invaginations. Note enamel lining inside the lumen.

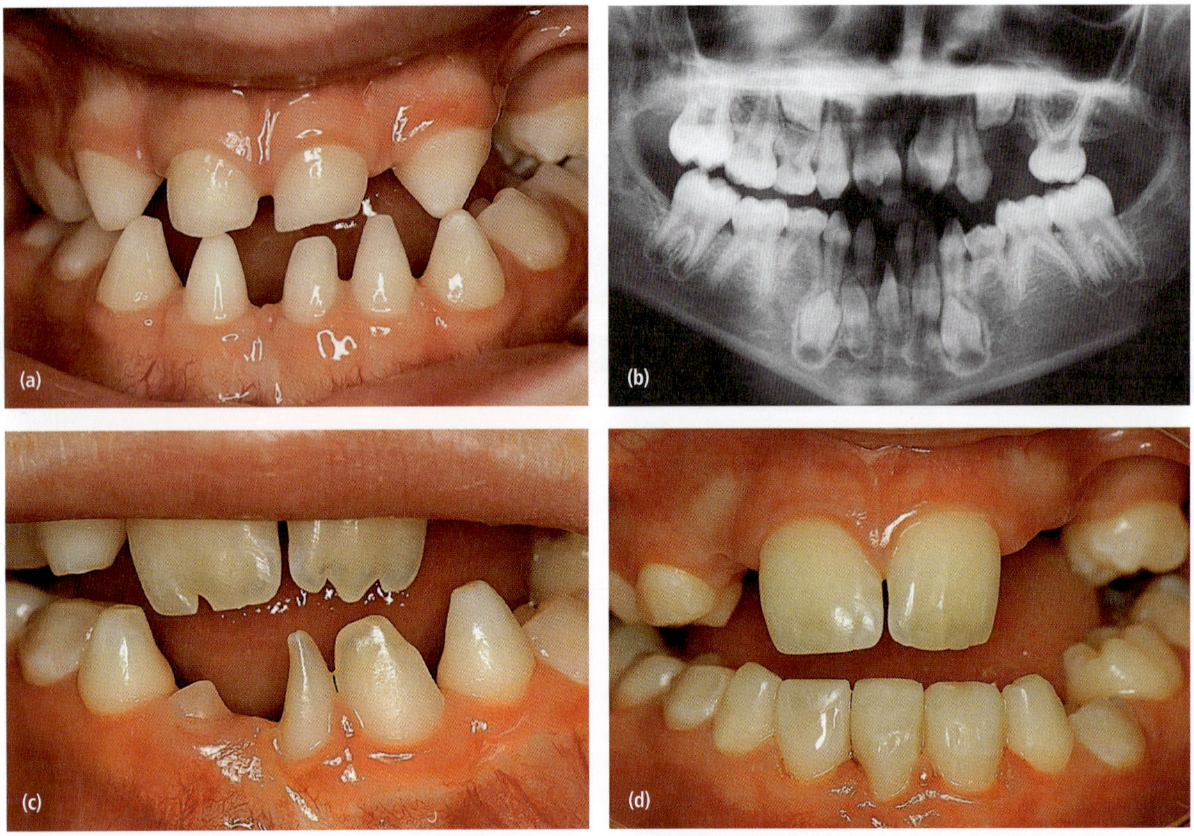

Figure 14-14 (a) A 4-year-old girl with incontinentia pigmenti. Observe the peg-shaped primary incisors. (b) Orthopantomogram at the age of 8 years. Observe the missing premolars and molars. (c) At the age of 9 years, thin peg-shaped permanent incisors are erupting in the mandible. (d) The same girl after rebuilding the mandibular incisors with composite resin.

Box 14-7 Double formations of teeth

Concrescence
Two normal appearing crowns are present and the fusion involves only the cementum.

Fusion
Union in dentin and/or enamel between two or more normal teeth. The fusion may also involve the pulp. Fusion most often leads to reduced number of teeth in the area.

Gemination
Incomplete division of a tooth germ or a union between a normal tooth and a supernumerary tooth. Thus there is no reduction in number of teeth.

than in the permanent dentition. Double formations are mostly found in the front teeth area and are rare in the premolar and molar area (Box 14-7, Fig. 14-10). The prevalence of double formations in the primary dentition is approximately 0.5–0.8%. In general, fusions are more common than gemination. Double formations in the primary dentition are often followed by aplasia of the permanent successor (20–75%). The anomaly is often observed in connection with Down syndrome, thalidomide embryopathy, and cleft palate.

Treatment of teeth with morphologic aberrations

Most of the teeth with morphologic abnormalities are easily reshaped and built up with composite resins by using the acid-etch technique. Small peg-shaped teeth, for example, can be transformed to normal size and appearance by such treatment (Fig. 14-14).

The invagination requires special treatment attention because of the risk of poor quality and permeability of the dental hard tissues in the bottom of the invagination. Thus, the risk of pulpal involvement is obvious after eruption of the tooth.

Due to retention of food and plaque in the fossa, caries may attack the tooth before complete eruption. Therefore, sealing of all lingual pits in incisors should be undertaken as soon as possible after eruption. True invaginations should be treated as deep carious lesions. Softened or carious tissues should be removed. The risk of accidental pulp exposure of the buccal side during excavation is obvious due to improper inclination of the drill. Extra long drills should thus be used to avoid guidance of the incisal edge of the tooth (Fig. 14-15). If the dentin at the bottom is hard and the tooth is without any pulpal symptoms, it is not necessary to extend the excavation into the frequently occurring canal seen as a small black spot at the bottom of the cavity. The bottom should be covered with a calcium hydroxide base and then filled with a composite resin material. If the pulp is exposed or if there are pulpal complications further treatment is dependent on root development, morphology and accessibility of the canal.

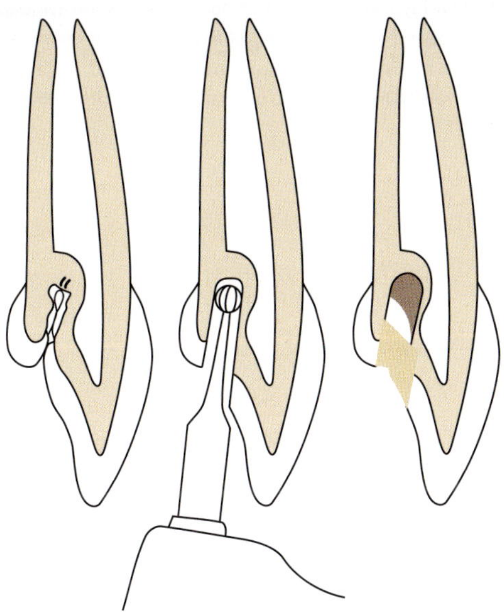

Figure 14-15 The treatment of dens invaginatus. The lumen is reamed out with an elongated round drill. The bottom and buccal walls of the lumen are covered with calcium hydroxide compound.

Odontomas

Odontomas may develop from disturbances in dental organogenesis varying from malformation of a tooth to odontogenic hamartomous tumors. Odontomas are the most common odontogenic "tumor". They occur mostly in the permanent dentition and can vary in size from some millimeters up to several centimeters. They are often revealed in radiographic examination with late tooth eruption or retentions. The odontomas can occur in compound or complex form. The compound odontoma consists of a varying number of tooth-like formations where the different dental hard tissues can be clearly distinguished (Fig. 14-16). The pathogenesis of compound odontomas may involve activation of the Wnt signal pathway since they are frequent in familial adenomatosis coli patients (caused by mutations in the Wnt inhibitor APC) and since structures resembling compound odontomas formed in transgenic mice as a result of Wnt signal activation (3). The complex odontoma is a more or less hazardous arrangement of dental hard tissue (Fig. 14-17). Odontomas are often well encapsulated and surgical removal is uncomplicated.

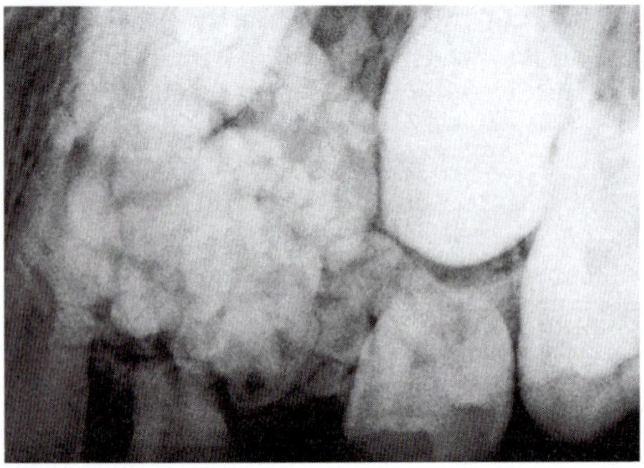

Figure 14-16 Radiographic examination of a compound odontoma.

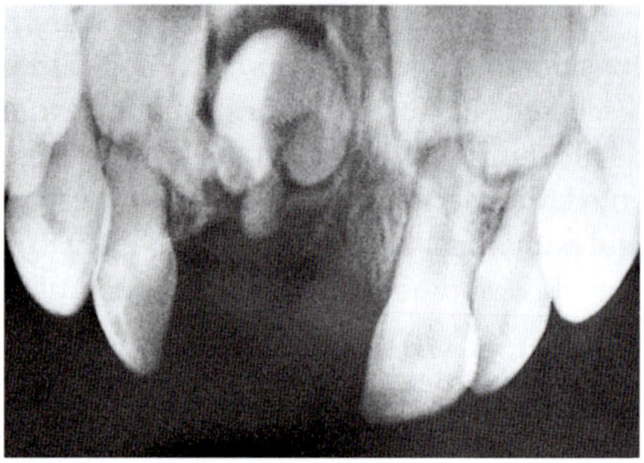

Figure 14-17 Radiographic examination of a complex odontoma in a 2-year-old girl as a result of trauma.

Background literature

Gene expression in teeth: http://bite-it.helsinki.fi/ (accessed August 2008).

Nanci A. *Ten Cate's oral histology: development, structure, and function*, 7th edn. St Louis, MO: Mosby, 2007.

Thesleff I, Nieminen, P. Tooth induction. In: *Encyclopedia of life sciences.* Chichester: John Wiley, 2005. http://www.els.net/ (doi.wiley.com/10.1038/npg.els.0004183) (accessed August 2008).

Thesleff I, Pirinen S. Dental anomalies: genetics. In: *Encyclopedia of life sciences.* Chichester: John Wiley, 2005. http://www.els.net/ (doi.wiley.com/10.1038/npg.els.0006088) (accessed August 2008).

Thesleff I. The genetic basis of tooth development and dental defects. *Am J Med Genet* 2006;**140**:2530–5.

References

1. Bergendal B, Koch G, Kurol J, Wänndahl G, eds. *Consensus Conference on Ectodermal Dysplasia with special reference to dental treatment.* Stockholm: Förlagshuset Gothia, 1998.
2. Bergendal B, Bergendal T, Hallonsten A-L, Koch G, Kurol J, Kvint S. A multidisciplinary approach to oral rehabilitation with osseointegrated implants in children and adolescents with multiple aplasia. *Eur J Orthod* 1996;**18**:119–29.
3. Järvinen E, Salazaar-Ciudad I, Birchmeier W, Taketo MM, Jernvall J, Thesleff I. Continuous tooth generation in mouse is induced by activated epithelial Wnt/βcatenin signalling. *Proc Natl Acad Sci USA* 2006;**103**:18627–32.
4. Lexner MO, Bardow A, Hertz JM, Nielsen LA, Kreiborg S. Anomalies of tooth formation in hypohidrotic ectodermal dysplasia. *Int J Paediatr Dent* 2007;**17**:10–18.
5. Rølling S. Hypodontia of permanent teeth in Danish schoolchildren. *Scand J Dent Res* 1980;**88**:365–9.
6. Schalk van der Weide Y. Oligodontia. A clinical, radiographic and genetic evaluation. Thesis. University of Utrecht, 1992.

15

Eruption and shedding of teeth

Göran Koch, Sven Kreiborg and Jens O. Andreasen

Chronology of normal tooth eruption

Primary dentition

The chronology of eruption of primary teeth for Swedish children is given in Box 15-1. The sequence of eruption and the timing of eruption for each tooth are similar for both sexes. The variability in the age of the children at emergence of the individual teeth is relatively small, with standard deviations of 2–3 months. On average, the eruption of primary teeth begins at about the age of 8 months with the mandibular central incisors, and ends at the age of about 30 months with the maxillary second molars. Thus, in most children the total period of eruption of primary teeth spans about 2 years.

Permanent dentition

The chronology of eruption of permanent teeth (except for the third molars) for Danish children is given in Box 15-2. The sequence of tooth eruption is almost identical for both sexes. However, all teeth erupt significantly earlier in girls than in boys. The sex difference in eruption times averages approximately 6 months. There is, however, no appreciable difference in the variability of the eruption times between the sexes. In general, the variability in eruption times for the permanent dentition is much larger than the variability observed in the primary dentition, with standard deviations of 8–18 months (about five times greater than in the primary dentition). The smallest variability in time of emergence is observed for the first molars and incisors, whereas the largest variabilities are found for the canines and premolars in each jaw. The eruption of the permanent dentition begins with eruption of the mandibular central incisors at 6 years of age and ends with the eruption of the maxillary second molars at 12 years. Thus, in most children, the total period of eruption of permanent teeth (except for the third molars) spans about 6 years. In both sexes, a tendency for grouped emergence is noted, the teeth within a group showing similar mean times of emergence. The following groups are distinguishable:

- first molars in each jaw and the mandibular central incisors
- maxillary central and mandibular lateral incisors
- mandibular canines and the first premolars in both jaws
- maxillary canines and the second premolars in both jaws
- second molars in both jaws.

Mechanism and theories of tooth eruption

Tooth eruption is defined as the movement of a tooth, primarily in the axial direction, from its site of development in the jaw bone to its functional position in the oral cavity. This process continues, in principle, until the tooth meets the teeth in the opposing jaw. However, with the subsequent growth of the jaws and alveolar processes the teeth will exhibit continued vertical, mesial, and transverse drift until adult age. In addition, even through the second to fifth decade of life very slow but continuous eruption and alveolar growth have been documented.

The eruption phase has been divided into the following stages: *pre-eruptive*; *intraosseous*; *mucosal penetration*; *preocclusal*; and *postocclusal*.

In the pre-eruptive stage, the tooth crown is formed and the position of the tooth in the jaw bone is relatively stable. When the root begins to form, the tooth starts moving inside the jaw bone towards the oral cavity (the *intraosseous stage*). The eruption path is, for most teeth, not only through the bone, but also through the roots of the primary teeth. The *mucosal penetration stage* occurs, in general, when half to three-fourths of the root of the erupting tooth is formed. The *preocclusal stage* is relatively short (a few months), whereas the *postocclusal stage* is much longer (several years) and is characterized

Box 15-1 The chronology of eruption of primary teeth for Swedish children

Primary teeth: boys

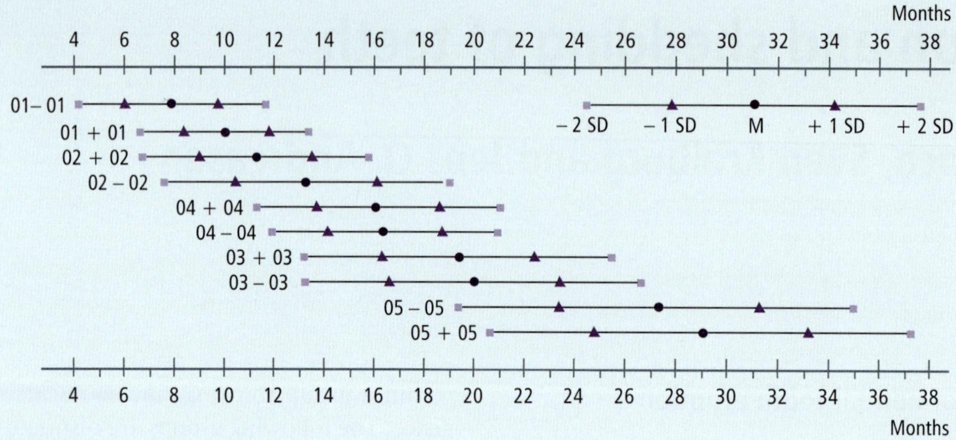

Primary teeth: girls

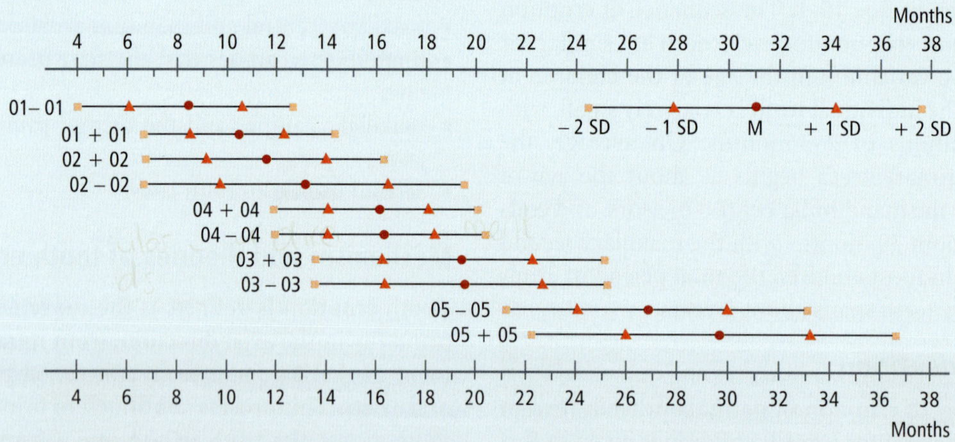

Mean times and standard deviations of primary tooth emergence. The Haderup system of dental designation is used: + signifies maxillary teeth, – mandibular teeth. 01 +0 1 and 01 – 01 represent maxillary and mandibular central incisors. Likewise 05 + 05 and 05 – 05 represent maxillary and mandibular second molars. Based on data from Lysell *et al.* (6).

by much slower tooth movement. Although the movement of teeth during eruption primarily occurs in the axial direction, the teeth actually move in all three planes of space. Apart from the rather precise eruption pattern of various tooth types there appears to be an individual very precise eruption time for homologous teeth, i.e., that left–right-side eruption should not deviate by more than 2–4 months. If that is the case then an eruption obstacle may be present (1).

Until recently, clinical studies of tooth eruption have been based on two-dimensional X-rays. However, with newer medical imaging techniques, such as computed tomography and magnetic resonance scanning, three-dimensional analysis of tooth eruption has become possible (Fig. 15-1a, b). With these technologies more accurate determination of the eruption path of individual teeth is now possible.

The eruption path is determined by genetic and local environmental factors. One of the most important local environmental factors is crowding among the developing and erupting teeth (7).

Tooth eruption is a biological process which is still not fully understood. The process is accompanied by multiple tissue changes, such as resorption and apposition of the alveolar bone, and development of the root and periodontium.

The eruption mechanism has for a long time been under investigation and several theories have been proposed, including eight different explanations of how eruption takes place (7,8). At present, the "polarized

Box 15-2 The chronology of eruption of permanent teeth (except for the third molars) for Danish children

Permanent teeth: boys

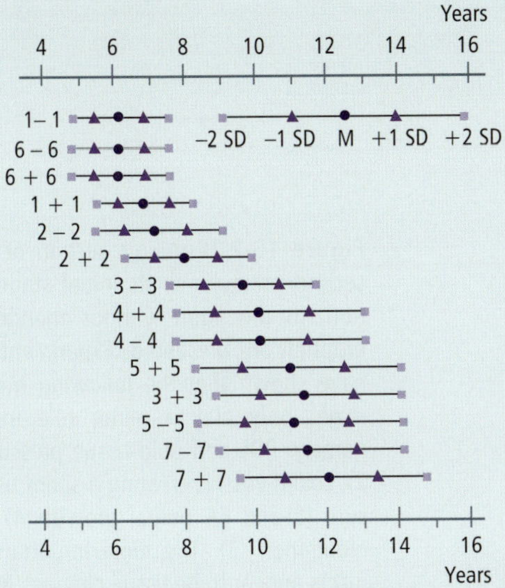

Permanent teeth: girls

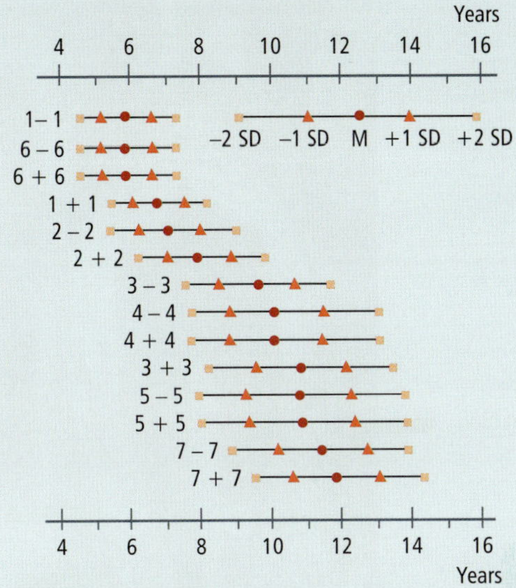

Mean times and standard deviations of permanent tooth emergence. Data from Helm and Seidler (2).

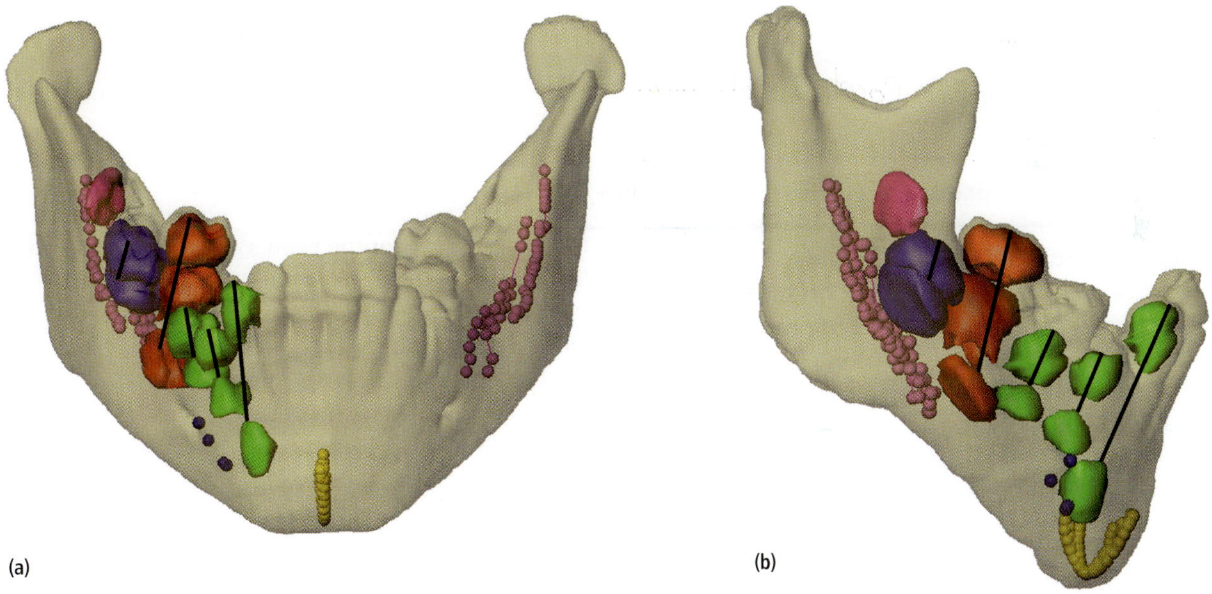

Figure 15-1 Transparent mandible at age 10 years. (a) Frontal view. Mental foramina, and segmented teeth (posterior to the incisors) from four different ages (0, 1, 7, and 10 years) are aligned automatically on the symphisis menti and the mandibular canals. Only the teeth and the mental foramen on the right side are illustrated. Lines indicate the eruption paths of the individual teeth. Tooth color code: purple = permanent third molar, blue = permanent second molar, red = permanent first molar, green = permanent premolars and the permanent canine. The mental foramen = blue. The symphysis menti = yellow. The mandibular canals = pink. (b) Lateral view. Lines indicate the eruption paths of the individual teeth. Color coding is the same as part (a).

follicle theory" is possibly the one which can best explain the initial stages of tooth eruption in humans (Fig. 15-2). According to this theory, the coronal part of the follicle will start its resorbing activity when root formation starts. This process is coordinated by selective bone growth in the apical part of the follicle. Due to this coordinated osteoclast/osteoblast activity an eruptive movement of the tooth will take place. The direction of this

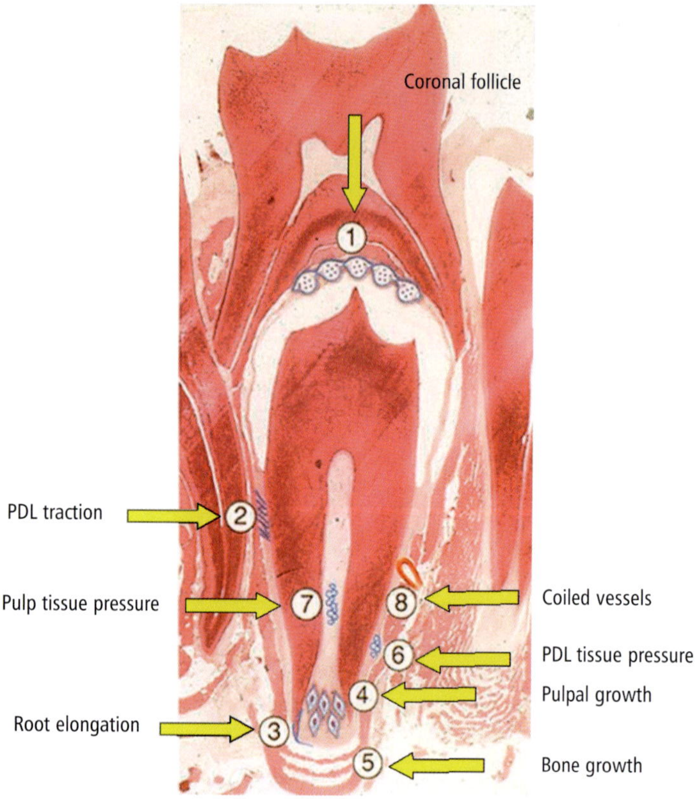

Figure 15-2 Histologic section of a human second premolar in its initial stage of eruption. In the figure various theories behind eruption are presented. Experimental studies have shown that the following mechanisms might only play a minor role in eruption namely: PDL and pulp tissue pressure (6 and 7), coiled vessels creating a slight tissue pressure (8 and 6), pulpal growth (4) and root elongation (3). The most important mechanisms appear to be tissue changes induced by the follicle namely induced coronal resorption and apical bone apposition (1 and 5). PDL traction (2) may play a role after penetration of the oral mucosa (8).

movement is apparently directed by the gubernacular cord, a tract in the bone filled with an odontogenic mesenchymal tissue with odontogenic epithelial islands. This cord will expand during eruption, and thereby guide the tooth into its right position in the jaw. When the erupting permanent tooth has resorbed the overlying primary tooth and/or bone, the next step is to penetrate the oral mucosa (usually when half to three-fourths of the root is formed). The coronal part of the follicle with the reduced enamel epithelium has been shown to possess the necessary collagenase activity to allow the permanent tooth germ to penetrate the mucosa (however, large amounts of fibrous tissue may present an obstacle to eruption; see later). After mucosal penetration, a fast extraalveolar eruption takes place, possibly related to periodontal ligament (PDL) traction and/or apical alveolar bone formation. Finally, when occlusion has been reached, vertical and horizontal changes can occur and the mechanisms for these events are largely unknown.

Longitudinal studies of aplasia sites with persistent primary teeth have shown that over a 10-year period, approximately 10% of the teeth showed very little resorption whereas the remaining teeth showed an average loss of approximately 5% root length each year (9).

Mechanism of shedding of primary teeth

Prior to shedding of primary incisors, canines and molars, the roots of the primary teeth are resorbed and their crowns shed. Dentinoclasts appear on the apical surface of the roots of the primary teeth, possibly initiated by the pressure created by the dental sac of the erupting permanent teeth. However, even if a permanent tooth is missing, the primary predecessor usually undergoes root reresorption, although commonly at a much slower pace. The role of pulpal dentinoclasts in this process is still being investigated.

Figure 15-2 illustrates the histologic picture during resorption of the roots of a primary mandibular second molar in connection with eruption of the second premolar. Figure 15-3 shows the histologic picture of the resorption of the palatal part of the root in a primary maxillary central incisor during eruption of the permanent maxillary central incisor.

Systemic disturbances affecting tooth eruption and shedding

A number of systemic diseases and syndromes affect tooth eruption and shedding of primary teeth. Premature tooth eruption and shedding of primary teeth are

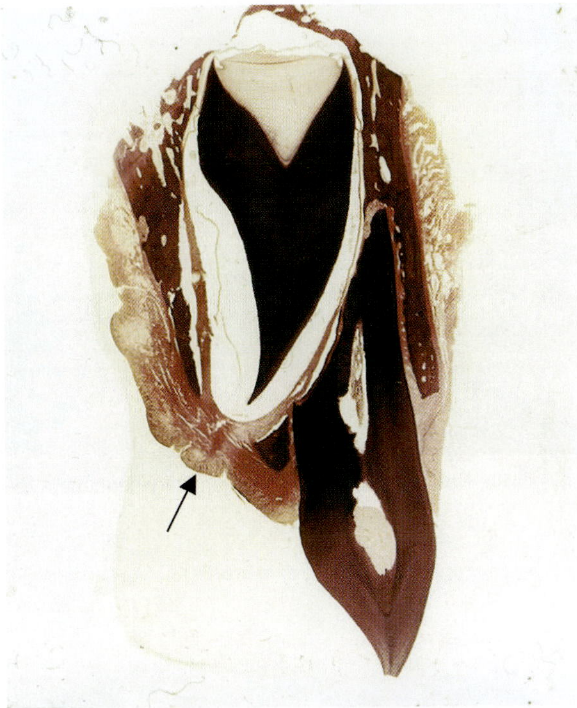

Figure 15-3 Histologic findings associated with the palatal resorption of a primary maxillary central incisor during eruption of the permanent incisor. Note also the presence of the gubernacular tract (arrow).

far more common than delayed eruption and shedding. In general, delay in eruption in the primary dentition is associated with delay in the permanent dentition, and the delay in the permanent dentition is mostly more pronounced than in the primary dentition.

Premature tooth eruption

Natal or neonatal teeth have been shown to occur in about 50 different syndromes. Of these, about 10 syndromes are associated with chromosomal aberrations, e.g., trisomy 13. Among other syndromes are Hallermann–Streiff syndrome and Ellis–van Creveld syndrome.

Delayed tooth eruption

In general, children with chronic diseases show delay in both physical and dental development, and will, consequently, show delayed tooth eruption. Several general diseases, including more than 150 different syndromes, have been shown to exhibit delayed tooth eruption (10).

Endocrinopathies and chromosomal aberrations

Endrocrinopathies, such as hypopituitarism, hypothyroidism, and hypoparathyroidism, often result in retardation of dental emergence in both the primary and the permanent dentition. Many chromosomal aberrations, including trisomy 21 (Down syndrome), are associated with delayed tooth eruption.

Syndromes

Many syndromes, and especially those involving skeletal dysplasias with disturbed bone metabolism, show severely retarded or arrested tooth eruption.

In the following, a few relevant examples will be given.

Subjects with *cleidocranial dysplasia* (CCD) are characterized by short stature, aplasia or hypoplasia of the clavicles, and severe disturbances in cranial ossification. These patients often develop numerous supernumerary permanent teeth occlusal to the normal permanent teeth. Tooth eruption is delayed in both the primary and permanent dentitions, but the delay is most severe in the permanent dentition, often with arrest of eruption and multiple retentions of both normal and supernumerary teeth. The disturbances in tooth eruption are related both to the skeletal pathology with retardation of osteoblast, osteoclast, and odontoclast differentiation, and to the presence of supernumerary teeth. Thus, even in regions without supernumerary teeth, shedding of primary teeth and eruption of permanent teeth can be extremely delayed or arrested (Fig. 15-4). Therefore, children with CCD should be monitored for disturbances in tooth eruption (and other dental abnormalities) from early childhood, and treatment should be instituted as early as possible (3–5).

Subjects with *tricho-dento-osseous syndrome* (TDO) are characterized by disturbances in the development of hair, teeth, and bones. The patients are of normal height, but the skeleton, including the craniofacial skeleton, is dense and reveals disturbed bone remodeling with reduced osteoclastic activity. Tooth eruption is delayed in both dentitions, but most severely so in the permanent dentition, which may also show arrested eruption leading to retention of several permanent teeth (Fig. 15-5). The cause of the eruption problems is related to the reduced osteoclastic activity. Therefore, children with TDO should be monitored for disturbances in tooth eruption (and other dental abnormalities) from early childhood, and treatment should be carried out as early as possible (11).

Subjects with *pycnodysostosis* are characterized by short stature, caused by shortening of the extremities. The skeleton, including the craniofacial skeleton, is characterized by osteopetrosis with increased bone fragility. The increased bone density of the jaws, combined with pronounced crowding, leads to delayed eruption in both dentitions, but is most pronounced in the permanent

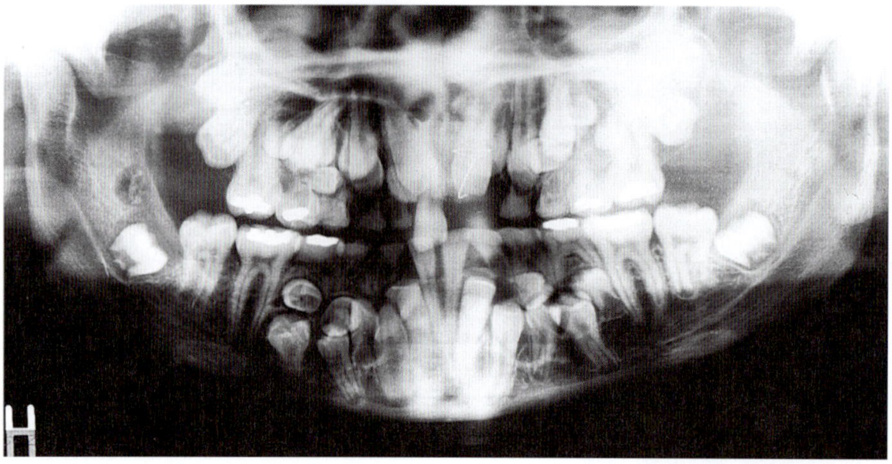

Figure 15-4 Orthopantomogram of a 16-year-old boy with cleidocranial dysplasia. Note the numerous supernumerary permanent teeth and the arrested eruption of many of the normal permanent teeth.

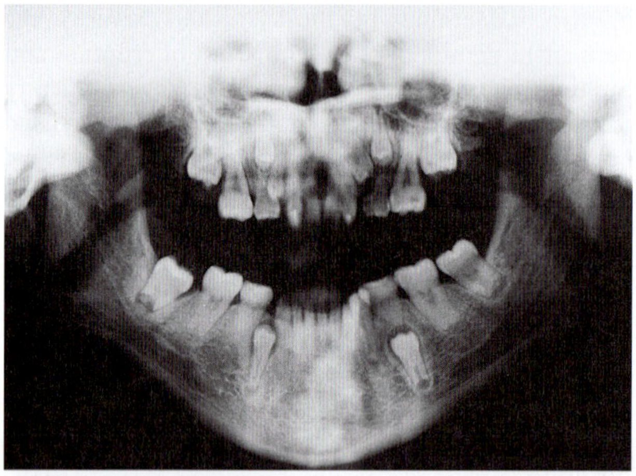

Figure 15-5 Orthopantomogram of a 13-year-old girl with tricho-dento-osseous syndrome. Note the severely delayed eruption of several permanent teeth and the dense jaw bones.

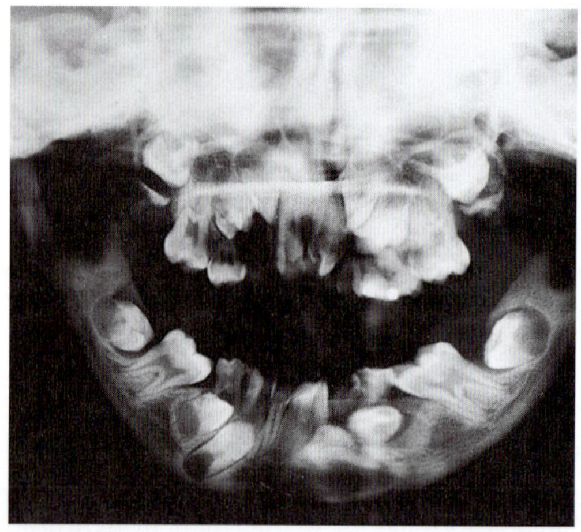

Figure 15-6 Orthopantomogram of a 10-year-old boy with pycnodysostosis. Note the delayed eruption of several permanent teeth and the ostepetrotic bones.

dentition. Thus, the permanent dentition may even show arrested tooth eruption and several other dental abnormalities (Fig. 15-6). These children should be monitored for disturbances in tooth eruption from early childhood, and treatment should be performed as early as possible (12).

Premature shedding of primary teeth

Systemic diseases that are associated with premature shedding of primary teeth include histiocytosis, hypophosphatasia, and neutropenia.

Histiocytosis is a symptom complex, which includes multiple eosinophilic granulomas, Hand–Schüller–Christian disease, and Letterer–Siwe disease. Early loss of posterior primary teeth is frequently observed, whereas the anterior teeth are less commonly involved.

Hypophosphatasia is a metabolic disease with impaired bone mineralization. The activity of alkaline phosphatase in plasma and tissues is reduced. Premature loosening and shedding of primary teeth are often seen. The anterior teeth are most frequently affected, whereas the primary molars are rarely involved. The teeth have a defect in cementum. There is often severe loss of alveolar bone with no or little gingival inflammation. The teeth are often shed without any signs of root resorption.

In *neutropenia*, the decrease in circulating neutrophils leads to lack of resistance to infection, which may predispose the children to gingivitis and periodontitis.

Premature shedding of primary teeth can occur in other diseases where the periodontium undergoes pathologic breakdown as seen in Papillon–Lefèvre syndrome (hyperkeratosis palmoplantaris with periodontoclasia), Down syndrome, and Ehlers–Danlos syndrome.

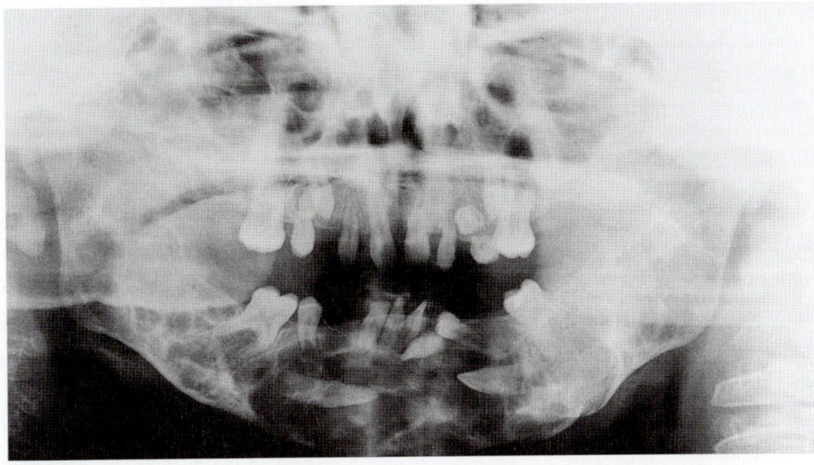

Figure 15-7 Orthopantomogram of 10-year-old boy with cherubism. The large cystic lesions in the maxilla and mandible have caused premature loss of primary teeth.

Other causes of premature shedding of primary teeth can be cystic lesions of the jaws, as seen in cherubism (Fig. 15-7).

Local disturbances affecting tooth eruption and shedding

It is essential to diagnose where the obstacle for the eruption process is located. The overwhelming cause is crowding, which may lead to impaction, and if this is the case, dental arch expansion or extraction is indicated. Crowding often leads to follicle collisions where one follicle is placed on top of the other thereby leaving both teeth unerupted. Another frequent cause is an ectopic eruption path, and in these cases extraction of primary predecessors and/or surgical creation of a new eruption path are the treatments of choice. Sometimes orthodontic traction must be used. In case of follicle and PDL pathology, arrest of eruption may occur; this condition is termed retention. Retention has further been divided into *primary retention* and *secondary retention*. Primary retention means that the eruption is arrested in the intraosseous stage due to pathology of the follicle and sometimes an ankylosis affecting either the crown or the root. Secondary retention means that an already erupted tooth due to ankylosis of the root is prevented from further eruption and thereby gradually comes more and more in to infraocclusion. In case of primary retention, the treatment of choice will normally be denudation of the tooth. In case of secondary retention, the tooth is ankylosed, and should be surgically removed. Finally, an eruption disturbance can be diagnosed to be a delayed eruption. In asymmetric cases where expected eruption time on one side is exceeded by more than 4 months, surgical exposure is indicated.

In Table 15-1 various causes for noneruption of permanent teeth are listed according to tooth type.

Local aberrations in primary dentition

Natal and neonatal tooth eruption

The frequency of natal or neonatal teeth is estimated at one case per 2000–3000 births and is equally common in boys and girls. Most of these premature erupting teeth are mandibular central incisors belonging to the normal dentition and they have a normal shape. The root has not yet developed and the tooth is loosely attached to the gingiva (Fig. 15-8). The symptoms related to natal/neonatal teeth include gingivitis, extreme mobility, self-mutilation of the tongue, and trauma to the mother's breasts. Natal and neonatal teeth should be extracted only if they are loose enough to involve risk of aspiration or if feeding is severely disturbed.

Symptoms associated with "teething"

Often, the primary teeth pierce the gums without causing any symptoms. However, in some children local symptoms such as redness and swelling in the oral mucosa overlying the erupting tooth is found. These symptoms appear a few days before clinical eruption. The child may also show signs of local irritation, drooling, and sometimes slight fever. Treatment for teething troubles was formerly directed at both local and supposed general symptoms. Since local massage of the gum pads obviously relieves the discomfort, various remedies with which the gums can be rubbed have been proposed. A bite-ring of rubber may be recommended because it is easy to clean, cannot be swallowed, and does not injure the gums.

Table 15-1 Most frequent causes of noneruption for various types of permanent teeth and suggested treatment

	Cause	Treatment
Maxillary incisors	Dilaceration (trauma)	Surgical exposure
	Supernumerary teeth	Surgical removal of supernumerary teeth
Maxillary canines, palatal impaction	Unknown	Surgical exposure and orthodontic traction
Maxillary canines, labial impaction	Crowding	Expansion of dental arch or removal
Mandibular canines, ectopic position	Unknown	Surgical removal or transplantation
Maxillary second premolar	Crowding	Expansion of dental arch or removal
Mandibular second premolar	Unknown	According to tilting extraction of primary molar, surgical exposure or transplantation
Maxillary first molar, mesial tilt	Unknown	None or distalization of first molar
Mandibular first molar, mesial tilt	Unknown	None or distalization of first molar
Maxillary first molar, infraocclusion	Ankylosis	Extraction
Mandibular first molar, infraocclusion	Ankylosis	Extraction
Second maxillary molar	Follicle collision with third molar	Remove third or second molar (usually third molar)
Second mandibular molar	Follicle collision with third molar	Remove third or second molar (usually third molar)

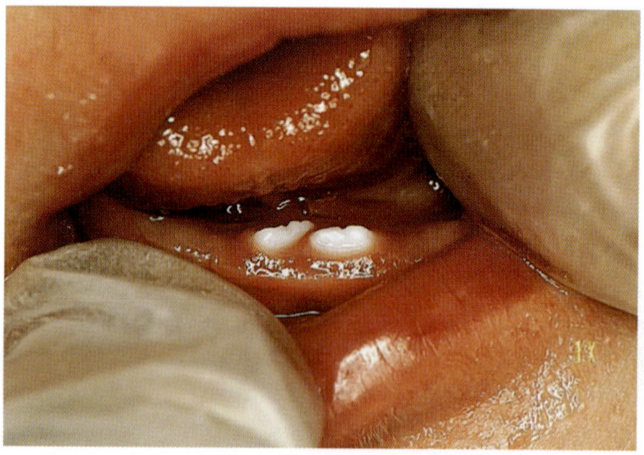

Figure 15-8 Natal teeth in a 2-day-old girl.

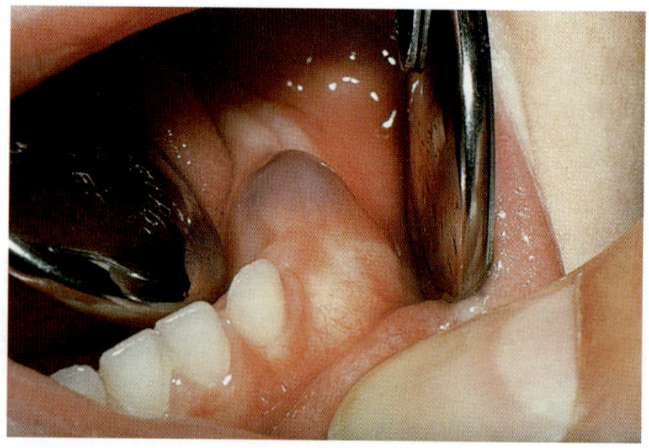

Figure 15-9 Fibrous gingival tissue delaying eruption of primary molars.

Fibrotic mucosa and eruption cysts

Changes in the oral mucosa overlying the erupting tooth may cause eruption disturbances. If the child is chewing intensively on hard objects, the alveolar mucosa may turn more fibrotic and cause delayed eruption (Fig. 15-9). In some cases surgical removal of the changed tissues might be necessary due to pain at chewing. A common finding in small children is eruption cysts. They are often swellings overlying an erupting tooth and may vary in size. They contain tissue fluid and sometimes some blood (eruption hematoma) accumulated superficially to the reduced enamel epithelium. In most cases no treatment is indicated since the changed mucosa will delay the eruption by only a few weeks. However, if the cyst is causing discomfort or the alveolar mucosa is pathologically thickened, surgical exposure of the tooth may be necessary. Similar changes are also found in the permanent dentition (Fig. 15-10).

Infraocclusion of primary molars

The definition of infraocclusion is that a tooth is positioned 1 mm or more below the normal occlusion plane/level. Infraoccluded primary molars mostly reach occlusal contact before they develop ankylosis. Following vertical growth of the surrounding alveolar bone, the ankylosed tooth seems to gradually be submerged into an infraoccluded position. The diagnosis of ankylosis is difficult to verify by radiography but easy to establish by percussion test and the clinical picture. Infraocclusion of primary molars can be found as early as 3–4 years of age

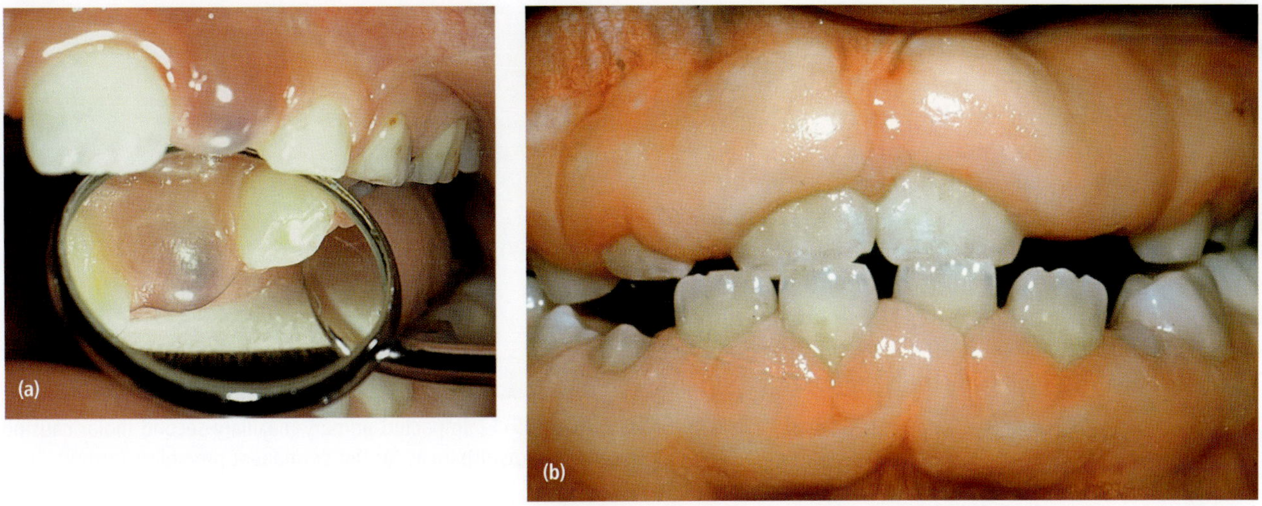

Figure 15-10 (a) Eruption cyst. (b) Gingival overgrowth caused by phenytoin medication influencing tooth eruption.

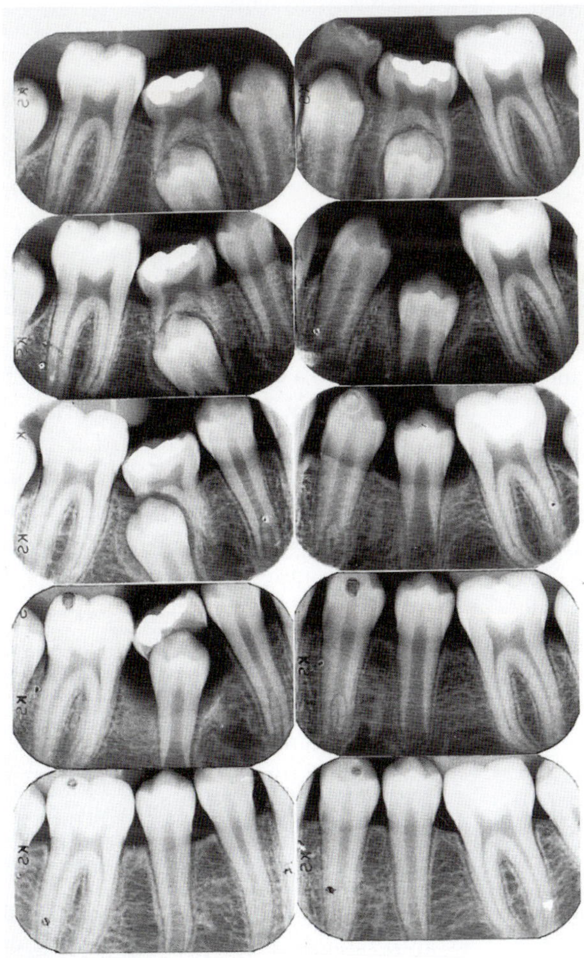

Figure 15-11 Infraocclusion of primary molars. Periapical radiographs of a boy followed from 11 years 7 months to 14 years 2 months of age. Left side, extraction side. Extraction resulted in the eruption 1 year earlier of the successor compared to the nonextraction side. Normal marginal alveolar bone height at end of observational period (J. Kurol, Thesis, 1984).

but is more predominant at 10 years of age; the aberration is then found in about 10% of the children. Infraocclusion has been found to be genetically influenced. The treatment depends on the presence of permanent successors to the infraoccluded tooth. If there is a permanent successor, normal exfoliation can be expected with a delay of 6–12 months (Fig. 15-11) without removal of the ankylosed tooth. If the neighboring permanent tooth is severely tilting over the ankylosed tooth, early orthodontic correction may be indicated. In cases with no successor, the therapy planning must be based on the conclusion that normal exfoliation cannot be expected.

Retention of primary teeth

The primary tooth that is most commonly involved is the maxillary second molar. The tooth anlage is malpositioned and often the roots bend and follow the wall of the sinus during development (Fig. 15-12). This means that spontaneous eruption cannot be expected. The impacted tooth can cause tilting of the permanent molar and disturbance in eruption of the permanent premolars. The impacted primary tooth has to be surgically removed. Also the primary second molar in mandible may become retained and thereby lead to severe eruption problems for the permanent successor.

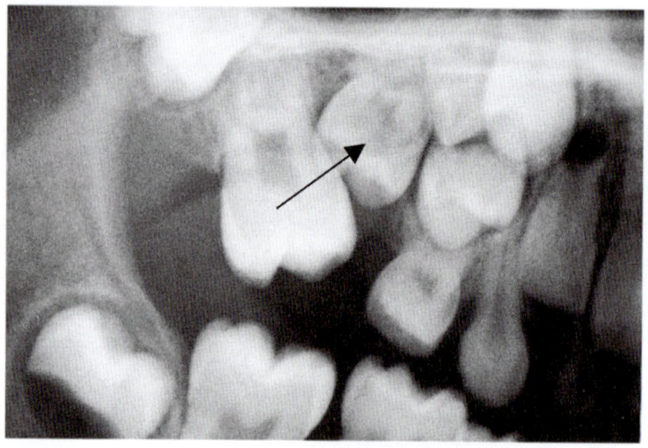

Figure 15-12 Impacted primary maxillary second molar causing eruption disturbances for the permanent premolars (arrow).

Local aberrations in permanent dentition

Disturbances in eruption are common in the permanent dentition. Besides the normal variation in eruption time a number of genetic disorders, diseases, and syndromes can affect tooth eruption as has been described earlier in this chapter. However, the most frequent disturbances in tooth eruption in the permanent dentition are local in origin (Box 15-3).

Box 15-3 Common local disturbances in tooth eruption in permanent teeth

- Ectopic eruption position often in combination with lack of space:
  - maxillary first molar
  - maxillary canine
  - maxillary central incisor
  - second premolar.
- Malpositions.
- Sequelae to trauma.
- Supernumerary teeth, mesiodentes, odontomas.
- Ankylosis.
- Developmental disturbances.
- Cysts.

Ectopic eruption

In crowded arches the maxillary first molar may be impacted by the distal surface prominence of the primary second molar (Fig. 15-13). The primary molar will be resorbed at the distal root surface, the permanent molar gets stuck and the eruption stops. However, it has been reported that spontaneous correction occurs in about half of the cases. A reasonable observational period is therefore recommended before extraction of the primary tooth or orthodontic treatment is performed.

Ectopic eruption of maxillary canines occurs in about 2% of children. It has been reported that 12% of these ectopically erupting canines will cause different degrees of resorption of the root of adjacent incisors (Fig. 15-14). It is therefore important, as a matter of routine, always to palpate buccally and palatinally for the canine when the child is 9–10 years old. If the canine cannot be palpated buccally, a detailed radiographic examination has to be carried out to reveal any resorptions or risk for resorptions of neighboring teeth. The treatment in case of resorption will be to change the eruption direction of the canine. This can in most cases be achieved by extraction of the primary canine. In severe cases, orthodontic intervention is necessary, including surgical exposure of the canine and a fixed appliance to place the tooth in a proper eruption path (see also Chapter 16).

Ectopically, labial late eruption of maxillary central incisors can occur as a result of early trauma in the region, odontomas or supernumerary teeth. Due to positioning and root angulation they sometimes tend to erupt in the vestibulum mucosa. After surgical exposure the incisor often erupts unaided and will end up in the right position and with reinstituted mucosa (Fig. 15-15). In children with crowded arches it is common that the second premolar in the maxilla will be displaced and erupt palatinally (Fig. 15-16) while the mandibular second premolar has a tendency to be impacted in a central position in the jaw. The treatment in the maxilla is

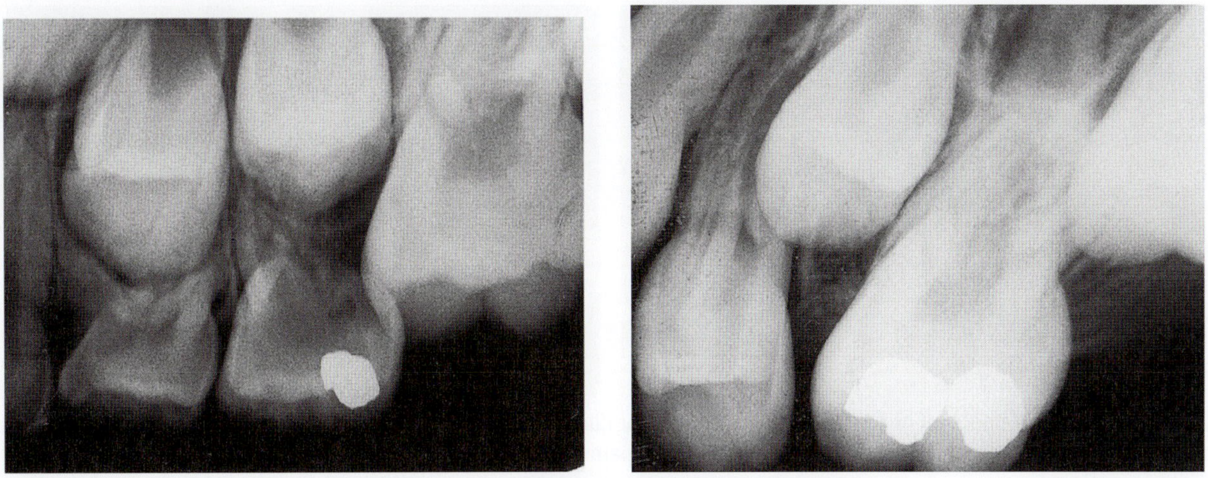

Figure 15-13 Retention of permanent maxillary first molar caused by the primary second molar. After extraction/exfoliation of the primary tooth, loss of space will often occur.

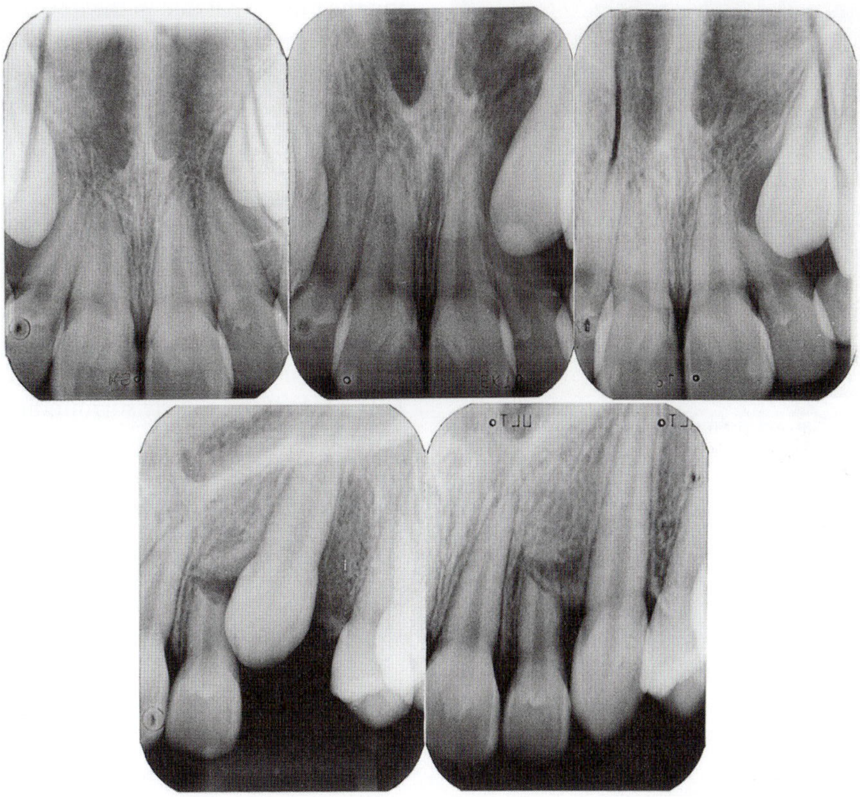

Figure 15-14 Ectopic eruption of left maxillary canine which has resorbed the root of the left maxillary lateral incisor. Extraction of the primary left maxillary canine result in a changed path of eruption of the permanent canine. The resorption stopped and a normal periodontal condition was established.

mainly extraction of the ectopically erupting tooth, while in the mandible the first premolar may often be extracted and the impacted second premolar will erupt. Alternatively, a persistent second primary molar should be extracted which in many cases will lead to eruption of the ectopic premolar.

Ectopic malpositions

In children with malposition of teeth, e.g., premolars or canines horizontally situated in the jaw, the most common treatment is surgical removal. However, if there is space enough, a surgical exposure can result in a spontaneous eruption in the occlusal line (Fig. 15-17).

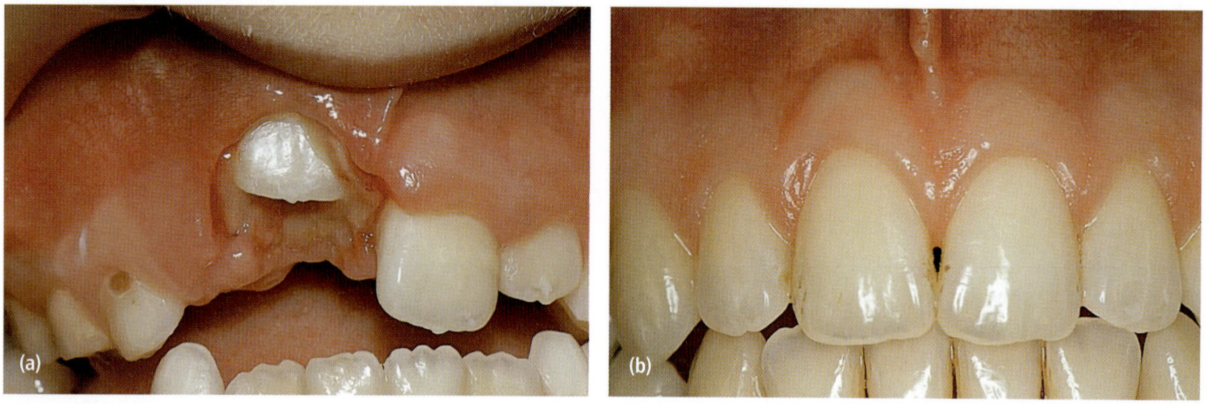

Figure 15-15 (a) Ectopic position of right maxillary central incisor due to a supernumerary tooth in the region causing root angulation and displacement of the central incisor. After removal of the supernumerary tooth and surgical exposure the central incisor erupted. (b) Eight years later.

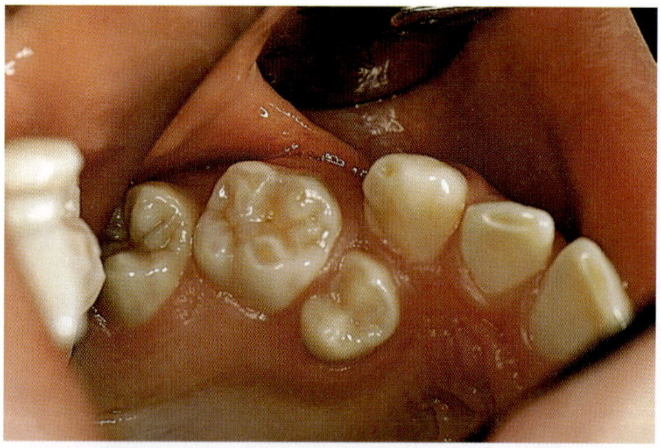

Figure 15-16 Maxillary second premolar erupting in the palate due to crowding.

Sometimes a malpositioned tooth may cause eruption disturbances of surrounding teeth. In children this can occur when a malpositioned third molar interferes with the eruption of the second molar (Fig. 15-18).

Sequelae to trauma

Traumatic injuries to the teeth involving intrusion of primary incisors may cause extensive damage of the developing permanent successor (see Chapters 18 and 19). The resulting dilaceration can cause severe disturbances in eruption. In approximately half of the cases there will be no eruption and the deformed tooth has either to be surgically removed or undergo a denudation procedure which will result in spontaneous eruption. Soon after this has occurred it is important to remove the dilacerated part of the crown and restore the tooth with composite. This will prevent bacteria from invading the pulp canal due to the invagination found in relation to the crown dilaceration. On the other hand, dilaceration might cause premature development and eruption (Fig. 15-19).

Supernumerary teeth, mesiodentes, and odontomas

Supernumerary teeth, mesiodentes, and odontomas constitute major reasons for disturbances in tooth eruption (Figs 15-20 and 15-21). However, it has to be understood that not all supernumerary teeth, mesiodentes, or odontomas will have an influence on eruption. Only if the follicle surrounding the tooth element is located in the eruption pathway will impaction (follicle collision) occur. Early diagnosis based on clinical and radiographic examinations is important to decide on the treatment and when it should be performed with an optimal result. In most cases the treatment involves surgical removal of the supernumerary teeth, mesiodentes, and odontomas.

Ankylosis

Infraocclusion and ankylosis of permanent *incisors* and *first molars* constitute a major clinical problem for the pediatric dentist. The ankylosis of incisors is often caused by traumatic injuries to the teeth and the treatment is discussed in Chapter 18. Diagnosis of ankylosis of a permanent molar is made following percussion test and the increasing infraposition of the tooth following growth (Fig. 15-22). A typical radiographic feature is an interradicular sign of ankylosis affecting the furcation area. Attempts to orthodontically extrude the ankylosed tooth will fail. The treatment of teeth with severe infraocclusion caused by ankylosis is surgical removal as soon as the diagnosis is made.

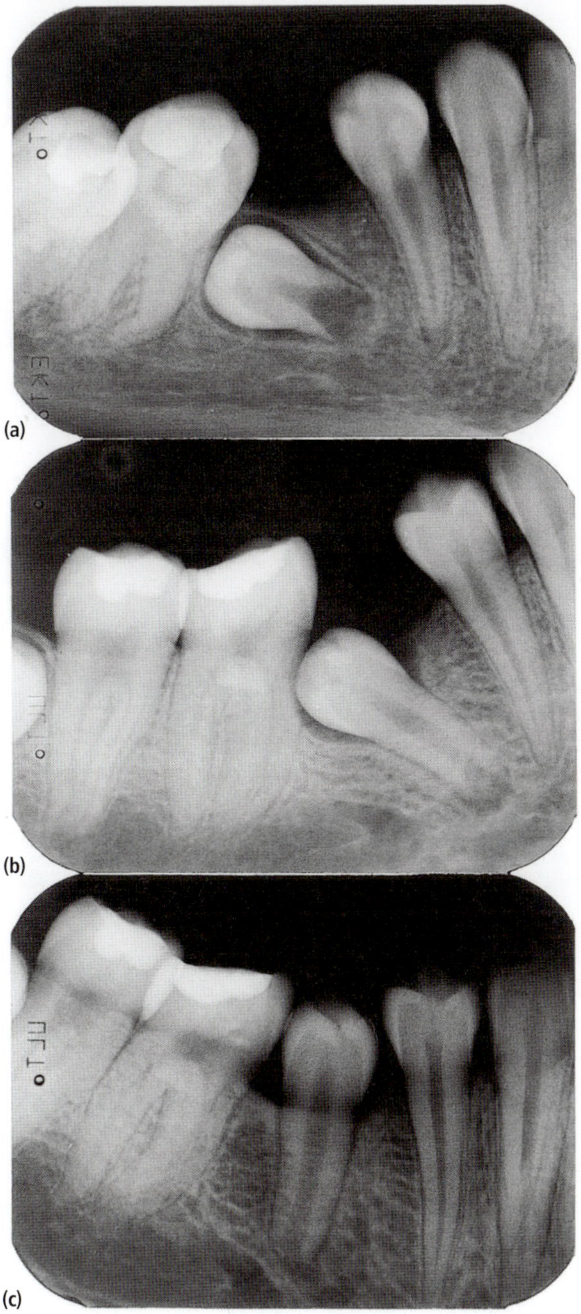

(a) (b) (c)

Figure 15-17 (a) Late development of impacted mandibular second premolar in a 14-year-old boy. (b) Two years later and after surgical exposure. (c) After another 2 years, spontaneous eruption and completed root development had occurred.

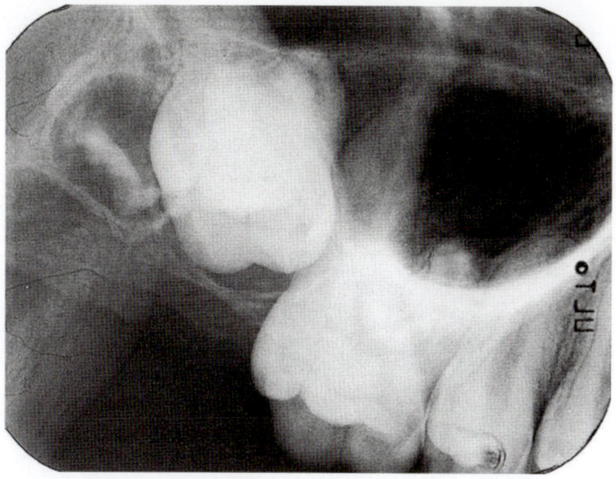

Figure 15-18 Ectopically positioned maxillary third molar disturbing eruption of the second molar in a 15-year-old boy. Observe the curved roots of the impacted tooth close to the sinus.

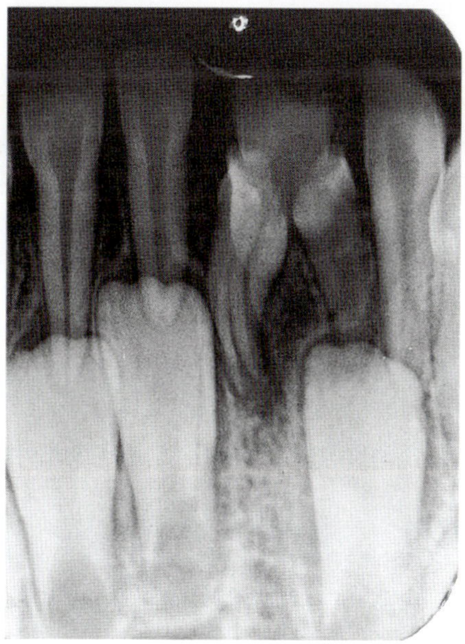

Figure 15-19 Premature development and eruption of a dilacerated mandibular central incisor caused by intrusive trauma against the primary incisors at the age of 1 year.

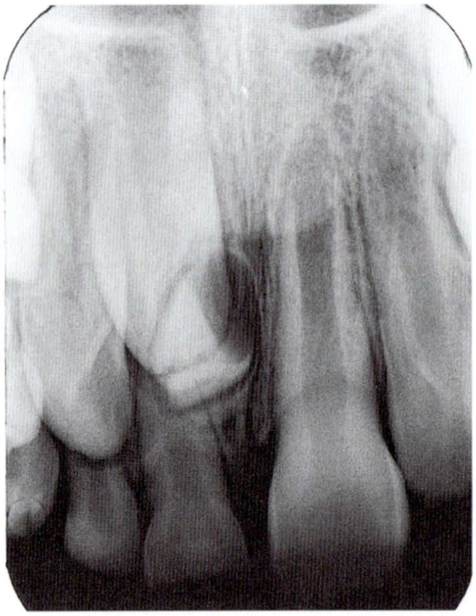

Figure 15-20 Mesiodens interfering with eruption of a central incisor in a 10-year-old boy.

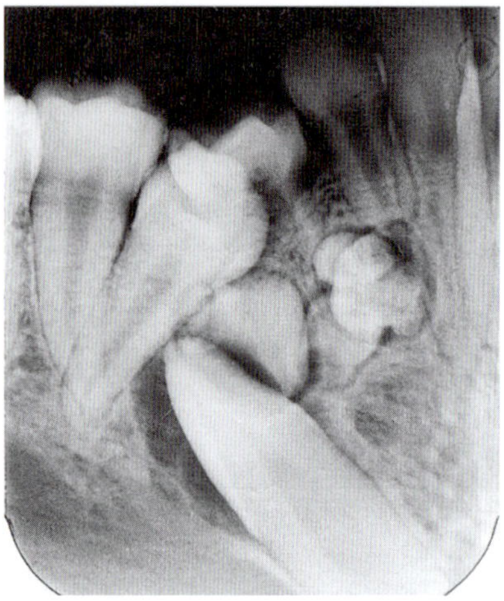

Figure 15-21 Odontoma interfering with eruption of a permanent mandibular canine.

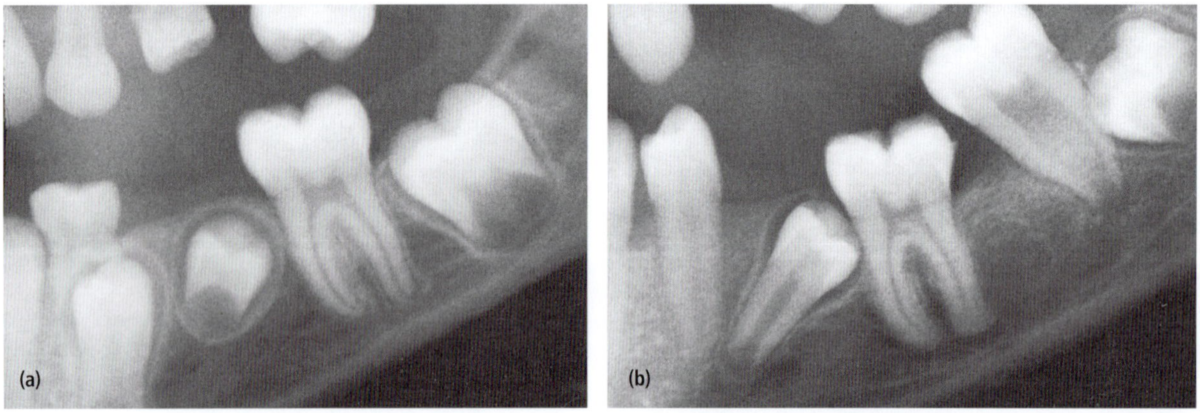

Figure 15-22 (a) An 8-year-old girl with history of several teeth in ankylosis. Percussion test revealed slight suspicion of ankylosis of permanent left mandibular first molar. (b) Four years later severe infraocclusion and ankylosis were verified.

Developmental disturbances

Tooth developmental disturbances such as morphologic aberrations and severe mineral disturbances can delay or inhibit the tooth eruption process possibly due to defects in the coronal follicle. In cases with, for example, local odontodysplasia ("ghost teeth") eruption will often not take place (Fig. 15-23).

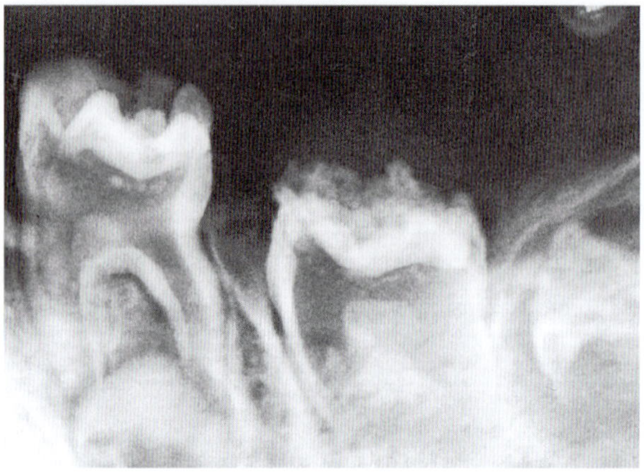

Figure 15-23 Odontodysplasia resulting in ceased eruption both in the primary and in the permanent dentition.

Background literature

Andreasen JO, Petersen JK, Laskin DM, eds. *Textbook and color atlas of tooth impactions.* Copenhagen: Munksgaard, 1997.

Gorlin, RJ, Cohen MM Jr, Levin LS. *Syndromes of the head and neck,* 3rd edn. New York: Oxford University Press, 1990.

Hall RK. *Pediatric orofacial medicine and pathology.* London: Chapman & Hall, 1994.

Kurol J. Infraocclusion of primary molars. Thesis. *Swed Dent J* 1984; Suppl 21.

References

1. Haavikko K. The formation and the alveolar and clinical eruption of the permanent teeth. *Suom Hammaasläk Toim* 1970;**66**: 103–70.
2. Helm S, Seidler B. Timing of permanent tooth emergence in Danish children. *Community Dent Oral Epidemiol* 1974;**2**:122–9.
3. Jensen BL, Kreiborg S. Development of the dentition in cleidocranial dysplasia. *J Oral Pathol Med* 1990;**19**:89–93.
4. Kreiborg S, Jensen BL, Larsen P, Schleidt DT, Darvann T. Anomalies of craniofacial skeleton and teeth in cleidocranial dysplasia. *J Craniofac Genet Dev Biol* 1999;**19**:75–9.
5. Kreiborg S. Syndromer med alvorlige dentitionsafvigelser. In: Hjørting-Hansen E, ed. *Odontologi '89.* Copenhagen: Munksgaard, 1989; 161–76.
6. Lysell L, Magnusson B, Thilander B. Time and order of eruption of the primary teeth. A longitudinal study. *Odontol Rev* 1962; **13**:217–34.
7. Marks SC, Schroeder HE. Tooth eruption: theories and facts. *Anat Rec* 1996;**245**:374–93.
8. Marks Sc, Svendsen H, Andreasen JO. Theories of tooth eruption in humans. In: Andreasen JO, Kølsen Petersen J, Laskin DM, eds. *Textbook and color atlas of tooth impactions.* Copenhagen: Munksgaard, 1997; 20–43.
9. Rune B, Sarnaes KV. Root resorption and submergence in retained deciduous second molars. *Eur J Orthod* 1984;**6**:123–31.
10. Suri L, Gagari E, Vastardis H. Delayed tooth eruption: pathogenesis, diagnosis, and treatment. A literature review. *Am J Orthod Dentofacial Orthop* 2004;**126**:432–5.
11. Østergaard RL, Kreiborg S, Niebuhr E. Trikodentoossøst syndrom. En oversigt og præsentation af et tilfælde. *Tandlægebladet* 1999;**103**:326–9.
12. Østergaard RL, Kreiborg S, Niebuhr E. Pycnodysostosis. En oversigt og præsentation af et tilfælde. *Tandlægebladet* 1999;**103**: 508–11.

16

Occlusal development, preventive, and interceptive orthodontics

Jüri Kurol and Bengt Mohlin

Dental occlusion, the interdigitation of maxillary and mandibular teeth, is dependent on developmental processes in three dimensions involving the cranial base, the jaws, and tooth eruption. The processes are strongly influenced by genetic as well as functional factors.

The main principles involved in the growth and development of the craniofacial skeleton are displacement and surface remodeling of bones. The mean growth at the various growth sites is indicated in Fig. 16-1. Since the maxilla is attached to the anterior cranial base, whereas the mandible is suspended under the middle cranial fossa, growth of the cranial base is of major importance for the intermaxillary relations and, thus, for the development of the occlusion. The maxilla is displaced downward and forward in relation to the anterior cranial base by growth and adaptation in the maxillary sutures. The sagittal relation between the jaws is maintained by marked growth of the mandible (Fig. 16-2).

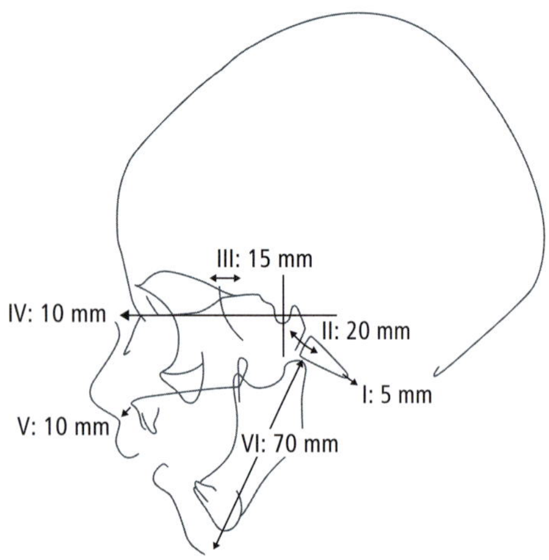

Figure 16-1 Average incremental growth (mm) of the cranial base and the jaws from birth to adult age. I: anterior margin of foramen magnum. II: spheno-occipital synchondrosis. III: spheno-frontal suture. IV: glabella. V: maxillary sutural displacement. VI: mandibular growth.

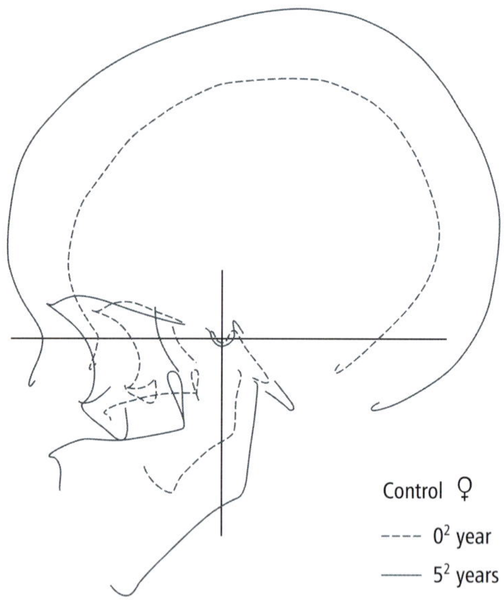

Figure 16-2 Facial growth in a normal girl from 2 months to 5 years 2 months of age. Superimposition was made on the nasion-sella line registered at sella. Note the magnitude of mandibular growth from a marked retruded position.

The transverse growth of the cranial base is characterized by lateral displacement of the temporal bones and thereby by the glenoid fossae.

Within the framework of this complex facial development, the erupting teeth come into interdigitation. However, individual variability in growth of the cranial base and the jaws is wide and the coordination of development in the various components is not always perfect. This is partly compensated for by dentoalveolar mechanisms that serve to bring the dental arches into a normal relationship.

The dentoalveolar compensatory mechanisms are dependent on normal oral function and normal tooth eruption. The space conditions in the dental arches and the function during occlusion and mastication are also important factors.

Occlusal development of the primary dentition

At birth the crowns of the primary teeth to a great extent have been formed, but root development has not yet started (see Chapter 14). Thus, the gum pads are low and the palatal vault is flat. When the jaws are closed there is normally contact only in the posterior region of the gum pads, and the mandible is retruded in relation to the maxilla. During the first year of life, however, the sagittal jaw relationship improves, allowing the incisors to erupt in a normal sagittal relation.

Occlusion in the posterior segments is first established around 16 months of age, when the primary first molars come into occlusal contact. Once a good intercuspidation in all three planes is achieved, the jaws are normally closed to the same position each time and normal development occurs. The established occlusion has a guiding role in the interrelation between the jaws and thereby for the proper positioning of later erupting permanent teeth (canines and second molars). Further stabilization of the occlusion is achieved by the occlusion of the large mesiopalatal cusps of the maxillary second molars.

With the eruption of primary teeth the alveolar processes develop, and there is a considerable increase in facial height (Fig. 16-3). The growth of the maxillary alveolar process also results in an increase in palatal height. The primary teeth erupt almost perpendicular to the jaw bases. The interincisal angle is approaching 180°, and the occlusal plane is flat. During development, the dentoalveolar segments generally move anteriorly in relation to basal structures of the jaws.

The primary dentition is characterized by half-circular dental arches. The most conspicuous feature is the space surplus in the front region of both jaws, needed later to accommodate the broader permanent front teeth. Especially marked diastemata are often found between the lateral incisors and the canines in the maxilla and the canines and first molars in the mandible. These diastemata are referred to as "primate spaces". The primary second molars erupt without proximal contact with the primary first molars. However, in most children these molars drift into proximal contact between the third and fourth years of life.

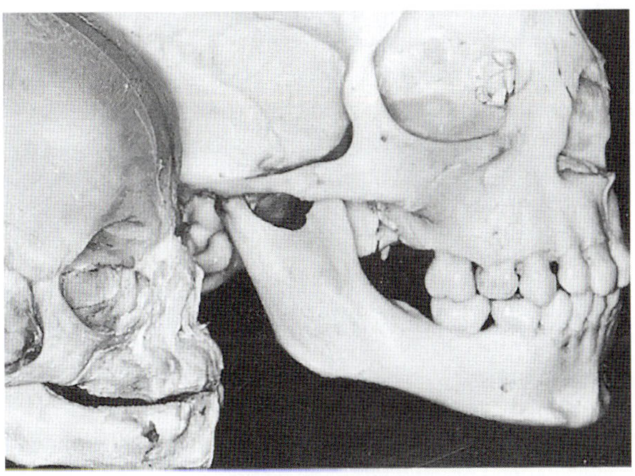

Figure 16-3 The eruption of primary teeth is accompanied by the development of the alveolar processes with considerable increase in facial height (from birth to 3 years of age).

As to the basal relationships of the jaws, young children differ from older children and adults by being more maxillary prognate and mandibular retrognate. At 2 years, the overjet is on average 4 mm, with a range of 2–6 mm. With attrition of the teeth and growth of the mandible, the overjet shows a steady decrease up to the age of 5 years, where an edge-to-edge incisor relationship is common.

The primary incisors generally erupt into a rather deep overbite if there is no obstacle to hinder them. The individual variation is, however, wide. On average, the overbite decreases up to the age of 5–6 years as an effect of attrition.

The molar relations in the primary dentition may be divided into two types:

- the primary dental arches end in a mesial step, i.e., the distal surface of the second molar in the mandible is mesial to the corresponding surface in the maxilla (Fig. 16-4, left)
- the dental arches end in the same vertical plan (Fig. 16-4, right).

Both situations are favorable for the later guidance of the permanent first molar into normal occlusion. It should, however, be noted that the occlusion undergoes dynamic changes with jaw growth, with dental attrition, mesial drift of the dental arches on the jaw bases, and increased sagittal mandibular growth (Fig. 16-2). At the time of eruption of the permanent first molar, a mesial step between the dental arches as shown in Fig. 16-4 left, is the most favorable.

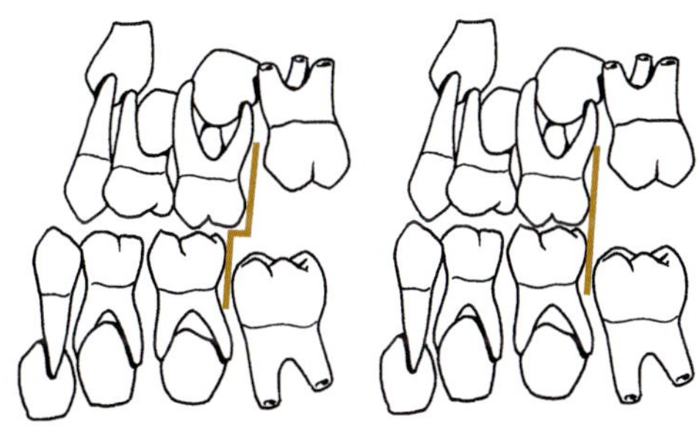

Figure 16-4 With a mesial step in the terminal plane of the primary dentition, the permanent molars may erupt directly into normal occlusion (left). If the primary dental arches end in the same vertical plane, the permanent molars will erupt into a cusp-to-cusp relation (right).

Malocclusions in the primary dentition

The role of the primary dentition for the establishment of permanent occlusion is well documented. The significance of the primary teeth as "space maintainers" for the permanent teeth is evident, especially after early loss of the primary second molars because of caries or ectopic eruption of permanent first molars. However, the primary dentition also has its own malocclusions, which, if untreated, may be transferred to the permanent dentition. Some of the malocclusions, especially anterior and posterior functional cross bites and scissor bites, have the additional disadvantage that they may influence facial growth and occlusal development if left untreated. Anterior functional cross bites may interfere with the expected lengthening of the upper dental arch, thus possibly causing a decrease of space for the permanent teeth. Functional lateral cross bites may be an obstacle for the transversal development of the upper dental arch. This may contribute to a space deficiency. As well as that, a higher temporal muscle activity has been recorded on the cross bite side also indicating a displaced mandibular position at rest. This displacement may contribute to an asymmetrical craniofacial and occlusal development. However, evidence in this area is still insufficient. If treatment of malocclusion is considered in the primary dentition, the patient's need for further treatment in the permanent dentition as well as the cooperation of the patient and parents has to be taken into consideration.

Etiology of malocclusion in the primary dentition

The genetic factors determining the size and position of the jaws are present from conception. Therefore, many of the genetically determined skeletal deviations manifest themselves in the primary dentition. This is especially true for Angle Class II and III, but also for deviations in the transversal dimension, which later are seen as posterior cross bite and scissors bite.

Functional factors such as chewing habits and the chewing resistance of the diet probably play a role in the development of malocclusions. This is based on observations of skull materials, people living with primitive feeding habits, and on animal experiments with a soft and a hard diet. The evidence is, however, still limited (6,17). Breathing habits play a role for facial growth and dental arch morphology. A study has been presented where 21 children aged 3–9 years were tonsillectomized because of sleep apnea. Of 13 open bites (63% of the children) 11 normalized, and of six lateral cross bites (29% of the children) three normalized at recall 2 years later (5). It should be remembered, however, that a large proportion of open bites spontaneously correct themselves (13,16).

Habits, mostly dummy and finger sucking, still rank high as etiologic factors for the development of malocclusions in the primary dentition (9) (Box 16-1, Figs 16-5 and 16-6).

Prevalence of malocclusions in the primary dentition

Malocclusions may be divided into four main groups (Box 16-2):

- deviations in available space
- deviations in the vertical plane
- deviations in the sagittal plane
- deviations in the transversal plane.

Box 16-1 Sucking habits and their influence on the primary dentition

- Dummy sucking is much more prevalent in Scandinavian children than finger sucking. Sucking habits vary a lot between different ethnic groups. In developing countries sucking habits in children are less common. The sucking habit is more prevalent in urban than in rural areas, and in girls than in boys according to Scandinavian studies (12).
- Dummy sucking often leads to posterior cross bite and open bite, and less often to overjet (Fig. 16-5). Finger sucking more often leads to overjet and proclination of the maxillary front, and more seldom to posterior cross bite (Fig. 16-6).
- The mechanism behind the development of cross bite caused by dummy sucking is the narrowing of the maxilla by frontal pressure, also believed to be caused by the lowering of the tongue, negative pressure in the mouth, and increased muscular pressure from cheeks and lips, in the canine region. The effect is especially great if the maxilla has in addition has a genetically conditioned narrow pattern.
- The benefit of the dummy sucking compared to finger sucking is that the children are weaned from the dummy sucking at an earlier age than from the finger sucking, usually by the age of 3–4 years, and very few proceed with the habit into the mixed dentition. A limited number of finger suckers (about 10%) continue with the habit into the mixed dentition period.
- After the dummy sucking habit has ceased in the primary dentition there will be a high grade of self-correction of the open bite created by the habit. However, the possibilities for self-correction of the posterior cross bite will depend on how large the discrepancy in width of the maxilla and mandible is, and how locked the intercuspidation is.

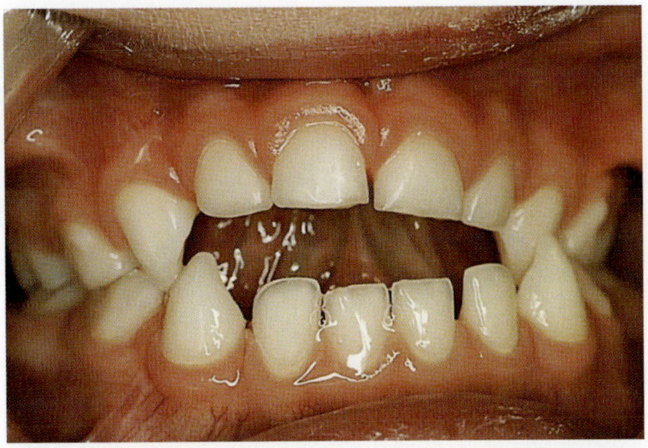

Figure 16-5 Posterior cross bite (patient's left side), midline deviation and mandibular lateral shift, and frontal open bite in a dummy sucker.

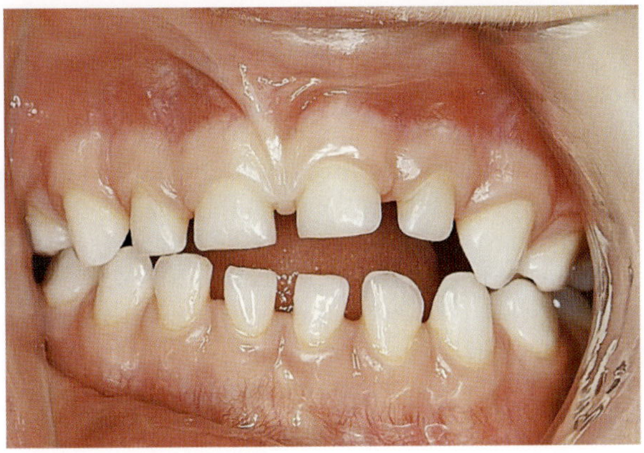

Figure 16-6 Results of finger sucking. Asymmetrical left side open bite and overjet.

Box 16-2 Prevalence of malocclusions in the primary dentition (%)

	Boys	Girls
Space conditions		
Crowding in the maxilla	1.5	2.9
Crowding in the mandible	0.5	1.9
Spacing in the maxilla	51.0	43.3
Spacing in the mandible	41.9	39.9
Vertical malocclusions		
Frontal open bite >0 mm	21.8	23.9
Frontal deep bite >3 mm	18.1	18.9
Frontal deep bite >5 mm	3.6	2.0
Sagittal malocclusions		
Maxillary overjet	35.8	23.9
Maxillary overjet >6 mm	11.9	11.9
Distal molar relations	49.5	49.0
Negative overjet >0 mm[a]	0	0
Mesial molar relations	1.0	0.5
Transversal malocclusions		
Posterior cross bites	10.6	17.3
Scissors bite[a]	0	0.5

[a] Cases not recorded in these investigations.

Space conditions

Space conditions (Box 16-2) have a somewhat different meaning in the primary dentition than in the permanent dentition. As the spacing of the front teeth in the primary dentition is a natural anatomical feature, small spaces or crowding will indicate that crowding also may appear in the permanent dentition. Crowding with rotated and displaced teeth occurs most often in the permanent mandibular front, but is seldom seen in the primary dentition.

Lack of space as such should not be treated in the primary dentition but should be a reminder to monitor the eruption of the permanent incisors carefully. With no or little spacing, the permanent central incisors will most often resorb both primary central and lateral incisors during eruption, thus shifting the lack of space further distally in the dental arch.

Malocclusion in the vertical plane

Malocclusions in the vertical plane (Box 16-2) do not constitute a large problem in the primary dentition. There is a high prevalence of frontal open bite, but it is nearly always dentoalveolar, and often the result of sucking habits. It will most often close when the sucking habit ceases (12). There is also a high prevalence of moderate deep bite, but this has little practical significance unless combined with forced cross bites. Severe deep bite is often combined with overjet and distal occlusion or sometimes scissors bite in lateral segments (Fig. 16-7) and will be corrected if these malocclusions are to be treated.

Malocclusions in the sagittal plane

Malocclusions in the sagittal plane (Box 16-2) are usually or traditionally measured as deviations in molar relationships and/or size of overjet/negative overjet. However, in the primary dentition we will often find that

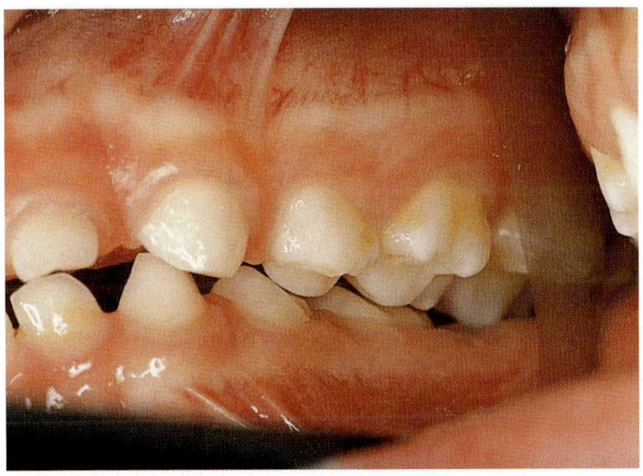

Figure 16-7 Unilateral scissors bite in the primary dentition.

molar relationships do not give any exact expression for future relations of either jaws or dental arches. Thus, it is more valid to use the canine relations when judging the sagittal relationships in the primary dentition.

Distal molar

Distal molar relations in combination with large overjet is prevalent (19). In the primary dentition this will be a small problem, but very often this malocclusion will also appear in the permanent dentition. Only in extreme cases where the mandible is held in a distal position, as with a scissors bite or very deep bite, will treatment in the primary dentition be indicated (Fig. 16-8).

Mesial molar

Mesial molar relations (Angle Class III) with or without negative overjet have a very low prevalence. Negative overjet may exist in neutral molar relation, and we may have mesial molar relation without negative overjet. The malocclusions are divided into three main groups. In reality, most cases present a mixture of skeletal and dentoalveolar deviations:

- skeletal
- dentoalveolar
- functional (forced bite).

In skeletal class III malocclusions, the size of the maxilla and mandible and/or their positions are disproportional. This may occur in three combinations (Fig. 16-9):

- the maxilla is small and/or distally placed
- the mandible is large and/or mesially placed
- a combination of these.

Whether there will be a normal overjet in the front, an edge-to-edge bite, or a negative overjet will depend on the dental compensation, which is the degree of labial inclination of incisors in the maxilla and the lingual inclination of the incisors in the mandible.

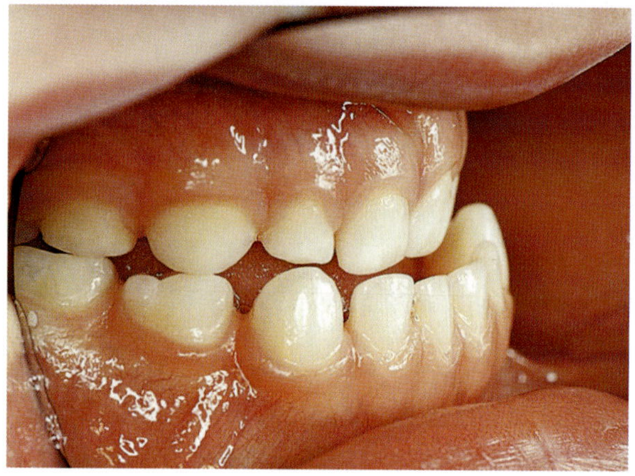

Figure 16-9 Skeletal class III without compensation. Note mesial relations between canines.

In cases of dentoalveolar negative overjet there may be a normal relation between the dental arches (best judged at the canines), and the negative overjet is then due to lingual inclination of incisors in the maxilla and labial inclination of incisors in the mandible (Fig. 16-10).

With forced negative overjet the patient can often bite edge to edge in the retruded contact position of the mandible, but slides forward into negative overjet (pseudo Class III) for full occlusion.

Treatment

The treatment needed for Class III occlusions and anterior cross bite will depend on the severity of the malocclusion and to what extent it causes dissatisfaction for the patient. In cases of skeletal Class III it was a common procedure in the past to use chin caps to try to restrict the growth of the mandible. The opinion now is that it is questionable whether this effect can be obtained. Furthermore, the strong and long-lasting pressure against the chin may also have adverse effects on the temporomandibular joints. If the basal malocclusion is caused by

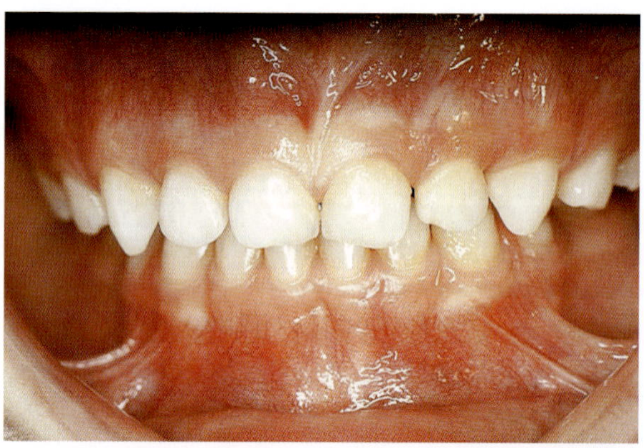

Figure 16-8 Bilateral scissors bite in combination with forced distal occlusion.

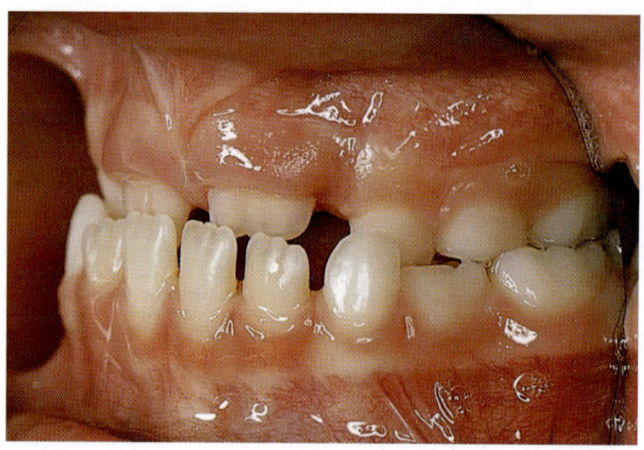

Figure 16-10 Dentoalveolar anterior cross bite. Neutral relations between canines. No forced anterior bite.

maxillary retrognathia, anterior protraction of the maxilla by means of a reversed headgear, i.e., Delaire mask, is a better solution. The mask may be used in the primary dentition, but since good cooperation is needed, the treatment may better be postponed until the early mixed dentition. One of the major reasons to treat is to create a dental compensation in order to reduce the influence of a deviant growth pattern. The evidence for good long-lasting effects of such treatment is still insufficient. However, the effect of the reversed headgear may be positive in cleft lip and palate patients.

The dentoalveolar anterior cross bites can usually be left untreated in the primary dentition unless they are forced. The main aim of treatment is to remove obstacles for the lengthening of the maxillary dental arch that occurs when the permanent incisors erupt. Treatment can be performed when the child is motivated and cooperative, normally at 5 years of age. The maxillary incisors will then be in position before eruption of the permanent incisors, which otherwise may erupt into anterior cross bite. Treatment alternatives will be grinding or a frontal expansion plate. Grinding should only be performed if the bite is not too deep. The grinding will "move" the incisal edges of the maxillary incisors labially and the mandibular incisors lingually (Fig. 16-11). The frontal expansion plate should be used if the bite is too deep for grinding (Fig. 16-12).

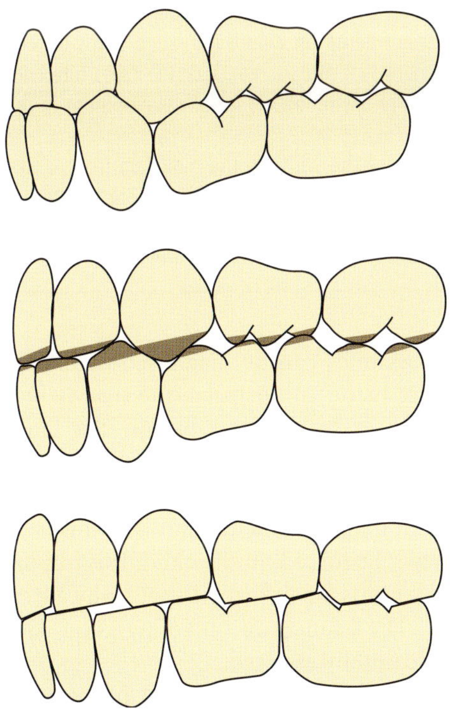

Figure 16-11 Grinding technique in forced anterior cross bite. The inclined plane is 45°, which brings the maxillary incisal edges into the frontal and the mandibular incisal edges into the distal direction.

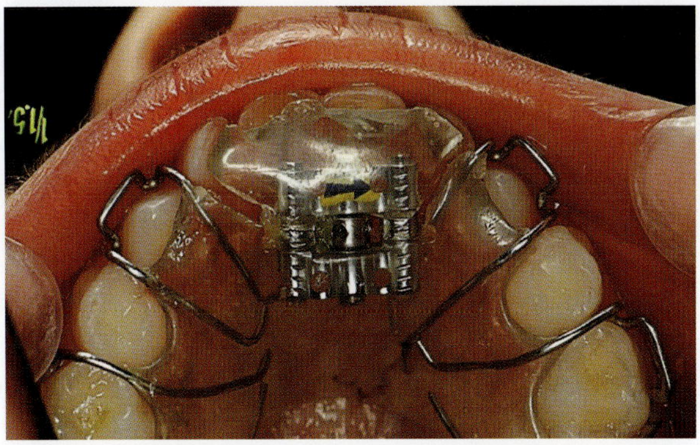

Figure 16-12 Removable appliance for frontal expansion of the maxillary front.

Malocclusions in the transversal plane

Malocclusions in the transversal plane (Box 16-2) are dominated by the unilateral forced posterior cross bites; the prevalence is between 10 and 23% (8). The large range is due to differences in the populations studied, in prevalence of dummy sucking, but also in differences in diagnostic technique. The prevalence of bilateral cross bite and scissors bite seems to be below 1%.

Definitions and diagnosis of posterior cross bites

The unilateral forced cross bite is characterized by a narrow, but symmetrical maxilla (Fig. 16-13a). In the retruded contact position, the molars will meet cusp to cusp. To find a stable occlusion, the mandible has to slide to one of the sides, creating a unilateral forced cross bite (Fig. 16-13b). The cusps on the cross bite side are often deeply locked into each other, and with little

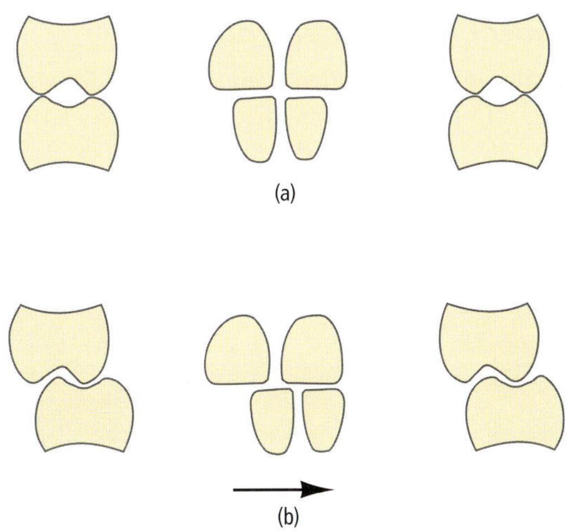

Figure 16-13 Forced posterior cross bite. The jaws are symmetrical, but the maxillary jaw is narrow. In the retruded position, the molars occlude cusp-to-cusp (a). Full occlusion needs forcing of the bite to the left (b).

chance of self-correction (full cross bite) (Fig. 16-14). In some patients the maxilla is wider, and the teeth on the cross bite side will meet cusp-to-cusp (half cross bite). If the maxilla is very narrow, a bilateral cross bite may be the result. These occlusions are normally not forced and occlude without midline deviation. A bilateral cross bite may be associated with an Angle Class III relation.

Cross bites normally establish at eruption of the primary canines and primary second molars. Thus, they may be diagnosed at about 3 years of age. It is important to decide whether the cross bite should be treated in the primary dentition, whether it could be expected to self-correct or whether treatment can be postponed until the early mixed dentition (Box 16-3).

Box 16-3 Posterior cross bite decisions

- Check for deviation between the retruded contact position and the intercuspal position.
- Check if there are obstacles towards increase in transversal width in the canine area.
- Check if an asymmetric occlusal and or craniofacial development can be expected.

Clinically:

- Check the retruded contact position for any midline deviation between this position and intercuspal position.
- Check if there are any primary contacts in RCP usually found between primary canines.
- Decide if grinding is appropriate or if transversal expansion should be preferred.
- Decide about the proper time for grinding and/or expansion.

Treatment need and cost-benefit for treatment of posterior cross bites

Treatment need and cost-benefit of treatment of posterior cross bites in the primary dentition have been discussed in several reports because some cross bites will self-correct, some treated cross bites will relapse, and some cross bites are combined with other malocclusions and thus their treatment may be postponed until a complete treatment later (Box 16-4). The economic aspects of early treatment have also been discussed (4). Two major reasons for correction of posterior cross bites have been stated. The first is that the cross bite (functional and nonfunctional) may be an obstacle to the expected gain in transversal width until eruption of the upper canines. This may contribute to a space deficiency at a later stage for the maxillary teeth. The second reason is a risk for asymmetrical craniofacial growth and occlusal development. The scientific evidence for both these treatment reasons is still insufficient.

Box 16-4 Arguments for early treatment of forced unilateral posterior cross bites

- Can probably prevent the asymmetric facial growth with the change of position of the glenoid fossa.
- May prevent unilateral chewing and marginally decrease the risk for temporomandibular disorders.
- May decrease the risk to establish an atypical neuromuscular movement pattern.
- Will prevent the cross bite from being transferred to the permanent dentition where the steep cusps of the permanent first molars may lock the cross bite even more.
- May hinder asymmetrical facial development in the frontal plane.
- Will increase the width in the maxillary front, and thus also improve the space condition before eruption of the wider permanent incisors.
- May prevent traumatic biting of the cheeks and tongue.

Treatment of posterior cross bites

In the literature it has often been stated that forced cross bites should be treated "as early as possible". However, even if cross bites can be diagnosed before the age of 3 years, it is better to postpone the treatment until the child reaches at least 5 years of age. The child should have stopped sucking habits before treatment of the cross bite. Also, it is important that child and parents are motivated for the treatment. An orthodontic treatment should never be forced on the child. It is important that child and parents are informed about why a treatment is beneficial. The chances of obtaining good cooperation should be carefully assessed.

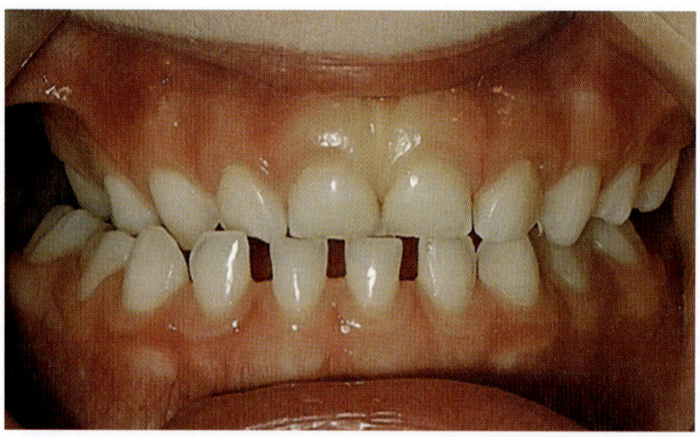

Figure 16-14 "Classical" unilateral posterior cross bite. Narrow maxilla with the mandibular midline forced to the cross bite side. Note lack of space in the maxilla.

The first and simplest treatment of forced posterior cross bite is grinding therapy (8). This is a good solution in cases where the intercuspidation is not too locked. The grinding does not solve the basic problem, the narrow maxilla, but it removes the early tooth contacts which

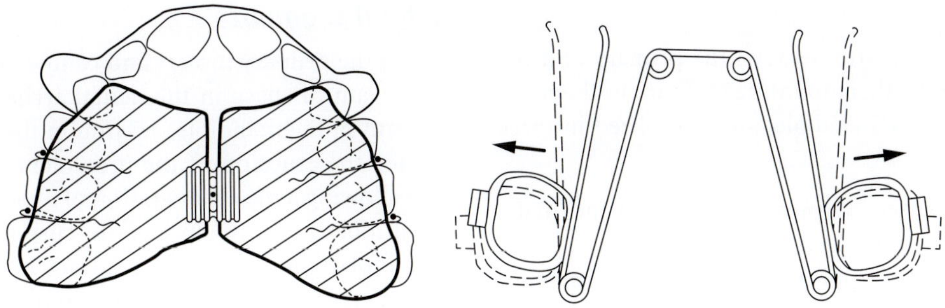

Figure 16-15 The most commonly used appliances for transversal expansion of the maxilla: the removable plate with an expansion screw and the Quad Helix appliance.

lead the mandible into the forced position. The grinding technique "moves" the cusps buccally in the maxilla, and lingually in the mandible. Usually, the occlusal interferences are most pronounced for the primary canines. The grinding is performed with continuous checks of the retruded contact position.

If expansion appliances are preferred, a removable plate with palatal screw or Coffin coil may be used. Another useful appliance requiring less strict cooperation is the Quad Helix lingual arch which is often used today (Fig. 16-15). The plate has to be worn at all times, except during meals and toothbrushing. The expansion may be about 5 mm, and if 0.5 mm (half a turn) is activated each week, the cross bite will be corrected in about 10 weeks. After the active expansion, the plate is used for retention for a couple of months.

There are different designs of Quad Helix appliances. In one type, the lingual arch is directly soldered to the bands. Another type has square palatal tubes, making activations outside the mouth possible. The orthodontic bands are cemented to the teeth, and thus the appliance does not require patient cooperation. Often, all the expansion may be done by the first activation. Thus, the Quad Helix requires fewer visits, and is therefore claimed to have a better cost-benefit than plates (4).

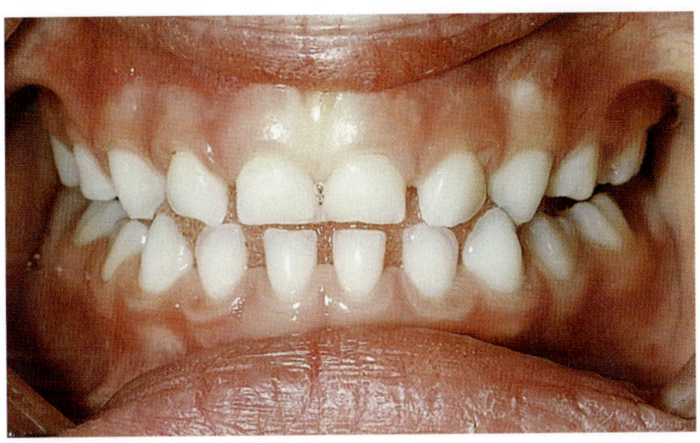

Figure 16-16 The same patient as in Fig. 16-14. Expansion was carried out by a removable plate. The width of the maxilla is satisfactory, but the occlusion is resting on premature contacts and grinding is needed. The midline is corrected and spaces are created in the maxilla.

After the expansion period, some adjustment and grinding of the teeth will be needed, especially on the canines. The cusps will not fit into occlusion, as the normal attrition has not occurred (Fig. 16-16).

The neuromuscular pattern for lateral guiding of the mandible may persist. If so, the child has to learn by self-training in front of a mirror how to guide the mandibular midline into alignment with the maxillary midline. The treatment time with a Quad Helix is around 6 months followed by a retention period of equal length.

Occlusal development through the mixed to permanent dentition

The mixed dentition lasts from the eruption of permanent mandibular first incisors and first molars (about 6.5 years of age) until shedding of the last primary tooth (about 12 years of age) (see Chapter 15). The first molars erupt in contact with the primary second molars. Thus, the establishment of molar sagittal relation will depend of the type of "step" between the distal surfaces of the maxillary and mandibular primary molars (Fig. 16-4). The permanent first molars frequently establish a cusp-to-cusp relation. This relation normally turns into an Angle Class I after shedding of the primary second molars because of the greater leeway space in the mandible. In lateral segments the combined widths of the primary molars and canines are larger than the erupting successors and this extra space is called leeway space.

Sufficient space for the permanent molars is created by the sagittal growth of the jaws. Most important is the growth in the distal direction by apposition of bone on tuber in the maxilla and by the resorption at the anterior border of the mandibular ramus. Dental development and tooth eruption are not always coordinated in time with the growth of the jaws. Thus, the molars may erupt into an ectopic position.

Front teeth

The discrepancies in size between the primary and the permanent front teeth, amounting to 7 mm in the maxilla and 5 mm in the mandible, are neutralized in three ways:

- by utilizing space surplus (diastemata) normally present in the primary dentition
- by the proclined eruption path of the permanent incisors (Fig. 16-17), which may add about 5 mm to the arch perimeter
- by an transversal increase in intercanine distance, which may add about 3 mm to the arch.

Thus, the space for the permanent maxillary incisors is normally sufficient. However, in cases of insufficient diastemata between primary incisors, crowding may develop. In cases with anterior forced bite the proclination of the maxillary incisors is likely to be reduced. This may also contribute to development of crowding of the teeth. The mandibular incisors need less space (5 mm), but the diastemas are also smaller and the eruption path is steeper. Thus, a temporary crowding may exist until it is corrected by the increase in transversal width. However, lack of space at eruption of mandibular front teeth often occurs, and the amount of the spacing in the primary dentition is a good indicator for the prognosis of the accommodation of the front teeth later. Crowding is generally more pronounced in girls than in boys (18).

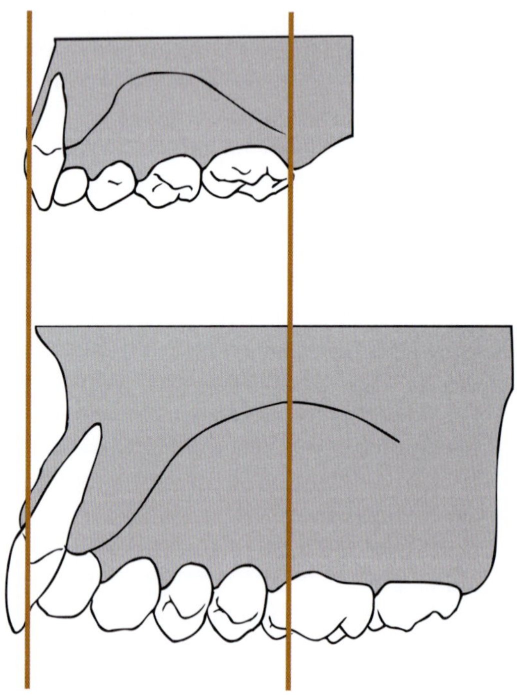

Figure 16-17 The permanent maxillary incisors erupt at a more labial inclination than their primary predecessors. Consequently, the dental arch becomes wider and longer.

Lateral segment

When the primary molars and canines are shed, there is a net gain of space in the dental arches (leeway spaces 2.5 mm in the mandible, 1.5 mm in the maxilla) available for the eruption of the premolars and canines and also allowing a mesial migration of especially the mandibular molars to turn any cusp-to-cusp relations between first molars into a neutral relation. In the maxilla, the leeway space is needed to accommodate the canines, which are 2 mm larger than their predecessors (Fig. 16-18). The increase in maxillary intercanine width in connection with eruption of the canines may also add some space. In the mandible, there is no corresponding gain in intercanine width related to canine eruption. The premolars will normally have sufficient space for eruption unless space is lost because of lack of space in the front, or because of early loss of primary molars due to caries or ectopic eruption of permanent first molars.

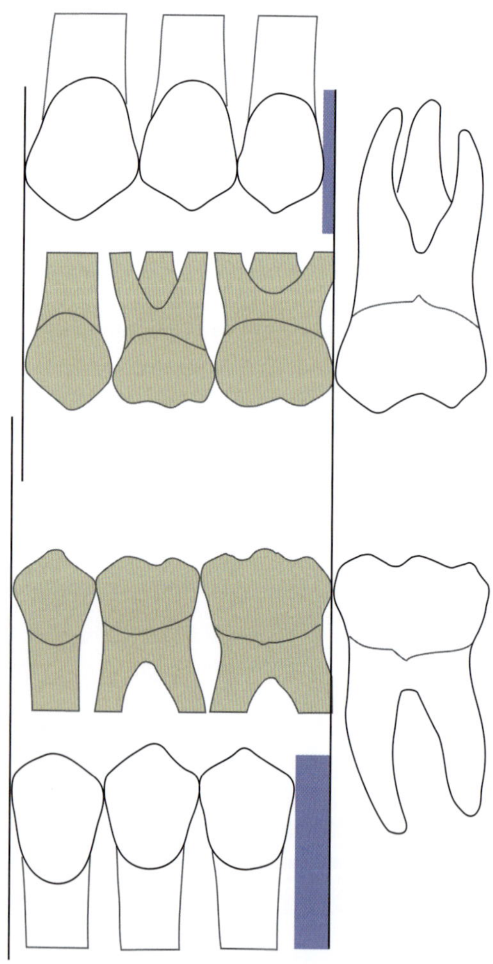

Figure 16-18 The primary canines and molars occupy more space than is necessary for the corresponding group of permanent teeth. The difference is called the "leeway space" and is greater in the mandible (2.5 mm) than in the maxilla (1.5 mm).

Even after completion of the permanent dentition (third molars excluded) dynamic changes continue in conjunction with the growth of the jaws and the alveolar processes. On average, the overjet decreases and the dental arches become shorter through mesial drift in the lateral segments, often resulting in a "physiological" crowding in the lower anterior front of an average of 0.5–1 mm from 12 to 20 years of age. The mean overbite decreases slightly up to the age of 18 years. The alveolar processes increase in height until late adolescence, more posteriorly than anteriorly. Clinical consequences of that growth will be that ankylosed teeth and implants will be left in an increasing infraposition. The transverse dimension of the dental arches, however, tends to remain relatively stable from the early permanent dentition.

Malocclusions in the mixed (and permanent) dentition

A large proportion of malocclusions in the primary dentition will, unless they are treated, persist in the permanent dentition. However, the most prevalent malocclusion in the primary dentition, the unilateral forced posterior cross bite, may self-correct in up to 45% of the cases (8) in the mixed dentition. The main groups of malocclusions in the permanent dentition and their prevalences are listed in Box 16-5.

Etiology of malocclusions

A malocclusion may develop as a result of genetic and/or environmental factors. The environmental factors may include oral habits (Box 16-1), reduced activity in jaw muscles, hypertrophic tonsils and adenoids, dental trauma, early loss of primary teeth, and severe chronic disease in childhood. However, dentoalveolar compensatory mechanisms may reduce the effects of aberrant jaw relations. A stable interdigitation between upper and lower teeth may preserve a normal relation between mandibular and maxillary teeth even in subjects with less favorable growth. In conclusion, the development of malocclusions will most often be caused by a non-functioning, incomplete, or impaired dentoalveolar compensatory mechanism rather than by the actual discrepancy in jaw relationships.

Box 16-5 Prevalence of malocclusions in the permanent dentition (%)

	Boys	Girls
Space conditions		
Crowding in the maxilla	20.6	26.3
Crowding in the mandible	33.0	31.7
Spacing in the maxilla	8.1	4.3
Spacing in the mandible	5.1	2.5
Vertical malocclusions		
Frontal open bite >0 mm	2.3	1.8
Frontal deep bite >5 mm	22.7	14.5
Sagittal malocclusions		
Maxillary overjet >6 mm	15.9	12.5
Distal molar occlusion	23.2	25.8
Mandibular overjet >0 mm	0.7	0.2
Mesial molar occlusion	4.1	4.5
Transversal malocclusion		
Posterior cross bite	9.4	14.1
Scissors bite	7.1	7.9

Sagittal malocclusion

An increased maxillary overjet may be the result of protrusion of the maxillary alveolar process, retrusion of the mandibular alveolar process, increased labial inclination of the maxillary incisors, lingual inclination of the mandibular incisors, protrusion of the maxilla and retrusion of the mandible (Fig. 16-19). Oral habits, especially finger sucking, may have an adverse effect on incisor inclination. Incompetent lip closure with the lower lip resting behind the maxillary incisors may also be associated to large overjet and further increase of the overjet. Mandibular prognathism is often genetically determined. Retrusion of the maxilla, occurring in some syndromes, may cause pseudomandibular prognathism. Mesial molar occlusion often occurs as a result of skeletal mandibular prognathism.

Distal molar occlusion may arise because of mesial migration of permanent maxillary molars due to early loss of primary second molars, inappropriate adjustment of the permanent first molars in the mixed dentition, retrusion of the mandible and protrusion of the maxilla. Mandibular retrusion is usually caused by genetic factors in otherwise healthy children.

Vertical malocclusion

Frontal open bite of dentoalveolar origin may be due to incomplete eruption of incisors or reduced vertical

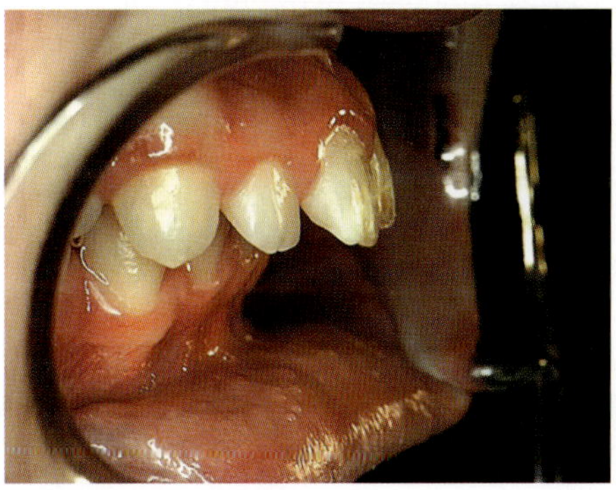

Figure 16-19 Maxillary overjet, incisor proclination, distal occlusion, and deep bite is a common combination.

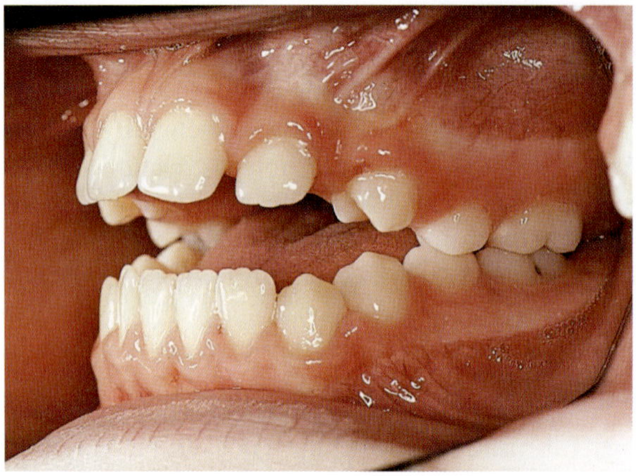

Figure 16-20 Dentoalveolar frontal open bite.

development of the anterior alveolar processes, usually due to a sucking habit (Fig. 16-20). Frontal open bite is common in the primary and the mixed dentition. In those ages, it is very often a transient phenomenon. A major contributing factor is an anterior tongue position at rest in order to allow the child to breathe normally. In this period, there is a discrepancy between tongue volume and available space in the oral cavity. The adenoids are often large. By reduction of adenoids and increased oral space due to growth a large proportion of these frontal open bites closes spontaneously. Skeletal open bite may be due to a posterior rotation of the mandible during growth.

Dentoalveolar deep bite may develop in cases with increased overjet. Excessive eruption of the incisors may occur when normal contact between maxillary and mandibular incisors is absent, for instance in Angle Class II.2 malocclusions with steep incisor inclination. Skeletal deep bite may develop if the mandible has an anterior rotation during growth. This is often associated with strong masticatory muscles.

Transversal malocclusion

Dentoalveolar cross bite or scissors bite of single teeth is often the result of crowding. Total forced unilateral posterior cross bite with mandibular midline deviation is often a consequence of a narrow maxilla (Fig. 16-21).

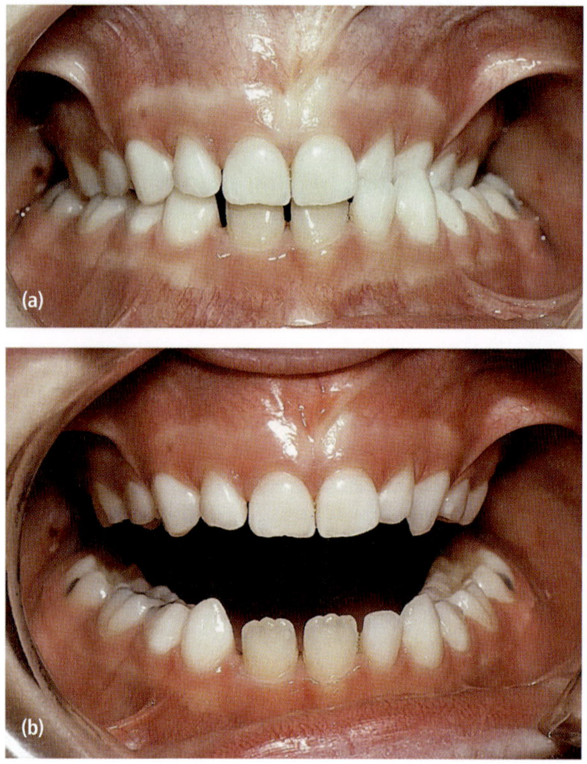

Figure 16-21 (a) Unilateral cross bite in the early mixed dentition. (b) Note the narrow maxilla in retruded position which needs active transversal expansion.

Skeletal unilateral cross bites or scissors bite may be associated with asymmetry in the cranial base, the maxilla or the mandible. Bilateral cross bite and scissors bite are rare types of malocclusion. They are most often of a skeletal origin and in many cases they are combined with deviations in the sagittal and vertical dimensions. Bilateral cross bite may, for instance, be associated with Angle Class III malocclusion.

Spacing anomalies

Crowding and spacing in the dentition depend on available space in the dental arches and mesiodistal diameter of the teeth (Fig. 16-22). Both size of jaws and size of teeth are strongly genetically influenced. Also, the minimal interproximal and occlusal dental wear in modern

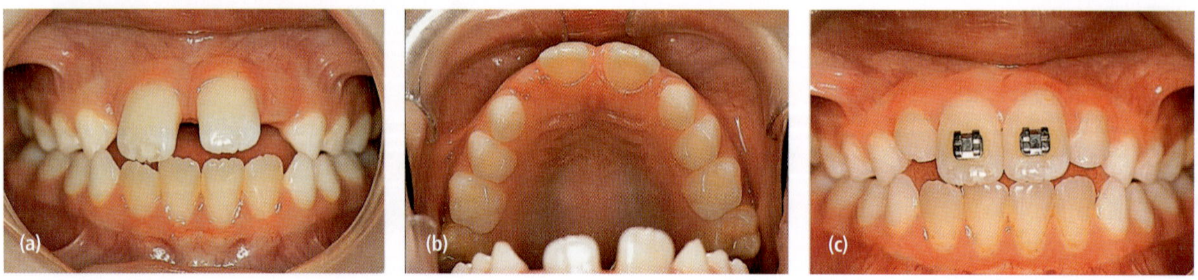

Figure 16-22 (a) Spacing in the maxillary front with a midline deviation to the right side. (b) If no treatment is given, the laterals will erupt in a frontal cross bite. (c) Early interceptive treatment results in normal eruption.

humans may partly explain the marked increase in occlusal anomalies. Observations from ancient skull materials, populations with primitive dietary habits, and from animal experiments using soft or hard diet, indicate an association between oral function and morphology. A high functional activity in jaw muscles changes mandibular morphology and contributes to more available space for the teeth. The prevalence of impacted wisdom teeth has been found to be much lower in skulls from earlier periods compared to modern populations (6,17). Early loss of primary teeth is also a cause of dentoalveolar crowding in the permanent dentition, depending on the region involved, the stage of occlusal development, the general space conditions in the dental arches, and the interdental locking, which may prevent tooth migration. Loss of second primary molars and primary canines seems to have the most negative consequences. Another effect of early loss of primary teeth may be delayed eruption of permanent successors.

The pediatric dentist's approach to orthodontic problems

The pedodontic approach to orthodontic problems is:

- to *prevent* the development of malocclusions
- to *intercept* malocclusions that have started to develop
- to *correct* malocclusions associated with increased risk for tooth damage, ectopic eruption or dysfunction
- to refer *extensive malocclusions* to specialists in orthodontics when treatment is indicated (11,16,22).

Prevention of malocclusions

As the major part of the etiologic factors are of genetic origin such malocclusions cannot be prevented to any large extent, and we have to focus on the environmental causative factors and eliminate them with preventive measures.

Loss of space

The loss of necessary space for the accommodation of the permanent teeth is still an important cause of malocclusions within Angle Class I. Every effort to maintain the mesiodistal dimension of the arches is important, first of all to reduce the need for early extraction of teeth, especially the "key teeth" – the primary second molars and canines. Thus, caries prevention and appropriate caries restoration are of the greatest importance for occlusal development. Space may occasionally be needed if primary molars are lost early. An important requirement for space maintainers is that they should not impair function, they should not interfere with alveolar growth or eruption of permanent teeth, and they should be cost-effective and not cause damage such as caries due to poorly fitted bands and loose appliances. A long-term orthodontic treatment plan should always precede the decision to use a space maintainer (Figs 16-23 and 16-24). In an individual with, for instance, general lack of space for the teeth to a degree that later extraction therapy is likely, the benefit of a space maintainer is very limited or none. Space maintainers are the most difficult to use where they are most needed.

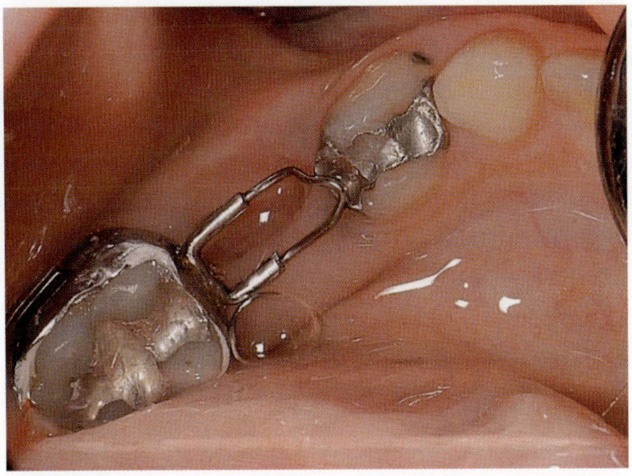

Figure 16-23 Gerber's space maintainer (band-tube-loop maintainer).

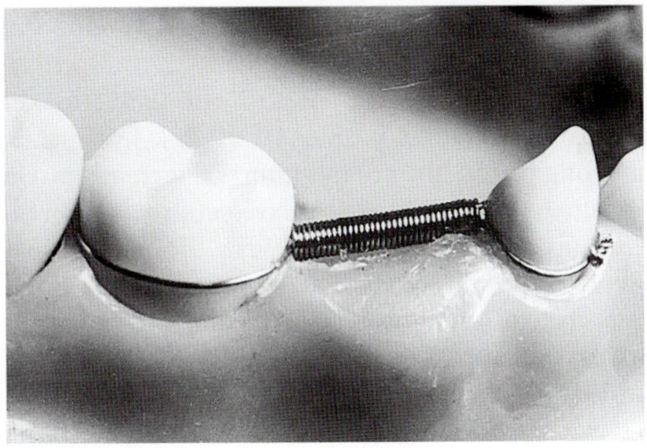

Figure 16-24 Sannerud's space maintainer.

Sucking habits

Sucking is believed to give rise to several malocclusions (Box 16-1) (12). It may be beneficial to break pacifier or finger sucking habits to prevent the development of a functional cross bite. Cross bites will often persist and will need active treatment. The treatment itself (removable plates, Quad Helix) will usually stop the habit. Before active treatment the child should be motivated and give consent for the habit breaking and have understood and accepted the procedure. A good question to ask the child is: "Do you want to stop the sucking habit?" A negative response usually means postponed treatment.

Another situation when breaking the habit is motivated is when it contributes to an increase of overjet and thus an increased risk for traumatic tooth injuries. Anterior open bite is usually corrected spontaneously if the habit is broken. Finger sucking is a more long-lasting and "deep-seated" habit than the use of a pacifier. About 10% of children continue with the habit into their mixed dentition. Helping these children to stop the habit could be psychologically well motivated.

Shedding of primary teeth and the eruption of permanent teeth

Monitoring the shedding of the primary teeth and the eruption of the permanent teeth is very important as many malocclusions manifest themselves during these processes (see Chapter 15). Primary retention is seldom observed in the primary dentition, but there is a high prevalence of secondary retention, caused by temporary ankylosis, in primary molars (up to 12%). Normally, such teeth will loosen and be shed with the permanent successor in a normal position. If the ankylosis persists for a long period, the infraposition will increase, leaving a greatly reduced height of the alveolar process. On rare occasions the neighboring teeth may tilt into the space (Fig. 16-25). Presence of the permanent successor should always be checked radiographically. If the tooth is missing in a young individual and there is expected to be a considerable vertical reduction of the alveolar process, this can motivate an early removal of the ankylotic tooth.

Primary teeth may also persist in the jaw without being ankylosed and without being in infraposition (Fig. 16-26). That happens regularly to teeth with agenesis of their permanent successors. In such cases the fate of the persisting tooth should be discussed with an orthodontist. In cases where the occlusion otherwise is excellent

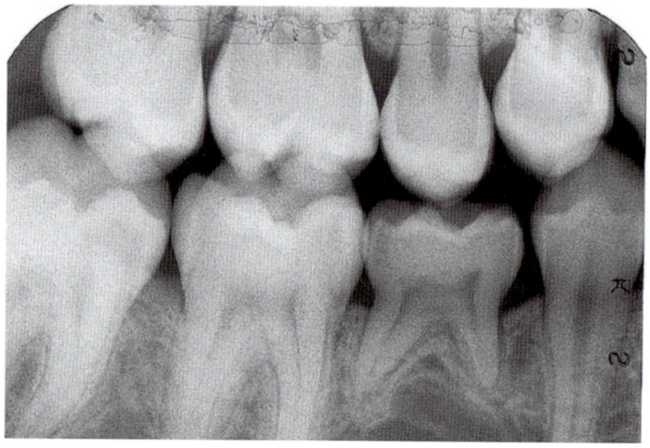

Figure 16-26 Boy at 18 years of age with persisting 85 and agenesis of 45. The tooth is in good condition and may be functioning for many years.

and the persisting tooth is in good condition (negligible caries, no infraposition, no significant resorption of roots, etc.), the primary tooth may be maintained, and may function for many years. If the occlusion and the condition of the persisting tooth are less favorable, the tooth should be extracted and the space closed by natural mesial drift, by orthodontic means or, more seldomly, by autotransplantation, implants or prosthodontic reconstructions. The prognosis for space closure is most favorable in the maxilla and in cases with crowding.

Primary teeth may also persist even if their successors are present. That may occur to the primary second molars in both jaws if the position of premolars does not allow resorption of all roots at the same time. In the maxilla especially, the palatal root may be left unresorbed and keep the tooth longer in place even if buccal roots are completely resorbed (Fig. 16-27).

Ectopic eruptions are a substantial problem during eruption of permanent teeth (Figs 16-28 and 16-29).

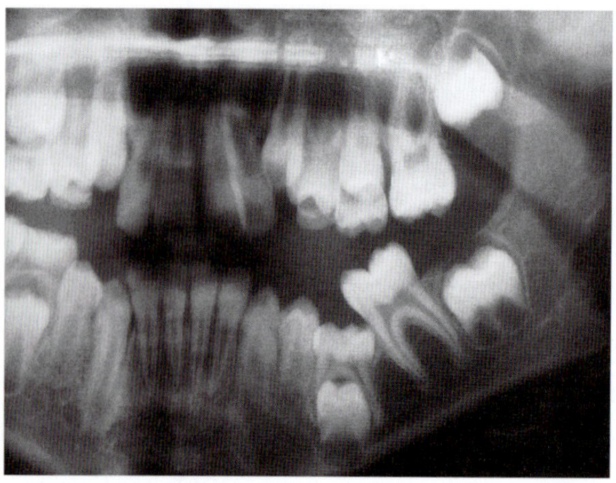

Figure 16-25 Ankylosis of primary molars resulting in infraposition of 75 (secondary retention) and tipping of 36.

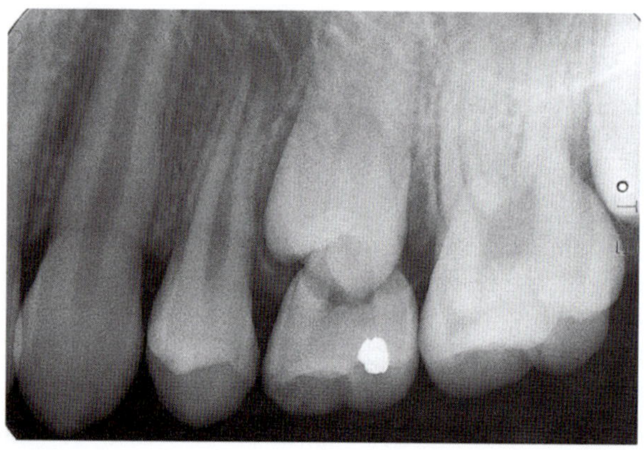

Figure 16-27 Persisting 65 due to a slight ectopic position of 25. The buccal roots are resorbed, while the palatal root is still intact.

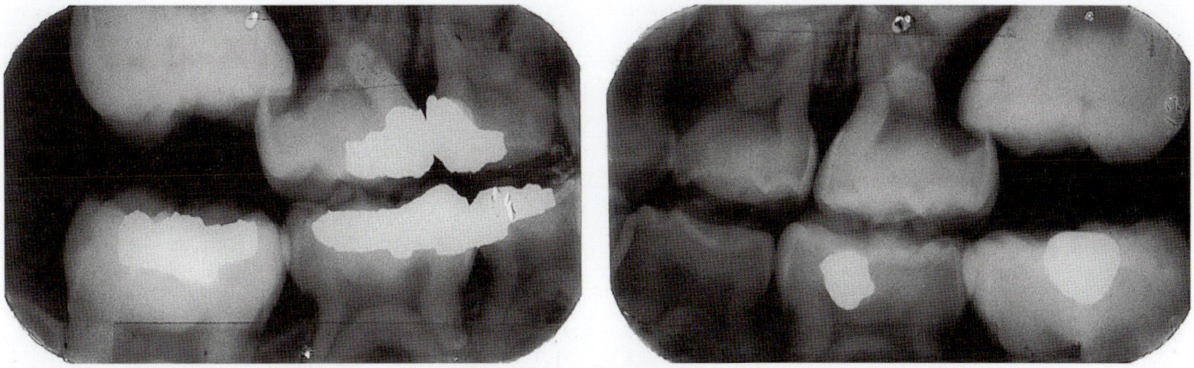

Figure 16-28 Ectopic eruption of 16,26 (hold cases) locked in the deep resorption cavity.

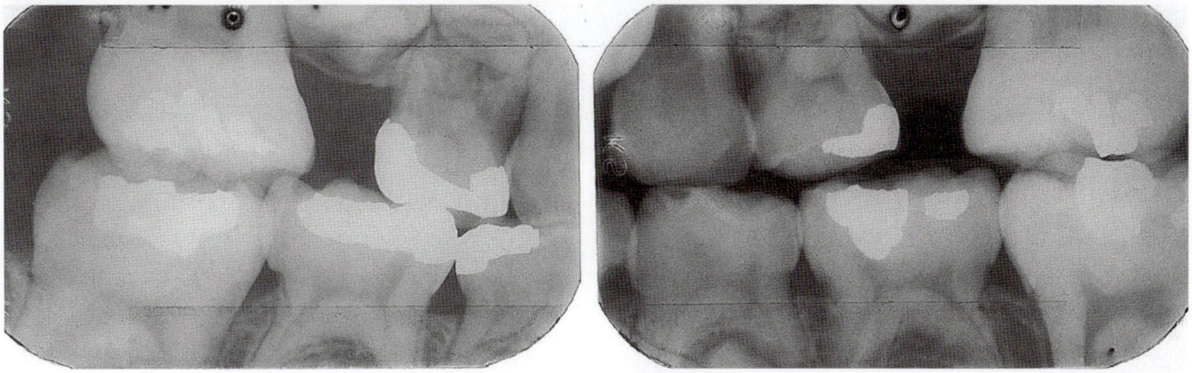

Figure 16-29 Same case as in Fig. 16-28 after extraction of 55,65. Severe loss of space for 15,25. Space was regained by means of headgear which distalized the permanent first molars to create space for 15,25.

The "classic" ectopic eruption is that of the first molars, especially in the maxilla, where the mesial part of the crown is locked beneath the distal curvature of the primary second molar. However, investigations show that in 60% of cases the ectopic teeth are released (jump cases). In the other 40% of cases (hold cases) distal movement of the ectopic molar to allow it to erupt normally is indicated. Even severely resorbed primary second molars usually persist and function as space maintainers (Figs 16-28 and 16-29). Also the maxillary canines may show ectopic eruption (or be retained). Ectopically erupting canines in a labial position and with none or small mesial displacement will probably not mean an increased risk for resorption of permanent incisors. The tooth can be allowed to erupt in a buccally displaced position and can, if treatment is requested for aesthetic reasons, be corrected in the permanent dentition period. Buccal displacement of a canine is probably often caused by lack of space for the tooth.

The palatally positioned canines may be more complicated to bring into normal position, depending on the degree of deviation in position. Extraction of a persisting primary canine and increase of available space by, for instance, distal movement of the lateral segments may normalize the eruption of a palatal canine. While they are in ectopic positions, the canines may cause resorption of the lateral and even the central incisors (Figs 16-30 and 16-31). Early detection of such cases is an important responsibility of the pediatric dentist.

Palpation of the buccal area of the canines will with normal eruption reveal a bulge/swelling about 1.5 years before eruption (in boys at 11.5 years and in girls at 10.5 years of age). About seven out of 10 impaction cases are unilateral and are easily distinguished as a clear difference between the sides. With bilateral impaction or ectopic eruption the clinician must use his or her clinical experience and feelings to decide whether the tooth should be palpable according to the individual's somatic and dental development. The prevalence of ectopic maxillary canines is approximately 2%; 85% of the ectopic eruptions are palatal; and girls are more affected than boys (13–15). In almost 50% of cases with ectopic eruptions incisor resorption will occur, often severely into the pulp. Therefore, early supervision, starting not later than 10 years of age, with palpation of the buccal canine area is most important to avoid severe complications and more prolonged orthodontic treatment with fixed appliances.

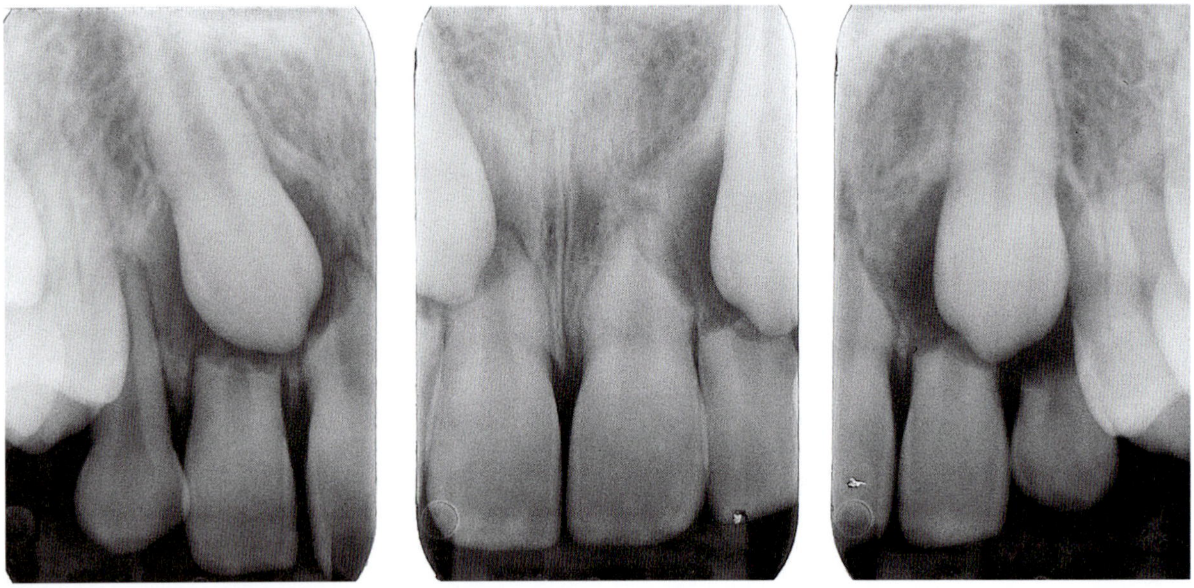

Figure 16-30 Ectopic eruption of 13,23 has almost completely destroyed the roots of 12,22 and also resorbed the roots of 11,21. Extraction of 12,22 was needed.

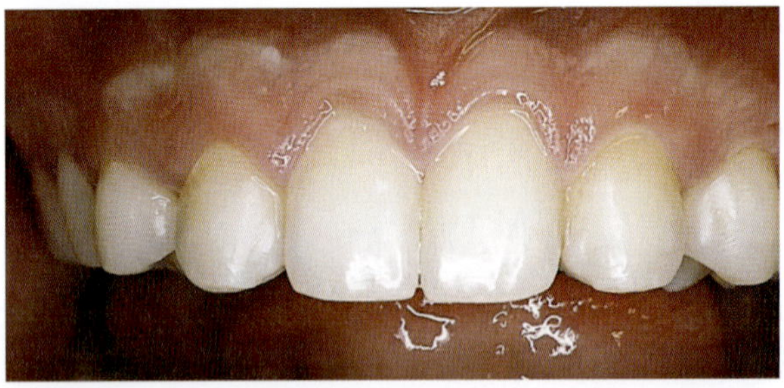

Figure 16-31 Same case as in Figure 16-31 after extraction 12, 22 and orthodontic treatment and grinding of canine cusps.

Trauma prevention

Prevention of trauma is also prevention of malocclusion because trauma to teeth may cause exarticulation or loss of teeth due to primary or secondary pulp necrosis, ankylosis, etc. Permanent teeth may also be severely damaged in crown development because of trauma to primary teeth, and also root dilacerations may occur. Studies (16,22) have shown a highly significant correlation between large overjet and incompetent lip posture and traumatic tooth injuries. There is also an association between the size of the overjet and prevalence and severity of tooth injuries. So far, no study specifically looking at the effect of overjet on traumatic tooth injuries has been presented. Nevertheless, the strong correlation between overjet and tooth injuries justifies correction of large overjets in late primary or early mixed dentition. An early treatment is motivated by the fact that many injuries occur before the age of 10 years.

Interceptive orthodontics

Interceptive treatment aims to break a negative developmental path. This deviation could be due to environmental factors. An example is a sucking habit causing reduction in the width of the upper dental arch. The discrepancy in width between the arches may force the individual to occlude in a lateral position in comparison to retruded contact position (RCP) in order to establish reasonably good interdigitation. As described above, the child often learns to keep the mandible laterally displaced at rest. This may cause an asymmetric occlusal and craniofacial development. The cross bite can also be an obstacle to the expected gain in width of the maxillary dental arch up to and including eruption of the canines. The result may be an increased lack of space for the teeth. Likewise, an anterior forced cross bite can interfere with the expected proclination of the maxillary incisors on eruption. Again, if left untreated this may contribute to increased crowding.

It is important to distinguish the forced cross bites interfering with optimal occlusal development from correction of primary crowding, usually of a genetic origin. Treatment of crowding with resulting displacement of teeth is usually motivated if the individual is clearly dissatisfied with the appearance. Such treatment decisions should normally be postponed to the permanent dentition period allowing the individual to be mature enough to be able to decide (21). A young individual cannot be expected to be able to make a decision until occlusal development is, at least, almost completed. Attempts to influence space by approximal grinding or even worse by so-called serial extraction have no scientific support and should be avoided. In general, treatment in the mixed dentition should be restricted to removal of obstacles for normal occlusal development and to correct malocclusions that may increase the risk for tooth damage. Early extractions such as serial extractions have probably more negative than positive effects and may also be a traumatic experience for the child. There also seems to be a risk for negative influence on the development of the alveolar process.

In summary, orthodontic treatment in the primary and mixed dentition periods should focus on ensuring optimal occlusal development and to reduce risks for tooth damage, i.e., root resorptions and traumatic injuries. A complete treatment plan including expected growth, occlusal development, and space conditions should always precede treatment. There is otherwise a great risk of focusing on details in deviation from ideal occlusion. It is also important to remember that malocclusion primarily means a biologic variation which very often is completely acceptable. Orthodontic diagnosis should not be confused with pathology. Orthodontic treatment should only be considered when obvious negative consequences of malocclusions can be identified and if the individual is clearly aware of the possible benefit of treatment. For a few individuals with a pronounced dissatisfaction with visible tooth malpositions, early treatment may be motivated. Normally, orthodontic treatment to improve aesthetics should be postponed to the permanent dentition period.

Supervising occlusal development in the primary and mixed dentition

In pediatric dentistry the diagnosis and supervision of dental and occlusal development are very important. The responsible dentist should know what to look for in certain developmental stages and also when preventive, interceptive, or corrective measures are indicated and most effective.

The eruption of teeth and the developmental status in the jaws may vary by about 5–6 years within the same age-group of individuals. Therefore, a description of dental stages can be made instead of age for describing physiological maturity. This means counting the teeth. The dental age can, for example, be used to estimate the age of children with unknown dates of birth. Instead of age, individuals can be described and grouped according to their tooth emergence status (Box 16-6).

Box 16-6 Dental age stages (Björk *et al.*, 1964)

DS 01	Primary dentition erupting.
DS 02	Primary dentition complete.
DS 1	Early mixed dentition (incisors erupting).
DS 2	Intermediate mixed dentition (incisors fully erupted).
DS 3	Late mixed dentition (canines or premolars erupting).
DS 4	Adolescent dentition (canines and premolars fully erupted).

Box 16-7 Common problems in the early mixed dentition, 6–9 years

- Habits causing malocclusions.
- Tooth eruption disturbances.
- Functional malocclusions.
- Obstacles to normal development of space for the teeth.
- Agenesis of permanent teeth.
- Large overjet increasing the risk for traumatic injuries.

The primary dentition

The consequences of oral habits and trauma ought to be followed up. Major malocclusions and space problems in the dental arches should be registered. Also, breathing disorders due to sleep apnea together with marked facial asymmetries may be noticed.

Early mixed dentition (6–9 years)

Box 16-7 contains examples of problems identified during supervision and guidance of the developing dentition. For more detailed reading see Kurol *et al.* (11). Tooth formation and tooth eruption times and sequences have been described earlier (Chapters 14 and 15).

Impacted incisors

Only one central incisor has erupted. Where is the other one? (Fig. 16-32).

Radiographic examination may reveal an eruption obstacle, e.g., odontoma. Extraction of the primary predecessor, surgical exposure and space maintenance may be indicated.

Early intervention is important.

Mesiodens

Moderate spacing of maxillary incisors is not uncommon in the early mixed dentition. A more pronounced medial diastema may indicate the presence of an extra tooth mesial to the central incisor roots: a mesiodens (Fig. 16-33). If active closure is planned, and also to

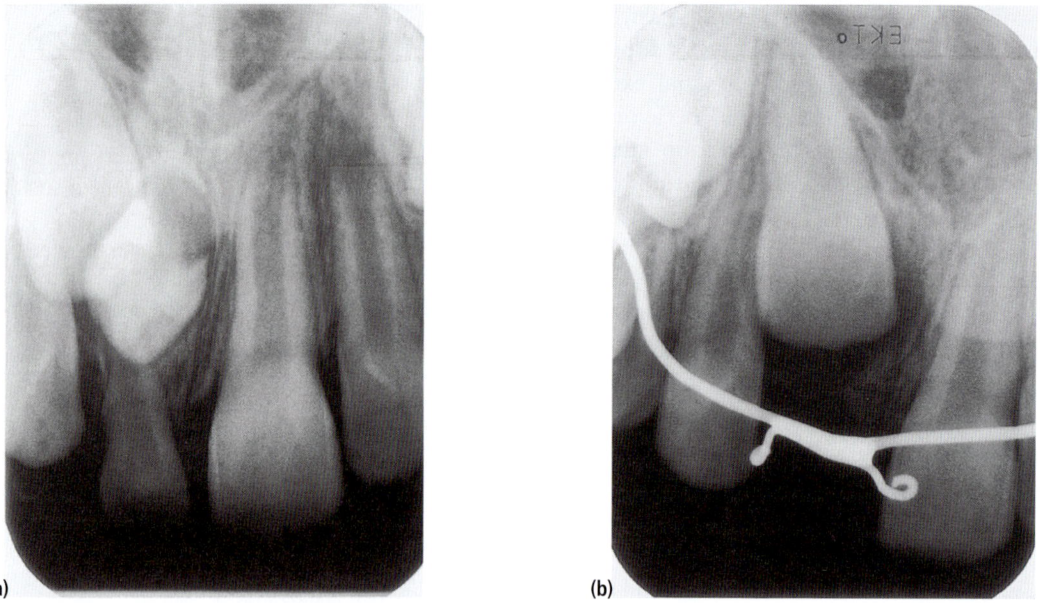

(a) (b)

Figure 16-32 (a) Only one central incisor (21) has erupted. After surgical removal of the supernumerary tooth, hindering eruption, a space maintainer is placed. (b) The lingual arch holds the space.

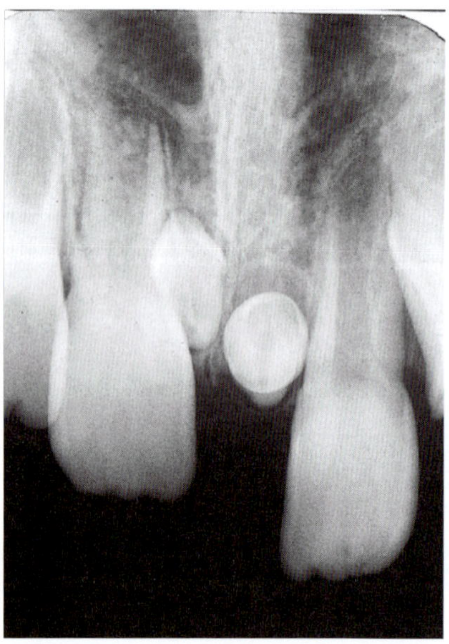

Figure 16-33 Radiograph showing two mesiodens as the cause of large median diastema.

allow for closure in connection with the eruption of lateral incisors and canines, removal may be necessary. Otherwise, half of the mesiodens will erupt in a palatal position and can easily be removed. Most of those which do not erupt may be left in place and could, if necessary, be supervised radiographically. There is no need to routinely remove mesiodens (7).

Ectopic first molars

The ectopic first molar resorbs the distal part of the primary molar and may be locked during eruption. The mesially tipped permanent molars may be moved distally with a spring on a removable appliance or with a sectional wire. The use of orthodontic appliances or separating elastics is preferred instead of earlier recommended brass wire. The resorption of the primary molar will then stop.

Ankylosed primary molars

With a successor present in a normal position supervision only is necessary. Normal shedding will occur, however, about 6 months later than normal (Chapter 15). If ankylosis occurs early, before the age of 6–7 years, the vertical eruption of neighboring teeth and vertical development of the alveolar process will leave the ankylosed primary molar in a position near or sometimes below the gingival margin. If the permanent first molar shows a pronounced tendency to tip in over the infraoccluded primary molar, this tipping should be treated early. With agenesis of the successor, the treatment should be planned together with an orthodontist according to space conditions and occlusion (10) (Chapter 14). Early removal of the primary molar is often beneficial, otherwise there may be a considerable reduction of the height of the alveolar process making later replacements far more difficult. Early removal of the primary molar also allows the permanent molar to move forward, thus completely or partially closing the gap.

Agenesis of teeth

Maxillary laterals. This situation is usually detected radiographically when the tooth is not erupting and occurs in 2–3% of children. Space closure is usually the first choice (20). In patients with a pronounced excess of space the treatment is often directed towards space maintenance and later replacement with implants. Both space closure and replacement by implants are usually well accepted by treated individuals.

Mandibular premolars. These are usually detected from bitewing radiographs, preferably early, at the age of 8–9 years. The prevalence is 4–5%. The primary molar, which is approximately 11 mm wide, may be left in the dental arch or extracted depending on space conditions and occlusion (Fig. 16-26).

Spontaneous space closure, orthodontic space closure and, on rare occasions, autotransplantation and prosthetic rehabilitation including oral implants are possibilities to discuss with the orthodontist.

Median diastema

This may be seen in the presence of mesiodens, congenital absence of lateral incisors, or a fibrous frenulum. With time the diastema will close with mesially directed forces from erupting lateral incisors and later maxillary canines. Frenectomy is not commonly used nowadays.

Anterior cross bite

Some of the important questions to ask are: is it dental, dentoalveolar, or skeletal? Is there any family background? What is the retrusion to intercuspidation (RP–IP) distance and which teeth occlude in the retruded position of the mandible? Is grinding of primary teeth possible? Are there indications for growth supervision with cephalometry? Single teeth may be treated early with an appliance that raises the bite and pushes the incisors anteriorly provided there is sufficient space. If there is an overall space deficiency, treatment ought to be postponed to the permanent dentition period. With many incisors in frontal cross bite, a skeletal pattern may be suspected.

Anterior maxillary crowding

Visible crowding mainly influences satisfaction with appearance (21,23). In the primary and mixed dentition periods, obstacles to normal occlusal development should be identified and removed. Otherwise treatment of crowding ought to be postponed to the permanent dentition when the individual is mature enough to decide on treatment.

Lateral cross bites

Unilateral. These are usually forced bites (80–90%). Check the width of the maxillary dental arch and compare in the retruded position with the width of the mandibular arch. If the maxilla is narrow, additional active transversal expansion is needed. In mild forced bites the grinding of interferences on primary canines together with about 6 months' expansion with a removable plate or a Quad Helix, fixed or removable appliance will correct this malocclusion early.

Bilateral. Check craniofacial morphology, asymmetries and mode of breathing. What about adenoids and tonsils? Consult an orthodontist.

Frontal open bite

What is the cause? Habits (tongue or thumb sucking), or is it skeletal and influencing anterior face height? What about adenoids/tonsils and a possible anterior tongue position? Remember that there is a good chance of spontaneous correction in the mixed dentition period.

Deep bite

Is it the result of overeruption of maxillary incisors or due to a skeletal pattern? What about the profile, shape of the mandible, or lower face height indicating a skeletal deep bite? Fixed appliances are usually required in these cases. Treatment may be indicated in patients with vertically unstable incisor relation, i.e., pronounced Class II.2 cases where overeruption of incisors is likely to occur.

Protruding maxillary incisors

Early retraction treatment is recommended for trauma prophylactic reasons, especially if the upper lip is short and is not protecting the incisors. Activators or removable plates can be used.

Late mixed dentition (9–12 years)

Ectopic maxillary canines

If after clinical examination and judgment the supervising dentist suspects an ectopic eruption, an extended radiographic investigation is indicated and contact with an orthodontist is necessary. With early detection it is possible in almost 80% of cases to change the ectopic path of eruption by early extraction of the primary canines (2). The treatment should be planned together with an orthodontist (Fig. 16-34 and Box 16-8).

Space conditions

Spacing or crowding of teeth is diagnosed and treated according to need and demand.

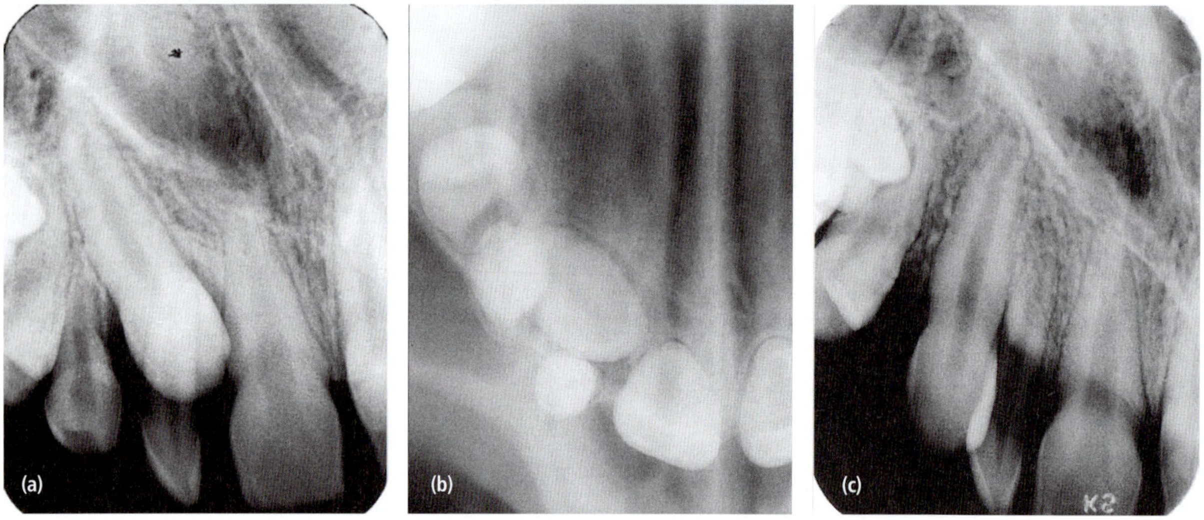

Figure 16-34 Early extraction (a, b) of the primary canine may spontaneously change the path of eruption (c) of palatal ectopic maxillary canines (2).

Box 16-8 Maxillary ectopic canines (2,9)

Facts
- Prevalence about 2%.
- 85% are palatal.
- More girls: two out of three.
- Seven out of 10 are unilateral.
- Age at eruption: girls 10.5 years, boys 11.5 years.
- Palpable bulge in the buccal sulcus about 1.5 years before eruption.
- With mesial migration of the canine, the risk for severe root resorptions increases.

Suggested policy
- Digital palpation should start at about 9–10 years of age depending on individual maturity.
- Early extraction of primary canines before 13 years of age may result in spontaneous correction of palatally ectopic canine cases (2).

Malposition of teeth

Scissors bite, cross bite, ectopic eruptions, ankylosed permanent molars are also diagnosed and treated according to need and demand.

Young permanent dentition (12–15 years)

By this age most tooth eruption disturbances and malocclusions should already have been diagnosed. Decisions may have been made earlier to supervise the development, assess the severity and consequences for the individual, and postpone the start of treatment, especially if the need for intervention is less pronounced and the benefit of treatment is limited.

General decisions for orthodontic treatment

As previously stressed, orthodontic treatment should only be considered if malocclusion causes pronounced problems for the individual. The presence of malocclusion is not *per se* an indication for treatment. It is important to identify and evaluate satisfaction of the patient. The patient is also entitled to a correct description of functional and health problems that may be related to the malocclusions. Generally, no major health risks have been associated with untreated malocclusions so far. The following areas ought to be evaluated and discussed with the patient. Preventive, interceptive treatment and treatment to prevent tooth damage have been discussed previously.

Dissatisfaction with appearance

This is no doubt the major reason for demand for orthodontic treatment (16,21–23). So far, there has not been found any profound psychological influence of malocclusions or orthodontic treatment. Teenagers, however, tend to relate self-esteem and influence on their relations with other teenagers to presence of malocclusion. Motivation to undergo treatment seems to be a social norm and relates to the beauty culture in teenagers' reference groups and society in general. Recent studies indicate a positive influence on quality of life by orthodontic treatment. Orthodontically treated subjects tend to express a higher level of satisfaction with appearance compared to those with untreated malocclusions. Follow-up into adult age indicates a higher tolerance to variations in tooth positions compared to younger individuals. On the other hand, untreated adults tend to rank their general appearance lower than individuals without malocclusions. An evaluation of the psychosocial benefit of an orthodontic treatment must always be individualized.

Caries and periodontitis

Subjects with malocclusions do not have more caries than those with ideal occlusion (16,22). There is insufficient evidence to establish an association between malocclusion and periodontitis. Studies of oral hygiene in relation to malocclusions have revealed that there is a slightly higher tendency for plaque accumulation in subjects with displacement of teeth or large overjet. This is only true, however, for those with an average level of oral hygiene. The influence of the dominant hand has, for instance, been found to have a greater influence than malocclusions.

Speech

Malocclusions such as frontal open bite, large overjet, mandibular overjet, or frontal spacing could be suspected to influence consonant articulation in a negative way. Available studies indicate that deviation of speech in relation to malocclusions usually is of a mild or, at most, moderate severity (16,22). In subjects with severe neuromuscular disturbances these can cause both speech deficiencies and severely altered craniofacial and occusal development. In children with cleft lip and palate there is often a nasality in the speech due to incomplete closure of the soft palate.

Chewing function

The effect of chewing is dependent on the size of the mastication surface. The food is more effectively broken into smaller particles in subjects with larger contact area between upper and lower teeth. The scientific basis to establish negative health effects related to limited chewing ability is still insufficient. It should not be forgotten, however, that a good ability to chew and to bite off the food can have a great psychological value.

Temporomandibular disorders

Most studies indicate that there is a week correlation between temporomandibular disorders (TMD) and malocclusions (16,22). It has been estimated that occlusal variables may explain 10–20% of TMD. Most studies have found no or only minor influence of malocclusions on TMD. Some studies present significant correlations, but the type of malocclusion studied differs between studies. Thus, few safe conclusions can be drawn. Longitudinally, it has been demonstrated that there are considerable variations in presence and severity of TMD in an individual over time (1,14). Functional variables such as cuspid protection or nonworking side interferences appear only to have a small influence on TMD. Psychological factors and muscular endurance, on the other hand, seem to have greater influence than malocclusions. In adults correlations have been found between class II and III malocclusions, open bite, and functional cross bites. Class II, III, and open bite malocclusions are often characterized by a steep mandibular plane angle. A steep angle has been associated with less strong masticatory muscles, which may make such subjects more vulnerable to overload of the muscles. In line with that, less TMD has been observed in subjects with a deep bite. Follow-up from teenage to about 30 years of age has revealed a pronounced reduction of signs and symptoms of TMD (1,14). In summary, malocclusions do not seem to have a major influence on development of TMD.

The selection of orthodontic patients

There is, unfortunately, a tradition to select subjects for orthodontic treatment on the basis of presence of malocclusions and on how much the occlusion deviates from the constructed norm for the ideal occlusion. Dentists often appear to be the ones who initiate treatment (23). Indices to prioritize for orthodontic treatment are constructed mainly in two ways. One includes a description of malocclusions and a ranking of malocclusion, i.e., the larger an overjet, the greater the treatment need. There seems to be an assumption of a relation between psychosocial dissatisfaction and oral health on one hand and the type and severity of malocclusions on the other. The other type is based on aesthetic evaluation by a panel of observers ranking photos of various clinical situations. There appears to be no scientific evidence for the validity of any available index (15,22). Instead, a treatment decision ought to be based on a thorough evaluation of the dissatisfaction of the patient. The patient should also be given good information of possible negative consequences for leaving the malocclusion untreated. The information should also include risks and discomfort of treatment and, not least, how extensive the treatment will be and how stable the treatment result is expected to be. Most of these discussions ought to take place in general dentistry.

References

1. Egermark I, Magnusson T, Carlsson GE. A 20-year follow-up of signs and symptoms of temporomandibular disorders and malocclusions in subjects with and without orthodontic treatment in childhood. *Angle Orthod* 2003;**73**:109–15.
2. Ericson S, Kurol J. Early treatment of palatally erupting maxillary canines by extraction of primary canines. *Eur J Orthod* 1988; **10**:283–95.
3. Ericson S, Kurol J. Resorption of incisors after ectopic eruption of maxillary canines. A CT study. *Angle Orthod* 2000;**70**:415–23.

4. Hermanson H, Kurol J, Rönnerman A. Treatment of unilateral crossbites with quad-helix and removable plates. A retrospective study. *Eur J Orthod* 1985;7:97–102.
5. Hultcrantz E, Larson M, Hellquist R, Ahlquist-Rastad J, Svanholm H, Jakobsson OP. The influence of tonsillar obstruction and tonsillectomy on facial growth and dental arch morphology. *Int J Pediatr Otorhinolaryngol* 1991;**22**:125–34.
6. Kiliaridis S. Masticatory muscle function and craniofacial morphology. *Swed Dent J* Suppl 36, 1986.
7. Kurol J. Impacted and ankylosed teeth: why, when, and how to intervene. *Am J Orthod Dentofacial Orthop* 2006;**129**:4, Suppl 1, 86–90.
8. Kurol J, Berglund L. Longitudinal study and cost-benefit analysis of the effect of early treatment of posterior cross-bites in the primary dentition. *Eur J Orthod* 1992;**14**:173–9.
9. Kurol J, Ericson S, Andreasen JO. The impacted maxillary canine. In: Andreasen JO, Kølsen Petersen J, Laskin D, eds. *Textbook and color atlas of tooth impactions. Diagnosis, treatment and prevention.* Copenhagen: Munksgaard, 1997; Chapter 6, 126–65.
10. Kurol J, Thilander B. Infraocclusion of primary molars and the effect on occlusal development. A longitudinal study. *Eur J Orthod* 1984;**6**:277–93.
11. Kurol J, Thilander B, Zachrisson B, Linder-Aronson S. Treatment of dentoalveolar and skeletal anomalies. In: Thilander B, Rönning O, eds. *Introduction to orthodontics*, 2nd edn. Solna: Förlagshuset Gothia, 1995; Chapter VI, 112–68.
12. Larsson E. The prevalence and aetiology of prolonged dummy and finger-sucking habits. *Eur J Orthod* 1985;**7**:172–6.
13. Mason R. Tongue thrust. In: *Oral motor behavior: impact on oral conditions and dental treatment.* NIH Publication No. 79–1845, USA, 1979; 32–48.
14. Mohlin B, Derweduwen K, Pilley R, Kingdon A, Shaw WC, Kenealy P. Malocclusion and temporomandibular disorder: a comparison of adolescents with moderate to severe dysfunction with those without signs and symptoms of temporomandibular disorder and their further development to 30 years of age. *Angle Orthod* 2004;**74**:319–27.
15. Mohlin B, Kurol J. A critical view of treatment priority indices in orthodontics. *Swed Dent J* 2003;**27**:11–21.
16. Mohlin B, Kurol J. To what extent do deviations from an ideal occlusion constitute a health risk? *Swed Dent J* 2003;**27**:1–10.
17. Mohlin B, Sagne S, Thilander B. The frequency of malocclusion and the craniofacial morphology in a medieval population in Southern Sweden. *OSSA* 1979;**5**:57–84.
18. Moorrees CFA. *The dentition of the growing child. A longitudinal study of dental development between 3 and 18 years of age.* Cambridge, MA: Harvard University Press, 1959.
19. Ravn JJ. Longitudinal study of occlusion in the primary dentition in 3- to 7-year-old children. *Scand J Dent Res* 1980;**88**:165–70.
20. Robertsson S, Mohlin B. The congenitally missing upper lateral incisor. A retrospective study of space closure versus restorative treatment. *Eur J Orthod* 2000;**22**:697–710.
21. Shaw WC. Factors influencing the desire for orthodontic treatment. *Eur J Orthod* 1981;**3**:151–62.
22. Malocclusions and orthodontic treatment in a health perspective. A systematic literature review. The Swedish Council on Technology Assessment in Health Care, 2005.
23. Trulsson U, Strandmark M, Mohlin B, Berggren U. A qualitative study of teenagers' decisions to undergo orthodontic treatment with fixed appliance. *J Orthod* 2002;**29**:197–204.

17

Developmental defects of the dental hard tissues and their treatment

Ivar Espelid, Dorte Haubek and Birgitta Jälevik

This chapter focuses on the diagnostic process and classification of disturbances in the dental hard tissues. General treatment principles and treatment planning are discussed. Then different types of dental defects are described as localized and generalized dental defects including those of genetic origin. The most common and important diseases or conditions are given most attention in the chapter. To cover the topic in its entirety, many conditions with low prevalence are mentioned in the boxes. More specific treatment aspects related to severe types of defects are given in the final part of the chapter.

Aspects related to tooth development

In contrast to bone, enamel and dentin are not remodeled. Therefore disturbances in the function of ameloblasts and/or odontoblasts during tooth development result in permanent defects. The tissues under development and mineralization can be reduced in either quantity or quality or both. As development of the first primary tooth begins in the fourth week *in utero* and the development of the roots of the wisdom teeth is completed around the age of 20 years, teeth serve a role similar to a "flight recorder" that covers a long time period. From this "record" the clinician can roughly judge when the disturbance occurred and the appearance of the defects may in some cases give clues as to the etiologic factor. But one major diagnostic challenge associated with developmental defects of teeth is that they frequently are not pathognomonic. The findings are often consistent with many possible etiological factors and the anamnesis is of crucial importance to achieve the correct diagnosis. On the other hand, there are some clinical findings which are pathognomonic or highly suggestive for a specific condition such as dental changes due to tetracycline medication during tooth formation.

In the body, enamel is the only mineralized tissue of epithelial origin. Once formed, it loses contact with living cells. The basic unit of the enamel is the prism, each prism being the product of four ameloblasts. The prisms are bundles of crystallites which are much bigger and better organized than other mineralized tissues in the body. Enamel is formed at three stages: (a) deposition and (b) mineralization of the matrix occur simultaneously, and (c) maturation, involving final degradation and transport of the organic constituents, does not begin until the full thickness of enamel has been achieved at a given site. *Amelogenins*, constituting the major enamel matrix protein species during the secretory stage, are progressively degraded and lost.

The striae of Retzius are incremental growth lines seen in enamel. These striae are results of a stop or a slowing down in enamel growth and end on the enamel surface as perikymata. Microscopically in cross-sections, striae of Retzius appear as concentric rings or as a series of dark bands in longitudinal sections. These are incremental lines similar to the annual rings on a tree. The cross-striations are created by the daily, incremental enamel matrix production. The long-period incremental growth lines are striae of Retzius. These lines are made with a periodicity of 6–11 days (33) (Figs 17-1 and 17-2). The neonatal line is an incremental line which is particularly pronounced due to the stress associated with birth and makes a distinction between the prenatal and postnatal enamel.

Dentin is mineralized connective tissue produced by odontoblasts, which are continually functional cells. The nonmineralized predentin, contiguous with the mineralized dentin, faces the coherent layer of odontoblasts located at the periphery of the pulp. Dentin is traversed by radial tubules, with each tubule housing an odontoblastic process. The main constituent of the organic dentin matrix is type I collagen.

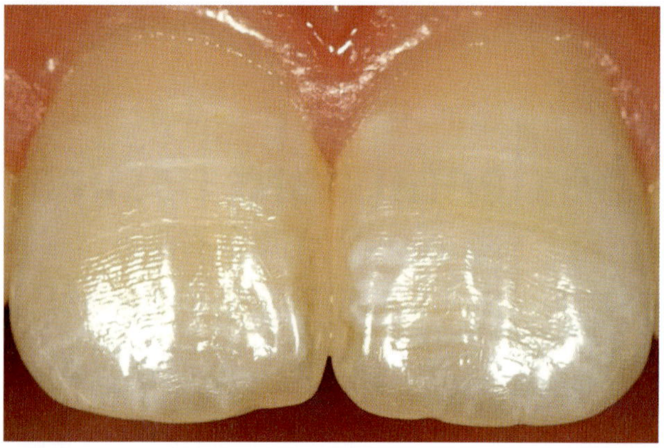

Figure 17-1 Perikymata shown as horizontal lines on buccal surfaces of central incisors. White, opaque patches and lines represent enamel disturbances (mild dental fluorosis). Seven-year-old child.

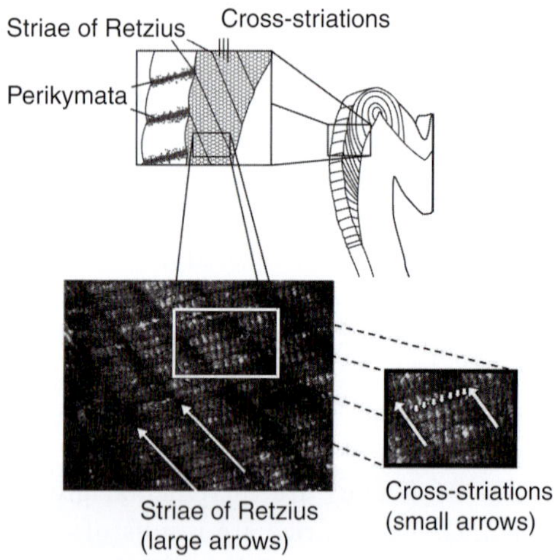

Figure 17-2 Schematic drawing and micrograph of perikymata (large arrows) and cross-striations of enamel (small arrows) indicating daily increments of enamel formation. The striae of Retzius represent incremental lines of enamel formation of about a week's duration and perikymata on the enamel surface are associated with these lines where they reach the outer surface. The figure is reproduced with minor changes with permission from the publisher and author.

Like dentin, cementum, which is formed by cementoblasts, is mesenchymal in origin. Morphologically, it is divided into the acellular cementum, which covers the cervical portion of the root and the cellular cementum overlying the apical portion. Cellular cementum is slowly deposited throughout the life of the tooth.

Etiology of developmental dental defects

Defects can be environmental or genetic. Often their cause for a given patient remains unknown. Genetic defects can be restricted to dental tissues or the dental defect can be a manifestation of generalized tissue/organ involvement. Environmental (also called acquired) dental defects can be divided into those caused by local factors and those caused by systemic factors. Typically, a local factor can be suspected when the enamel defect affects a single tooth or a group of neighboring teeth, or has an asymmetric distribution in the dentition. General symmetric defects are related to the timing of the insult and thus to the sequence of the development of the teeth and are called chronological defects. Etiology of general defects not related to any particular time period during tooth formation is either genetic or due to nongenetic, longstanding environmental influence. Figure 17-3 gives a systematic approach to the collection and classification of findings. Boxes 17-4, 17-11, and 17-12 list diseases and etiologic factors which can lead to developmental disturbances in the dental hard tissues.

Collection of information and treatment planning

Anamnestic information

The medical history is of utmost importance for disclosing the etiology of the dental aberration. Often, the nature of the symptoms is not specifically related to a certain cause and differential diagnostic considerations have to be made to form the final diagnosis. Keywords regarding history taking are mapping of family and childhood diseases, previous and current intake of medication, and environmental contamination level during childhood, fluoride exposure, dental history, and symptoms. Important questions to ask are listed in Box 17-1.

Extraoral examination

A brief examination of the features of the head and face is recommended to record indications of abnormal development. Also, inspection of skin, hair, and nails may in some cases give useful information since they develop from the ectoderm like enamel.

Clinical characteristics of developmental dental defects

The classification of abnormalities of the dental hard tissues is governed by clinical characteristics of the affected tooth. However, with the expanding knowledge of the molecular basis of genetically determined dental defects, the need for classifications relying on specific molecular defects has become increasingly evident. The most apparent defects are those seen in the enamel, namely enamel opacity and enamel hypoplasia (Fig. 17-4). Since dentin is less available to inspection, the fact that dentin may also be involved is often unappreciated and the defects are described and referred to as defects of the enamel (Box 17-2).

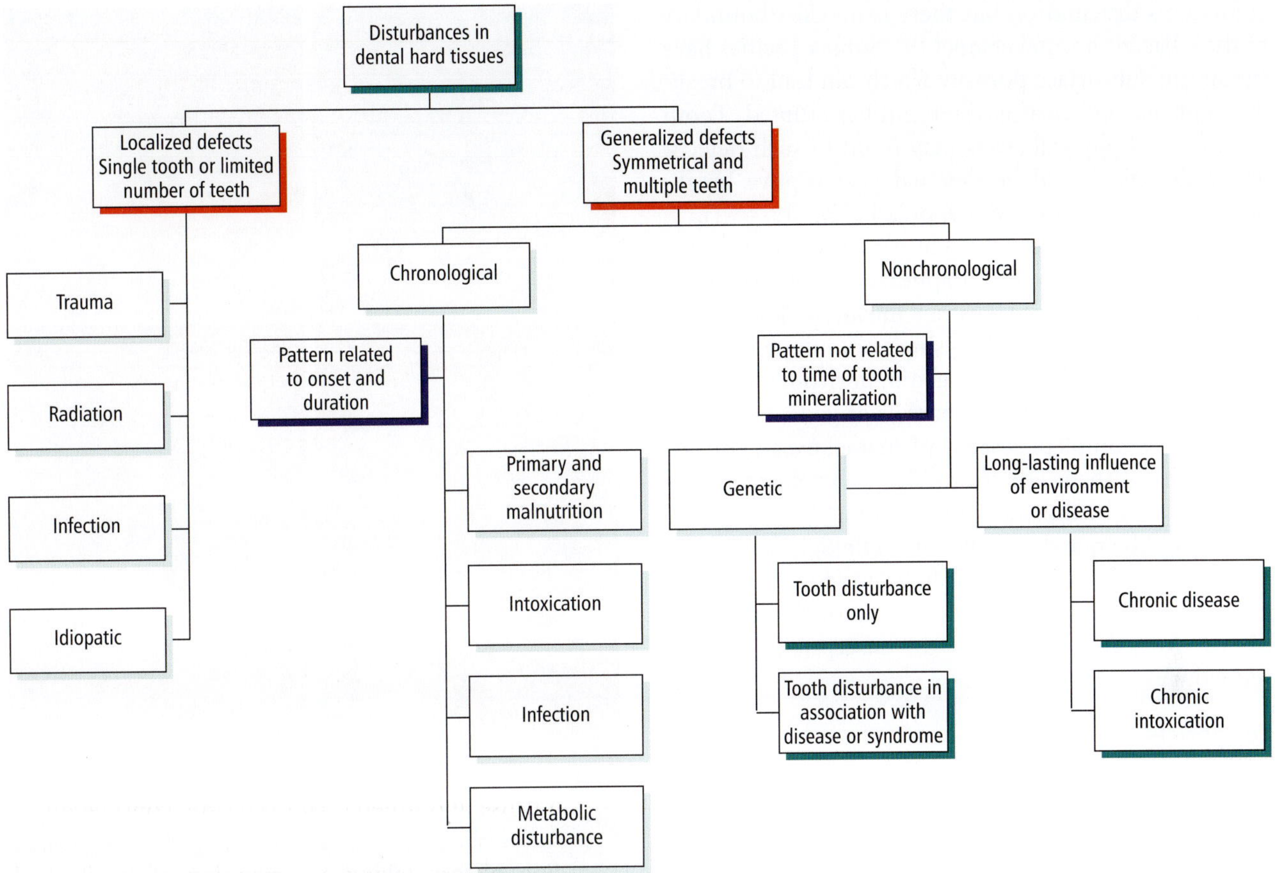

Figure 17-3 Schematic overview showing a systematic approach to the collection of data and classification of findings related to developmental disturbances of the dental hard tissues.

Box 17-1 Important questions when examining a patient with mineralization disturbances of teeth

- Which teeth are affected?
- Are both primary and permanent teeth affected?
- Are the teeth sensitive?
- Do siblings or relatives have any dental disturbances?
- What are the findings in the radiographic examination?
- What do the hair and nails look like?
- How was the general health of the mother during pregnancy?
- Were there any complications at birth?
- What was the gestational age of the child?
- Was the child breastfed or fed with a formula?
- Did the child receive fluoride or vitamin supplementation?
- Did the child drink fluoride-containing water during childhood?
- How was the general health in early childhood?
- Were there any severe illnesses?

Box 17-2 Opacity and hypoplasia

Qualitative defects
- Opacity (see Fig. 17-4b, c):
  - incomplete mineralization below an enamel surface which is intact at the time of eruption
  - change in the color and translucency of enamel
  - enamel surface may break secondary to trauma from masticatory forces, leaving sharp boundaries.
- Discolored enamel (see Fig. 17-4d).

Quantitative defects
- Hypoplasia (see Fig. 17-4e, f):
  - deficient enamel matrix formation
  - the enamel is thin throughout, or pitted, or grooved or missing over substantial areas
  - the defect has rounded boundaries
  - opacities are also frequently present in combination with hypoplastic lesions (see Fig. 17-19h).

An enamel opacity results from incomplete mineralization and is a qualitative defect. Another term frequently used synonymously for this condition is enamel hypomineralization. Opacities are often divided into demarcated and diffuse lesions. Demarcated opacities have a clear and distinct boundary to the adjacent normal enamel and they can be white, yellow, or brown in color. Diffuse opacities can have a linear, patchy, or contiguous distribution but there is no clear boundary to the adjacent normal enamel (9). Some opacities have significant subsurface porosity which can lead to breakdown of the surface after the tooth has erupted. Tooth attrition and physical stress may result in such defects. These defects should be denoted posteruptive breakdown (Fig. 17-4g) and not hypoplasia (Fig. 17-4e–f).

Enamel hypoplasia is a consequence of deficient enamel matrix formation. It appears as a surface defect resulting from reduced enamel thickness. Hypoplasia can occur in the form of pits – single or multiple, shallow or deep, or scattered or arranged in horizontal rows; or grooves – single or multiple, narrow or wide, or evident as partial or complete absence of enamel over a considerable area of the tooth crown. The enamel of reduced thickness may be translucent or opaque (9).

It should be noted that the same etiologic factor may cause an opacity or hypoplasia, the end result depending on the timing, duration, and severity of the influence of the disturbing agent and the susceptibility of the individual.

Diagnosis

To make a final diagnosis it is necessary to combine the information from the patient history and medical record and clinical and radiographic findings from the dental examination. In some cases it might be impossible to reach a final diagnosis or there is more than one likely diagnosis. For example, mild degrees of dental fluorosis and some cases of amelogenesis imperfecta (AI) have similar appearance.

Classification

Historically, symptoms and newly discovered diseases were named and more or less arbitrarily classified according to the current knowledge and beliefs. As medicine and dentistry progress continuously more knowledge of the etiology and genetics is acquired. Classification of hereditary enamel and dentin diseases primarily based on molecular etiology will be an absolute necessity for genetic counseling, but so far not enough knowledge of the genetics for proposal of new classifications describing the relationship between genotype and phenotype is available (4,22,40,49).

A classification based primarily on the genetics and secondarily on phenotypic expression has been proposed (4). The first criterion is information on the defective gene locus and then the biochemical consequences of this failure. This systematic approach is more common in medicine; however, it may over time also lead to reclassification of hereditary dental defects as well.

For hereditary dentin defects, the classification of dentinogenesis imperfecta (DI) and dentin dysplasia (DD) by Shields *et al.* from 1973 (37) is commonly used (Box 17-3). However, newer studies indicate that the entities DI-II and DI-III are different phenotypic expressions of the same defect in the gene 4q13-21. Similar gene defects are found in DD-II indicating that this is a

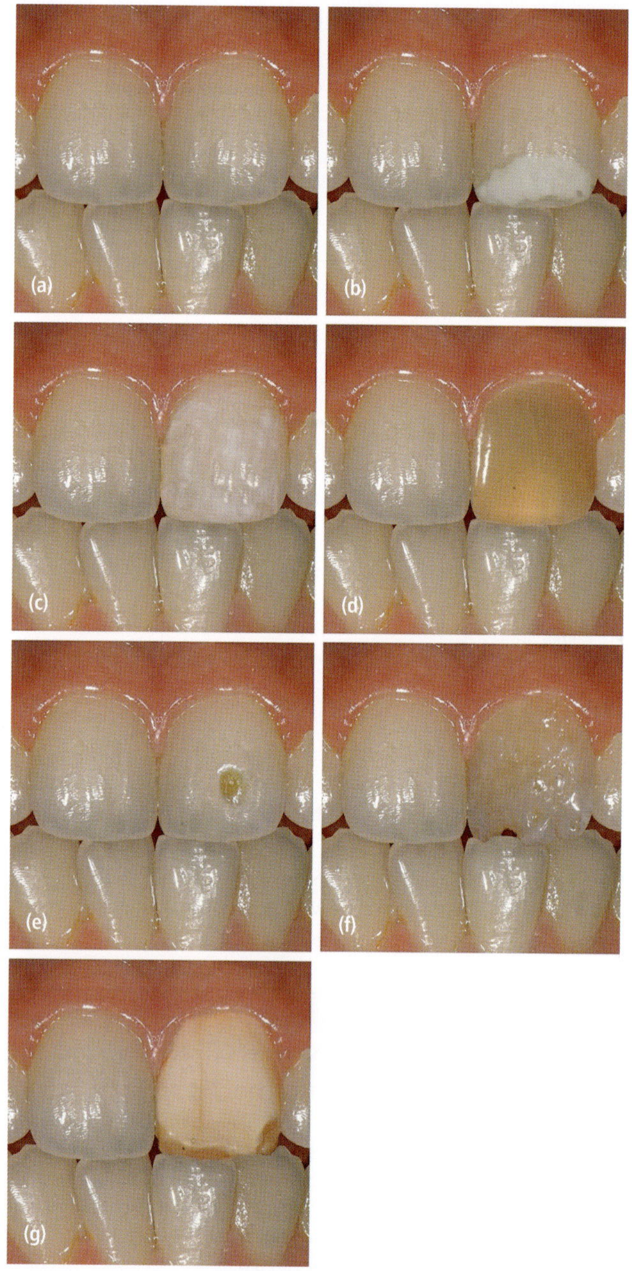

Figure 17-4 Classification and examples of types of enamel defects due to disturbances in the tooth formation. The natural appearance of the incisor 21 (a) is manipulated to illustrate (b) demarcated opacity (white), (c) diffuse opacities (white) with no well-defined margins, (d) discolored enamel which has some translucency, (e) single hypoplasia (single deep pit), (f) multiple hypoplastic defects, and (g) posteruptive breakdown due to hypomineralized enamel. Note that very often in cases with enamel defects, several teeth in the dentition will be affected.

Box 17-3 Classification of dentinogenesis imperfecta and dentin dysplasia according to Shields *et al.* (37)

Dentinogenesis imperfecta (DI)

- *Type I (DI-I).* DI seen in patients with osteogenesis imperfecta (syndromic form of DI). Discoloration of teeth, enamel chipping, and extreme attrition of dentin are common features.
- *Type II (DI-II).* Hereditary opalescent dentin not associated with any other disease. The dental changes are similar to type I.
- *Type III (DI-III).* Brandy wine isolate hereditary opalescent dentin. A very rare entity found in a special population in Maryland, USA. Two typical findings in DI-III are multiple pulp exposures and shell teeth. These findings are used to differentiate from DI-II, but they are not always unique to DI-III because shell teeth can sometimes be seen in DI-II (22).

Dentin dysplasia (DD)

- *Type I (DD-I).* DD characterized by radicular dentin dysplasia or rootless teeth.
- *Type II (DD-II).* Anomalous dysplasias of dentin with frequent discoloration of primary teeth; permanent teeth often appear normal clinically but have thistle-tube formed pulp chambers. Pulp stones may occur.

similar entity. Another problem with Shields' classification is the DI-I diagnosis. This is based on dentin alterations in a syndrome while other syndromes such as Ehlers–Danlos (EDS) are not included. EDS may have phenotypes with dysplastic dentin and obliterated pulp which can mimic DD-I and DI-II with variable expressivity and similar findings may appear in some other syndromes as well (22).

Similar difficulties in the classification of AI and in the distinction between AI and tricho-dento-osseous syndrome (TDO) exist. For example, it has been questioned whether an autosomal dominant hypoplastic hypomaturation type of AI (ADHHAI) with taurodontism is a true distinct clinical entity of AI or if it is TDO syndrome (13,35). TDO syndrome is associated with a four-base deletion in the *DLX3* gene (30). Later, another two-base deletion in the *DLX3* gene was demonstrated and associated with ADHHAI (14). New studies of a family with the *DTX3* two-base deletion revealed mild expression of typical traits of TDO syndrome (hair and teeth) but either no or very mild affection of bone. Therefore, it appears that TDO syndrome is associated with deletions in the *DLX3* gene and that the molecular defect of ADHHAI with taurodontism still remains undiscovered (49).

All known diseases with a genetic component are catalogued and described in the electronic database Online Mendelian Inheritance in Man (OMIM). This can be accessed with the Entrez database searcher of the National Library of Medicine in USA (http://www.ncbi.nlm.nih.gov/sites/entrez?db=OMIM). The database contains updated genetic information about all the hereditary diseases including those with dental implications.

General treatment principles

Patients with developmental disturbances of the teeth constitute a very heterogeneous group with respect to treatment needs. The opinions and instruction from general practitioners as to when and to what extent developmental defects of enamel need treatment vary considerably. The perception of dentists is influenced by type, size, and color of the defects, and in addition dentist-related factors such as the age of the dentist (48). There is no common standard showing when it is correct to perform operative treatment. In relation to cases with mainly esthetic problems, the self-perceived opinion of the patient is of paramount importance with respect to the treatment need.

The appearance of normal enamel may vary from one individual to another with respect to color, texture, and morphology. Teeth constitute an important part of an individual's appearance and satisfaction with teeth contributes to well-being for many people. As professional health workers it is important not to strengthen the tendency in the society to judge people by the appearance of their teeth and dentists should be aware that perceptions of desirable tooth color vary among parents, dentists, and children (38). On the other hand, the dentist has to accept that the "owner" of the teeth has his or her right to dislike the appearance, but the task for the dentist is to decide whether it is within the ethics of the health profession to do the specific treatment considered. The concept of normality has a wide range also with respect to tooth color.

Treatment planning

It is important to identify and address the particular needs of each individual patient. Rapport with parents and child is essential for establishing a long-term relationship, particularly in cases with an extended treatment and follow-up period. Systematic collection of clinical experience in relation to rare dental conditions can be made in larger, more specialized clinics in which dentists treat a number of these patients. But there is also reason to claim that the general practitioner can do much of the treatment, but preferably under supervision in complex cases to ensure that the patient will receive proper treatment.

The period from diagnosis of the defect through childhood and adolescence can be divided into three phases: acute treatment, observational period, and long-term treatment.

Acute treatment

The treatment of teeth with developmental disturbances that cause pain, teeth with marked disintegration of enamel (chipping), exposed dentin, and/or extreme wear has to be taken care of as soon as possible after eruption. The overall goals of acute treatment are to relieve symptoms and prevent further disintegration of teeth and consequential problems. Diseases where such conditions can be encountered could be severe AI or DI, which as soon as the first tooth has erupted may have problems due to a heavily affected primary dentition. Exposed dentin should be protected to avoid pain and the choice of restorative materials differs with the type of dental problems. Temporary materials as intermediate restorative material (IRM) may be useful and conventional glass-ionomer cement (GIC) may also be used as semi-permanent restorations. The eruption of the permanent dentition starts at 5–7 years of age and introduces a new treatment period for the permanent first molar and the permanent front teeth in severe cases. Acute treatment will include handling of the extreme sensitivity of teeth and covering of the exposed dentin.

Young individuals who are severely affected with developmental disturbances are sometimes very sensitive to pain, and it is important to provide proper pain control which often is combined with sedation. Patients with extensive treatment need are in danger of developing dental fear (18). General anesthesia is recommended when young patients have to undergo extensive treatment. A caring attitude with respect for the integrity of the child combined with good pain control and feeling of control will help in prevention of dental fear (see Chapters 4 and 5).

Observational period

After the acute treatment is taken care of there is a transitional period when the permanent front teeth and permanent first molar should be kept under supervision and restorations are maintained according to the individual needs. In this period from about 7 to 11 years of age the major lines in the final treatment are planned. In complicated cases it is necessary to have contributions from a multidisciplinary team of specialists. In addition to the pediatric dentist, the team could consist of an orthodontist, an oral surgeon, a prosthodontist, a maxillofacial radiologist, or other specialists relevant for the specific condition. During the planning it is important to find the most appropriate time for various treatments such as tooth extractions and prosthetic therapy.

In cases where the need for treatment is extensive and may result in partial or complete prosthetic reconstruction, the child may often go through a lot of early, intermediate treatment in the primary and young permanent dentition during childhood. This may include provisional or permanent fillings, microabrasion in an attempt to remove tooth discoloration, insertion of a partial denture to replace teeth extracted early, or missing due to hypodontia, tooth retention, or eruption disturbances. In many cases there is no need for further treatment, but the teeth with disturbances have to be paid particular attention at the dental check-ups due to increased risk for caries, chipping of enamel, or attrition (Fig. 17-5).

Long-term treatment

The long-term treatment goals are a combination of a well-functioning dentition, no pain or sensation from teeth, and good aesthetics. Prosthetic work has a limited durability and a lifelong period with regular dental check-ups is needed. In cases with generalized severe disturbances full crown therapy as early as in teenage

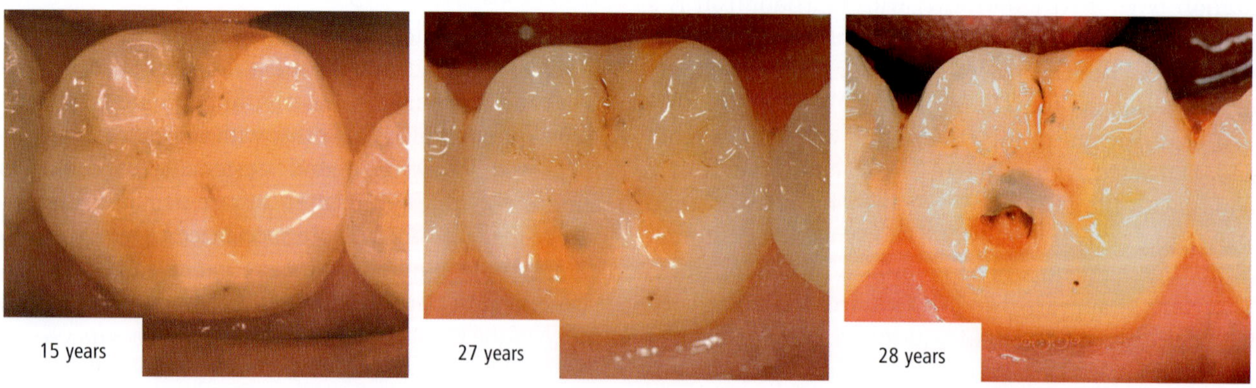

Figure 17-5 Tooth 46 with enamel disturbances probably due to preterm birth and associated health problems. Photos show 46 at three different ages illustrating that hypomineralized enamel is susceptible to wear and when dentin was exposed at 27 years of age deep caries developed during the next year. As for the rest of the dentition the patient was caries free.

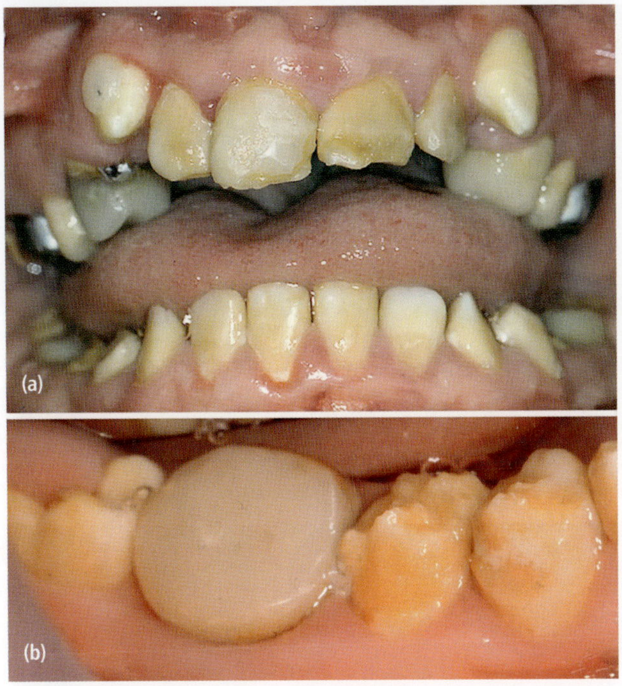

Figure 17-6 A 16-year-old boy with hypomaturation type of amelogenesis imperfecta. He has received much dental treatment and had many consultations with several general practitioners and an orthodontist without much success. Upper (a) shows gingivitis, plaque, chipping of enamel, imperfect restorations, and buccally erupting canines indicating suboptimal treatment. Lower (b) illustrates the chipping of enamel and an attempt to restore 46 which was not very successful. During the treatment, the patient developed odontophobia which partially explains the findings. Patients like this would probably be better off treated in a more specialized clinic which could take care of both the teeth and the person.

years may represent the optimal treatment. In patients with less severe tooth disturbances, a tooth-saving philosophy using adhesive techniques might be the best alternative. A good relationship between the dentist and the patient is beneficial for the clinical results, and the pediatric dentist should put particular effort into the avoidance of dental fear in these patients. In cases with complicated and extensive treatment needs it is important to be aware relative early on of the need to consult specialists within the field to obtain the best possible treatment outcome (Fig. 17-6).

Environmentally determined dental defects

Localized defects of the dental hard tissues

External damage to developing teeth

A common local *trauma* to the permanent tooth germ occurs often with avulsion or intrusive luxation in very young children when the primary incisor penetrates the unmineralized or still poorly mineralized permanent tooth (Fig. 17-7). It is useful to think of the three-dimensional localization of the primary teeth in relation to the permanent tooth buds. The root apices of the primary front teeth are placed in a more buccal position compared to the permanent teeth. A trauma to the primary teeth, which bring these into physical contact during trauma or creates an infection in the area is likely to create some kind of damage to the permanent tooth. The severity may vary from a minor opacity to a hypoplasia with missing enamel and altered morphology of crown and/or root. Another, local trauma to developing teeth may result from dental mutilation. Dental mutilation has long been an important cultural tradition in various ethnic groups around the world. Enucleation of the primary canine bud is reported among British-born Somali children, raising important health issues (34). Removal of primary teeth or attempts to remove tooth germs from their follicles with improper instruments may often damage the developing teeth (Fig. 17-8). In the study from the UK 32% of the subjects showed dental features that could indicate previous removal of canine buds.

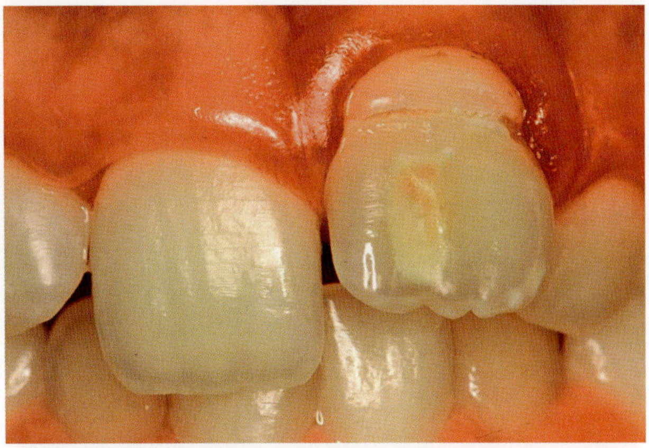

Figure 17-7 Hypoplasia of permanent maxillary left central incisors due to intrusion trauma of primary incisor at the age of 30 months (the child is now 10 years old) (courtesy of G. Koch).

A long-lasting periradicular *infection* of a primary molar may result in a range of developmental disturbances of the permanent successor (Fig. 17-9). These vary from enamel opacities to enamel hypoplasia and to arrest of development of the permanent tooth germ (10). Which of these possible and various changes in the permanent tooth occur is determined by the interaction of a number of factors, including the timing, severity, and duration of the insult in relation to the development of the permanent tooth, and the susceptibility/resistance of the host. Therapeutic *irradiation* or high-dose chemotherapy can severely disturb dental development resulting in enamel defects, microdontia, arrested root development, and agenesis of some teeth (Fig. 17-10).

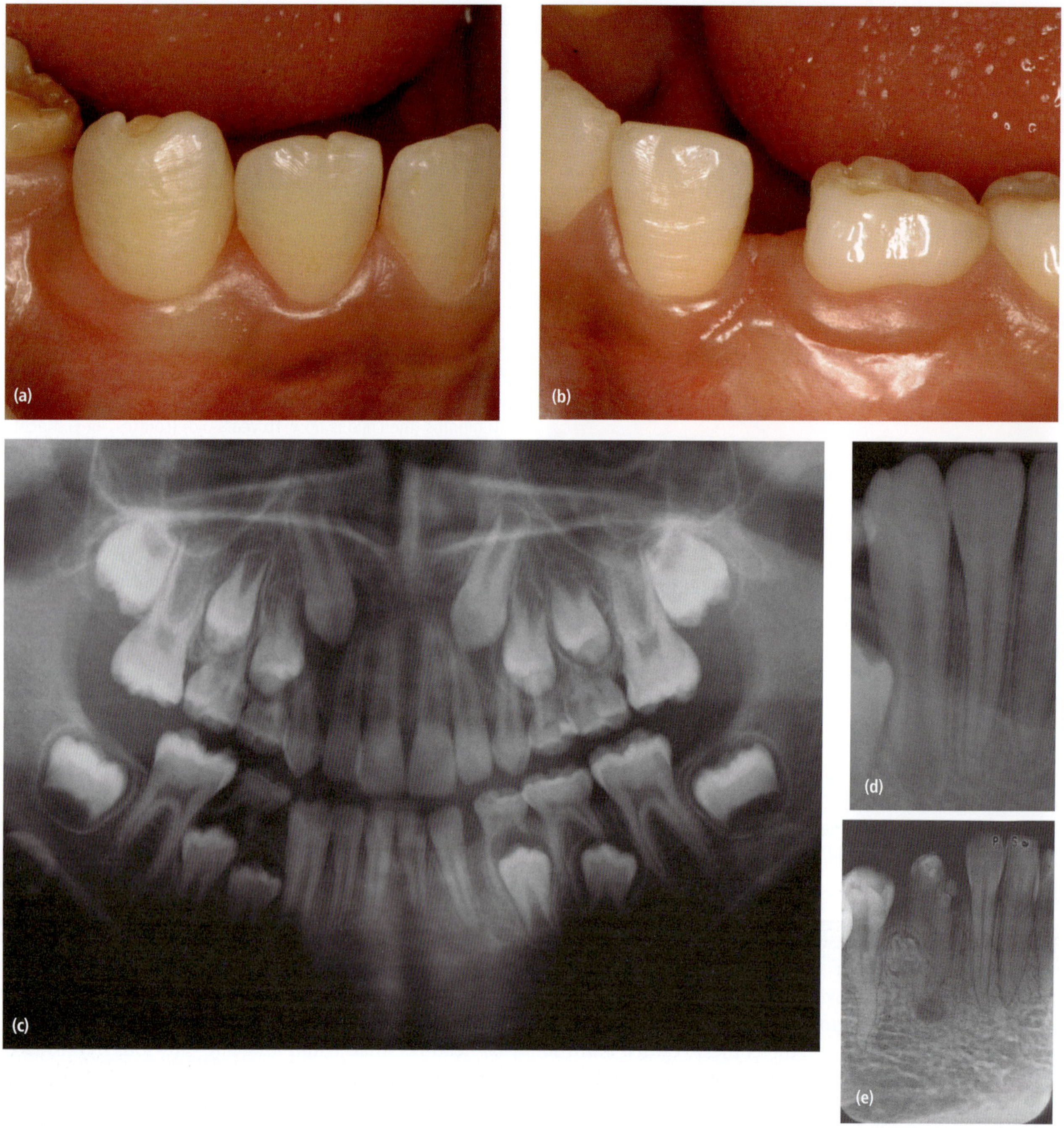

Figure 17-8 Dental mutilation resulting in (a) hypoplasia with exposure of dentin of the right lower permanent canine and (b) absence of the left lower permanent canine due to removal of the tooth germ (germectomy). (c) Panoramic radiograph shows absence of the permanent left canine. (d) Radiograph of the right lower permanent canine shows apparently normal development of the root despite the malformed tooth crown due to the damage previously performed towards the tooth germ. (e) Intraoral radiograph of a malformed and hypoplastic permanent mandibular canine in a 14-year-old Ethiopian girl as a result of dental mutilation. An odontoma on the root surface and periapical destruction are present.

Generalized defects of the dental hard tissues

Disturbances in the development of the dental hard tissues of systemic origin can occur prenatally, perinatally, postnatally, during infancy, or during early childhood. At birth, even the normal change from intrauterine to extrauterine life may have an adverse effect on amelogenesis and dentinogenesis as evidenced by the so-called neonatal line (Fig. 17-11). This pronounced incremental line is seen histologically in all primary teeth. Any stressful event during birth is likely to accentuate this line, resulting in clinically evident enamel defects.

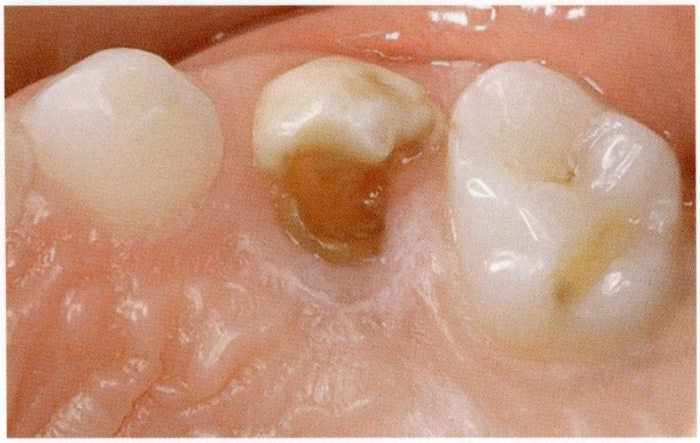

Figure 17-9 Erupting defective 24 in a 6-year-old girl who had 64 extracted 6 months earlier. The extracted tooth had a long-standing, chronic periapical periodontitis.

Other factors associated with developmental defects include ingestion of chemicals (fluoride, tetracycline, thalidomide, aromatic hydrocarbons such as polychlorinated biphenyls and dioxin); prematurity/low birthweight (Fig. 17-12); severe malnutrition, neonatal hypocalcaemia, vitamin D deficiency; bilirubinemia, thyroid and parathyroid disturbances; maternal diabetes; neonatal asphyxia; certain viral infections; and metabolic disorders.

Box 17-4 Diseases/etiologic factors which may cause chronological, symmetric distributed defects

- High-dose radiation (total body irradiation, TBI). Typically, irradiated teeth under development form V-shaped roots, and have early apical closure, and reduced root size. Combination of TBI and chemotherapy in young children lead to more severe dental disturbances (Fig. 17-10).
- Drugs:
  - chemotherapy in cancer treatment may lead to microdontia and enamel defects in some individuals
  - tetracyclines[a] given during tooth formation period result in discoloration of teeth and sometimes hypoplasia (Fig. 17-13)
  - fluoride[a] (dose dependent). Enamel changes from nearly invisible white opacities to marked discoloration and posteruptive breakdown (Figs 17-14 and 17-15).
- General infections. Dental defects typically related to stage of development. Disturbances can be hypomineralized enamel, hypoplastic defects, or combinations of these.
- Very preterm delivery (<34 weeks) and very low birthweight (<1500 g) may cause hypoplastic enamel in some individuals (Fig. 17-12).

[a] See the main text for more details about this condition.

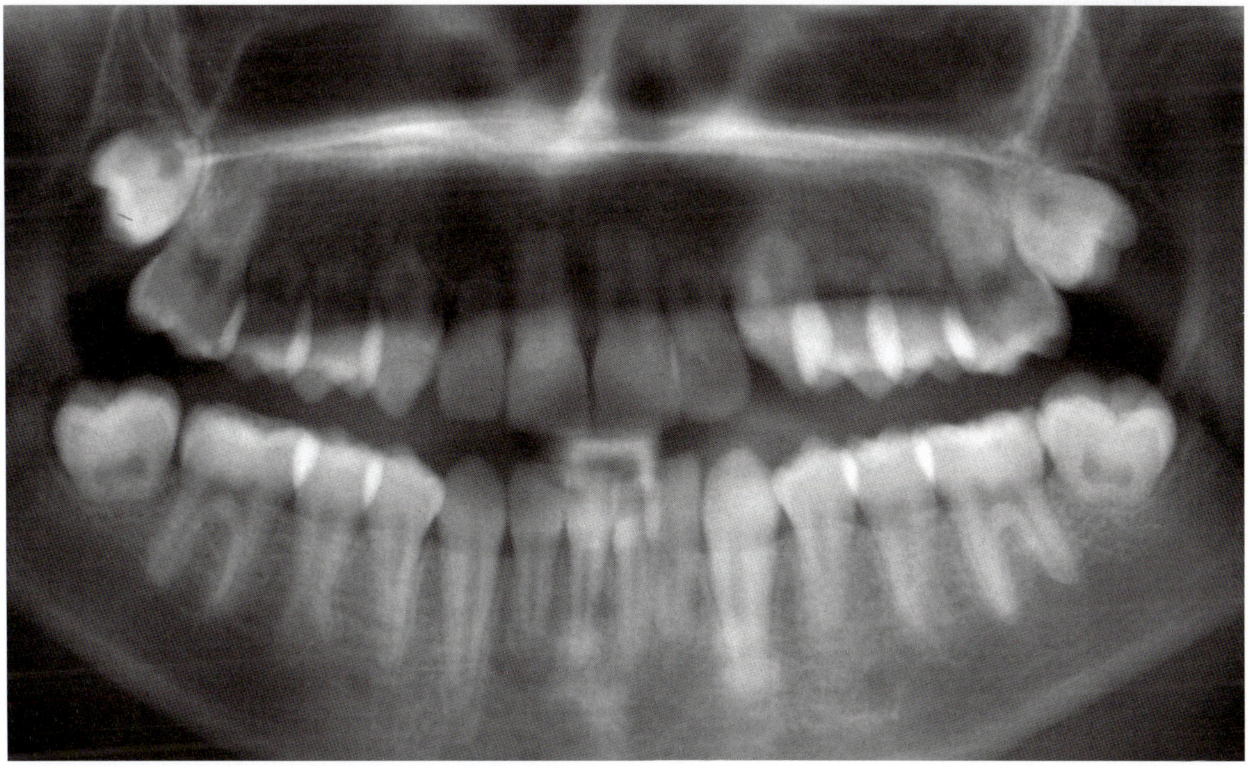

Figure 17-10 Arrested root development in a 13-year-old boy who was treated by irradiation at 7 years of age because of a rhabdomyosarcoma in nasopharynx.

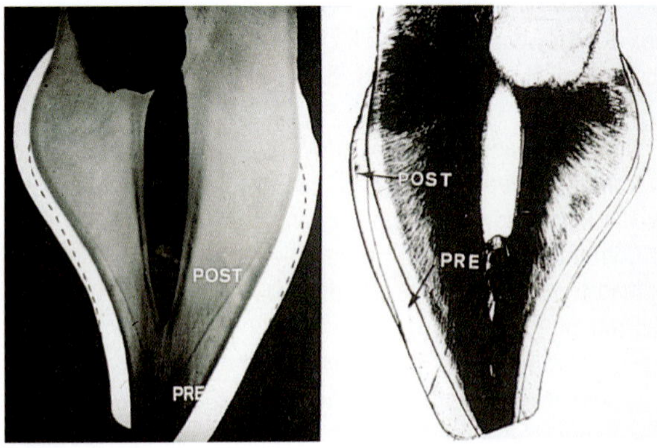

Figure 17-11 Neonatal lines of dentin (left) and enamel (right) demarcate the respective hard tissues formed/mineralized before and after birth.

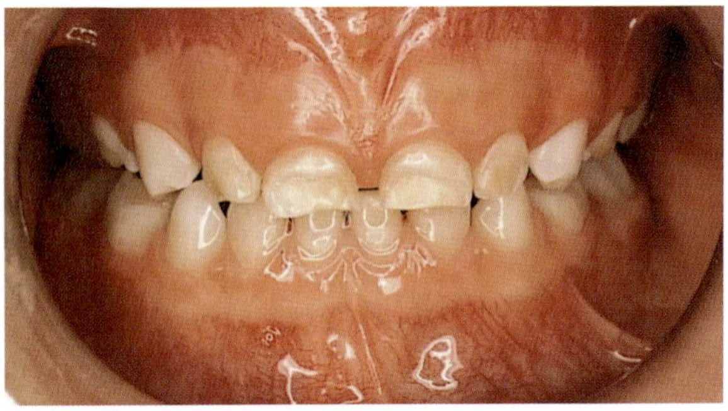

Figure 17-12 Hypoplasia of enamel of a preterm child.

This list by no means includes all the generalized environmental conditions that have been described as associated with developmental defects of the dental hard tissues. The resultant defect is generally not specific to the generalized environmental insult but depends, as with localized defects, on the timing, severity, and duration of the insult, the stage of development of the dentition, and the susceptibility of the host; and the same insult may result in different responses in different individuals. However, there are a few exceptions and among those are discolorations of teeth caused by tetracycline given during the tooth-forming period (Fig. 17-13).

Fluoride-induced defects

The presence of appropriate concentrations of fluorides in the oral environment, whether it originates from naturally occurring fluorides in the water supply or added as part of a public health program, or in oral hygiene products, e.g., toothpastes and mouthrinses, has contributed significantly to the major reduction in dental caries in industrialized countries over the past three decades. However, excess fluoride ingestion can result in enamel disturbances. Clinically, mild fluorosis appears as thin white lines following the perikymata (Fig. 17-14). In more severe cases the enamel is chalky, stains easily, and has areas of posteruptive breakdown due to the forces of abrasion or attrition (Fig. 17-15). The teeth erupt with an intact surface and the breakdown is related to areas of subsurface porosity.

It has been suggested that fluoride outside the ameloblasts decrease the concentration of free calcium ions and thereby reduces the activity of the proteases. Thus, fluoride interferes with the degradation of amelogenin, which leads to a higher content of protein in the enamel (5).

Fluoride defects have been studied in areas with naturally occurring high concentrations of fluoride in the water supply. Children who swallowed fluoride toothpaste during early infancy, when the amelogenesis was still proceeding, can also have enamel opacities. This is also seen in populations where fluoride tablets are used frequently. The differential diagnosis of these opacities can be difficult as some hypomaturation types of AI may clinically resemble fluorosis. Anamnestic information is crucial for a correct diagnosis.

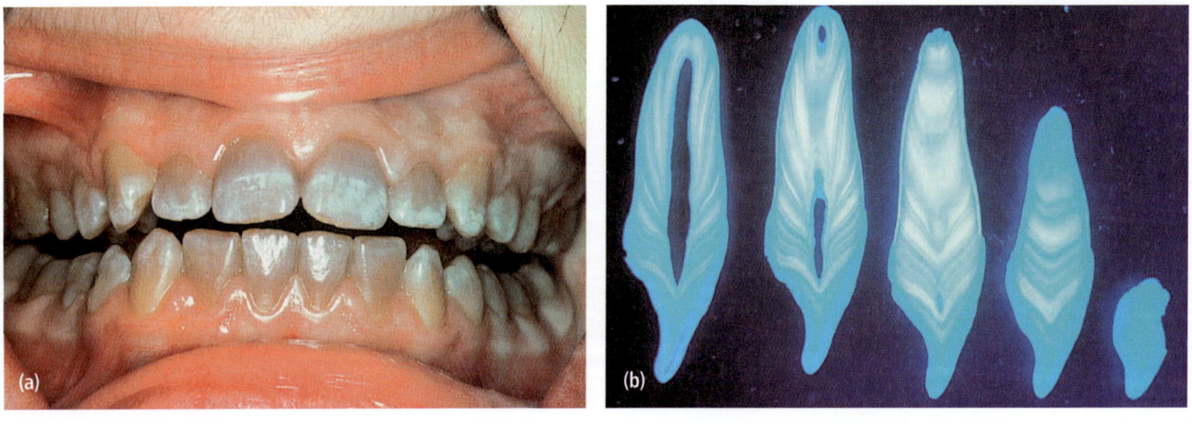

Figure 17-13 (a) A 14-year-old girl with cystic fibrosis who was treated with repeated courses of tetracyclines for recurrent chest infection. (b) Histologic sections of a tooth showing the bands of tetracycline staining (courtesy of R.W. Fearnhead).

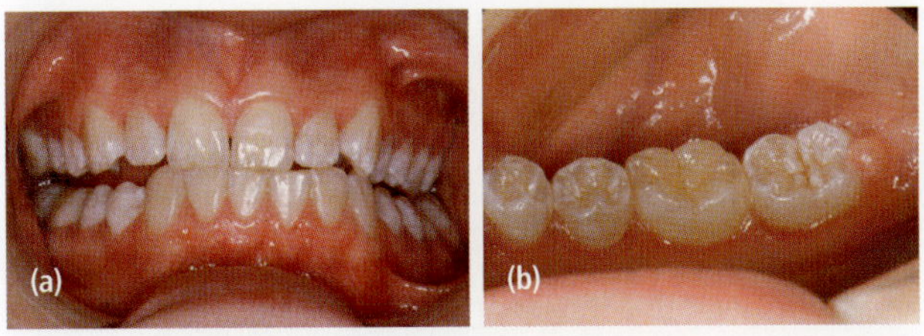

Figure 17-14 Mild fluorosis in a 15-year-old girl.

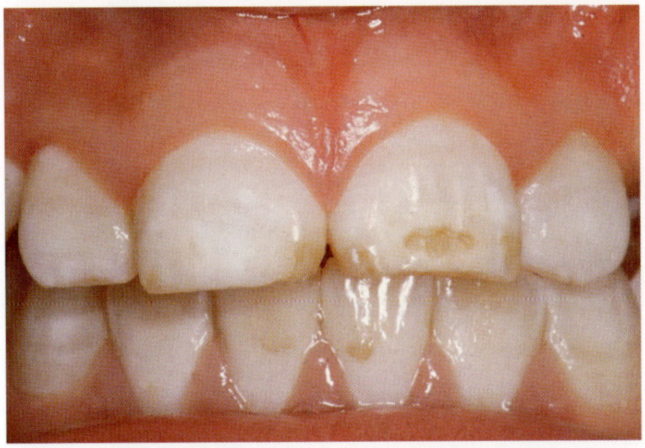

Figure 17-15 Dental fluorosis with posteruptive breakdown of the enamel and tooth wear in a 12-year-old boy with natural high (≈5 ppm) fluoride concentration in the drinking water.

Tetracycline defects

Tetracycline has a strong affinity to mineralized tissues, primarily to dentin and bone. Tetracycline oxidation occurs on exposure to light. Since dentin is not remodeled, the dentin defects are persistent. The discolored horizontal bands may appear gray, bluish, or, in natural light, the teeth may all have grayish appearance. The discolored enamel usually has some translucency left. The severity of the defect depends on the time of exposure in relation to the stage of tooth development, duration of exposure, dosage, and the type of tetracycline preparation. Repeated exposure gives rise to series of bands of tetracycline bound to dentin and within the enamel (Fig. 17-13). As tetracycline may cause discoloration of teeth these antibiotics should not be prescribed to children below the age of 8 years, pregnant women, and lactating mothers.

Molar–incisor hypomineralization

Demarcated opacities in the permanent first molars are common in many child populations. Epidemiological studies have found prevalence estimates up to 20–25%. The first permanent molars are particularly affected, but the permanent incisors are often also involved. In the literature, this condition has had many denominations as hypomineralized permanent first molars, idiopathic enamel hypomineralization, nonfluoride hypomineralization in permanent first molars, and cheese molars. In 2001, the denomination molar–incisor hypomineralization (MIH) was proposed and is currently widely used, even though the logic of the terminology of the condition may be disputed (43).

The enamel defects can be present in one to four first molars and one or more incisors are often also affected concomitantly. Similar lesions can be seen in the second deciduous molars and in the cuspal parts of the permanent canines, as these teeth are mineralizing in the same period of time as the molars and incisors. The degree of disturbance in the molars varies from creamy-white spots, with a hard, well-mineralized surface, to yellowish-brown discoloration and enamel disintegration. The defects in the incisors are described as creamy-white, sometimes yellowish-brown spots. The number of affected teeth varies and the enamel spots do not always appear symmetrically (Fig. 17-16). Histomorphological studies of the enamel in affected permanent first molars reveal areas of porosity in the occlusal half of the crown of varying degrees. The enamel in the cervical half of the crown is most often well mineralized (20). The yellowish-brown defects are more porous than the creamy-white demarcated opacities and extend through the whole enamel layer, while creamy-white demarcated opacities are situated in the inner parts of the enamel (Fig. 17-17).

The most severely affected molars often show disintegration of the enamel in the occlusal parts (Fig. 17-18). These teeth create problems for the patients as well as for the dentists. Children often report shooting pain when they are brushing their teeth or even breathing cold air, often already shortly after the eruption of the affected teeth has started. At dental examination, the children most often open their mouths reluctantly, and react intensely to air blowing. The severely affected teeth are in need of restoration soon after eruption due to disintegrated enamel and subsequent caries (18,24).

The etiology of MIH has not yet been fully understood. There have been some suggestions of possible etiologic factors. The clinical appearance indicates some specific environmental influence on the development of enamel during a limited period of time. Exposures to dioxins from breast milk as well as medical problems related to birth, and to respiratory diseases during the first 3 years of life have been reported to be related to the frequency and severity of enamel defects in permanent first molars. However, those factors cannot explain all cases (2,21).

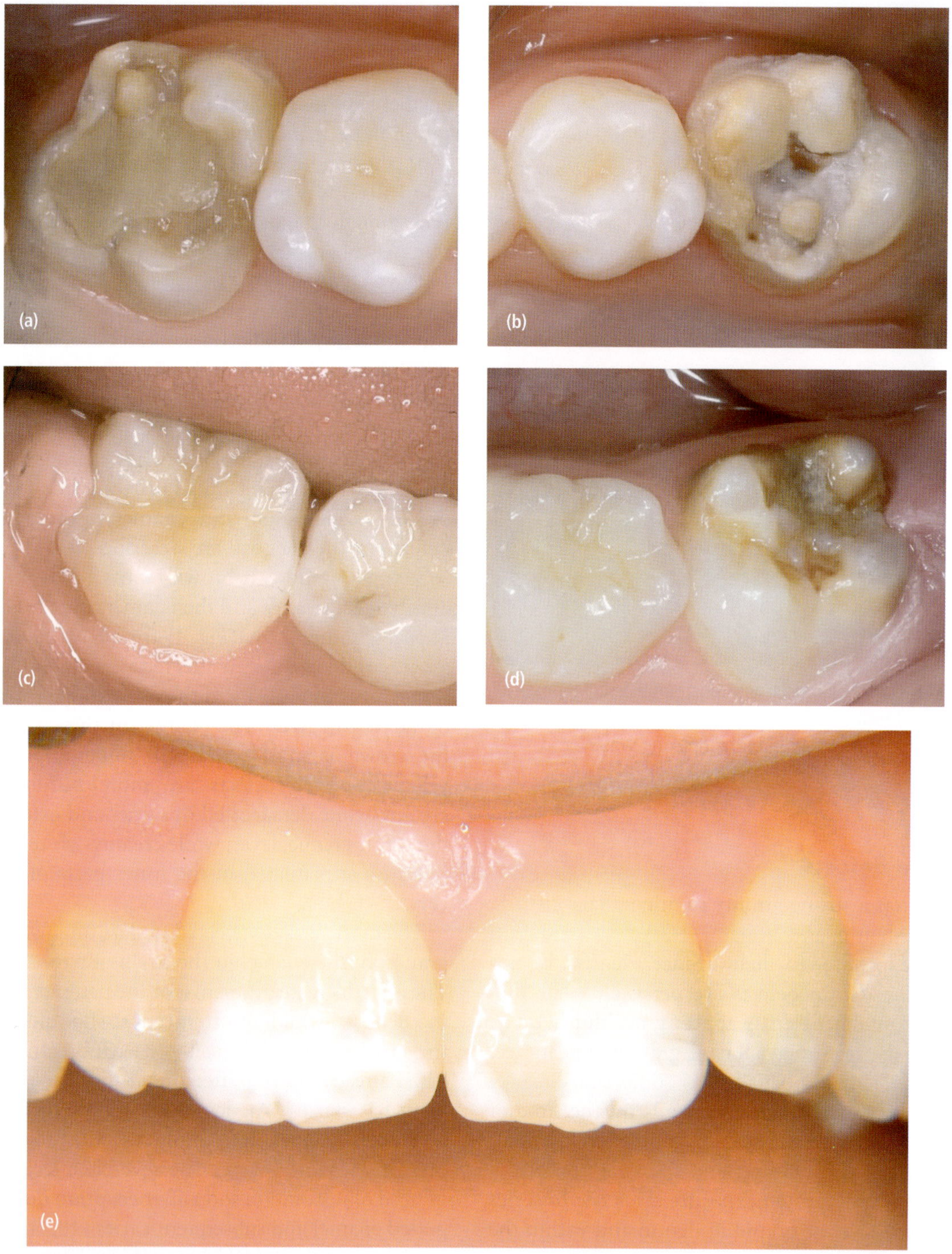

Figure 17-16 MIH in an 8-year-old boy showing different manifestations in similar teeth: (a) 16 with a defective restoration; (b) 26 with seriously disintegrated enamel and caries; the tooth is very sensitive and toothbrushing is impossible; (c) 46 healthy; (d) 36 disintegrated enamel, but no frank cavitation; (e) demarcated white opacities in the upper front teeth.

Inherited defects of the enamel

Amelogenesis imperfecta

AI is a genetic disease characterized by clinical as well as genetic heterogeneity (11,16,40,49) (Fig. 17-19 and Box 17-5). Crawford *et al.* (11) have defined the disease: "AI represents a group of conditions, genomic in origin, which affect the structure and clinical appearance of the enamel of all or nearly all the teeth in a more or less equal manner, and which may be associated with morphologic or biochemical changes elsewhere in the body. AI is a developmental condition of the dental enamel

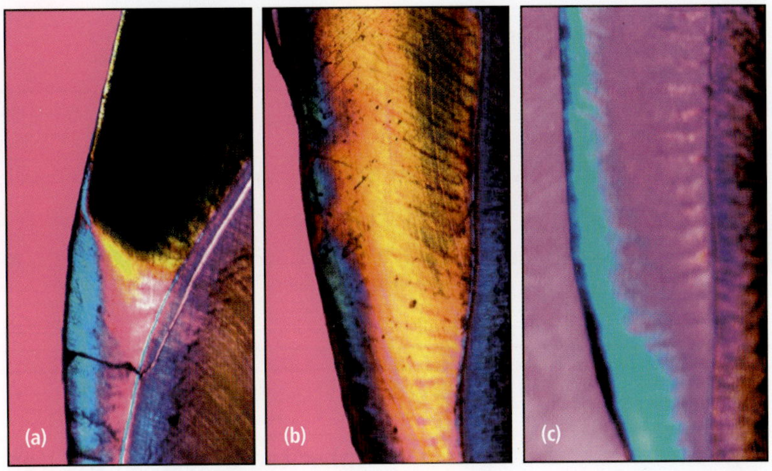

Figure 17-17 Ground sections of permanent first molars in polarized light microscopy: (a) clinically yellow–brown defects extending through the whole enamel layer; (b) clinically white–cream opacities are situated in the inner parts of the enamel; (c) clinically normal enamel.

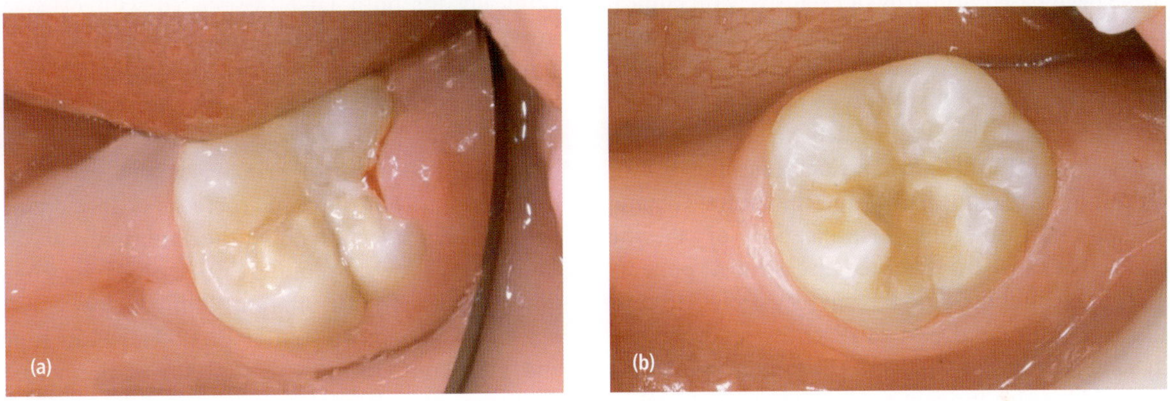

Figure 17-18 (a) A severely hypomineralized lower first molar is erupting. Normal morphology. (b) Heavy disintegration 6 months later.

(characterized by hypoplasia and/or hypomineralization) that shows autosomal dominant, autosomal recessive, sexlinked and sporadic inheritance patterns, as well as sporadic cases."

AI is caused by mutations in the genes controlling the amelogenesis and follows patterns of autosomal dominant, autosomal recessive, or X-linked inheritance (Box 17-6). Occasionally, new mutations occur in genes controlling the amelogenesis and in such cases a family history or pattern of inheritance relevant to the disease may not be possible to identify. AI is seen in both the primary and the permanent dentition (Figs 17-19 and 17-20). The disease may be less clinically evident in the primary dentition in some AI variants.

Different prevalence figures have been reported in different parts of the world, from one in 14,000 in Michigan, USA, to one in 700 in the north of Sweden. The majority of reports in the literature are descriptions of cases and only a few epidemiological studies providing prevalence data are available (7,41,46).

The clinical picture of AI is highly variable and numerous variants have been described (47). Dental literature has focused on three main types, one named hypoplastic type (Fig. 17-19e–g) and two hypomineralized types, called hypomaturated (Fig. 17-19a–c) and hypocalcified types (Fig. 17-19d). Further, a fourth type mixing hypoplastic and hypomaturated traits (Fig. 17-19h) and, in addition, characterized by taurodontism has been mentioned in the literature (45,47). The characteristics of the three main types of AI are given in Boxes 17-9–17-11. In the majority of teeth with AI the mineral content is lower than in unaffected teeth. Even in AI teeth characterized by hypoplasia, various degrees of hypomineralization in areas of the enamel are found (6). As mentioned above, taurodontism may be a feature in some variants of AI. There is an association between AI and anterior

Box 17-5 Genes with mutations associated with amelogenesis imperfecta

Causative gene	Gene encoding	Component	Role	Association between inheritance patterns and mutations in genes
AMELX	Amelogenin	Enamel matrix protein	Essential for normal enamel formation	X-linked
ENAM	Enamelin	Enamel protein	Structural protein secreted by ameloblasts	Autosomal dominant
MMP20	Enamelysin	Matrix metalloprotease	Expressed by ameloblasts and involved in development of enamel	Autosomal recessive
KLK4	Kallikrien four	Serine protease	Involved in development of enamel	Autosomal recessive

open bite of skeletal origin, but no exact reason for this co-occurrence has been found. In some cases of AI delayed eruption and/or retention of teeth are seen (Box 17-7).

The numerous classification systems suggested over time have been based primarily or exclusively on clinical manifestation (phenotype). In the 1990s, classification of AI based on the molecular defect, biochemical results, mode of inheritance, and phenotype was suggested (3). The intense research activity related to understanding the genetics of AI will inevitably increase the use of genetic testing in diagnostics of AI in the future. Genetic counseling and molecular identification of specific mutations that cause the inherited disease in AI patients and their families may be more easily accessible and turn out to be an integrated part of diagnosis of AI in the future. The increasing body of information on the genetics of AI is also thought to be an integrated part of the classification of AI in the future (49).

A number of mutations in genes involved in the amelogenesis have been described, and data on phenotype–genotype correlations are increasing even though each genotype is not correlated to a specific phenotype, meaning that more than one genotype can result in apparently undistinguishable phenotypes. To date, mutations associated with AI have been identified in four genes (AMELX, ENAM, KLK4, and MMP20) known to be involved in enamel formation (Box 17-5) (11,16,40,49). The relatively high number of mutations and deletions in genes involved in the amelogenesis demonstrated so far displays the complexity in the genetic heterogeneity and phenotypic diversity of AI. Further, more genes than the ones already described are most likely to contribute to the etiology of AI (23).

Inherited defects of the dentin

Dentinogenesis imperfecta

Shields *et al.* (37) have subgrouped three different types of DI (Box 17-10). Dentinogenesis is affected in all types. Clinically for both DI-I (associated with osteogenesis imperfecta, OI) and DI-II, primary teeth tend to be more severely affected than permanent teeth. Later formed permanent teeth are less severely affected than early formed ones. The teeth are opalescent with bluish-brown discoloration of primary as well as permanent teeth. Enamel has often microcracks or infractions and tends to chip away, exposing the abnormal, soft dentin. Thus, the teeth wear rapidly. Primary teeth may be worn down to the gingival margin within a few years after eruption if not protected (Fig. 17-21). Pulp exposure and pulp complications may occur. In the permanent dentition, pulpal involvement is rare due to the rapid obliteration of the pulp chambers. The crowns appear bulbous and the roots are often short and thin on radiographs (Fig. 17-22). Initially, normal pulp chambers obliterate soon after eruption and root canals are gradually narrowed. Among patients with mild signs of OI, examination for dental defects may contribute towards establishing the final, medical diagnosis (27).

DI is a single-gene disorder. Even though the phenotypes of DI-I and DI-II are similar, the genetics associated with the respective types differ. While DI-II has an inheritance pattern which is autosomal dominant with high penetrance, OI (DI-I) is a genetically heterogeneous group of generalized connective tissue diseases. The vast majority of known mutations related to OI are located in the genes encoding the two type I procollagen chains. The main clinical symptom of OI is bone fragility, but

Figure 17-19 (opposite) Clinical manifestation of amelogenesis imperfecta. (a) Hypomaturation type (generalized white opacities with brownish discolorations on upper central incisors). (b) Hypomaturation type (generalized yellowish opacities). (c) Hypomaturation type. (d) Hypocalcified type. (e) Hypoplastic type (rough, pitted). (f) Hypoplastic type (rough, vertical grooves). (g) Hypoplastic type (rough, thin enamel) (courtesy of J. Daugaard-Jensen). (h) Combination of hypomaturation and hypoplastic type (courtesy of J. Daugaard-Jensen).

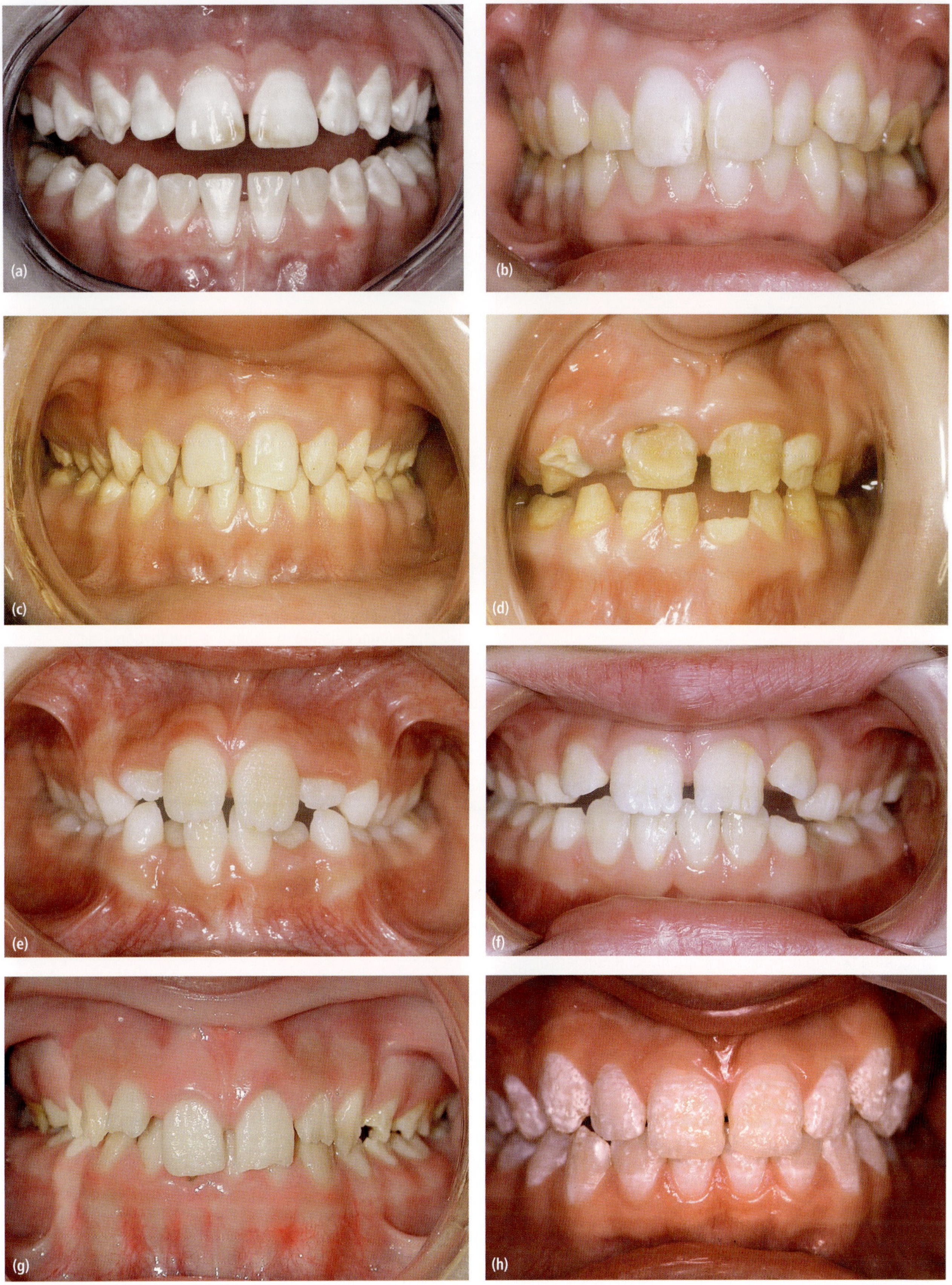
(a)
(b)
(c)
(d)
(e)
(f)
(g)
(h)

Box 17-6 Autosomal dominant inheritance

One of the parents will have the mutant gene (A) and will have the disease. Each child born will have a 50% risk of getting the disease. In autosomal dominant inheritance both males and females are affected in approximately equal numbers. Family members are affected in each generation and males can transmit the condition to males or females and vice versa. Unaffected people do not transmit the condition. Expression of the disease may vary in individuals carrying the same mutant gene.

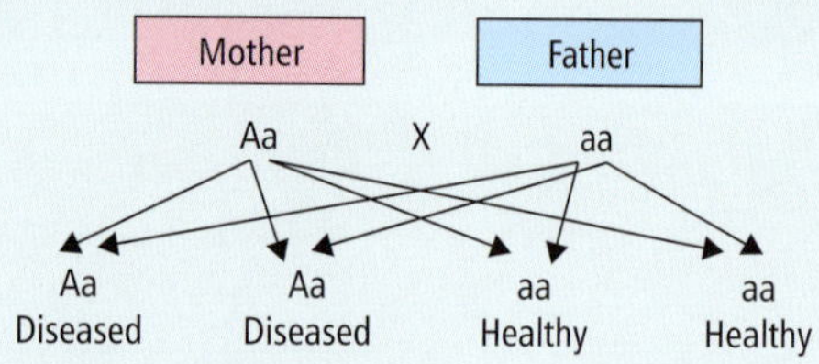

Autosomal recessive inheritance

Both parents have the mutant gene (b) (carriers), but do not have the disease. For each child there is a 50% risk for being carrier of the mutant gene without having the disease. There is a 25% risk for the child to be diseased (received the mutant gene from both parents) and 25% that the child is healthy and does not carry the mutant gene. In autosomal recessive inheritance each sex is affected with equal frequency and severity.

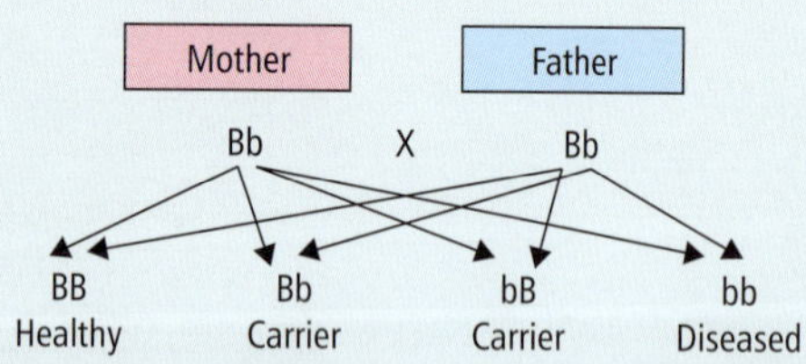

X-linked inheritance

This pattern of inheritance can be both recessive and dominant. Generally more males than females are affected. Males are uniformly affected while females affected will have the disease with varying expression due to the effect of lyonization (X-chromosome inactivation). All daughters of diseased males will be carriers if recessive inheritance and diseased if dominant inheritance. If the mother is carrying the diseased gene then 50% of daughters will be carriers if the inheritance pattern is X-linked recessive and 50% of daughters will be affected if the pattern is X-linked dominant.

Lyonization

In normal female cells, one of the X chromosomes is inactivated early in embryonic life, so that there is only one functional X chromosome per cell as in males. The outcome of this inactivation is that a woman is a mosaic of cells regarding expression of her X chromosome. Thus, the enamel may display alternating vertical bands of imperfect and normal enamel which can be found in X-linked forms of AI.

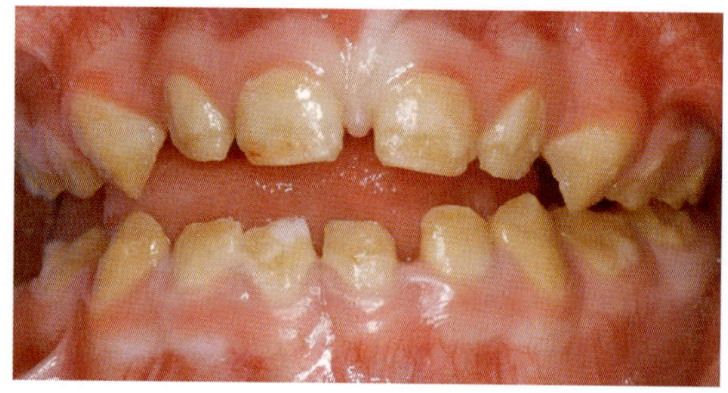

Figure 17-20 Hypocalcified AI in the primary dentition of a 3-year-old girl.

Box 17-7 Characteristics of hypoplastic AI

Hypoplastic enamel is pathologically thin enamel varying from some pits/grooves to generalized thin enamel in the dentition:

- it is a quantitative defect of enamel, i.e., enamel that does not reach normal thickness either locally or generally
- enamel may be rough, smooth, pitted, grooved, locally hypoplastic or the complete tooth crown appears with thin enamel
- teeth often do not meet in an approximal contact point if the enamel mantle in general is thin (hypoplastic)
- eruption disturbances may occur, i.e., delayed eruption or impacted teeth are seen
- an anterior open bite of skeletal origin may occur
- radiographically, most often normal radiographic contrast of enamel and dentin
- in families with X-linked inheritance, females may show normal and hypoplastic enamel alternating in a vertical pattern due to lyonization.

Box 17-8 Characteristics of hypomaturation AI

Hypomaturation forms of AI have enamel with increased content of proteins. This is clinically evident as deviant color (opaque enamel):

- it is a qualitative defect of the enamel, i.e., the enamel is insufficiently mineralized either locally or generally
- normal form of the teeth at the time of eruption, but enamel may chip away posteruptively, especially in the incisal–occlusal areas
- opaque white to yellow–brown discoloration of enamel
- radiographically there is reduced differentiation between enamel and dentin
- in families with X-linked inheritance, females may have vertical stripes of opaque enamel altering with bands of normal enamel due to lyonization.

Box 17-9 Characteristics of hypocalcified AI

Hypocalcified forms of AI have enamel with very high content of proteins, discoloration, and rough and soft texture:

- it is a qualitative defect of enamel, i.e., the enamel is insufficiently mineralized and soft
- more severely hypomineralized than the hypomaturated type
- yellow to yellow–brown color of enamel
- early loss of enamel due to severe hypomineralization
- normal amount of enamel at eruption, but wears quickly away posteruptively
- minimal contact between teeth
- teeth may erupt with delay
- an anterior open bite of skeletal origin may be seen
- often accumulation of a large amount of supragingival calculus
- pronounced thermal sensitivity
- radiographically there is a lack of contrast between enamel and dentin.

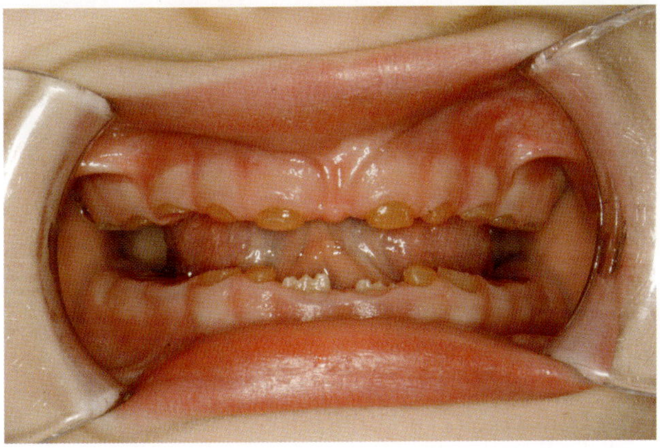

Figure 17-21 A 5-year-old child with DI showing extreme tooth wear in the primary molars. No operative treatment has been offered so far, although the child would have benefited from stainless-steel crowns in the molar regions to keep the occlusion. Permanent lower central incisors are in eruption.

Box 17-10 Hereditary dentin defects: genetic basis (15,22,25)

Highly specialized odontoblast cells secrete the dentin extracellular matrix. Important information about the genetic regulation of this process has been revealed during the past decade. Molecular analysis of humans with dentin disease and testing in transgenic gene knock-out models has given an insight into the role which major dentin extracellular proteins play in the formation of dentin. In addition to the production of different types of collagen, the dentin-forming odontoblast and the bone-forming osteoblast produce noncollagenous proteins. In the last group are also five glycoproteins (SIBLINGS: small integrin-binding ligand N-linked glycoproteins), which are involved in bone and dentin formation. They are the primary candidate genes for isolated, inherited defects of dentin and form a cluster on chromosome 4q21-q25.

In Box 17-3 based on Shields *et al.*'s (37) classification, two major groups (DI and DD) are defined. From a molecular etiological point of view these two entities are not logical because genetic studies have identified the human chromosome 4q21 as loci for DI-II, DI-III, and DD-II. It is suggested that these three dentin diseases are allelic. It is important to follow patients over time to observe radiographically the pulp chambers and root canals with respect to obliteration. MacDougall *et al.* (25) speculate that altered or abnormal levels of dentin sialoprotein (DSP), which is derived from DSPP, may cause abnormal dentin matrix mineralization and discolorations. These findings are related to both DI-II and DD-II.

The phenotypes seen in DI may also be seen in other conditions and syndromes (22). An example is Ehlers–Danlos syndrome (EDS) which is a heterogeneous group of inherited disorders of connective tissue. Major features are tissue fragility, bruising of the skin, and hypermobility of the joints. Some forms of EDS have dentin defects similar to DD-I and DI-II.

In humans with dentin defects, mutation only in dentin sialophosphoprotein (DSPP) has been demonstrated. So far all reports indicate an autosomal dominant pattern of inheritance. Nine different DSPP mutations, which are related to dentin disease, are reported (15,25) and clinically the associated phenotype represents a continuum from the mild end (DD-III) to the most severe defects (DI-III).

the disease may affect sclera, tendons, meninges, dentin, and dermis (Fig. 17-23). Bones may break spontaneously and for no known reason. OI can also cause weak muscles, a curved spine, and hearing loss. OI is subdivided into four types of different severity.

Dentin dysplasia

According to Shields' classification (Box 17-3) there are two types of DD. Type I (DD-I) is also called radicular dentin dysplasia or rootless teeth and is an incomplete tooth formation. Clinically, tooth crowns appear normal, but radiographic examination will often show incomplete root formation and a conical or missing root. In addition, periapical lesions in relation to teeth without caries are typical. Total obliteration of pulp chambers of primary teeth usually occurs. In permanent teeth crescent-shaped pulpal remnants of crown pulp may be seen on radiographs. Further, tooth exfoliation may occur.

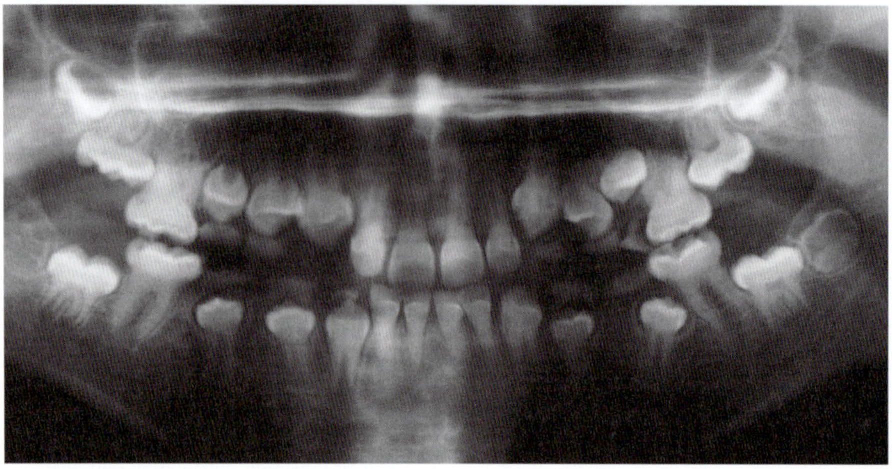

Figure 17-22 Panoramic radiograph of a 10-year-old boy with DI inherited as a single trait (type II). Note the obliterated pulp chambers and the cervical constrictions of the crowns.

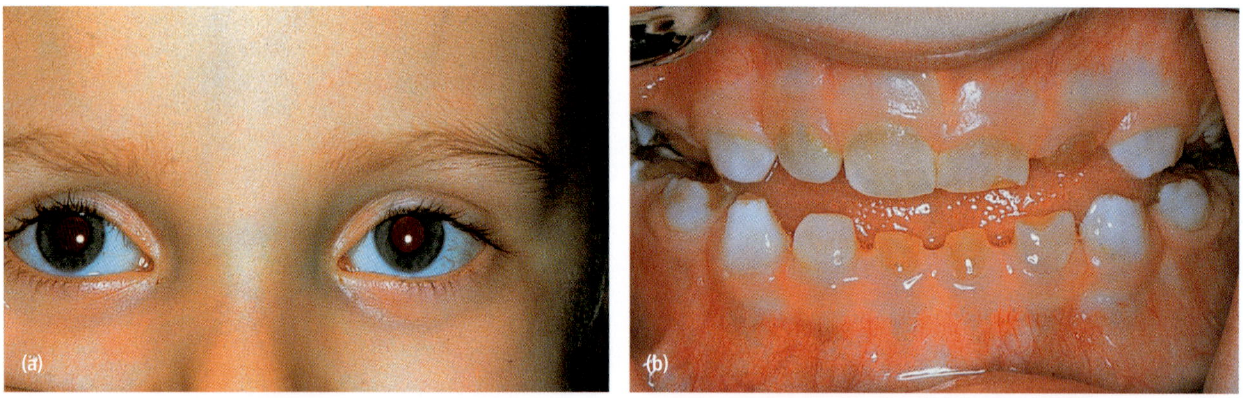

Figure 17-23 Osteogenesis imperfecta. (a) Blue sclerae in a 4-year-old boy. (b) Characteristic dentin defect (DI type I) in the same boy.

It is a rare autosomal dominant condition (one in 100,000), but so far it is unknown if the condition is also an allelic disorder of dentin sialophosphoprotein (DSPP) gene (22).

DD type II (DD-II) is a rare autosomal dominant condition which is also called coronal dentin dysplasia. The findings are different in the two dentitions. The primary dentition is opalescent with a gray or brownish discoloration as seen in DI. Pulp obliteration is seen on radiographs in primary teeth, while the permanent teeth appear to be normal. However, thistle-tube pulp chambers with pulp stones are seen radiographically (Fig. 17-24). There is reason to believe, from a genetic point of view, that DD-II and DI-II and III phenotypes are the same disease, but of different severity (22). DD-II is the mild form, and DI-III the most severe type. It is suggested that these three dentin defects (DI-II and III, and DD-II) should be called DSPP-associated dentin defects (15).

Disturbances in calcium/phosphate metabolism with relevance to mineralization of teeth

Rickets

Vitamin D deficiency has been called rickets. The sources of this fat-soluble vitamin (prohormone) are either diet or production in sun-exposed skin. Vitamin D regulates the absorption of calcium from the jejunum and is very important for the mineralization of bone and dental hard tissue. Hypocalcemia leads to skeletal and dental deformities, etc. Rickets affects the structural organization of enamel and the mineralization. Teeth have typical chronological symmetric hypoplastic defects related to the time period when the hypocalcemia was prominent. Dental hard tissue formed before and after that period is normal (Fig. 17-25).

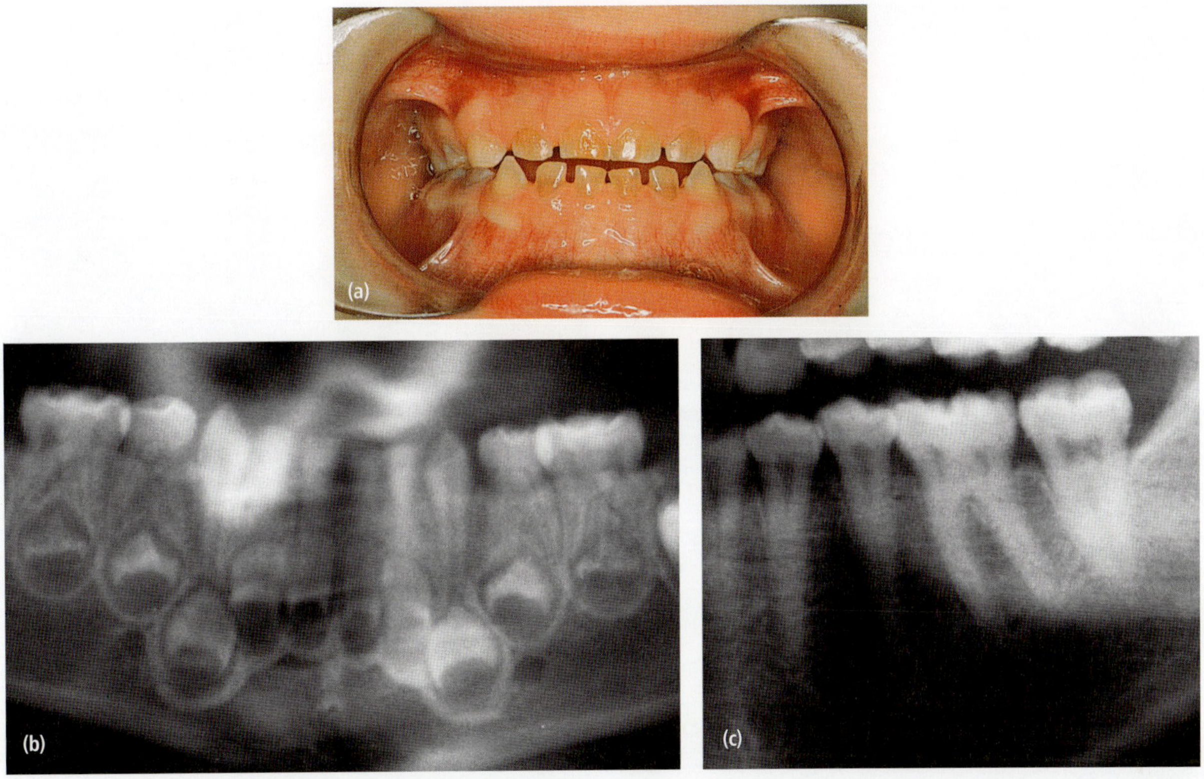

Figure 17-24 Dentin dysplasia type II. (a) A 3-year-old boy with DD type II. (b) Panoramic radiograph showing pulpal obliteration in the primary molars. (c) Radiograph of the mother showing characteristic thistle-tube-shaped pulp chambers and narrowed root canals.

Box 17-11 Some systemic diseases and genetically determined diseases and syndromes associated with defects of the dental hard tissues

- Osteogenesis imperfecta.[a]
- Disturbances in calcium and phosphate metabolism:
  - rickets[a] (vitamin D deficiency) (Fig. 17-25)
  - familial hypophosphatemia[a] (inborn error of metabolism) (Fig. 17-26)
  - celiac disease[a] (malnourishment and calcium deficiency due to malabsorption in the small intestine).
- Hypophosphatasia (inborn error of metabolism) is a rare autosomal recessive condition which results in low activity of alkaline phosphatase. Common symptoms include defective bone and teeth and higher chance of bone fracture. Hypophosphatasia may lead to premature loss of primary teeth, due to disturbed cementum formation (Fig. 17-40). Dentin is not affected (42).
- Hyperbilirubinemia may lead to irreversible brain damage (kernicterus) due to deposition of bilirubin in the brain and spinal cord, accompanied by nerve cell degeneration. Hyperbilirubinemia is associated with liver disease and biliary obstruction. Bilirubin may cause extensive discoloration while deposited in teeth. Often seen in combination with hypoplasia.
- Ehlers–Danlos syndrome is a rare, genetic disorder affecting collagen synthesis. The disease has several variants of different severity. Typical are loose joints (e.g., in the temporomandibular joint) and hyperextensible skin. Advanced periodontal disease is associated with type VIII. The dental changes are hypoplastic areas in the enamel and abnormal dentin, which may be similar to that of radicular dentin dysplasia. The dentin may have vascular inclusions and incorporated denticles. Radiographs show stunted and deformed roots and pulp calcifications, particularly at the midpoint of the root canal.
- Epidermolysis bullosa (EB) is a rare genetic, bullous disorder with extremely fragile skin and is characterized by blister formation in response to mechanical trauma. Generalized enamel hypoplasia is common; the highest prevalence is seen in junctional EB.
- Tuberous sclerosis is a rare, incurable genetic disorder. The disease leads to benign tumors in many vital organs such as brain, heart, kidneys, skin, lungs, and eyes. Mental retardation, autism, and seizure are other symptoms. Most patients have enamel pitting in their teeth (both dentitions).
- Tricho-dento-osseous syndrome. An enamel defect involving hypomaturation and hypoplasia associated with taurodontism has been described in association with tight curly hair and dense bone.

[a] See the main text for more details about this condition.

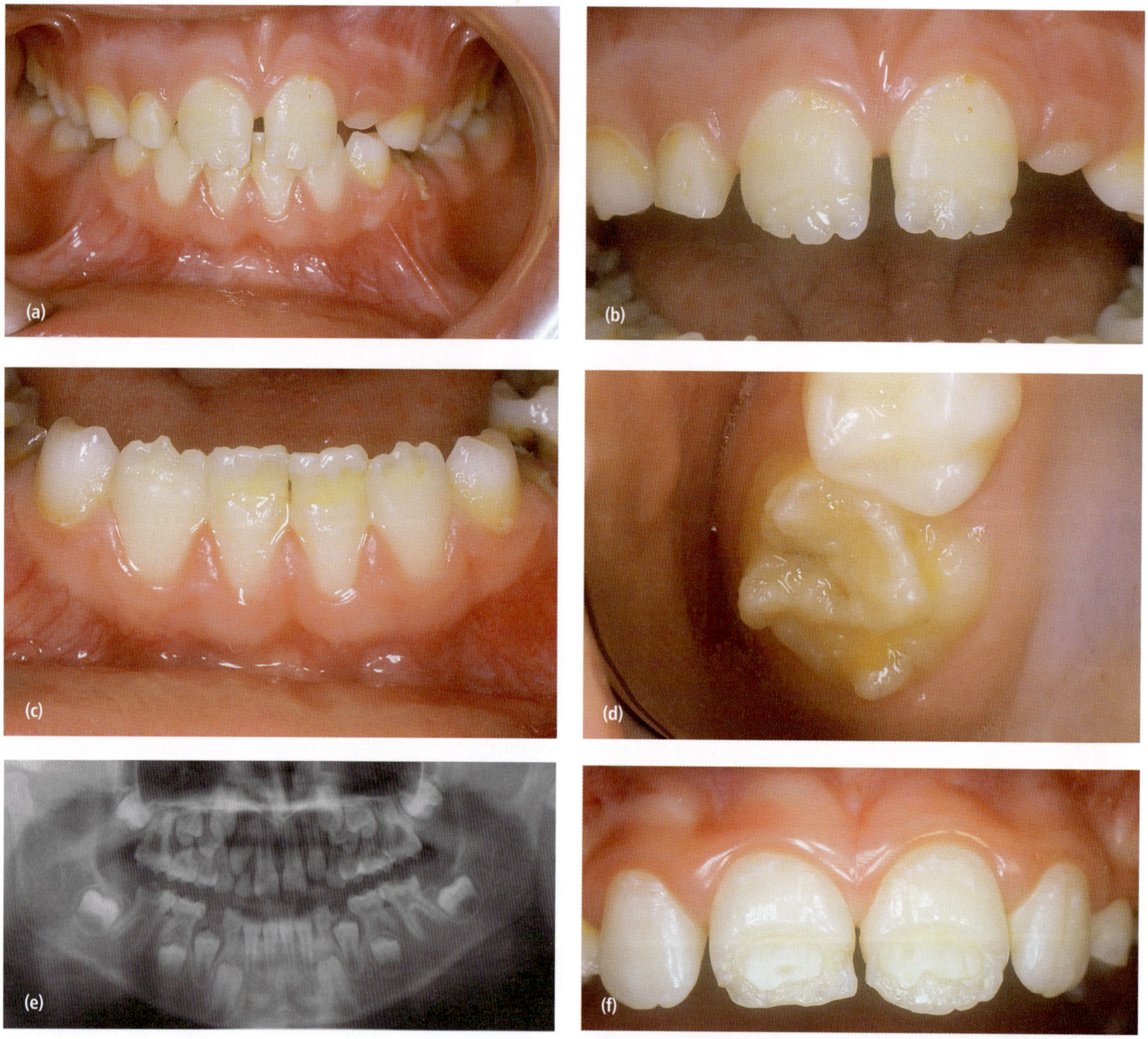

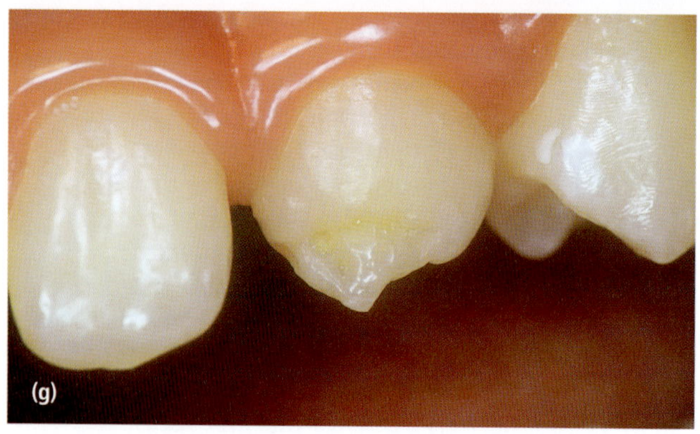

Figure 17-25 Vitamin D deficiency rickets (nutritional rickets). (a–d) Chronological and symmetrical hypoplasia in permanent incisors and first molars in a breastfed 8-year-old boy who was not given a vitamin D supplement in the first year of life. (e) Defects can often be seen on a panoramic radiograph. (f) An 11-year-old boy with severe hypoplasia on upper permanent incisors due to vitamin D deficiency rickets. Areas in the lesions are often white or yellow. (g) Often cusp tips of permanent canines are also affected.

Vitamin D-resistant rickets (familial hypophosphatemia)

Familial hypophosphatemia is a rare inherited disorder characterized by impaired reabsorption of phosphate in the kidneys leading to low levels of phosphate in serum. It is most often inherited as an X-linked trait. Dentin has globular defects and is hypomineralized with enlargement of the pulp. Bacterial invasion through enamel cracks and dentinal defects of the teeth may lead to abscesses arising from seemingly sound teeth (Fig. 17-26).

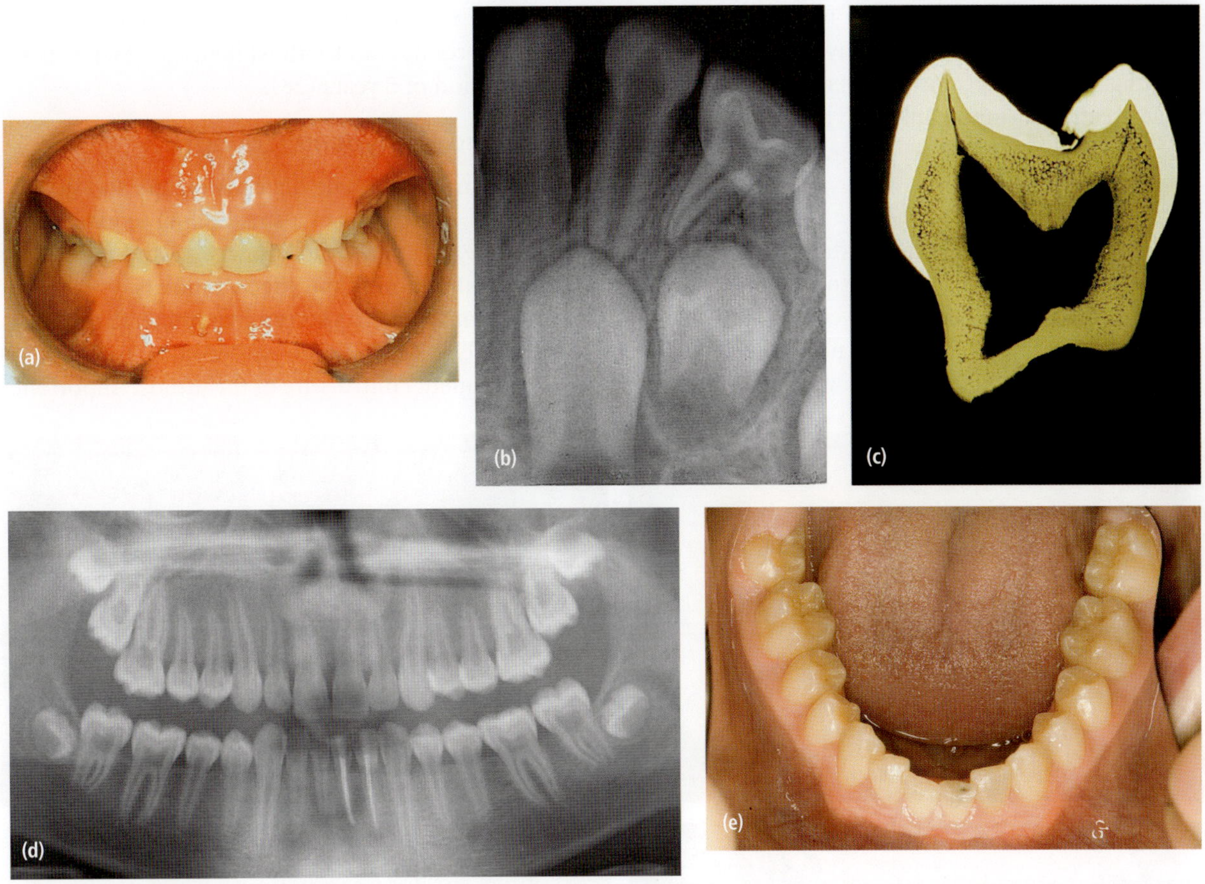

Figure 17-26 Familial hypophosphatemia. (a) A 6-year-old boy with several infected primary teeth. (b) Radiograph of mandibular primary teeth in a 4-year-old boy. Note the enlarged pulp chambers. (c) Microradiograph of a primary molar. Note the enlarged pulp chamber and pulp horns extending to dentinoenamel junction. Defective circumpulpal dentin, mantle dentin seemingly normal. (d) Panoramic radiograph showing periapical radiolucency in the lower incisor region and two lower incisors that have already been endodontically treated in a 14-year-old boy. Note also the enlarged pulp chambers and the extended pulp horns in the permanent dentition. (e) Clinical picture of the lower jaw of the same 14-year-old boy.

Abscess formation is seen particularly in the primary dentition and one abscess may predict future abscesses (29). It is difficult to prevent abscess formation.

Celiac disease

Celiac disease will in some cases give rise to hypoplastic enamel in permanent teeth formed during acute episodes of the disease at a very young age (32). The villi in small intestine are destroyed due to intolerance to gluten that is found in wheat, rye, and barley. The patient will be malnourished and too little calcium is absorbed. The treatment is a lifelong gluten-free diet. Susceptibility to celiac disease is associated with human leukocyte antigen genes. People with celiac disease tend to have other autoimmune diseases such dermatitis herpetiformis (DH). Symptoms are severe itching and the extensive eruption of vesicles and groups of papules which appear on the elbows, knees, and other pressure points. A gluten-free diet may also help to control this disease. There is a reported higher frequency of enamel defects in patients with DH (1) and the author suggests that it should be considered whether symmetric, unexplained dental defects may be the only detectable sign of a gluten-sensitive enteropathy. It is hypothesized that a gluten-induced immunological reaction during the tooth formation period may give rise to defective enamel (26). So far there is no scientific evidence which confirm this theory. The reported prevalence of dental defects in celiac disease patients varies from 10 to 96% in the literature (31). However, a recent case–control study of 50 celiac disease patients was not able to confirm a higher prevalence among them (31).

Treatment

Fluorosis

For mild and moderate cases the main problem is poor aesthetics affecting the front teeth especially in the upper jaw. The mild opacities are confined to the superficial area of enamel. The appearance of these can be improved by the technique of microabrasion (Fig. 17-27). More severe defects extend deeper and may require the use of restorations or veneers. Cases of severe fluorosis require extensive treatment comparable with treatment of severe AI (Fig. 17-28).

Tetracycline defects

Management of discolored teeth is difficult since much of the color originates from dentin. In cases of moderate or severe discoloration, composite veneers may be used as temporary treatment. They may need to be replaced by porcelain veneers or jacket crowns at a later age. However, recently it has been shown that extended bleaching resulted in tooth whitening, which was stable over a period of 5 years (28).

Molar–incisor hypomineralization

The treatment rationale depends on the severity of the lesion and it varies from a small filling to extensive restoration, e.g., onlays and crowns, to the radical treatment as extraction of the affected molars.

When moderate or severe hypomineralized areas in the enamel have been diagnosed in a newly erupted tooth, frequent controls are of the utmost importance in

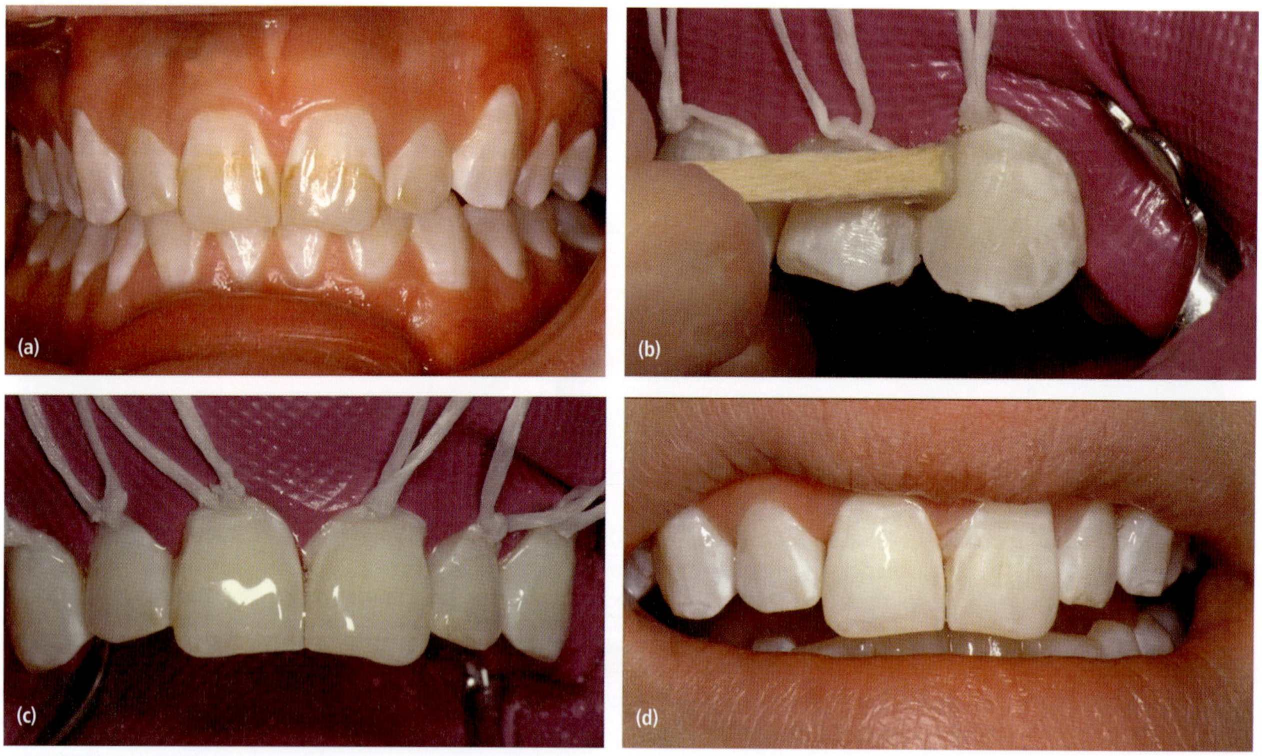

Figure 17-27 (a) Mild dental fluorosis in a 14-year-old girl. (b) The surface is rubbed using a wooden pin with 18% hydrochloric acid in pumice. (c) The surfaces are covered by 2% sodium fluoride gel. (d) Treatment result.

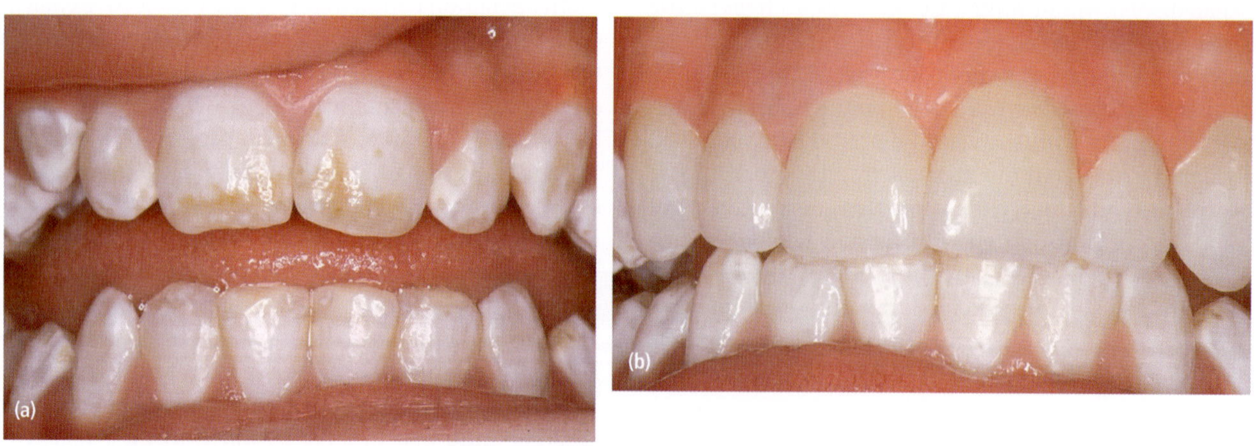

Figure 17-28 Porcelain veneers in a 13-year-old girl with moderate dental fluorosis.

order to determine the future fate of the tooth. Fluoride varnishing prevents caries and may also have some influence on preventing hypersensitivity.

The main clinical problems are the continuing enamel disintegration with subsequent caries and the frequently reported hypersensitivity of the affected tooth. When the lesions comprise large areas of the tooth surface, the filling often has to be surrounded by opaque porous enamel. Then, depending on the degree of porosity and the size of the opacity, continuous disintegration of enamel may occur and repeated filling therapy may be needed. Occasionally, an affected tooth is extremely sensitive when it erupts, preventing the child from toothbrushing and eating ice-cream, while other teeth become more and more sensitive, in particular after repeated filling treatment. It is a main treatment objective to cover exposed dentin to avoid sensitivity, caries development, and damage to the pulp. In cases like this with highly sensitive teeth, dentists frequently report considerable difficulties in anesthetizing.

In filling therapy, GICs are the material of choice, as microscopy studies of affected enamel have shown a poor etched surface not suitable for composite bonding (17,44) (Fig. 17-29). Resin-modified GICs appear to work well. Pretreatment with sodium hypochlorite can be a good idea, as there is indication of retained organic substance in the porous enamel. Painless treatment is important. In cases with difficult anesthetizing, sedation with nitrous oxide may help. Use of preoperative analgesics may also be considered.

In cases with extensive disintegration, troublesome hypersensitivity, and/or increasing dental anxiety, crown therapy or extraction of the tooth must be considered. The choice of treatment alternative should be made in collaboration with both the child and the parents after the permanent dentition has been mapped and the development of occlusion analyzed. When crown therapy is preferred, a stainless-steel crown can be used as a semipermanent restoration until the adjacent permanent teeth erupt to the occlusal plane, when it is replaced by a cast-metal crown. However, in many cases extraction is to be preferred, when, for example, crowding is expected, or when the child is not able to manage crown therapy. One advantage of extraction is that the troublesome treatment-consuming tooth is gone, since similar defects in the bicuspids or the second molars are seen rarely. Extraction of the permanent first molars generally presents no problems as regards the maxilla when performed prior to eruption of the second molar. In general, the best result was found when extractions were performed prior to eruption of the second permanent molar. Crowding in the relevant quadrant is also found to be favorable for a good orthodontic result as well as presence of the third molar. A careful follow-up and easy access to orthodontic expertise are mandatory in all cases of extraction of permanent teeth due to developmental defects (19).

The age of the child, the cooperative skills, and "dental age" are some of the factors necessary to take into consideration before extensive preparation of the teeth. The

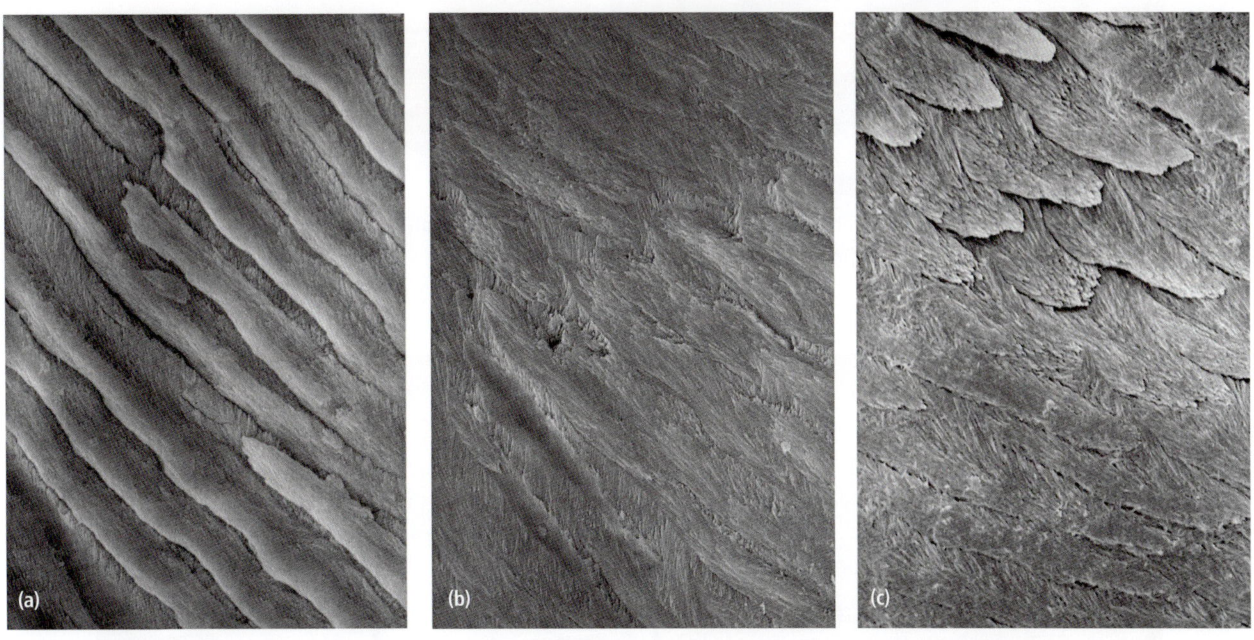

Figure 17-29 Scanning electron microscopy. The cut surface has been etched with 30% phosphoric acid for 30 s. (a) Normally mineralized enamel. (b) Hypomineralized enamel. (c) The border between normal and hypomineralized enamel.

exact age when it is possible to perform this type of treatment is difficult to establish on a general basis. In the treatment of young individuals the dentist may need to take intermediary types of treatment into consideration. Examples of this treatment plan could be the use of restorative materials and techniques requiring minimal preparation due to using an adhesive bonding technique (Figs 17-30–17-32).

Amelogenesis imperfecta

In general, the main clinical problems of AI are poor aesthetics, sensitivity of teeth, chewing difficulties, and the loss of tooth substance due to chipping and attrition often resulting in loss of occlusal vertical dimension (35). The severity of each symptom depends on the age of the patient, the type of AI, and the quality of the enamel. The psychosocial impact of AI on affected individuals has been studied (8). AI was found to have a marked impact on the overall psychosocial health, which should be kept in mind when treating AI patients.

Treatment of AI is ongoing during childhood and adolescence. Advanced restorative care and eventually complete prosthetic reconstruction are in some cases the only long-term treatment solution (Fig. 17-33). However, many intermediate phases in treatment, with special focus on "dealing with a child", may be necessary during childhood before the complete reconstruction can be performed.

Both before and after initiation of treatment of AI patients, the imperfect enamel necessitates well-functioning prevention. Professional prevention, including fluoride therapy and fissure sealing, should support the oral health care maintained at home.

With primary dentition, the severity of the enamel defects is often less extensive. In spite of that the sensitivity of primary teeth may in some cases be troublesome, occlusal attrition considerable, and restorative care complicated. In those cases the recommended and most long-lasting therapy is to cover the primary molars with stainless-steel crowns (Fig. 17-34). In less severe cases, regular supervision and fluoride treatment to reduce sensitivity can be an adequate therapy.

In the young permanent dentition the severity of the enamel defect influences the choice of treatment. Some patients with milder hypomaturation types of AI may not need other treatment than the one necessary to satisfy their cosmetic needs. In more severe cases with extensive degrees of hypomineralization of the enamel, more advanced treatment may be needed to ensure proper functioning, e.g., function-stabilizing treatment

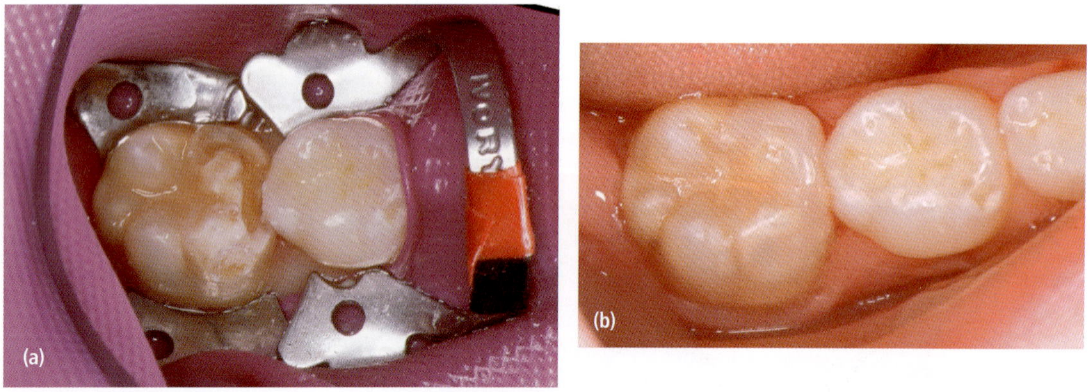

Figure 17-30 An 8-year-old girl with an MIH-affected molar to be restored. Porous, soft enamel was removed by a bur until hard, sound enamel appeared. After acid etch of the cavity walls, dentin–enamel bonding agent was applied and the tooth was restored with composite.

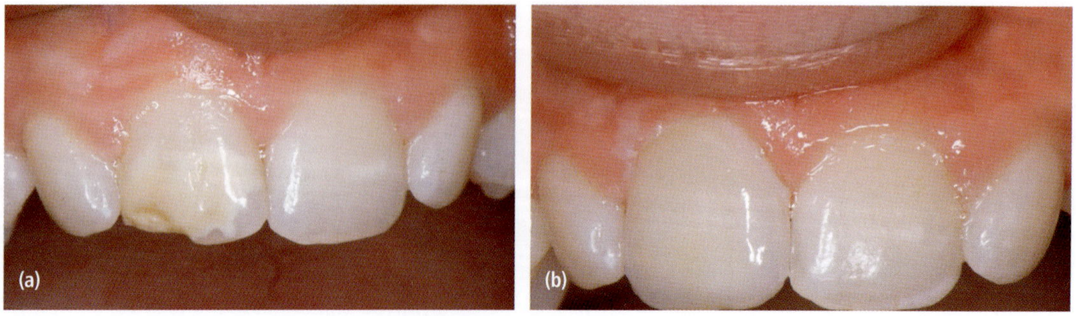

Figure 17-31 Thirteen-year-old boy with MIH. Enamel disintegration in 11 was restored with a porcelain veneer.

on permanent first molars, including stainless-steel crowns, composite or porcelain onlays, partial or full-cast gold crowns or copings with a need for minimum preparation. Apart from reducing thermal sensitivity these types of treatment serve to maintain normal vertical and mesiodistal dimensions. In less severe cases where the loss of vertical dimension is not as pronounced, dressing of the molars with composite or similar materials with adequate binding properties can be sufficient (Fig. 17-35). Not all forms of AI respond

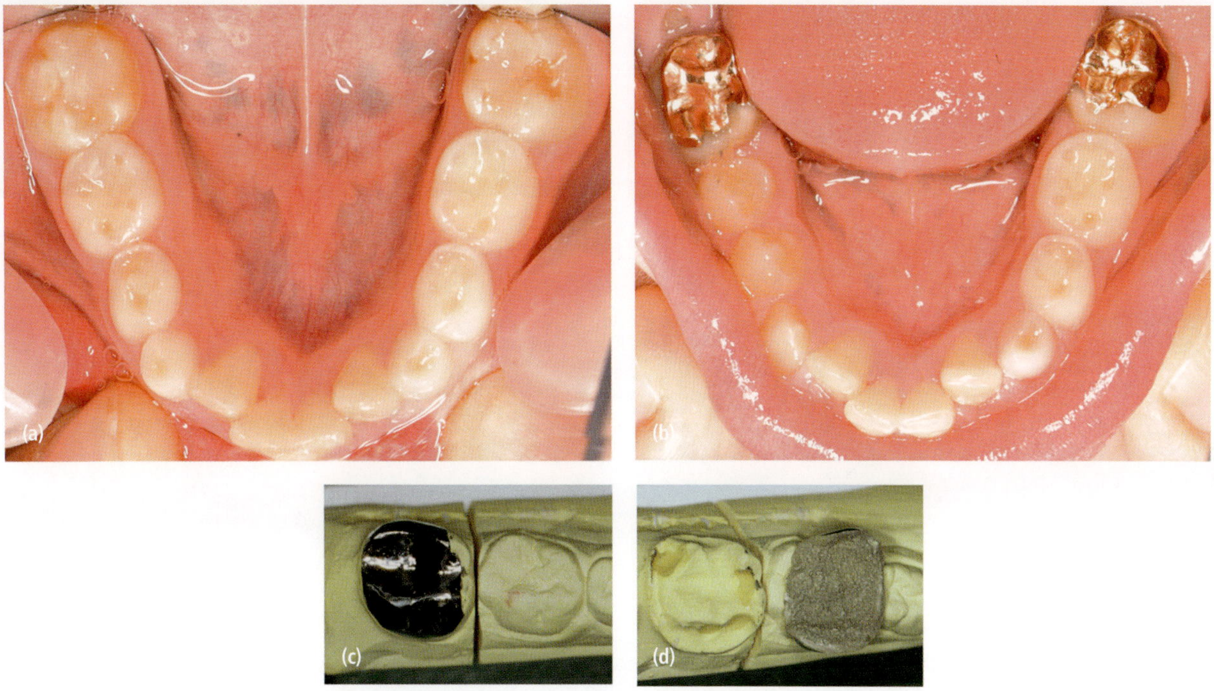

Figure 17-32 (a) Hypomineralized permanent first molars with opacities, posteruptive breakdown of enamel and insufficient conservative treatment, i.e., posteruptive enamel breakdown along the margins of composite fillings. (b) Treatment with cast-gold copings after minimal preparation due to the scarce thickness required to be able to make a cast-gold coping. (c) A gold-cast coping on the cast. (d) The gold-cast coping can be made with surface roughening by use of sugar crystal impression method with the purpose of improving the retention (courtesy of E. Gaardmand).

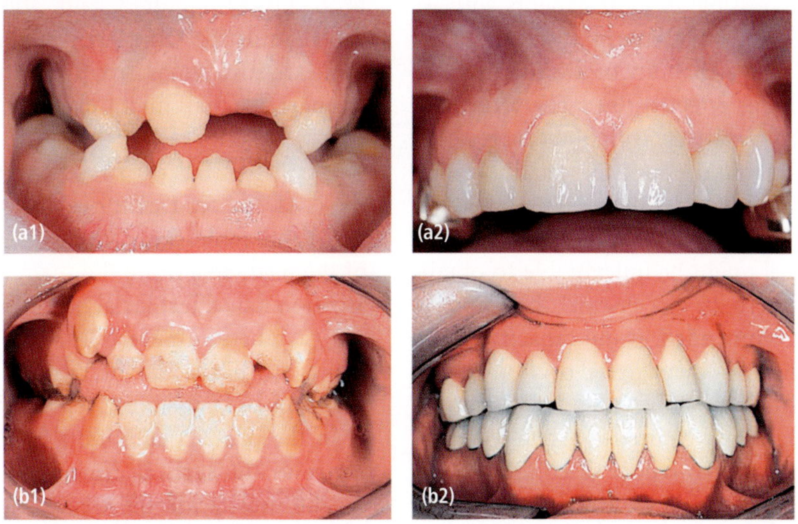

Figure 17-33 (a1) A 9-year-old girl with AI (hypoplastic type). (a2) Same girl at the age of 14 years. Maxillary incisors restored with ceramic veneers (courtesy of I. Andersson-Wenckert). (b1) Dentition of a 12-year-old boy with AI (hypocalcified type) before orthodontic treatment and placement of crowns. (b2) Same boy at the age of 20 years with single metalloceramic crowns in the mandible and single conventional gold crowns with composite facades in the maxillary teeth (courtesy of H. Holming).

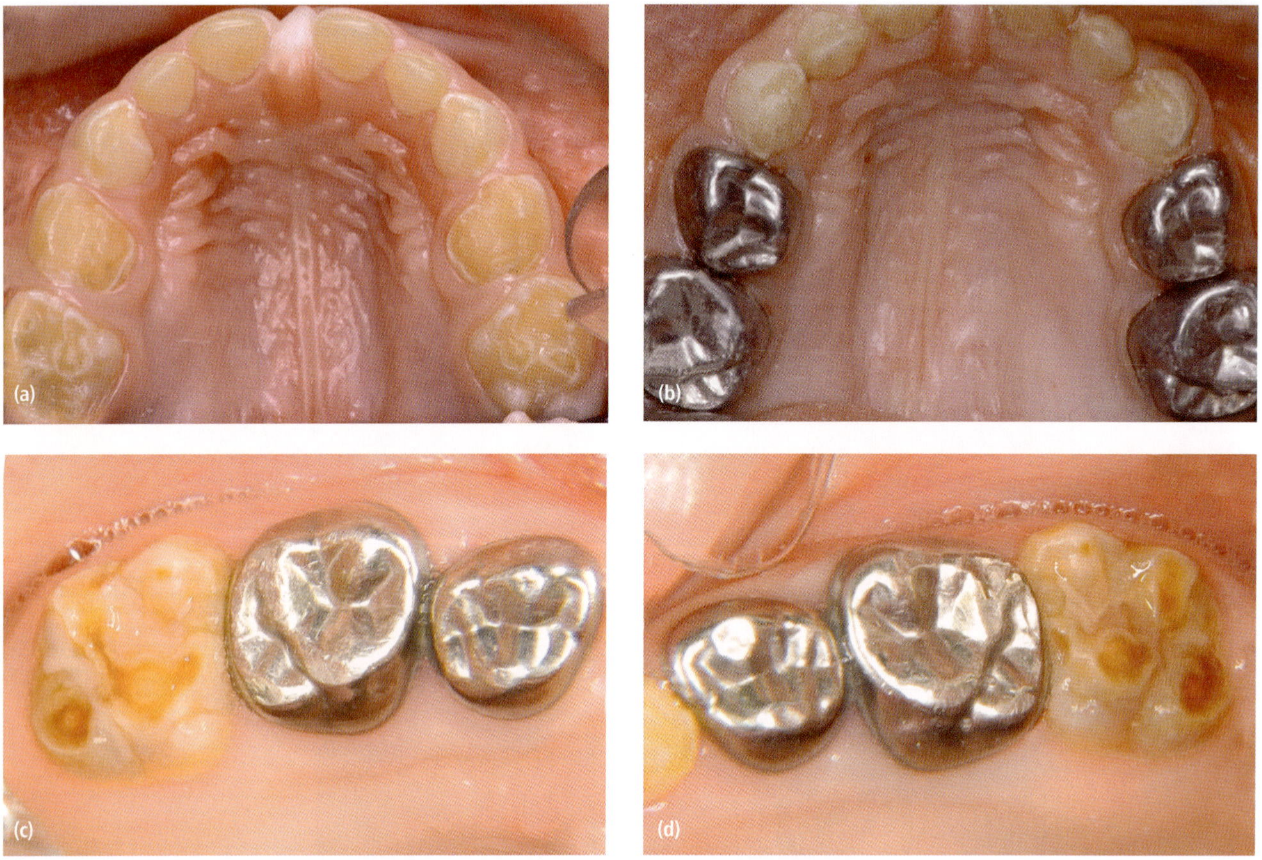

Figure 17-34 A boy with teeth affected by hypocalcified AI: (a) 3.5 years, problems with sensitivity and chipping of enamel; (b) 3.5 years, the molars are restored by stainless-steel crowns; (c, d) 9 years, time for dressing the permanent molars with steel crowns due to chipping and attrition of enamel.

favorably to enamel bonding and, for example, for the hypocalcified variety of AI, enamel bonding may not be sufficient to keep the filling in place (35). However, a bonding to enamel is possible in most patients with AI and, despite that, the etching patterns may vary in different AI variants (36). The etchability of the enamel may depend on which gene is affected (39). Therefore, the dentist should proceed tentatively with bonding restorative materials to enamel and check the quality of the restorations regularly. Sometimes there is not sufficient enamel to ensure proper retention of the filling. As the structure of the enamel might be unfavorable to obtain a reliable etching pattern in the enamel, bonding to exposed dentin is recommended. If the capacity of the child to cooperate is limited, the material of choice is the one that is least technique sensitive and demanding. Retreatment of the child may be needed as the cooperation of the child improves. To reduce discoloration, AI cases with severe hypoplasia should be sealed soon after eruption. As the child gets older, appearance becomes more important and poor aesthetics demand consideration. Direct restoration of the incisors with composites or, later on, porcelain veneers or crowns may be indicated to improve the aesthetics sufficiently. Continued eruption and discoloration of the filling margins necessitate continuous control and adjustment. The aesthetic problems of children and adolescents with enamel defects must be taken seriously and sometimes require that extensive restorative procedures are carried out at a younger age than might usually be considered.

Dentinogenesis imperfecta

As in AI, the treatment of DI is ongoing through childhood and adolescence. Poor aesthetics and the attrition of the teeth constitute the main problems. If untreated, attrition may affect facial height, appearance, and masticatory function. Severe attrition of the primary teeth allows attrition of the permanent first molars soon after eruption and a vicious circle is initiated (Fig. 17-34).

In the primary dentition for the long-term maintenance of the vertical dimension, stainless-steel crowns on the molars are the treatment of choice. Treatment should be started as soon as excessive attrition or spontaneous fractures of the enamel are observed, when there is still sufficient tooth substance left for retention of the crowns (Fig. 17-36a). An early diagnosis is there-

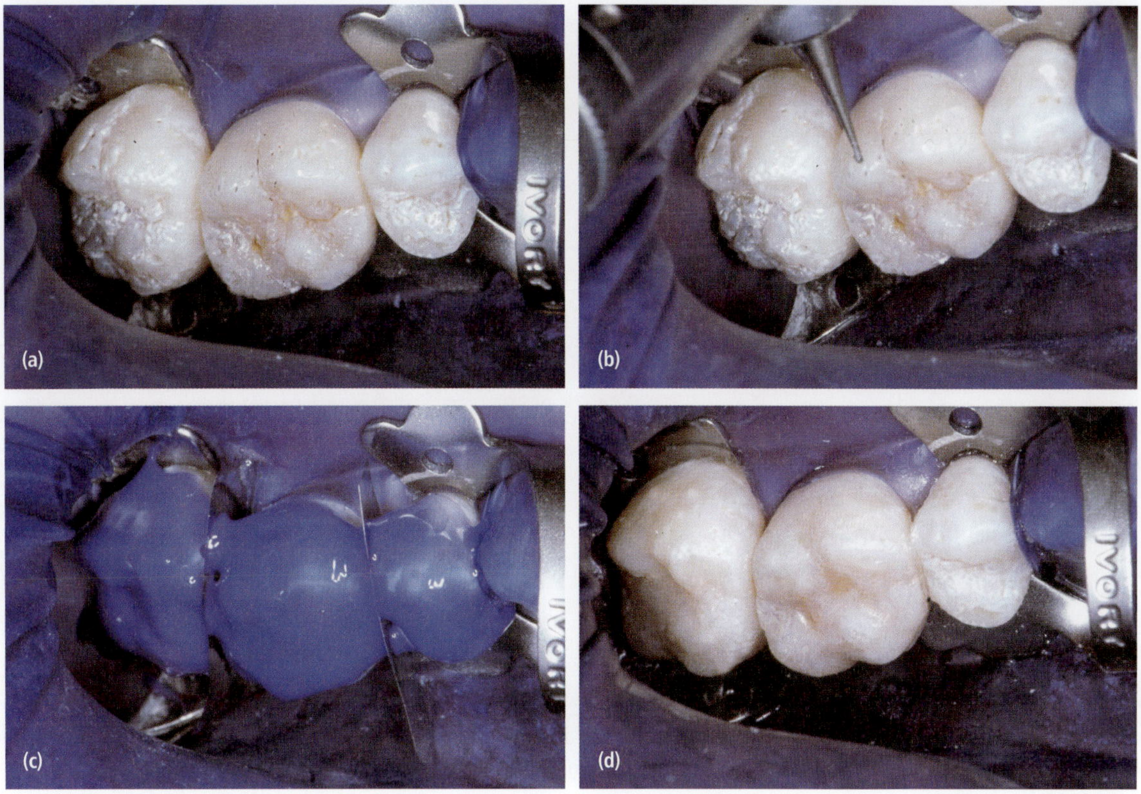

Figure 17-35 Treatment of hypoplastic, rough pitted AI. (a) Prior to treatment, (b) pits are cleaned by the bur, (c) etching, and (d) the teeth are dressed with flowable composite.

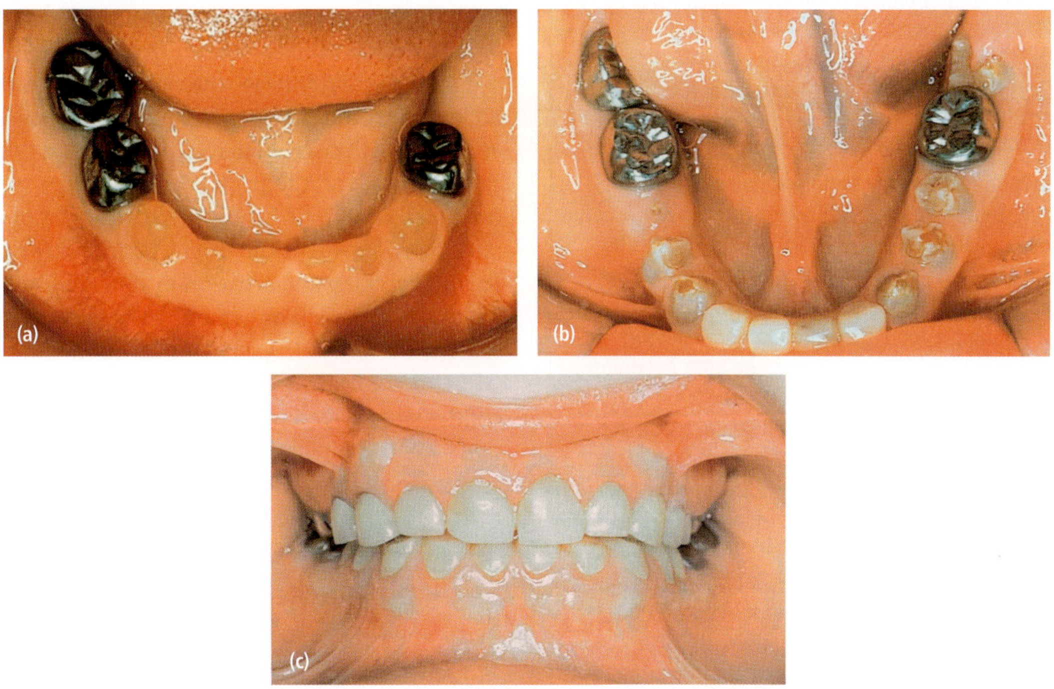

Figure 17-36 A boy with DI type II. (a) Mandibular teeth at the age of 3 years 5 months. The primary left second molar was infected due to attrition and had to be extracted. Stainless-steel crowns have been made to prevent further attrition. (b) The permanent molars have been fitted with stainless-steel crowns and the incisors with laboratory-made composite crowns (courtesy of J. Waltimo). (c) Same patient at the age of 10 years 4 months (courtesy of J. Waltimo).

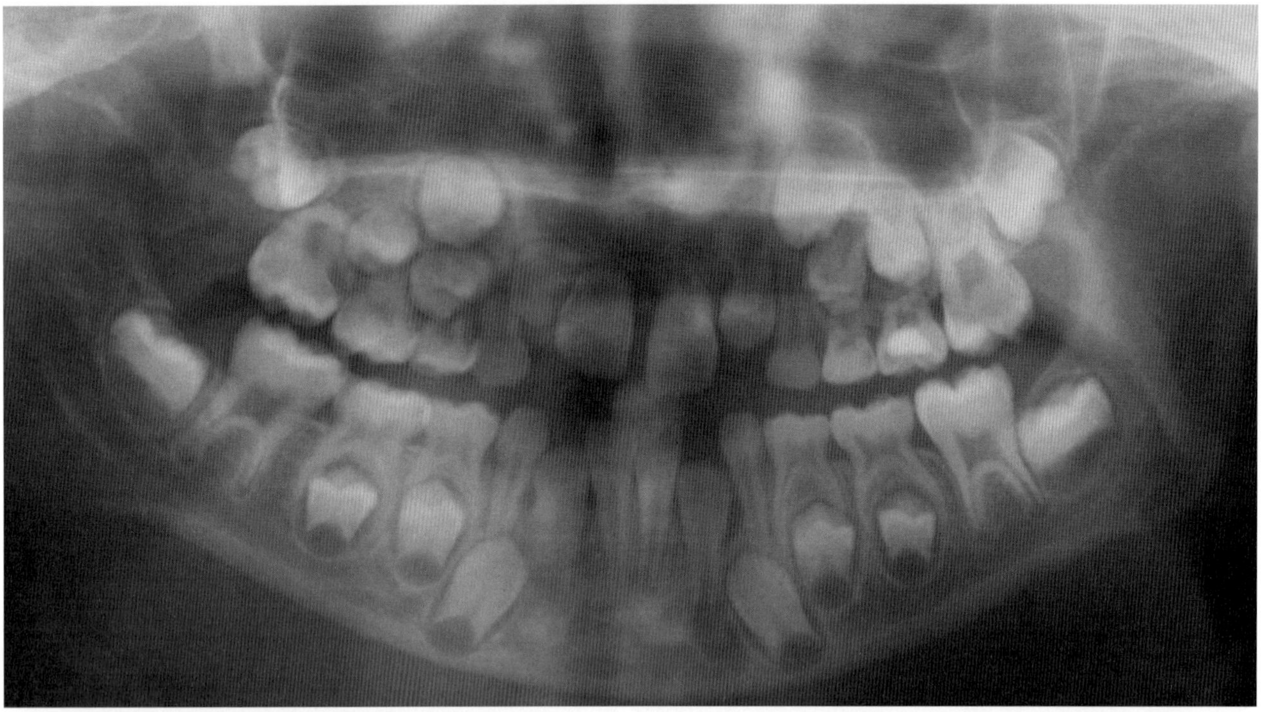

Figure 17-37 A 7-year-old boy with damage of permanent maxillary teeth after localized, high-dose radiation (56 Gy) at 3.5 years of age due to a tumor in the right maxilla. Very short roots in permanent teeth are seen in the affected area (courtesy of the craniofacial team, Rikshospitalet, Norway).

Box 17-12 Diseases/etiologic factors which may cause localized defects that are most often nonsymmetrically distributed

- Traumatic injury to a permanent tooth germ (Figs 17-7 and 17-8).
- Local infection in the jaw, which may be a sequela after a pulp infection in a primary tooth, can affect the permanent tooth bud (Fig. 17-9).
- High-dose radiation (localized irradiation) (Fig. 17-37).
- Traumatic laryngoscopy and prolonged endotracheal intubation during the first months after birth may cause damage to primary tooth germs, often upper incisors (crown dilacerations). The defects can be both hypoplasia and opacities.
- Regional odontodysplasia involves all dental tissue and is nonhereditary. Most often the affected teeth are within the same quadrant. Usually the anterior teeth are more severely affected. Possible etiologic factors have been suggested as vascular disorder, trauma, latent virus in tooth germs, metabolic disturbances, local infections, and somatic mutation (12). Affected teeth are twice as often seen in maxillary teeth as in mandibular teeth. The condition is often observed with eruption of the primary teeth. Affected primary teeth are usually succeeded by affected permanent teeth (Figs 17-38 and 17-39).

fore important as well as frequent follow-ups. Necrotic primary teeth should be extracted.

In the young permanent dentition, contradictory to AI, the defects are less severe. In cases with severe attrition of the primary teeth, the vertical dimensions have to be increased to allow permanent molars and incisors to erupt normally. To achieve this, stainless-steel crowns can be placed on the primary molars even in cases with extensive attrition of these teeth. The use of a customized guard at nighttime might be useful for preventing enamel cracking and attrition in young permanent teeth. In cases of cracking and/or attrition, stainless-steel crowns or cast-gold onlays with minimal preparation, GICs, or composites can be used (Fig. 17-36b, c). As the child matures, ceramic crowns are alternative restorations for the molars and direct composites or ceramic crowns for the front teeth.

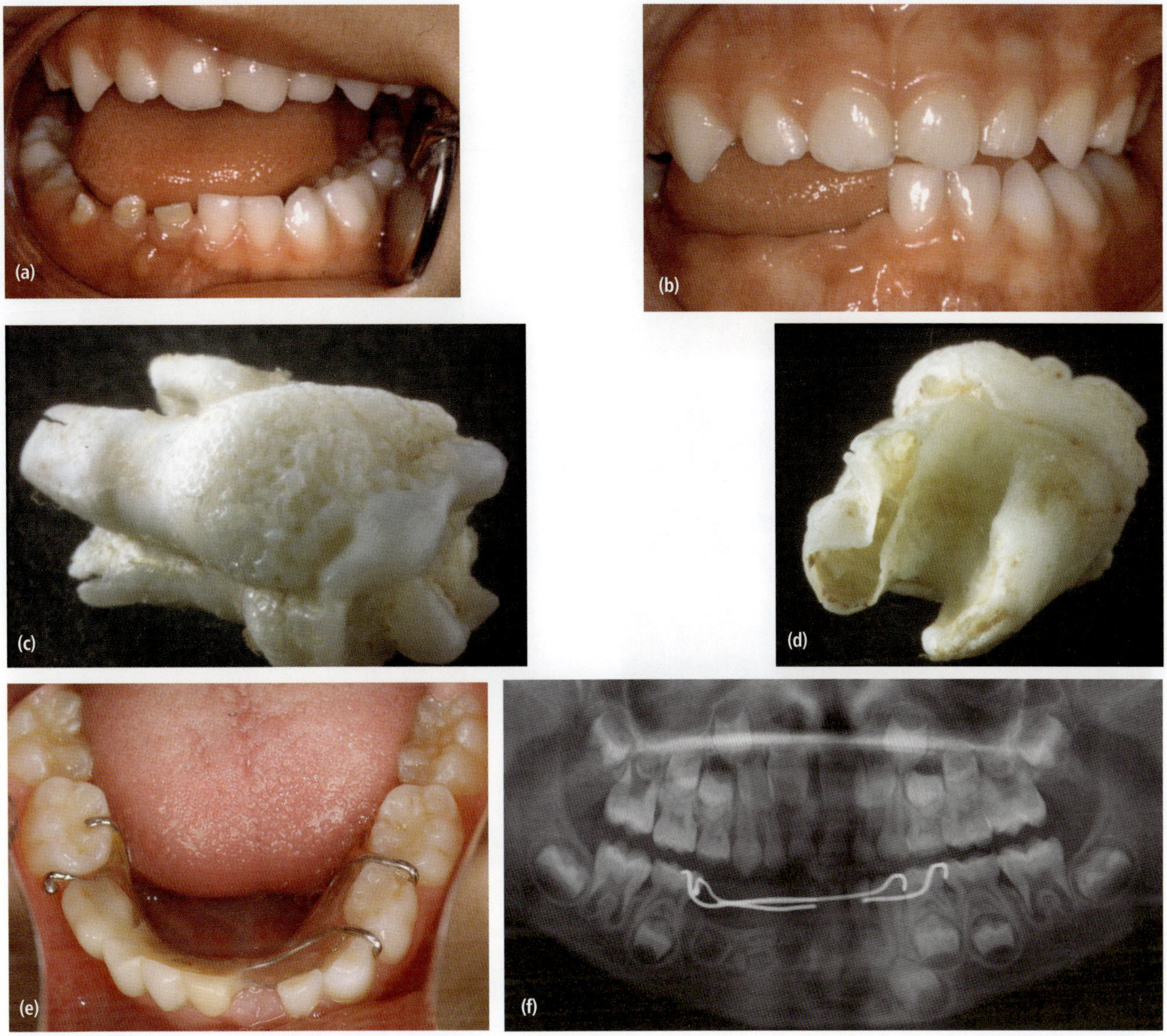

Figure 17-38 Regional odontodysplasia. (a) Malformed teeth in the lower right quadrant in a 3-year-old boy. An abscessed incisor is seen. (b) Dental treatment under general dental anesthesia consisted of extraction of all teeth in the lower right quadrant except a more robust lower right second primary molar which could contribute in maintenance of the functional height of the primary dentition and in continuation of some alveolar growth in the region. (c) First primary molar after tooth extraction showing enamel hypoplasia of the tooth crown. (d) The complete tooth is fragile, and the amount of tooth substance is scarce. The root complex has an open apex, and the pulp chamber is abnormally large. (e) A denture was inserted when the boy was 4 years old. As seen on the picture where the child is 6 years old, the denture may need adjustment when primary teeth are gradually lost due to shedding. (f) Panoramic radiograph shows that the successors are also affected. The denture was in place when the radiograph was taken as the retentive elements are visible on the photograph.

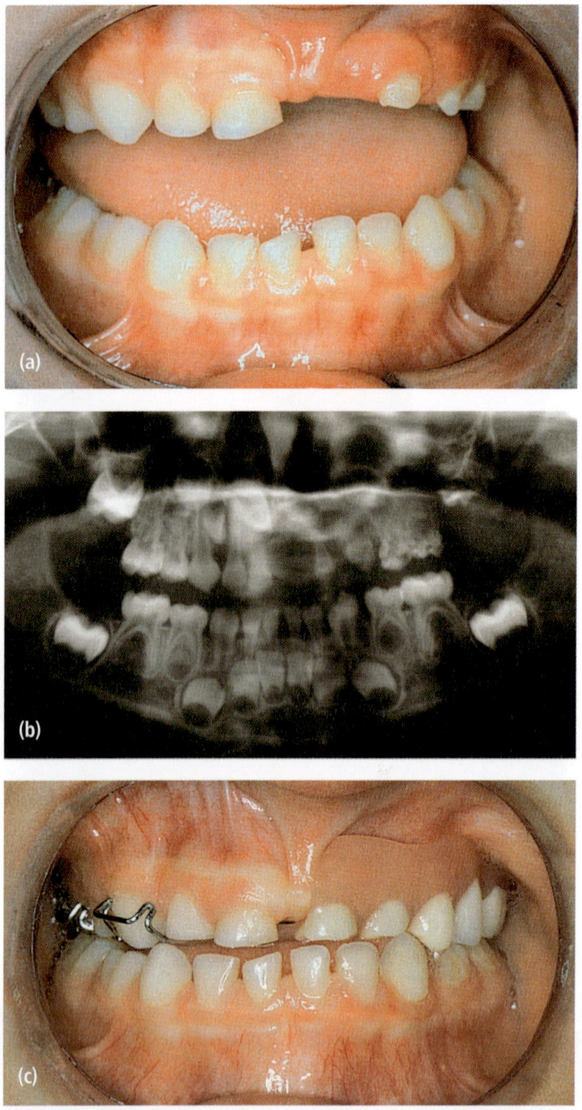

Figure 17-39 Regional odontodysplasia. (a) Abscessed incisors in the maxillary left quadrant. (b) Panoramic radiograph shows involvement of all the teeth in the quadrant. (c) The child was treated by extraction of the affected teeth except the permanent first molar, which was thought to maintain some alveolar growth in the region. The maxillary partial denture was placed after extractions at the age of 3 years.

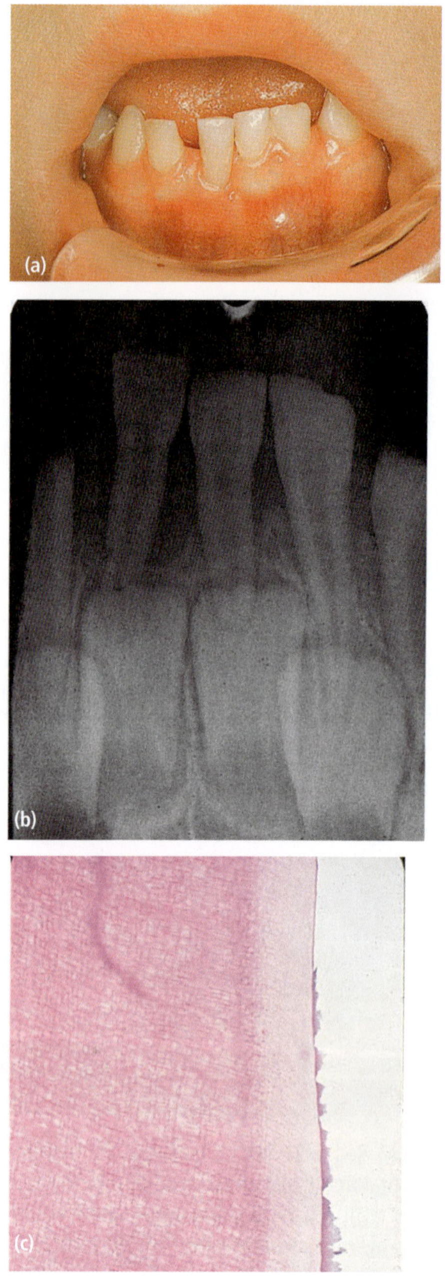

Figure 17-40 Hypophosphatasia. (a) A 3-year-old boy with a benign form of hypophosphatasia. Mandibular right central incisor is poorly attached and mobile. (b) Radiograph of incisor teeth showing severe alveolar bone loss in the lower incisor region. (c) Histological section showing thin cementum on the root surface.

References

1. Aine L. Coeliac-type permanent-tooth enamel defects. *Ann Med* 1996;**28**:9–12.
2. Alaluusua S, Lukinmaa PL, Koskimies M, Pirinen S, Holtta P, Kallio M, *et al.* Developmental dental defects associated with long breast feeding. *Eur J Oral Sci* 1996;**104**:493–7.
3. Aldred MJ, Crawford PJ. Amelogenesis imperfecta – towards a new classification. *Oral Dis* 1995;**1**:2–5.
4. Aldred MJ, Savarirayan R, Crawford PJ. Amelogenesis imperfecta: a classification and catalogue for the 21st century. *Oral Dis* 2003;**9**:19–23.
5. Aoba T, Fejerskov O. Dental fluorosis: chemistry and biology. *Crit Rev Oral Biol Med* 2002;**13**:155–70.
6. Backman B, Angmar-Mansson B. Mineral distribution in the enamel of teeth with amelogenesis imperfecta as determined by quantitative microradiography. *Scand J Dent Res* 1994;**102**: 193–7.
7. Backman B, Holm AK. Amelogenesis imperfecta: prevalence and incidence in a northern Swedish county. *Community Dent Oral Epidemiol* 1986;**14**:43–7.

8. Coffield KD, Phillips C, Brady M, Roberts MW, Strauss RP, Wright JT. The psychosocial impact of developmental dental defects in people with hereditary amelogenesis imperfecta. *J Am Dent Assoc* 2005;**136**:620–30.
9. Commission on Oral Health, Research & Epidemiology. A review of the developmental defects of enamel index (DDE Index). Report of an FDI Working Group. *Int Dent J* 1992;**42**:411–26.
10. Cordeiro MM, Rocha MJ. The effects of periradicular inflamation and infection on a primary tooth and permanent successor. *J Clin Pediatr Dent* 2005;**29**:193–200.
11. Crawford PJ, Aldred M, Bloch-Zupan A. Amelogenesis imperfecta. *Orphanet J Rare Dis* 2007;**2**:17.
12. Crawford PJ, Aldred MJ. Regional odontodysplasia: a bibliography. *J Oral Pathol Med* 1989;**18**:251–63.
13. Crawford PJ, Aldred MJ. Amelogenesis imperfecta with taurodontism and the tricho-dento-osseous syndrome: separate conditions or a spectrum of disease? *Clin Genet* 1990;**38**:44–50.
14. Dong J, Amor D, Aldred MJ, Gu T, Escamilla M, MacDougall M. DLX3 mutation associated with autosomal dominant amelogenesis imperfecta with taurodontism. *Am J Med Genet A* 2005;**133**:138–41.
15. Hart PS, Hart TC. Disorders of human dentin. *Cells Tissues Organs* 2007;**186**:70–7.
16. Hu JC, Chun YH, Al Hazzazzi T, Simmer JP. Enamel formation and amelogenesis imperfecta. *Cells Tissues Organs* 2007;**186**:78–85.
17. Jalevik B, Dietz W, Noren JG. Scanning electron micrograph analysis of hypomineralized enamel in permanent first molars. *Int J Paediatr Dent* 2005;**15**:233–40.
18. Jalevik B, Klingberg GA. Dental treatment, dental fear and behaviour management problems in children with severe enamel hypomineralization of their permanent first molars. *Int J Paediatr Dent* 2002;**12**:24–32.
19. Jalevik B, Moller M. Evaluation of spontaneous space closure and development of permanent dentition after extraction of hypomineralized permanent first molars. *Int J Paediatr Dent* 2007;**17**:328–35.
20. Jalevik B, Noren JG. Enamel hypomineralization of permanent first molars: a morphological study and survey of possible aetiological factors. *Int J Paediatr Dent* 2000;**10**:278–89.
21. Jalevik B, Noren JG, Klingberg G, Barregard L. Etiologic factors influencing the prevalence of demarcated opacities in permanent first molars in a group of Swedish children. *Eur J Oral Sci* 2001;**109**:230–4.
22. Kim JW, Simmer JP. Hereditary dentin defects. *J Dent Res* 2007;**86**:392–9.
23. Kim JW, Simmer JP, Lin BP, Seymen F, Bartlett JD, Hu JC. Mutational analysis of candidate genes in 24 amelogenesis imperfecta families. *Eur J Oral Sci* 2006;**114** Suppl 1:3–12; discussion 39–41, 379.
24. Leppaniemi A, Lukinmaa PL, Alaluusua S. Nonfluoride hypomineralizations in the permanent first molars and their impact on the treatment need. *Caries Res* 2001;**35**:36–40.
25. MacDougall M, Dong J, Acevedo AC. Molecular basis of human dentin diseases. *Am J Med Genet A* 2006;**140**:2536–46.
26. Maki M, Aine L, Lipsanen V, Koskimies S. Dental enamel defects in first-degree relatives of coeliac disease patients. *Lancet* 1991;**337**:763–4.
27. Malmgren B. *Clinical, histopathologic and genetic diagnosis in osteogenesis imperfecta and dentinogenesis imperfecta.* Stockholm: Karolinska Institutet, 2004.
28. Matis BA, Wang Y, Eckert GJ, Cochran MA, Jiang T. Extended bleaching of tetracycline-stained teeth: a 5-year study. *Oper Dent* 2006;**31**:643–51.
29. McWhorter AG, Seale NS. Prevalence of dental abscess in a population of children with vitamin D-resistant rickets. *Pediatr Dent* 1991;**13**:91–6.
30. Price JA, Bowden DW, Wright JT, Pettenati MJ, Hart TC. Identification of a mutation in DLX3 associated with tricho-dento-osseous (TDO) syndrome. *Hum Mol Genet* 1998;**7**:563–9.
31. Procaccini M, Campisi G, Bufo P, Compilato D, Massaccesi C, Catassi C, *et al.* Lack of association between celiac disease and dental enamel hypoplasia in a case-control study from an Italian central region. *Head Face Med* 2007;**3**:25.
32. Rasmussen P, Espelid I. Coeliac disease and dental malformation. *ASDC J Dent Child* 1980;**47**:190–2.
33. Risnes S. Growth tracks in dental enamel. *J Hum Evol* 1998;**35**:331–50.
34. Rodd HD, Davidson LE. 'Ilko dacowo:' canine enucleation and dental sequelae in Somali children. *Int J Paediatr Dent* 2000;**10**:290–7.
35. Seow WK. Taurodontism of the mandibular first permanent molar distinguishes between the tricho-dento-osseous (TDO) syndrome and amelogenesis imperfecta. *Clin Genet* 1993;**43**:240–6.
36. Seow WK, Amaratunge A. The effects of acid-etching on enamel from different clinical variants of amelogenesis imperfecta: an SEM study. *Pediatr Dent* 1998;**20**:37–42.
37. Shields ED, Bixler D, el-Kafrawy AM. A proposed classification for heritable human dentine defects with a description of a new entity. *Arch Oral Biol* 1973;**18**:543–53.
38. Shulman JD, Maupome G, Clark DC, Levy SM. Perceptions of desirable tooth color among parents, dentists and children. *J Am Dent Assoc* 2004;**135**:595–604; quiz 654–5.
39. Simmer JP, Hu JC. Dental enamel formation and its impact on clinical dentistry. *J Dent Educ* 2001;**65**:896–905.
40. Stephanopoulos G, Garefalaki ME, Lyroudia K. Genes and related proteins involved in amelogenesis imperfecta. *J Dent Res* 2005;**84**:1117–26.
41. Sundell S, Koch G. Hereditary amelogenesis imperfecta. I. Epidemiology and clinical classification in a Swedish child population. *Swed Dent J* 1985;**9**:157–69.
42. van den Bos T, Handoko G, Niehof A, Ryan LM, Coburn SP, Whyte MP, *et al.* Cementum and dentin in hypophosphatasia. *J Dent Res* 2005;**84**:1021–5.
43. Weerheijm KL, Jalevik B, Alaluusua S. Molar–incisor hypomineralisation. *Caries Res* 2001;**35**:390–1.
44. William V, Burrow MF, Palamara JE, Messer LB. Microshear bond strength of resin composite to teeth affected by molar hypomineralization using 2 adhesive systems. *Pediatr Dent* 2006;**28**:233–41.
45. Winter GB, Brook AH. Enamel hypoplasia and anomalies of the enamel. *Dent Clin North Am* 1975;**19**:3–24.
46. Witkop CJ. Hereditary defects in enamel and dentin. *Acta Genet Stat Med* 1957;**7**:236–9.
47. Witkop CJ Jr. Amelogenesis imperfecta, dentinogenesis imperfecta and dentin dysplasia revisited: problems in classification. *J Oral Pathol* 1988;**17**:547–53.
48. Wong HM, McGrath C, King NM. Dental practitioners' views on the need to treat developmental defects of enamel. *Community Dent Oral Epidemiol* 2007;**35**:130–9.
49. Wright JT. The molecular etiologies and associated phenotypes of amelogenesis imperfecta. *Am J Med Genet A* 2006;**140**:2547–55.

18

Traumatic injuries: examination, diagnosis, and immediate care

Ingeborg Jacobsen and Jens O. Andreasen

It is well known that the majority of dental injuries occur in children. Thus, in a Swedish study, 83% of all individuals with acute dental trauma were younger than 20 years of age (9). Injuries to primary or permanent teeth can appear rather severe, particularly when associated with trauma to supporting tissues (Figs 18-1 and 18-2). The situation is distressing for both the child and parents. It is important that the dentist and the other members of the dental team are well prepared to meet the many complex and challenging problems in the care of dental emergencies (Box 18-1).

Epidemiology

A study from Denmark showed that 30% of children had suffered traumatic dental injuries in the primary dentition and 22% in the permanent dentition (1). The incidence of injuries to primary teeth increases from 1 year of age, and most traumas involve children younger than 4 years of age. In the permanent dentition, the most accident-prone time is between 8 and 10 years of age (Fig. 18-3). Boys appear to sustain injuries to permanent teeth twice as often as girls. Even in preschool children, trauma in boys is reported to outnumber cases in girls. Dental injuries usually affect one or two of the anterior teeth, and especially the maxillary central incisors (Fig. 18-4) (14).

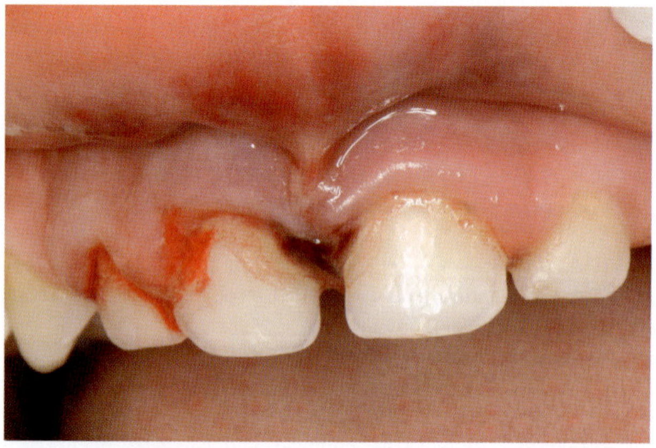

Figure 18-1 A 3-year-old boy with swollen upper lip, lacerated frenum, gingival bleeding, and palatal luxation of the right central and lateral incisors.

Etiology

In a young child learning to walk and to run, muscle coordination and judgment are incompletely developed and falling injuries frequently occur. Trauma to the orofacial area may also be part of child physical abuse. The characteristics of this unfortunate condition are presented in Box 18-2.

A Norwegian study of children aged from 7 to 18 years reported that 48% of all dental traumas occurred during school hours and 52% during leisure time. Nearly half of the leisure-time injuries occurred when children were playing. Ten percent happened in traffic, and half of these were bicycle accidents. Twenty-five percent occurred while partying or visiting bars and clubs.

In contrast to common belief, only 8% of all injuries were sports related. Finally, in the age group 16–18 years, 23% of all orofacial injuries resulted from violence (15).

Examination

To ensure that all relevant data are recorded, a standardized trauma form is recommended (4). This form serves as a checklist for the dentist at the initial visit and at subsequent appointments.

History

When the patient is received for treatment, the first step is to get an initial impression of the extent of the injury. Has a tooth been knocked out? Is the patient's general condition affected? Is there a need for immediate medical care? If not, the following questions should be asked to

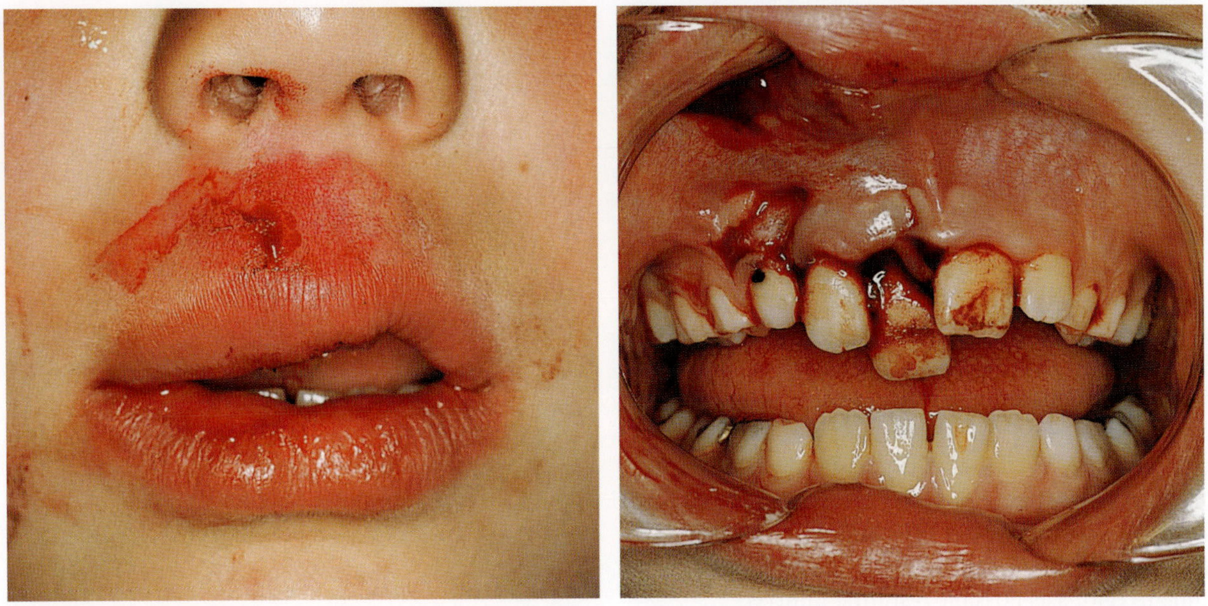

Figure 18-2 The patient has had an impact where the force has been transmitted through the upper lip to the teeth and the alveolar process. Note the lip laceration and abrasion and the displacement of the right central and lateral incisors.

Box 18-1 Care of dental injuries in children

The dental team must:

- Be aware of and understand the anxiety of both children and parents.
- Reduce the stress and anxiety by remaining calm and reassuring.
- Have the knowledge and skill to make an accurate diagnosis, and perform appropriate and prompt emergency treatment.
- Reduce pain as much as possible. Always consider the use of local anesthetics and analgesics.

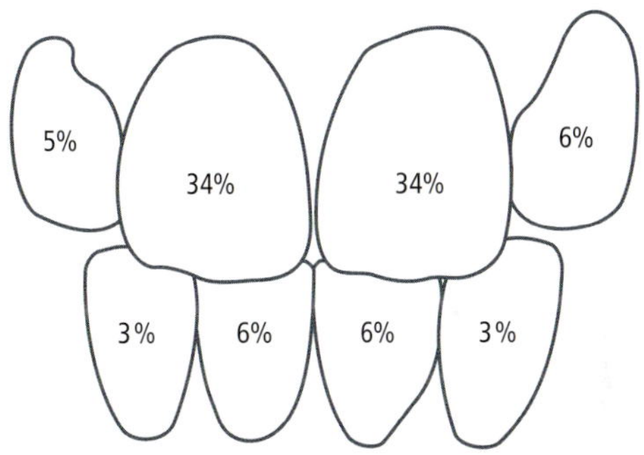

Figure 18-4 Distribution of injuries of the most frequently injured permanent teeth: 97% of all injuries affected the incisors (14).

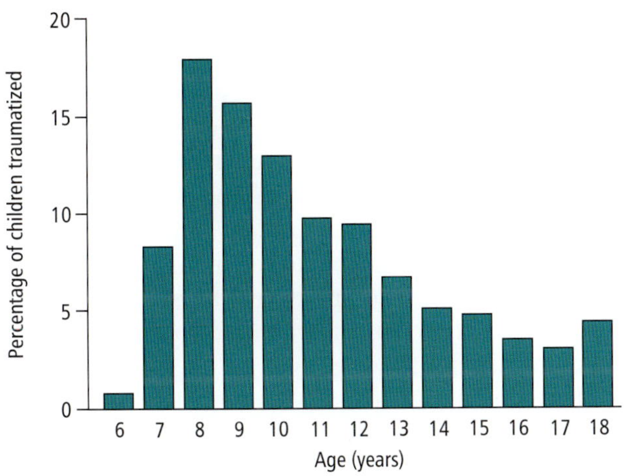

Figure 18-3 Percentage distribution of 1275 children with traumatic dental injuries related to age at the time of injury (14).

Box 18-2 Important aspects of child physical abuse

- Most often the child is between 1 and 3 years.
- There is usually a significant delay between injury and presentation at the clinic.
- There are often signs of multiple different bruises obviously sustained over a period of time.
- Approximately half of the children have orofacial injuries.
- The child's history differs from the parents', or history given by parents does not fit the clinical findings.
- In Scandinavian countries it is mandatory to report suspected cases.

end up with a correct diagnosis, and allow treatment planning:

- *When did the injury occur?* The time interval between injury and treatment can influence both the treatment procedure and the expected outcome. Thus, optimal repositioning of an extruded permanent tooth is difficult if treatment is delayed. The time factor is also very critical for the prognosis of replanted teeth.
- *Where did the injury occur?* This information is important for insurance and social security purposes. The place of accident also provides information on the need for tetanus prophylaxis in replantation cases.
- *How did the injury occur?* The nature of the blow may provide clues as to the type of injury to be expected. For example, when a blow hits the chin, the mandibular arch is forced against the maxillary arch, with jaw fracture or crown-root fracture in the premolar or molar regions as possible resulting injuries.
- *Was there a period of unconsciousness?* If so, for how long? Is there headache? Amnesia? Nausea? Vomiting? Excitation or difficulties in focusing the eyes? These are all signs of brain concussion and require medical attention.
- *Is there any disturbance in the bite?* Disturbance in the occlusion can imply luxation injury, alveolar fracture, jaw fracture, or luxation or fracture of the temporomandibular joint. Limitations of mandibular movement or mandibular deviation on opening or closing the mouth indicate that the jaw might be fractured.

Medical history

A short medical history should reveal possible allergies, blood disorders, and other information about conditions that could interfere with treatment.

Extraoral examination

Note is taken of swelling, bruises, or lacerations to the face and lips. Deep lip wounds are examined closely with respect to tooth fragments or other foreign bodies (Fig. 18-5).

Intraoral examination

The examination must be systematic and include the recording of:

- Swelling, laceration, and hemorrhage of the oral mucosa and gingiva.
- Abnormalities in occlusion.
- Missing, displaced or loosened teeth, fractured crowns, or cracks in the enamel.

It is important to examine all teeth within a traumatized area and, in close bite situations, also teeth in the opposite jaw. Particular note is taken of the following factors:

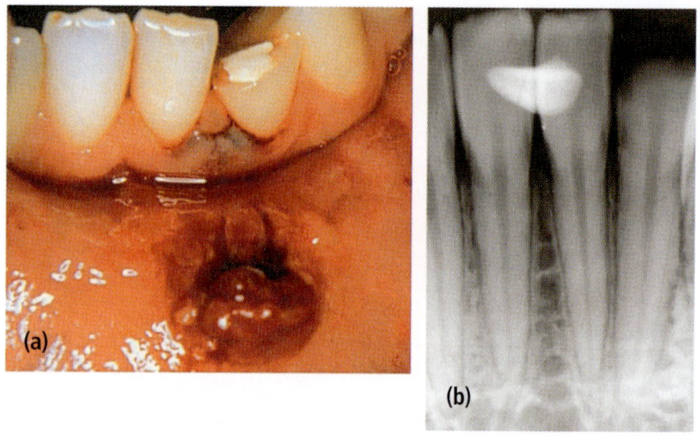

Figure 18-5 (a) Crown fracture of mandibular lateral incisor and mandibular lip lesion. (b) A radiograph reveals the fractured tooth fragment hidden in the lip lesion.

- *Displacement.* The direction as well as the extent (in millimeters) of displacement should be recorded. Minor displacement can be difficult to detect. In such cases it is helpful to examine the occlusion as well as radiographs taken at various angulations.
- *Mobility.* The degree of mobility is assessed in both a horizontal and vertical direction, keeping in mind that immature permanent teeth and primary teeth undergoing root resorption have quite extensive physiologic mobility. When several teeth move together *en bloc*, a fracture of the alveolar process is suspected.
- *Reaction to percussion.* The handle of a mouth mirror is tapped gently against the teeth in both a horizontal and vertical direction. Tenderness to percussion indicates damage to the periodontal ligament. A high metallic tone implies that the injured tooth is locked in bone.
- *Color of the tooth.* Discoloration may appear almost immediately after the injury. Special attention should be paid to the palatal surface in the gingival third of the crown.
- *Reaction to sensibility tests.* It is usually not possible to obtain reliable information from a young, frightened child. However, in the permanent dentition electrometric sensibility testing should be performed whenever possible. It gives important information about the neurovascular supply to the pulp, and provides a baseline value for comparison at follow-up examination. The contralateral uninjured tooth or another comparable tooth serves as a control. The most reliable response is obtained when the electrode is placed upon the incisal edge. It is important to explain the purpose of the test and the type of reaction to be expected. To avoid painful stimulation of the tooth, the rheostat should always be increased slowly.

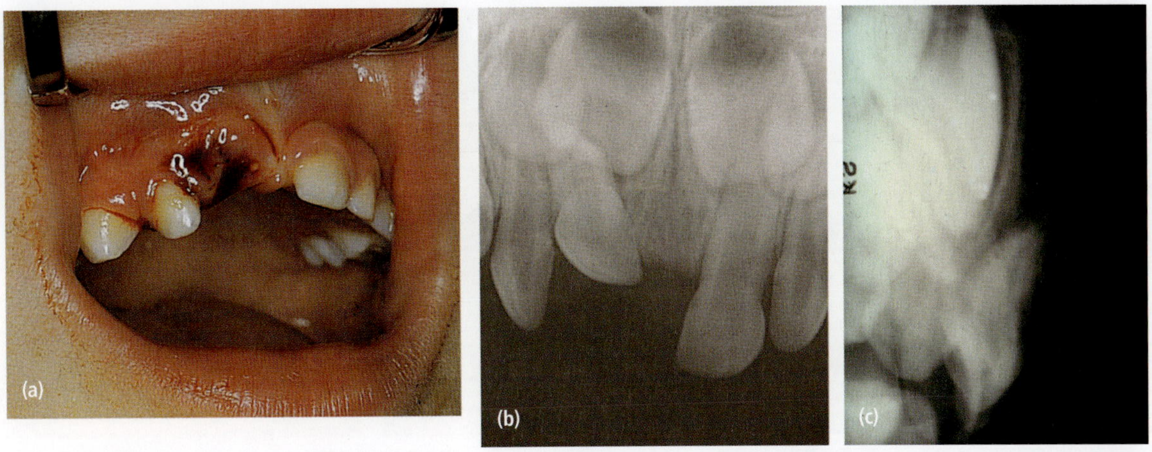

Figure 18-6 (a) Clinical condition immediately after severe intrusive luxation of the primary right central incisor. (b) The occlusal exposure shows foreshortening of the intruded tooth, indicating buccal displacement away from the permanent follicle. (c) This is evident in the lateral radiograph, since the apex of the intruded incisor is forced through the buccal bone plate.

Radiographic examination

A detailed radiographic examination is mandatory in order to get an impression of the injury to the supporting tissues, the stage of root development and, in the case of primary tooth injuries, the relation to permanent successors (Fig. 18-6).

Before a radiographic examination is carried out, a clinical examination should establish the extent of the trauma region. This area is then radiographed; ideally, the injury site should be viewed from different angulations.

Permanent teeth

For an injured anterior front with all incisors involved, four exposures should be taken (one occlusal and three 90° horizontal angle exposures), where the central beam is directed interdentally between the incisors. This combination of radiographs results in each traumatized tooth being seen from different angulations, which increases the likelihood of diagnosing even minor dislocations (Fig. 18-7).

In deep lip wounds a soft tissue radiograph is essential to diagnose tooth fragments or other foreign bodies. A film is placed between the lips and the alveolar process, and the exposure time should be approximately 25% of a dental exposure time.

Primary teeth

A young child is often difficult to examine radiographically because of fear or lack of cooperation. With the parents' help and the use of special film holders, it is usually possible to obtain a radiograph of the traumatized area (see also Chapter 8). In these instances an occlusal film held by the parents and a steep exposure angle should be used. It should also be noted that exposure time can be reduced by 30% for each 10 kVp increase.

Diagnosis

With combined information from the clinical and radiographic examination, a diagnosis is made and the injury is classified as a guide to the treatment required. In this chapter the classification recommended by the World Health Organization (WHO) will be used. The code numbers are according to the International Classification of Diseases (7).

Injuries to the hard dental tissues and the pulp

- *Enamel infraction (S 02.50).* An incomplete fracture (crack) of the enamel without loss of tooth substance.
- *Enamel fracture (uncomplicated crown fracture) (S 02.50).* A fracture with loss of tooth substance confined to the enamel.
- *Enamel–dentin fracture (uncomplicated crown fracture) (S 02.51).* A fracture with loss of tooth substance confined to enamel and dentin, but not involving the pulp.
- *Complicated crown fracture (S 02.52).* A fracture involving enamel and dentin, and exposing the pulp.

Injuries to the hard dental tissues, the pulp, and the alveolar process

- *Crown-root fracture (S 02.54).* A fracture involving enamel, dentin, and cementum. It may or may not expose the pulp (uncomplicated and complicated crown-root fracture).
- *Root fracture (S 02.53).* A fracture involving dentin, cementum, and the pulp. Root fractures can be further

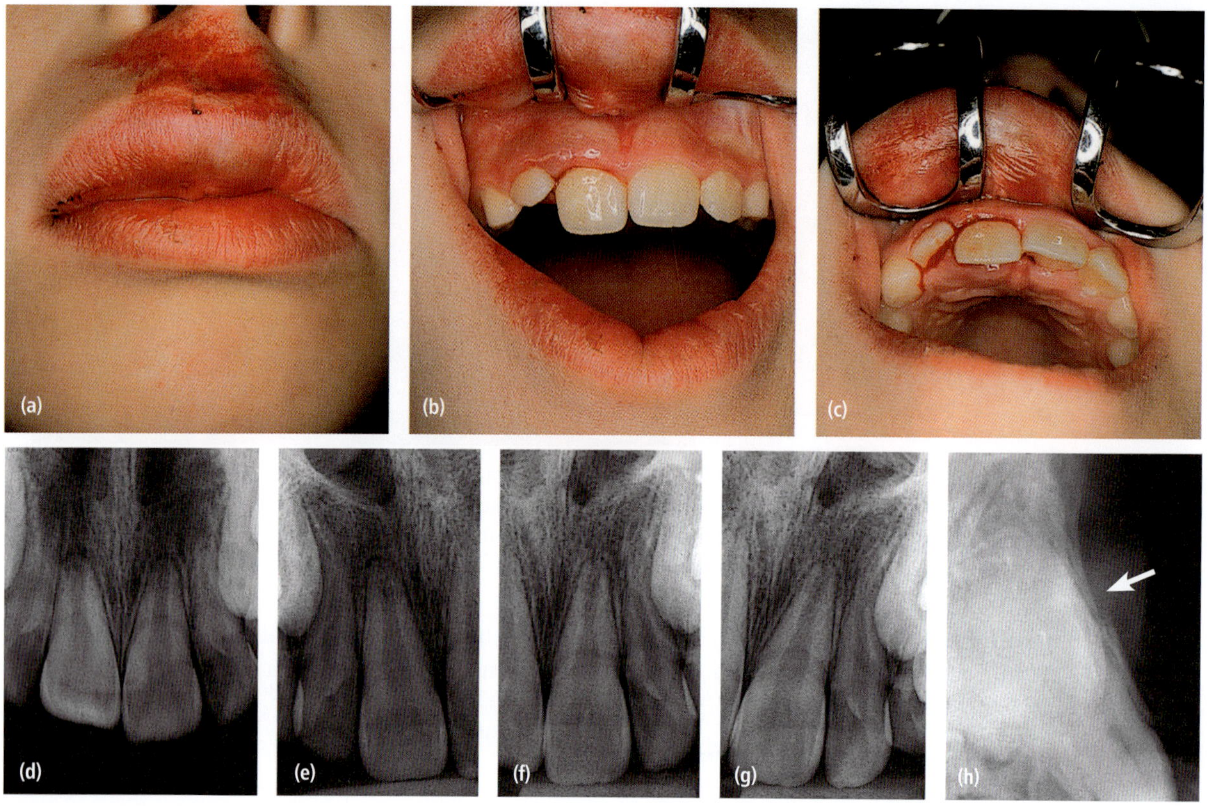

Figure 18-7 (a–c) Clinical appearance after lateral luxation of the right central incisor. (d–g) One occlusal and three periapical radiographs. Note that the occlusal exposure is optimal for showing the buccal displacement of the root. (h) The lateral radiograph illustrates where the fracture of the buccal bone plate has occurred (arrow).

classified according to displacement of the coronal fragment and localization of the fracture.

- *Fracture of the mandibular (S 02.60) or maxillary (S 02.40) alveolar socket wall.* A fracture of the alveolar process that involves the alveolar socket.
- *Fracture of the mandibular (S 02.60) or maxillary (S 02.40) alveolar process.* A fracture of the alveolar process that may or may not involve the alveolar socket.

Injuries to the periodontal tissues

- *Concussion (S 03.28).* An injury to the tooth-supporting structures without abnormal loosening or displacement of the tooth, but with marked reaction to percussion.
- *Subluxation (S 03.28).* An injury to the tooth-supporting structures with abnormal loosening, but without displacement of the tooth.
- *Extrusive luxation (S 03.21).* Partial displacement of the tooth out of its socket.
- *Lateral luxation (S 03.20).* Displacement of the tooth in a direction other than axially. This is accompanied by comminution or fracture of the alveolar socket.
- *Intrusive luxation (S 03.21).* Displacement of the tooth into the alveolar bone. This is accompanied by comminution or fracture of the alveolar socket.
- *Avulsion (exarticulation) (S 03.22).* Complete displacement of the tooth out of its socket.

Injuries to gingiva or oral mucosa

- *Laceration of gingiva or oral mucosa (S 01.50).* A shallow or deep wound in the mucosa resulting from a tear; usually produced by a sharp object.
- *Contusion of gingiva or oral mucosa (S 01.50).* A bruise usually produced by impact with a blunt object and not accompanied by a break in the mucosa, usually causing submucosal hemorrhage.
- *Abrasion of gingiva or oral mucosa (S 01.50).* A superficial wound produced by rubbing or scraping of the mucosa, leaving a raw, bleeding surface.

The distribution of various dental diagnoses in the primary and permanent dentition is shown in Figs 18-8 and 18-9, respectively. In the permanent dentition uncomplicated crown fractures are very common. In contrast, subluxations and luxations dominate in the primary dentition (16). This is probably due to resilience of the

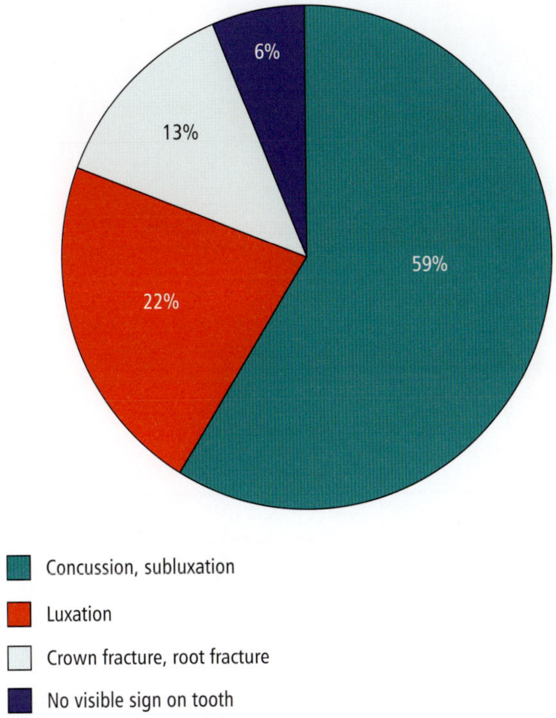

Figure 18-8 Percentage distribution of diagnoses for traumatized primary teeth (16).

alveolar bone in young children, favoring loosening or displacement rather than fractures of the hard dental tissues.

Immediate care: primary teeth

During its early development, the permanent incisor is located palatally and in close proximity to the apex of the primary incisor (Fig. 18-10). Consequently, with injuries to primary teeth, the dentist must always be aware of possible damage to the underlying permanent teeth.

A young child is often unable to cooperate, and the following procedure is suggested for clinical examination (Fig. 18-11):

- The parent is seated on a chair with the child on his or her lap, facing the parent.
- The dentist, who is seated behind the child, receives and steadies the child's head in the lap.
- The parent gently restrains the child's arms and legs.

In this way, a thorough examination of the oral structures can easily be done in a few minutes.

With the assistance of a parent or another adult, it is also possible to obtain radiographs of the traumatized area. However, active treatment such as splinting of loosened teeth or endodontic therapy may be extremely difficult. Therefore, in the majority of cases, the dentist has to decide whether the traumatized tooth is best treated by extraction, or whether it can be maintained without any extensive treatment. A primary incisor should always be removed if its maintenance will jeopardize the developing permanent tooth bud.

Enamel and enamel–dentin fracture

Most crown fractures consist of enamel or superficial enamel–dentin fractures. In both situations, slight grinding of sharp edges is sufficient. If the fracture is extensive, and the child cooperative, the tooth can be restored with glass-ionomer cement or composite.

Complicated crown fracture

Normally, extraction is the treatment of choice. However, if full cooperation of the child can be achieved, the same procedure as outlined for permanent teeth can be followed.

Crown-root fracture

These cases involve fracture of enamel, dentin, and cementum. Frequently, the pulp is also exposed. Restorative treatment is extremely difficult and the tooth is best extracted.

Root fracture

If the coronal fragment is severely dislocated, extraction is again the treatment of choice. No effort should be made to remove the apical fragment, as such intervention might damage the underlying permanent tooth. After removal of the coronal fragment, uncomplicated resorption of the apical fragment should be expected (Fig. 18-12). Without evident displacement, the coronal fragment may show little mobility, and no immediate extraction is required. The tooth should be kept under observation. Sometimes necrosis develops in the coronal fragment, whereas the apical portion nearly always remains vital. In these cases the coronal fragment only should be extracted.

Concussion, subluxation, and luxation injuries

These injuries dominate in the primary dentition. Most often, the patients also have extensive soft tissue damage such as swollen lips, lacerations, and hemorrhage of the oral mucosa and gingiva (Fig. 18-13). The parents are instructed to clean the traumatized area gently with 0.1% chlorhexidine solution, using cotton swabs (twice daily for 1 or 2 weeks). Normally the soft tissue heals quickly. Swelling will usually subside within a week.

Concussion

Most concussions are not seen by the dentist at the time of the accident. The parents may see no need to seek

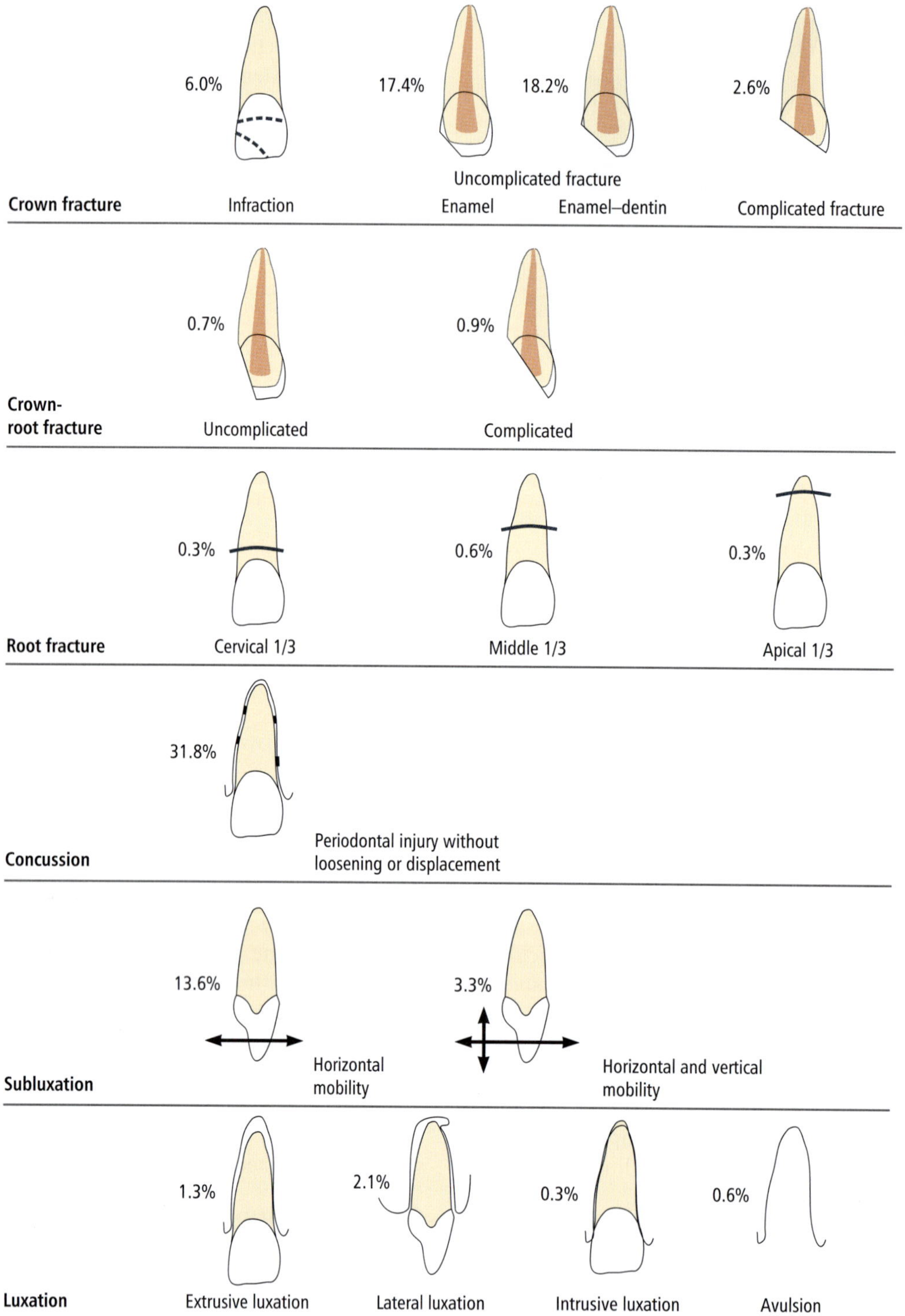

Figure 18-9 Distribution of 2019 traumatized permanent teeth according to diagnosis in 1275 children aged 7–18 years (14).

dental treatment, or they may not be aware of the injury until tooth discoloration appears.

Subluxation

The parents are advised to keep the traumatized area as clean as possible, and to feed the child on a soft diet for a few days. Mobility should diminish within 1–2 weeks.

Extrusive luxation

An extruded tooth shows considerable mobility, and the tooth is best treated by immediate extraction.

Lateral luxation

- *Palatal displacement of the crown* is most common. This implies that the apex is forced in a buccal direc-

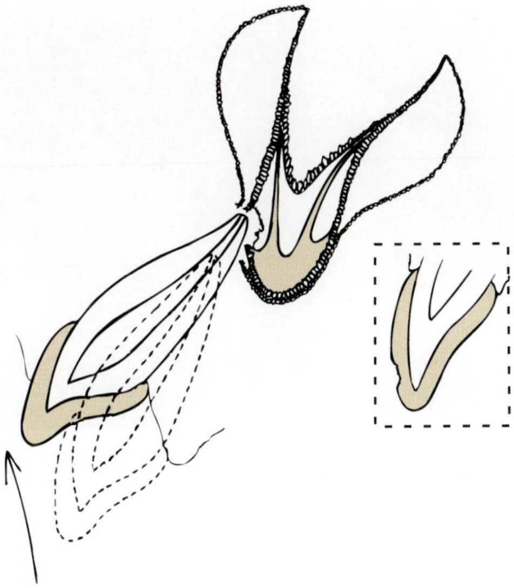

Figure 18-10 Schematic drawing illustrating developmental disturbance of permanent tooth bud at the age of 2 years. The crown of the primary incisor is displaced buccally, forcing the root into the crown of the developing permanent incisor.

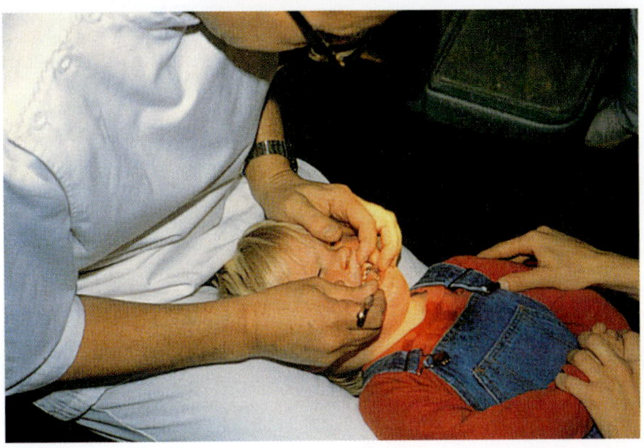

Figure 18-11 Procedure for examination of a young child's mouth (see text).

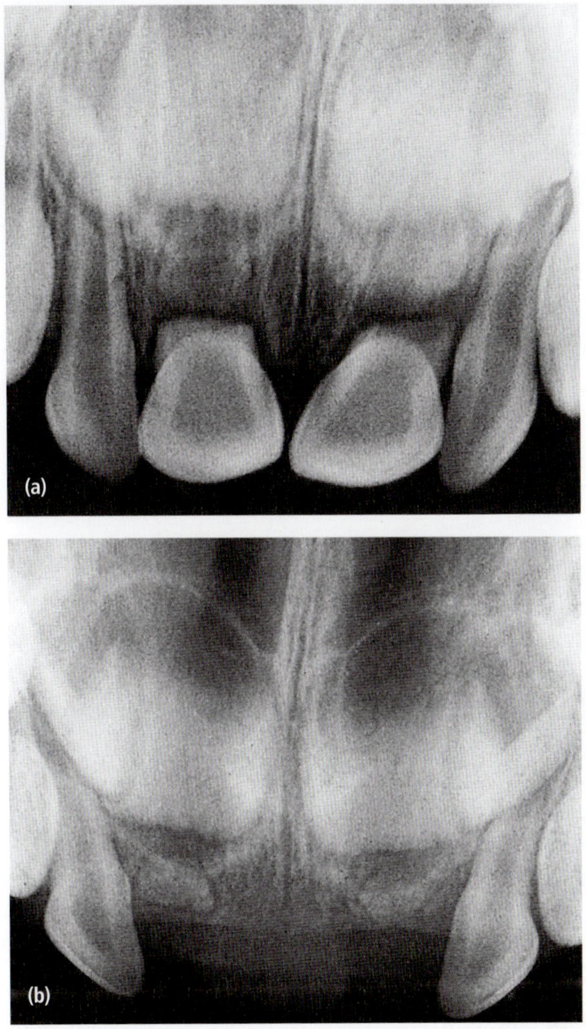

Figure 18-12 (a) Fractured roots of both central incisors with dislocation of the coronal fragments. (b) Normal resorption of the apical fragments after removal of the coronal fragments.

tion and thus away from the permanent tooth bud. These teeth can usually be left untreated. Over a period of 1–2 months, tongue pressure will usually reposition the tooth (Fig. 18-14).

- *Buccal displacement of the crown* (Figs 18-10 and 18-15). The root will be displaced palatally in the direction of the permanent tooth bud. Extraction is the treatment of choice to prevent further damage to the permanent tooth.

Intrusive luxation

An intruded tooth often shows severe displacement. Sometimes it will be completely intruded into the alveolar process and mistakenly assumed to be lost, until a radiograph shows the intruded position (Fig. 18-16).

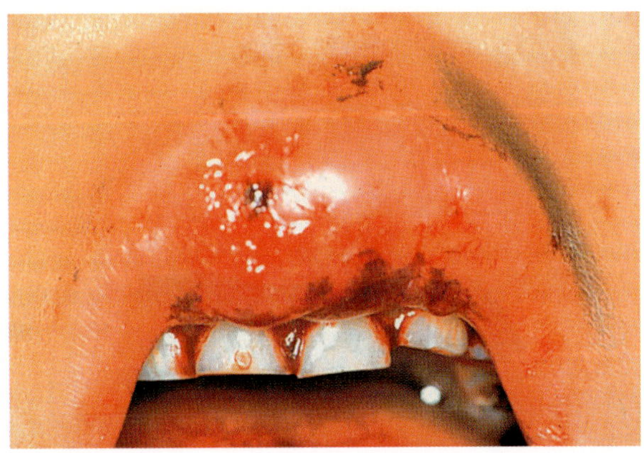

Figure 18-13 Severe soft tissue damage with extensive hemorrhage. Both central incisors and the right lateral incisor are extruded and extremely mobile.

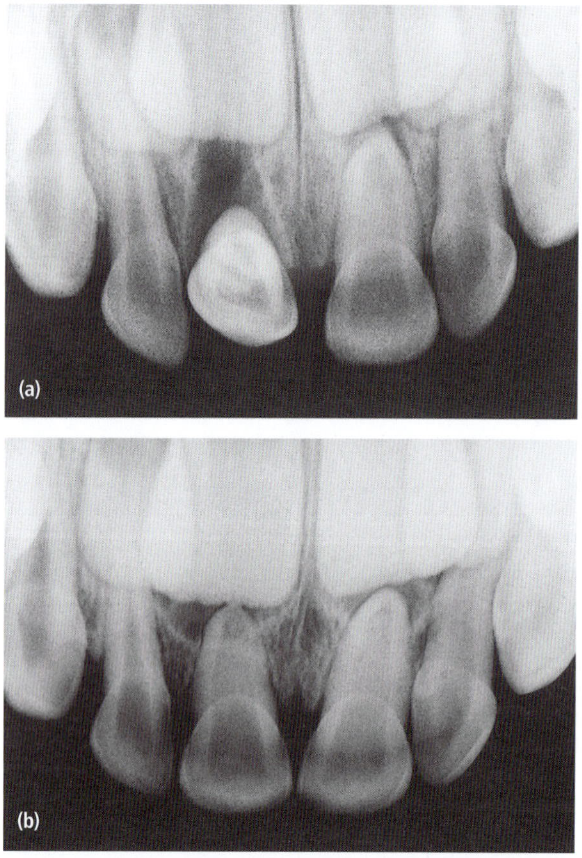

Figure 18-14 (a) Severe palatal luxation of the right central incisor. No treatment other than observation was performed. (b) Two months later, the tooth is back in normal position due to tongue pressure.

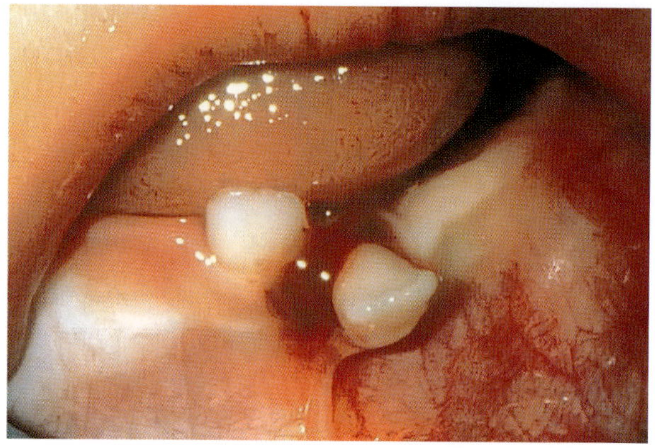

Figure 18-15 Clinical condition immediately after buccal displacement of the left central incisor in an 8-month-old girl.

With all intrusions, it is essential to clarify whether the root is forced in a palatal or buccal direction. The diagnosis should be based on a combined clinical and radiographic examination.

- *Clinical examination.* Due to a buccal curve of the apex, the primary root tends to be displaced through the buccal bone plate. It is advisable to palpate the buccal sulcus fold. If part of the crown is visible, the tooth crown axes will also indicate the direction.
- *Radiographic examination.* The foreshortened appearance of the intruded tooth implies buccal displacement of the root and thus away from the permanent tooth germ, whereas the elongated image suggests palatal displacement towards the permanent successor (Fig. 18-6).
- *Treatment.* If the primary root is displaced palatally, i.e., towards and possibly into the developing tooth germ, extraction is recommended. Extraction is performed to minimize further damage to the developing permanent tooth. Elevators should never be used to luxate the intruded incisors. Forceps should be the only instrument employed for this purpose. The intruded tooth should be grasped mesiodistally and lifted out of its socket in an axial direction. Thereafter digital pressure should be applied to the buccal and palatal aspects of the socket to reposition the displaced bone plates.

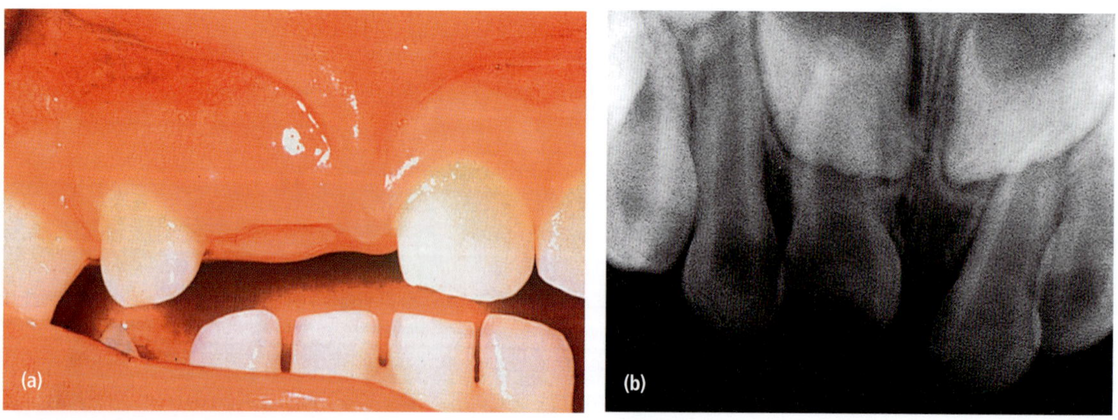

Figure 18-16 (a) Clinical examination after trauma of an 18-month-old child. The parents assumed that the right central incisor was lost. (b) The radiograph reveals severe intrusive luxation. Additional radiographs should be taken to disclose the exact direction of the intrusion (see Fig. 18-6).

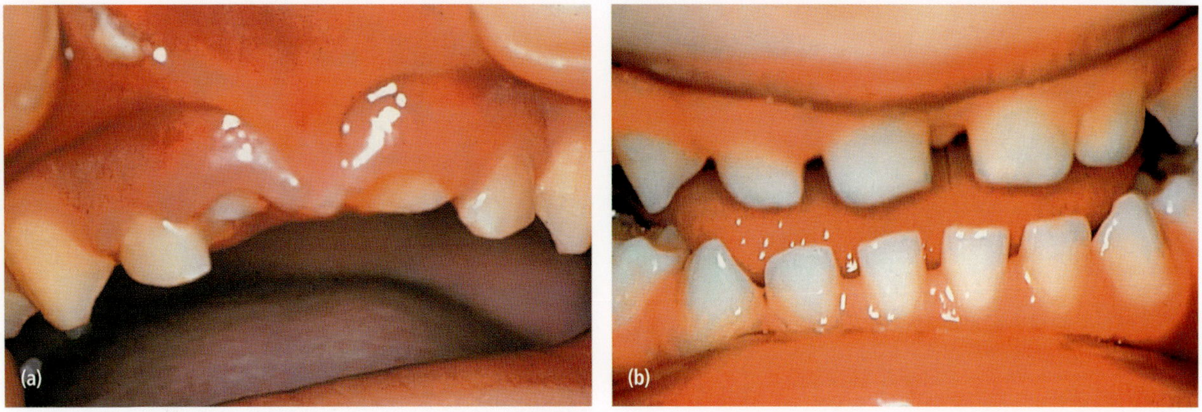

Figure 18-17 (a) Condition immediately after intrusive luxation of both central incisors. (b) Re-eruption is evident 6 months later.

With displacement of the root in a buccal direction, the intruded tooth can most often be allowed to re-erupt. The parents are instructed to clean the traumatized area with 0.1% chlorhexidine solution. During the re-eruption phase, there is always a risk of infection, and the patient should be seen once a week for the first 3–4 weeks. Signs of infection include swelling, spontaneous bleeding, and abscess formation. There may also be a rise in body temperature. In these cases, the traumatized tooth must be removed and antibiotic therapy instituted. Without signs of infection, re-eruption will generally take place within 2–6 months (Fig. 18-17). If re-eruption fails to occur, ankylosis should be suspected. If the ankylosed tooth interferes with eruption of the permanent successor, it must be removed.

Avulsion

A radiographic examination is essential to ensure that the missing tooth is not intruded (Fig. 18-16). Replantation is contraindicated, as pulp necrosis is a frequent complication. Moreover, there is a risk of further injury to the permanent tooth germ by the replantation procedure, whereby the coagulum from the socket can be forced into the follicle.

Immediate care: permanent teeth

As shown in Fig. 18-3, the most common age of trauma is between 8 and 10 years. This implies that a traumatized tooth most often has an open apical foramen, a wide root canal, and fragile dentinal walls in the cervical area. If pulp necrosis develops, no further dentin apposition occurs, and there is a considerable risk of spontaneous root fracture cervically with subsequent loss of the injured tooth (see Chapter 19). Consequently, the primary concern is to maintain pulp vitality to allow continued root formation including physiologic dentin apposition in the critical cervical area.

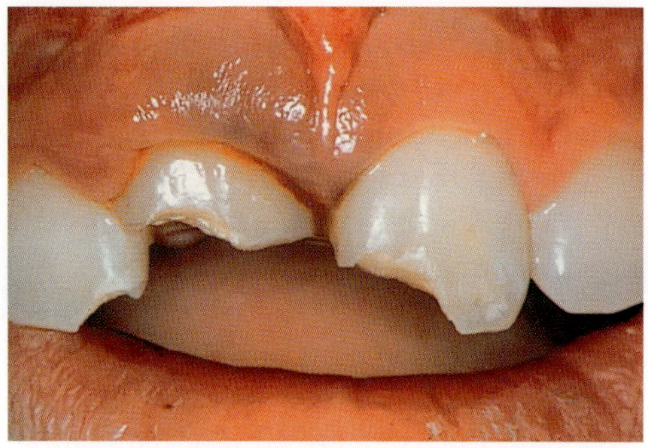

Figure 18-18 Uncomplicated crown fracture involving either mesial corners or entire incisal edge. The gingival bleeding indicates that intrusive luxation has also occurred in the right central incisor.

Crown fractures

It is most important to diagnose concomitant periodontal injuries, since the risk of complications to crown fractures is significantly increased with an additional luxation injury (Figs 18-18 and 18-19).

- *Enamel infraction.* Infractions are incomplete fractures without loss of tooth substance. The fracture line usually stops at the enamel–dentin junction. Infraction lines are best seen when the light beam is directed parallel to the long axis of the tooth. No active treatment is required. However, the energy of the impact may be transmitted to the periodontal tissues and the neurovascular supply at the apical foramen. Recalls are therefore necessary.
- *Enamel fracture.* Minimal tooth substance is lost, and restoration is normally not needed. Most often, a slight contouring of the fractured angle will provide an aesthetically satisfactory result. If necessary, the contralateral tooth can be rounded off similarly to make the teeth symmetrical.

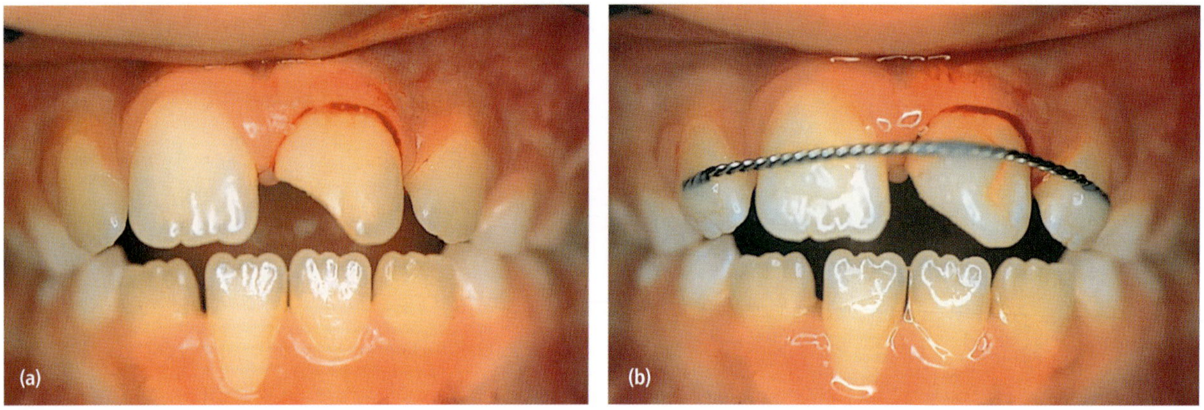

Figure 18-19 (a) Both subluxation and uncomplicated crown fracture have occurred in the left central incisor. (b) The tooth is stabilized with a splint, and a temporary crown restoration is applied.

- *Enamel–dentin fracture.* Some typical examples are shown in Figs 18-18 and 18-19. Crown fractures involving dentin result in exposure of dentinal tubules to the oral environment. If the dentin is left unprotected, bacteria or bacterial toxins may penetrate the tubules, resulting in pulpal inflammation. Although the inflammation may be reversible, pulp necrosis is also a possible outcome. The pulp should therefore be protected against external irritants as quickly as possible, and the tooth crown restored by one of the following restorations.
- *Temporary crown restoration.* There are situations in which a temporary restoration should be preferred over a period of time. One example is when the child's general health condition is also affected. A temporary restoration may then be the most practical solution until the child has recovered. Another example is when an associated luxation injury requires immediate fixation, as shown in Fig. 18-19. The procedure is to cover exposed dentin with calcium hydroxide. After etching, rinsing, and drying of the enamel, a layer of light-curing composite resin is applied. Alternatively the whole fracture surface can be covered with a glass-ionomer cement "bandage".
- *Reattachment of a crown fragment.* It is important to inform the public that a fractured fragment can be reattached. People should also know that dehydration of the fragment must be avoided. One advice is to place the fragment in a glass of water and to seek dental treatment as soon as possible. If a temporary restoration is indicated for a period of time, the fragment should be stored in physiologic saline in the delay period. The broken fragment can then be bonded to the tooth with a flowable composite (Fig. 18-20) (3).
- *Composite crown build-up.* If the fractured fragment is not found, or if it is too small to be reattached, a composite build-up has been shown to be successful both functionally and aesthetically in the young patient (Fig. 18-21). The treatment procedure is summarized in Box 18-3.
- *Complicated crown fracture.* This fracture involves enamel and dentin, with exposure of the pulp (Fig. 18-22). The overall aim of the treatment is preservation of a vital noninflamed pulp. The pulp must be sealed from bacteria so that it is not infected during the period of repair. In most cases this can be achieved by either pulp capping or partial pulpotomy. The indications and techniques for these two treatment

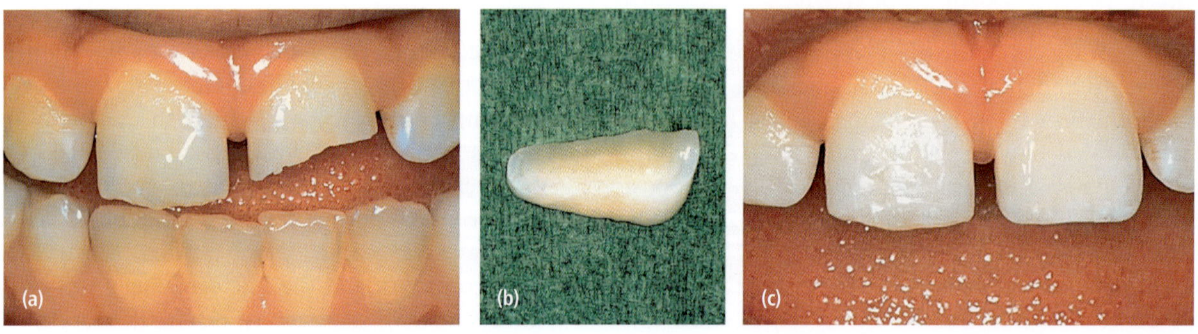

Figure 18-20 (a) Enamel–dentin fracture of the left central incisor in an 8-year-old boy. (b) The fractured crown fragment. (c) Condition immediately after reattachment of the fragment.

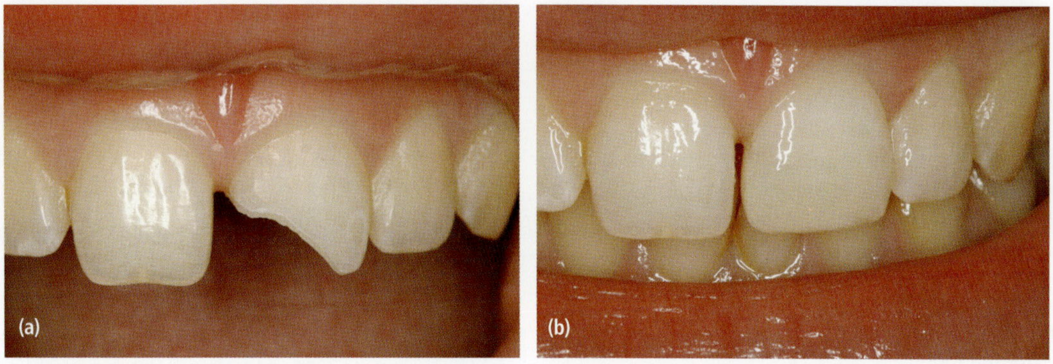

Figure 18-21 (a) A 12-year-old girl with enamel–dentin fracture of the left central incisor. (b) Condition shortly after the composite crown build-up.

Box 18-3 Composite crown build-up

- Make a 2-mm wide shallow preparation in the enamel surrounding the fracture area.
- Select and adapt a celluloid crown form, e.g., Odus Pella®. Place two holes incisally to allow air escape during insertion.
- Select the proper color shade of the composite material.
- Apply a rubber dam after application of topical anesthesia to the gingiva.
- Etch a 2–3-mm wide zone of the enamel around the fracture surface. Rinse thoroughly and dry.
- Apply the bonding resin.
- Fill the crown form with the composite material, and place it in correct position.
- Cure the material carefully buccally and palatally.
- Remove the crown form and the rubber dam. Finish with diamonds and discs.

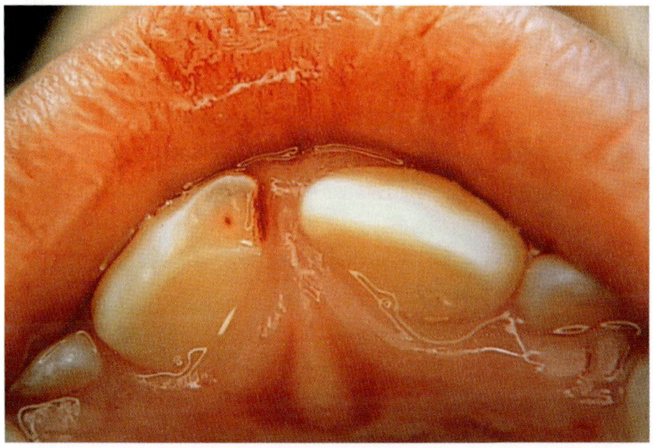

Figure 18-22 Right central incisor with a small pulpal exposure, but with loosening and marked tenderness to percussion. Partial pulpotomy was decided to be the treatment of choice.

procedures are presented in Boxes 18-4 and 18-5 (see also Chapter 12).

Both capping and partial pulpotomy have shown favorable prognoses. However, if in doubt as to the treatment of choice, partial pulpotomy should be performed, since it results in better wound control and ensures a bacteria-tight seal of the pulp cavity (8).

Crown-root fracture

These injuries involve enamel, dentin, and cementum, and are often complicated by pulpal exposures. The fracture is sometimes vertical with the fracture line in the same direction as the long axis of the root. A more typical finding is an oblique course of the fracture line, as shown in Fig. 18-23. The fracture is then usually located a few millimeters incisally to the gingival margin on the buccal surface. Palatally, the fracture is found to extend below the cementoenamel junction.

Box 18-4 Pulp capping

Indications

- Pulp status normal prior to trauma.
- No associated luxation injury with damage to the apical blood supply.
- Pulp exposure less than 1 mm.
- Interval between pulp exposure and treatment less than 24 hours.

Technique

- Isolate the tooth with a rubber dam.
- Clean the fracture surface with sterile cotton pellets moistened with saline or chlorhexidine.
- Dry the exposure site using sterile cotton pellets.
- Cover the perforation with calcium hydroxide cement.
- Apply the protective restoration (temporary restoration, crown fragment reattachment, or composite build-up).

Box 18-5 Partial pulpotomy

This treatment implies removal of inflamed pulp tissue. Usually, the level of amputation should be about 2 mm below the exposure site. Partial pulpotomy is indicated in both immature and mature teeth provided the pulp has a bright red appearance. Neither size of the exposure nor interval between injury and treatment is critical for the prognosis.

Technique
- Anesthetize the tooth.
- Isolate with a rubber dam and clean the fracture surface with sterile cotton pellets moistened with saline or chlorhexidine.
- Prepare a box-like cavity at the exposure site.
- Use high speed and a cylindrical diamond bur, ensuring copious water supply.
- Remove the pulp to a depth of about 2 mm.
- Achieve hemostasis either by irrigation with sterile saline or by slight pressure from cotton pellets.
- Cover the wound with a paste of calcium hydroxide (e.g., Calasept®). Over this, a hard-setting cement is applied.
- Apply the protective restoration (temporary restoration, crown fragment reattachment, or composite build-up)

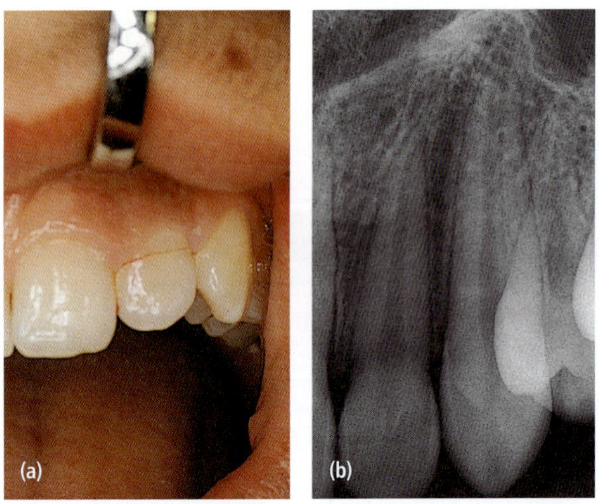

Figure 18-23 Crown-root fracture of the left lateral incisor. (a) Buccally, the fracture line is located close to the gingival margin. (b) The radiograph only demonstrates the position of the buccal part of the fracture, whereas the palatal part cannot be seen.

In some cases, loose fragments can be stabilized by bonding, as least as a temporary measure. However, the prognosis is rather doubtful. In fractures communicating with the oral cavity, periodontal breakdown is most likely to occur. Thus, with most crown-root fractures, the treatment is to remove the loose fragment or fragments. Any pulpal involvement must be determined. If the pulp is exposed, treatment should follow recommendations given in Chapter 12. Further treatment depends on how deeply the fracture extends into the root surface. The goal is to create a situation where the tooth can be restored after removal of the coronal fragment. If the root portion is of sufficient length, one of the following procedures is suggested:

- *Fragment removal and gingival reattachment.* The coronal fragment is removed and the gingiva is allowed to reattach to the exposed dentin (i.e., by formation of a long junctional epithelium). After some weeks, the tooth can be restored above the gingival level.
- *Fragment removal and surgical exposure of subgingival fracture.* After removal of the coronal fragment, the subgingival fracture is exposed by gingivectomy and/or osteotomy if the fracture extends below the alveolar crest. After gingival healing, the tooth is restored with a post-retained crown. While this procedure might appear to be most direct, long-term aesthetic success may be compromised due to an accumulation of granulation tissue in the gingival sulcus palatally, which can lead to buccal migration of the restored tooth.
- *Fragment removal and orthodontic extrusion.* The coronal fragment is initially stabilized to adjacent teeth. Pulp extirpation and canal obturation with guttapercha and sealer can be performed at a later appointment. The coronal fragment is then removed and the tooth extruded over a 4–6-week period. The tooth should be slightly overextruded (0.5 mm), due to risk of relapse (12). A buccal gingivectomy is performed, whereafter the tooth can be restored.
- *Fragment removal and surgical extrusion.* The coronal fragment is removed, then the root is loosened with elevators and forceps and repositioned in a more incisal position, so that the entire fracture surface is exposed above the gingival level (11). The root fragment is then stabilized with sutures or a nonrigid splint. The pulp is extirpated, a guttapercha point is placed loosely in the canal to later facilitate canal location, and the entrance to the root canal is sealed with a temporary cement. After 4 weeks, when the tooth is stabilized in its socket, endodontic treatment is completed; and after a further 4–5 weeks, the tooth can be restored.

Root fracture

A root fracture involves dentin, cementum, and the pulp. The coronal fragment may be extruded or displaced in a palatal direction (Fig. 18-24). Treatment consists of immediate repositioning of the coronal fragment and stabilization with a flexible splint (Box 18-6). Fixation should also be carried out in cases without dis-

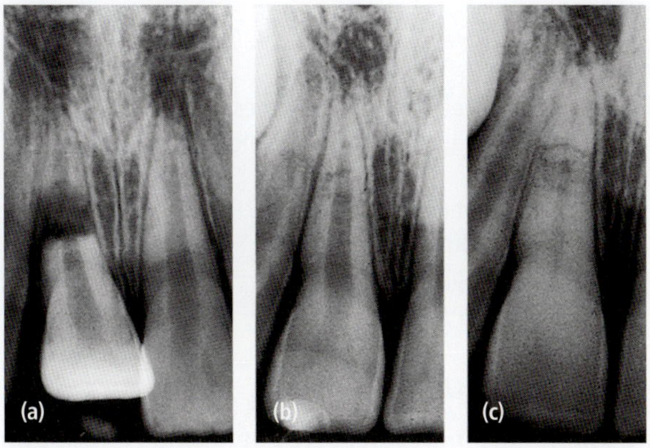

Figure 18-24 (a) Root fracture in the right central incisor with severe dislocation of the coronal fragment. (b) Optimal repositioning performed within 1 hour. (c) Condition 1 year later, with normal findings in the fracture area and partial pulp canal obliteration.

Box 18-6 Root fracture

- Consider the need for local anesthesia.
- Reposition the coronal fragment gently with digital pressure.
- If the buccal socket wall is also fractured, it is necessary to reposition the displaced bone before attempting to reposition the coronal fragment. This is done with a small, flat instrument inserted between the root surface and the socket wall.
- Take a control radiograph to ensure that the repositioning is optimal.
- Stabilize the tooth with a splint (Box 18-7).
- With middle or apical third fractures, a splinting period of 4 weeks appears sufficient to ensure healing. Fractures located near the cervical area may require stabilization for a longer period of time (up to 4 months) (5).

Box 18-7 Splinting (Figs 18-19, 18-25, and 18-28)

- An orthodontic wire (0.032 or 0.016 inches) or a TTS splint is bent to conform to the buccal surfaces (middle one-third) of the injured teeth and also to one or two uninjured teeth on either side of the teeth to be stabilized.
- Apply phosphoric acid gel for 15–20 seconds to the buccal surfaces of the selected teeth.
- Rinse thoroughly with a steam of water.
- Apply a thin layer of a light-curing composite resin.
- Attach the wire to the uninjured teeth and thereafter to the injured teeth. Ensure that they are in proper position.
- Instruct the patient to use 0.1% chlorhexidine mouthrinse twice daily for a week.

location, as close contact between the fragments is considered essential during the period of initial repair (19).

Splinting technique. An acceptable splint should be easy to construct. It should be flexible and neither add further trauma to the periodontal tissues nor interfere with occlusion. The splint should allow sensitivity testing and access to the root canal if endodontic treatment is required. Two simple methods based on the etch technique and fulfilling the above-mentioned requirements are presented in Box 18-7 and Figs 18-19, 18-25, and 18-28 (17).

Concussion

These lesions are defined as injuries to the periodontal tissue without displacement or loosening of the tooth. Marked tenderness to percussion is the characteristic finding. No immediate treatment is required, but follow-up examination is important to verify that no associated pulp injury has occurred.

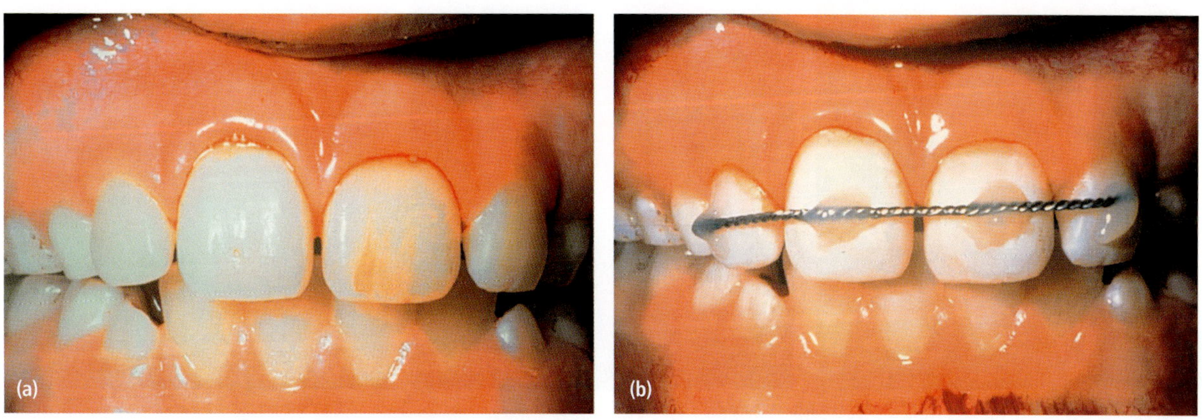

Figure 18-25 (a) Subluxation of both central incisors with mobility in both the horizontal and vertical directions. (b) The teeth are stabilized with an orthodontic twisted wire, resin material, and the acid-etch technique (see Box 18-7).

Subluxation

The involved teeth show varying degrees of mobility and there might be bleeding from the gingival margin.

It has not been proven that splinting will improve the chance of pulp survival or periodontal repair. However, in the case of mobility in both a horizontal and a vertical direction, the tooth may be splinted for 1–2 weeks for the comfort of the patient (Fig. 18-25). Should the tooth be only slightly loosened, it is sufficient to recommend a soft diet for 1–2 weeks. To achieve optimal plaque control in the healing period, the use of chlorhexidine solution is always recommended.

Extrusive luxation

A partial, axial displacement out of the alveolar socket has occurred. The tooth appears elongated and is extremely mobile. There is also bleeding from the gingival sulcus (Fig. 18-26).

The treatment principle implies immediate repositioning and fixation (Box 18-8). Repositioning will facilitate repair of the periodontal ligament. Optimal repositioning is also essential to allow pulp revascularization and continued root development of an immature tooth.

Lateral luxation

Lateral luxation implies displacement in a palatal, buccal, mesial, or distal direction accompanied by comminution or fracture of the alveolar socket. Most often, a palatal luxation occurs (Fig. 18-27). The apex is then displaced in the opposite direction and usually forced through the buccal bone. Repositioning requires disengagement of the apex from its bony lock (Box 18-9).

Box 18-8 Extrusive luxation (Fig. 18-26)

- Consider the need for local anesthesia.
- Reposition the tooth gently with finger pressure on the incisal edge.
- Check the position radiographically.
- Stabilize the tooth with a splint.
- Maintain the splint for 2 weeks.

Intrusive luxation

Intrusion is the most severe type of luxation and appears to be most frequent in the 6–12 years age group (18). The tooth is forced axially into the socket, resulting in damage to the alveolar bone, the periodontal ligament, the cementum, and the pulp (Fig. 18-29).

In the young permanent dentition with incisors under eruption, the diagnosis is sometimes difficult (Fig. 18-18). In these cases a high metallic percussion sound indicates intrusive luxation with the tooth locked in bone.

A variety of treatment methods are suggested for intruded teeth. One option is to leave the tooth to re-erupt. Another is to reposition the tooth by orthodontic forces. Immediate surgical repositioning is also recommended. However, divergence of opinion still exists concerning the best treatment (6).

External replacement resorption (ankylosis related) has recently been found to be the main reason for loss of intruded incisors (18). Moreover, replacement resorption was also found to occur more often in orthodontically and surgically repositioned teeth than in teeth allowed to re-erupt.

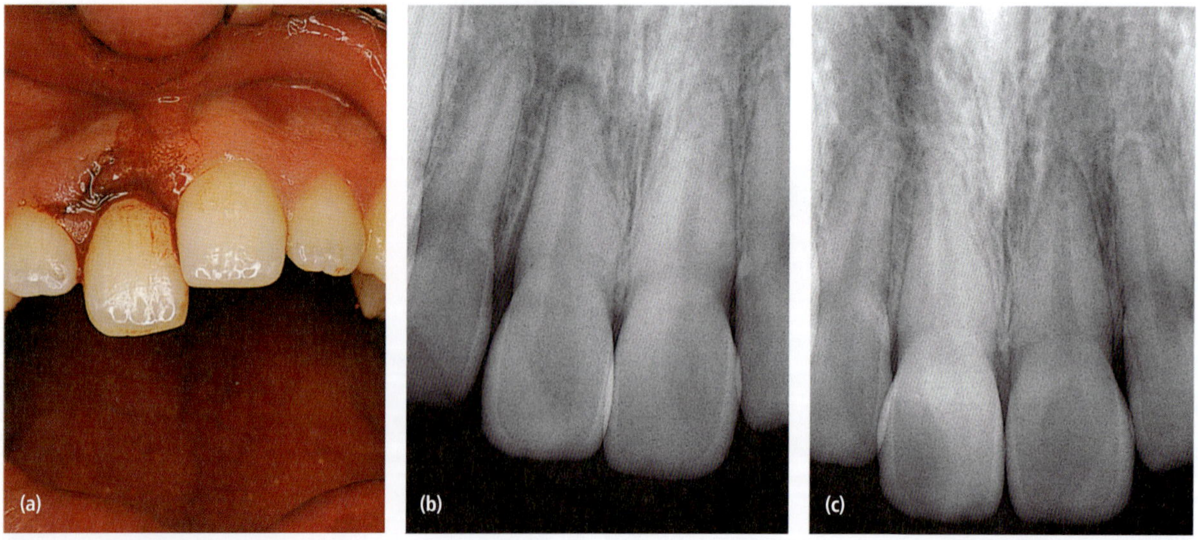

Figure 18-26 (a) Extrusive luxation of the right central incisor. The tooth appears elongated and is also very mobile. (b) The radiograph shows increased periodontal width apically. (c) A radiograph taken after repositioning illustrates optimal position of the tooth in its socket.

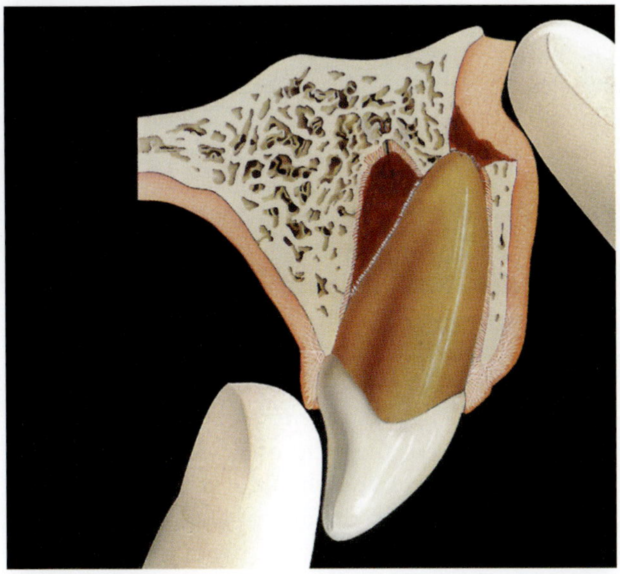

Figure 18-27 Palatal luxation of the crown. The apex is forced through the buccal bone. Repositioning requires disengagement of the tooth from its bony lock. Apply firm digital pressure in an incisal direction, and move the tooth back through the fenestration into the socket. Thereafter, axial pressure will bring the tooth back to its original position.

Box 18-9 Luxation in a palatal direction (Fig. 18-27)

- Administer local anesthesia.
- Palpate the vestibular sulcus, and localize the displaced root apex. Apply firm, digital pressure in an incisal direction and move the tooth back through the fenestration into the socket.
- Reposition the tooth back to its original position by axial pressure.
- Reposition fractured bone with finger pressure.
- Take a radiograph to verify correct position.
- Stabilize the tooth with a splint.
- Maintain the splint for a minimum of 4 weeks.
- Take a radiograph after about 4 weeks. If there are signs of marginal bone breakdown, the splint is maintained for another 3–4 weeks.

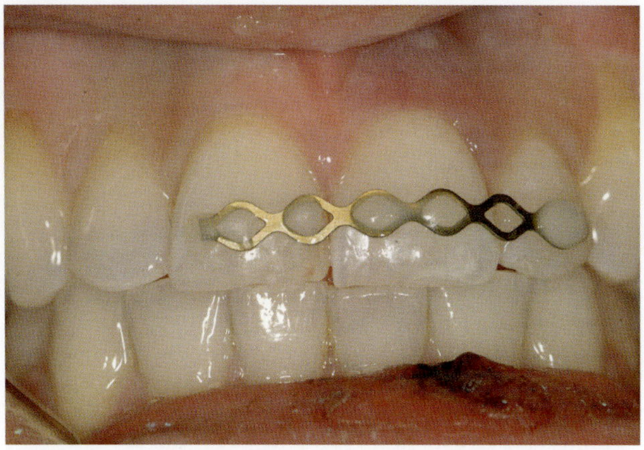

Figure 18-28 The left central incisor has been luxated 1–2 mm in a palatal direction. Repositioning was performed shortly after trauma and a Titanium Trauma Splint (TTS) was applied and maintained for 4 weeks.

Guidelines for the treatment are suggested in Box 18-10.

Avulsion

The alveolar bone, cementum, periodontal ligament, gingiva, and the pulp are all damaged when a tooth is totally displaced out of its socket.

Replantation. When avulsion occurs, replantation is the treatment of choice. Due to a frequent occurrence of external root resorption, it is not possible to guarantee long-term retention of a replanted tooth. However, even when resorption does occur, the replanted tooth can be maintained for years, serving as an ideal space maintainer (Fig. 18-30). Moreover, in the young permanent dentition, a replanted tooth prevents horizontal and vertical bone loss and facilitates later alternative treatment, e.g., orthodontic closure, premolar transplantation, or dental implants.

A number of factors are associated with complications seen after replantation. The most critical factor related to periodontal healing is the extraoral time. A Danish study reported that teeth replanted within

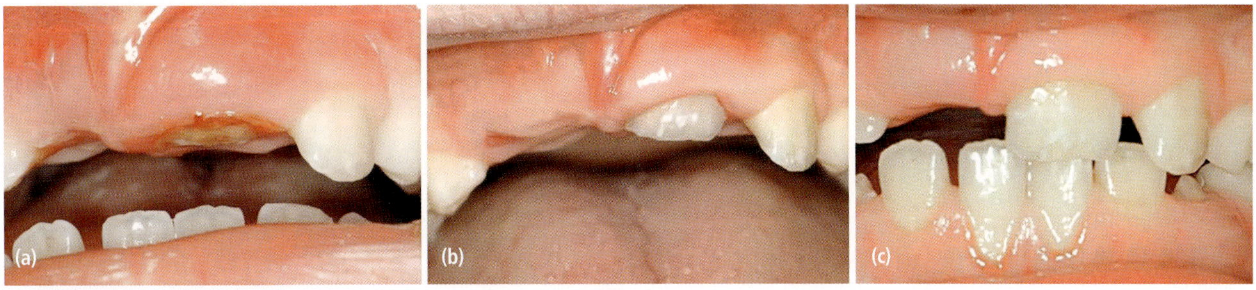

Figure 18-29 Complete intrusion of the left central incisor in a 9-year-old boy. (a) The incisal edge is barely visible 5 days after the accident. It was decided to await re-eruption. (b) Partial re-eruption is evident a month later. (c) Complete re-eruption 10 months after trauma. (Delayed eruption of the right incisor is due to a supernumerary tooth.)

Box 18-10 Intrusive luxation: treatment guidelines

In most intruded teeth re-eruption should be awaited.
- Instruct the patient to rinse twice daily with a 0.1% solution of chlorhexidine.
- Perform close clinical and radiographic control. In all likelihood re-eruption will take place over a period of 3–12 months (Fig. 18-29).
- Should endodontic treatment be required in a severely intruded tooth before re-eruption has occurred, a gingivectomy can be performed to gain access to the root canal.

Surgical repositioning is recommended if the tooth is driven up into the floor of the nose or out in the soft tissue of the vestibulum.
- Reposition the tooth with forceps.
- Stabilize the tooth with a splint, and instruct the patient to rinse with chlorhexidine.
- Maintain the splint until radiographs show satisfactory socket healing.

5 minutes had the best prognosis (2). Consequently, replantation should preferably be done at the site of injury in order to minimize the extraoral period. If immediate replantation is impossible, it is of utmost importance that the periodontal ligament attached to the root is kept moist. Studies have demonstrated that the number of viable cells in the periodontal ligament declines very rapidly with an increase in the drying time. Fifteen to 20 minutes seems to be the limit of drying of an avulsed tooth to avoid root resorption. An avulsed tooth should be stored in a physiologic storage medium until it can be replanted. The following storage media have been shown to permit both periodontal and pulpal healing: milk, physiologic saline, tissue culture media, and saliva. However, at the site of injury, only saliva is always available. Recommendations for the treatment of avulsed teeth are presented in Boxes 18-11–18-13.

Should endodontic treatment be performed? Pulp survival is not likely in the event of closed apical foramen, and endodontic treatment should always be started after 7–10 days and prior to removal of the splint. The canal is filled temporarily with calcium hydroxide paste.

In teeth with a wide-open apical foramen, revascularization of the pulp may occur and endodontic treatment is postponed. However, these teeth must be followed closely. With definite signs of necrosis such as apical radiolucency and/or external inflammatory root resorption, endodontic treatment should be started immediately. It is recommend that a replanted tooth with incomplete root formation is examined radiographically every second week until pulp necrosis is confirmed or continued root formation is evident (Fig. 18-31).

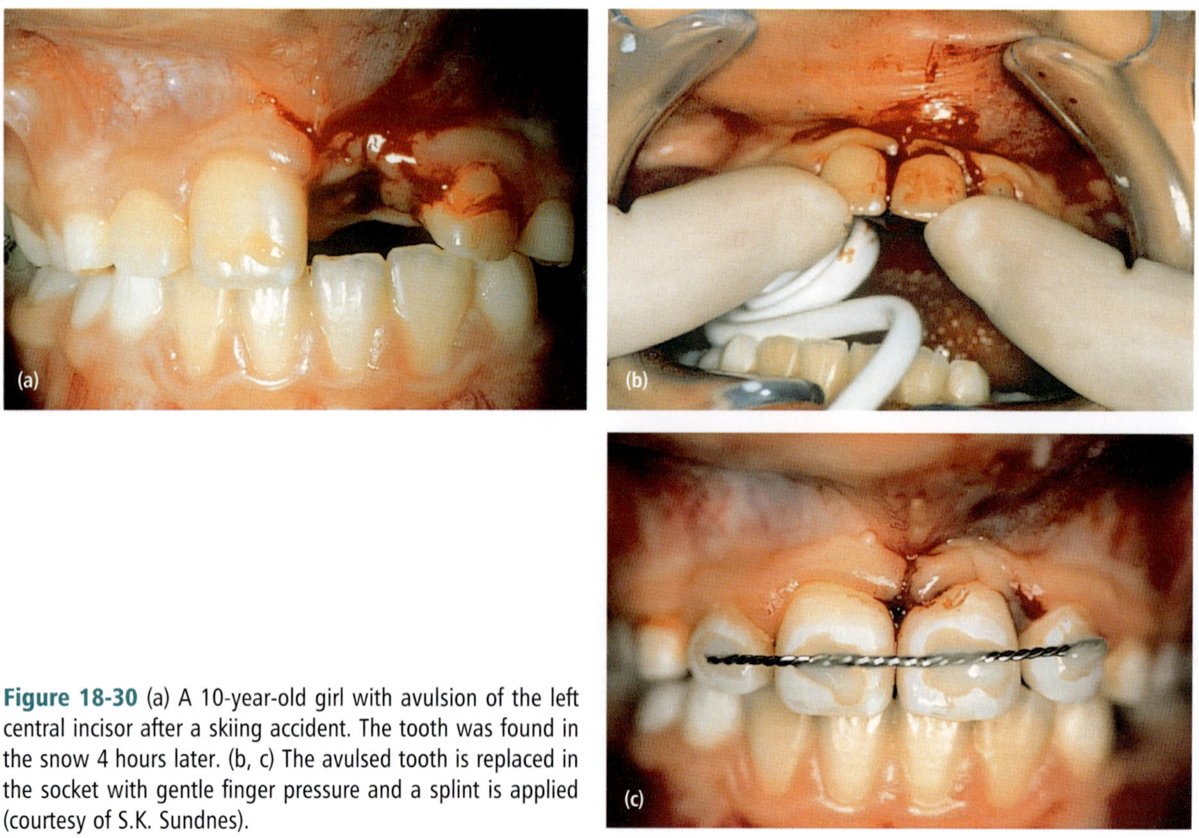

Figure 18-30 (a) A 10-year-old girl with avulsion of the left central incisor after a skiing accident. The tooth was found in the snow 4 hours later. (b, c) The avulsed tooth is replaced in the socket with gentle finger pressure and a splint is applied (courtesy of S.K. Sundnes).

Box 18-11 Avulsion: replantation at the site of injury

The public must be well informed about what to do if a tooth is knocked out.

The best advice

- Pick up the tooth by the crown.
- Avoid touching the root.
- Push the tooth back in place as quickly as possible.

The next best advice

- Place the tooth in the child's mouth between the teeth and the cheek, or if this is not possible put the avulsed tooth in a glass of milk.

In both instances dental aid should be sought immediately.

Box 18-12 Avulsion: replantation in a dental clinic. The extraoral dry time is less than 60 min

- Consider the need for local anesthesia.
- Rinse the root surface and the apical foramen with a stream of saline, and place the tooth in saline.
- Remove the coagulum from the socket with a stream of saline. Examine the socket. If there is a fracture of the socket wall, reposition it with a suitable instrument.

(In teeth with *open* apex, pulp revascularization is possible, and will be optimized with topical tetracycline treatment. If available, cover the root surface with minocycline hydrochloride microspheres (Arestin®, OraPharma Inc., Warminster, PA, USA.)

- Replant the tooth slowly with gentle finger pressure.
- Stabilize the tooth with a flexible splint.
- Check position of the replanted tooth both clinically and radiographically. Suture any gingival lacerations.
- Administer systemic antibiotics for a week. Tetracycline is the first choice for patients older than 12 years. Phenoxymethyl penicillin is recommended for children 12 years and younger due to a risk of tetracycline discoloration of young permanent incisors.
- Consult a physician for evaluation of the need for tetanus prophylaxis.
- Instruct the patient to use 0.1% chlorhexidine mouthrinse twice daily for a week.
- Remove the splint after 1–2 weeks. It appears that a short splinting time favors both periodontal and pulpal healing, whereas a rigid long-term splinting leads to dentoalveolar ankylosis.
- Endodontic considerations (see text).

Box 18-13 Avulsion: replantation in a dental clinic. The extraoral dry time is longer than 60 min

The long-term prognosis is poor. Ankylosis with subsequent root resorption is the expected outcome. However, fluoride treatment of the root surface will delay progress of the resorption.

- Remove attached necrotic soft tissue from the root surface with gauze.
- Immerse the tooth in a 2% sodium fluoride solution for 20 min.
- Administer local anesthesia.
- Remove the coagulum from the socket with a stream of saline. Examine the alveolar socket. If there is a fracture of the socket wall, reposition it with a suitable instrument.
- Replant the tooth slowly with gentle finger pressure.
- Stabilize the tooth with a flexible splint.
- Check position of the replanted tooth both clinically and radiographically. Suture any gingival lacerations.
- Administer systemic antibiotics. See Box 18-12.
- Consult a physician for evaluation of the need for tetanus prophylaxis.
- Instruct the patient to use 0.1% chlorhexidine mouthrinse twice daily for a week.
- Remove the splint after 4 weeks.
- Endodontic considerations (see text).

Injuries to the alveolar process

This trauma entity is defined as a fracture of the alveolar process, which may or may not involve the alveolar socket. The typical clinical appearance is where a segment containing one or more teeth is displaced axially or laterally, usually resulting in occlusal disturbance. When mobility testing is performed, the entire fragment is found to be mobile, and percussion test gives a dull sound. Gingival lacerations are frequent. Radiographically, a fracture line can usually be seen, depending on the angle of the central radiographic beam. The horizontal part of the fracture line may be found in all locations, ranging from the cervical to the apical or periapical region. A differential diagnosis must be made with root fracture. In the case of a root fracture, change in the angulation of the central beam will not alter the fracture position on the root surface. However, in the case of an alveolar fracture, the fracture line will move up or down in relation to the root surface according to the horizontal angulation. The bone fracture may disrupt vascular supply to the teeth, which can result in pulp necrosis. Due to the frequent concomitant luxation injury and damage to the periodontal ligament, root resorption can sometimes occur. The treatment principles comprise repositioning and immobilization of the displaced bone-tooth fragment and monitoring of pulp vitality. Using infiltration or, preferably, a regional block anesthesia, the fragment is repositioned. As with lateral luxation, it is sometimes necessary to disengage the apices of the

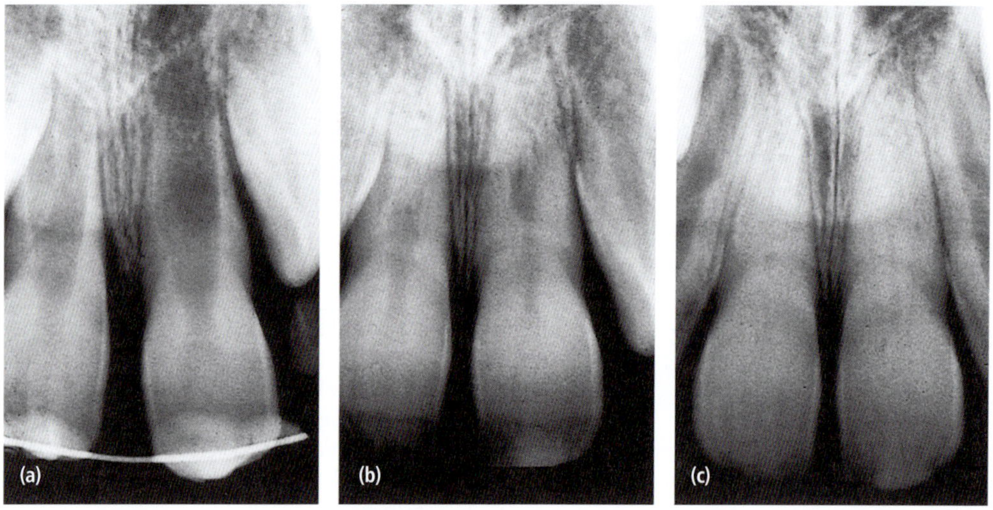

Figure 18-31 Successful replantation of the left central incisor in a 7-year-old boy. The avulsed tooth was immediately pushed back in place by the boy's father. (a, b) Six days and 1 year after replantation, respectively. (c) Four years after the accident with completed root formation and almost total pulp canal obliteration. Note also obliteration in the right central incisor after a subluxation injury (courtesy of S.K. Sundnes).

involved teeth from a bony lock. In the permanent dentition the fractured segment is splinted with a rigid or semi-rigid splint for 4 weeks.

Generally, no measures are taken to stabilize a mobile fragment in the primary dentition, due to lack of sufficient teeth for the splinting procedure. After repositioning of the displaced fragments, the parents are advised to feed the child on a soft diet during the first weeks after the injury. The parents are also instructed to wash the traumatized area twice daily with 0.1% chlorhexidine solution.

Injuries to the gingiva and the oral mucosa

Soft tissue lesions must be adequately treated and recalled for healing control. Minor lacerations of the mucosa, the lip or the tongue should be sutured after careful debridement and cleansing of foreign bodies. With gingival lacerations it is necessary to achieve good tissue positioning to ensure healing. Mouthrinsing or local treatment with 0.1% chlorhexidine solution is recommended to decrease the risk of infection during wound healing.

It is emphasized that if the wound has been contaminated with soil, prophylactic vaccination against tetanus should be given as soon as possible.

Submucosal hematomas in the vestibular region or the floor of the mouth may indicate a jaw fracture, and careful radiographic examination is indicated.

Prevention of traumatic injuries

The causes of orofacial injuries in children vary considerably, and there is no easy way to prevent the majority of these injuries. However, although sports are the cause of relatively few orofacial injuries, these are often severe and involve a greater number of teeth than other injuries.

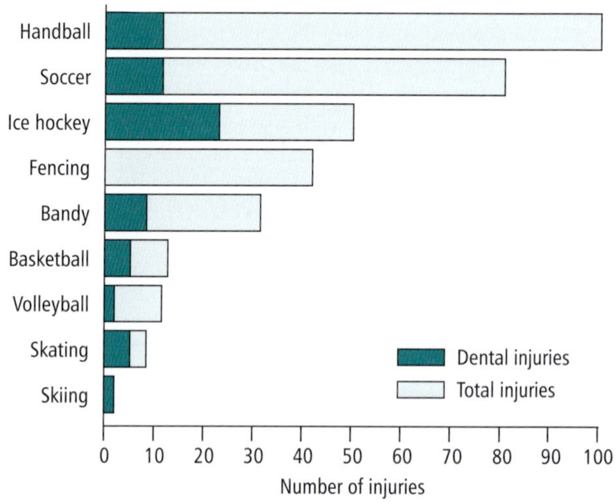

Figure 18-32 Frequency of dental and other sports injuries per 10,000 people from 1981 to 1983 in Norway (13).

Contact sports, such as ice hockey, football, handball, soccer, and basketball, with their high risk of collisions at high speed, are especially prone to resulting in dental and other injuries (Fig. 18-32) (13).

Use of mouth guards

The evidence for the effect of mouth guards for all types of contact sports is incomplete. However, it is apparent that a correctly made mouth guard can reduce both the frequency and the severity of the injuries in many instances. Thus, the use of mouth guards in ice hockey in Canada has reduced the annual rate of dental injuries from 8.3% to 1.2%. A North American study also reported a dramatic decrease in the frequency of orofacial injuries in basketball players using mouth guards (10).

Types of mouth guards include the following:

- *Stock variety protectors* are of latex rubber or polyvinyl chloride, usually made in three sizes, and are supposed to be universally fitting; the advantage being their low cost. However, they have been found to impede both speech and respiration, as they can only be kept in place by occlusion. There is no evidence that they can redistribute forces of impact.
- *Mouth-formed protectors.* Varieties are fitted from a manufactured kit consisting of a fairly rigid outer shell and a soft resilient heat-cured or self-cured lining. These protectors have the advantage of a better fit, while still being quite inexpensive.
- *Custom-made protectors* are individually processed by a dentist or dental technician on plaster study models of the athlete's dental arches. These protectors, while significantly more expensive than stock or mouth-formed protectors, have been found to be acceptable and comfortable for most athletes.

Face masks

Face masks are used in ice hockey. This device has been found to be very effective in protecting players from orofacial injuries and is now mandatory in organized ice hockey in many countries.

References

1. Andreasen JO, Ravn JJ. Epidemiology of traumatic dental injuries to primary and permanent teeth in a Danish population sample. *Int J Oral Surg* 1972;**1**:235–9.
2. Andreasen JO, Borum MK, Jacobsen HL, Andreasen FM. Replantation of 400 avulsed permanent incisors. 1. Diagnosis of healing complications. *Endod Dent Traumatol* 1995;**11**:51–8.
3. Andreasen FM, Norén JG, Andreasen JO, Engelhardtsen S, Lindh-Strømberg U. Long-term survival of fragment bonding in the treatment of fractured crowns: a multicenter clinical study. *Quintessence Int* 1995;**26**:669–81.
4. Andreasen JO, Andreasen FM, Bakland LK, Flores MT. *Traumatic dental injuries – a manual*, 2nd edn. Oxford: Blackwell Munksgaard, 2003.
5. Andreasen JO, Andreasen FM, Mejare I, Cvek M. Healing of 400 intra-alveolar root fractures. 2. Effect of treatment factors such as treatment delay, repositioning, splinting type and period and antibiotics. *Dent Traumatol* 2004;**20**:203–11.
6. Andreasen JO, Bakland LK, Andreasen FM. Traumatic intrusion of permanent teeth. Part 3. A clinical study of the effect of treatment variables such treatment delay, method of repositioning, type of splint, length of splinting and antibiotics on 140 teeth. *Dent Traumatol* 2006;**22**:99–111.
7. Application of the International Classification of Diseases to Dentistry and Stomatology. ICD-DA 3rd edn. Geneva: WHO, 1995.
8. Cvek M. A clinical report on partial pulpotomy and capping with calcium hydroxide in permanent incisors with complicated crown fracture. *J Endod* 1978;**4**:232–7.
9. Glendor U, Halling A, Andersson L, Eilert-Petersson E. Incidence of traumatic tooth injuries in children and adolescents in the county of Västmanland, Sweden. *Swed Dent J* 1996;**20**:15–28.
10. Heintz WD. Mouth protectors: a progress report. *J Am Dent Assoc* 1968;**77**:632–6.
11. Kahnberg K-E. Surgical extrusion of root-fractured teeth – a follow-up study of two surgical methods. *Endod Dent Traumatol* 1988;**4**:85–90.
12. Malmgren O, Malmgren B, Frykholm A. Rapid orthodontic extrusion of crown-root and cervical root fractured teeth. *Endod Dent Traumatol* 1991;**7**:49–54.
13. Nysether S. Dental injuries among Norwegian soccer players. *Community Dent Oral Epidemiol* 1987;**15**:141–3.
14. Skaare AB, Jacobsen I. Dental injuries in Norwegians aged 7–18 years. *Dent Traumatol* 2003;**19**:67–71.
15. Skaare AB, Jacobsen I. Etiological factors related to dental injuries in Norwegians aged 7–18 years. *Dent Traumatol* 2003;**19**: 304–8.
16. Skaare AB, Jacobsen I. Primary tooth injuries in Norwegian children (1–8 years). *Dent Traumatol* 2005;**21**:315–19.
17. von Arx T, Filippi A, Buser D. Splinting of traumatized teeth with a new device: TTS (Titanium Trauma Splint). *Dent Traumatol* 2001;**17**:180–4.
18. Wigen TI, Agnalt R, Jacobsen I. Intrusive luxation of permanent incisors in Norwegians aged 6–17 years: a retrospective study of treatment and outcome. *Dent Traumatol* 2008;**24**:612–18.
19. Zachrisson BU, Jacobsen I. Long-term prognosis of 66 permanent anterior teeth with root fracture. *Scand J Dent Res* 1975; **83**:345–54.

19

Traumatic injuries: follow-up and long-term prognosis

Jens O. Andreasen and Ingeborg Jacobsen

Due to the varying healing capability of dental tissue to a traumatic injury, a variety of healing complications may occur. The range of this may be exemplified by local accelerated dentin formation after a crown fracture to complete root resorption after an intrusion injury. In order to comprehend the wide spectrum of complications, the healing capacity of the pulp and periodontium should be considered.

A traumatic dental injury represents acute transmission of energy to the tooth and supporting structures, which results in fracture and/or displacement of the tooth and/or separation or crushing of the supporting tissues [gingiva, periodontal ligament (PDL), and bone]. In the case of separation injury (e.g., extrusive luxation), the major part of the injury consists of cleavage of intercellular structures (collagen and intercellular substance), while there is limited damage to the cells in the area of trauma. This implies that wound healing can arise from existing cellular systems with a minimum of delay (Fig. 19-1).

In contrast, in a crushing injury (e.g., intrusive luxation), there is extensive damage to both cellular and intercellular systems; and damaged tissue must be removed by macrophages and/or osteoclasts before the traumatized tissue can be restored. Such damage adds several weeks to the healing process and is reflected in the splinting period (Fig. 19-2).

Wound healing events

Wound healing events comprise revascularization of ischemic tissue or formation of new tissue in the case of tissue loss (Fig. 19-3). In both instances, wound healing takes place by a coordinated movement of cells into the traumatized area, where macrophages form the healing front, followed by endothelial cells and fibroblasts. Vascular loops are formed in a stroma of tissue dominated by immature collagen (Type III) and proliferating fibroblasts. These cells are synchronized via chemical signals released by the involved cells and the surrounding tissue. This phenomenon has been termed the *wound healing module*. This process appears to advance in the pulp and periodontium at a speed of approximately 0.5 mm a day.

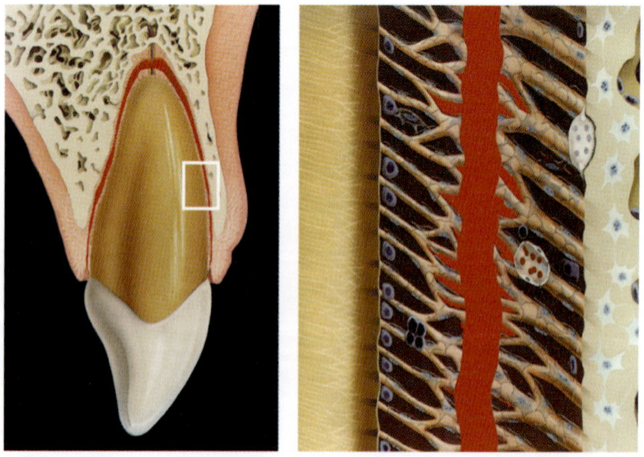

Figure 19-1 Nature of trauma in the case of separation injury [from Andreasen *et al*. (1)].

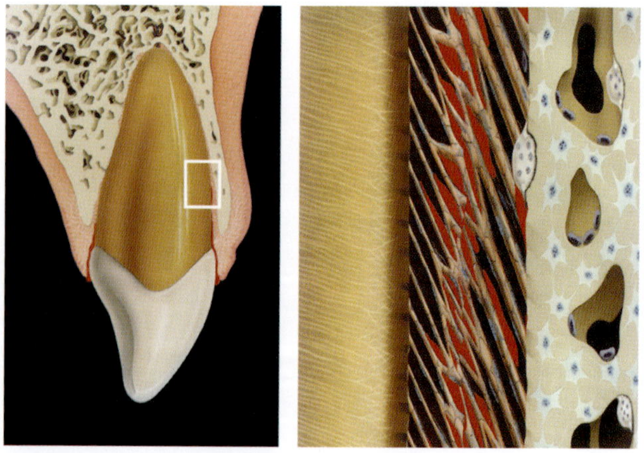

Figure 19-2 Nature of trauma in the case of crushing injury [from Andreasen *et al*. (1)].

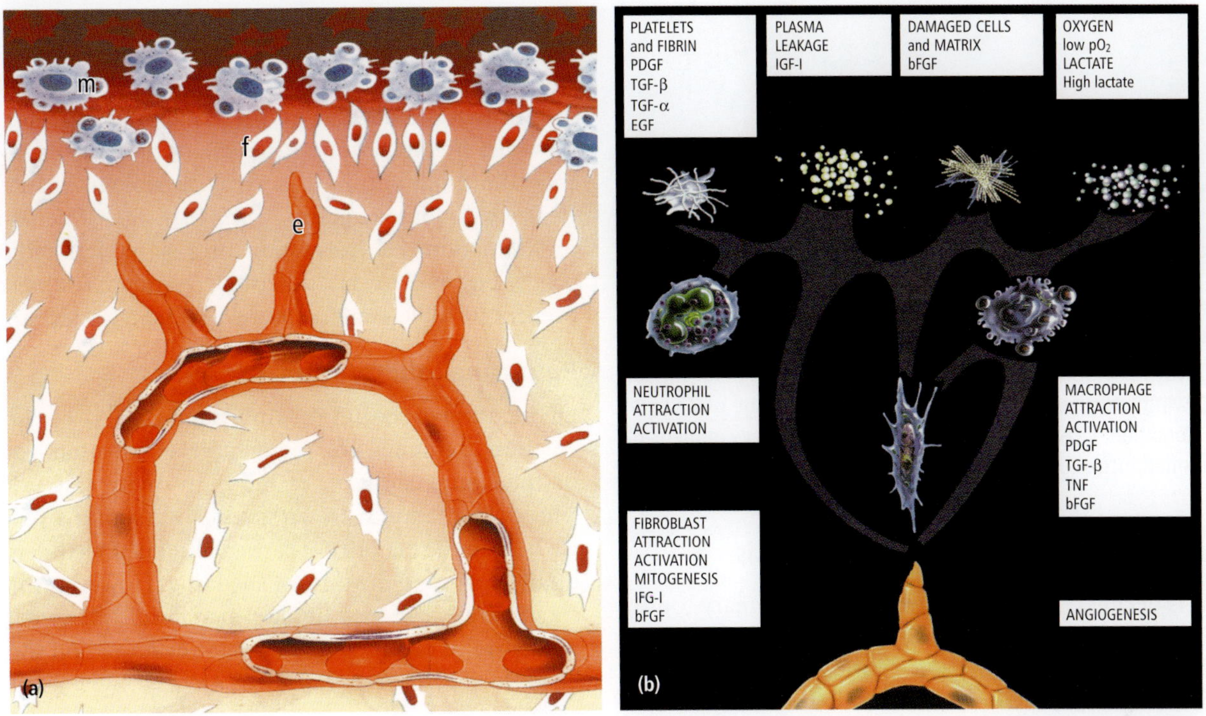

Figure 19-3 Later wound healing events; macrophages (m) form the healing front, followed by endothelial cells (e) and fibroblasts (f) [from Andreasen *et al.* (1)].

In the following, wound healing responses will be described as they appear in the case of simple luxation injuries, with only a separation injury of the PDL and the pulp, and subsequently with the complicated luxation injuries with crushing injuries.

- *Separation injuries.* After 1 week, new collagen formation starts to unite the severed PDL fibers and results in initial consolidation of a luxated or a replanted tooth. After 2 weeks, repair of the principal fibers is so advanced that approximately two-thirds of the mechanical strength of the PDL has been regained. In luxated teeth with a severed vascular supply, ingrowth of new vessels into the pulp starts 4 days after injury and proceeds at a speed of approximately 0.5 mm per day in teeth with open apices (5). Revascularization is usually markedly influenced by the size of the pulpo-periodontal interface, being almost complete and predictable in teeth with open apices (≥1.0 mm) and progressively decreasing in frequency below that diameter and becoming rare in teeth with a narrow apical foramen (<0.5 mm).
- *Crushing injury.* In complicated luxation injuries with crushing or other damage of the PDL (e.g., desiccation after avulsion), complicating sequelae may occur which result in root resorption (5). These processes occur due to the loss of the protecting cementoblast layer and the epithelial rests of Malassez along the root surface due to the traumatic events. When these cell layers disappear, there is free access of osteoclasts and macrophages to remove damaged PDL and cementum on the root surface that leads to root resorption.

To ascertain the progress of healing and/or the initiation of complications, detailed clinical and radiographic examination must be carried out at specific intervals where complications have become diagnosable. In that respect, clinical examination procedures such as inspection of color changes of the crown, mobility of the tooth, responses to percussion tests and sensibility testing, and radiographic examination are crucial. Radiographic imaging is especially important, as most significant complications can only be diagnosed radiographically. However, radiographic examination can easily lead to false-negative findings if a proper technique is not used. Thus, a standardized radiographic technique should be used whereby the tooth is visualized in several projection angles, which are identical from one examination to the next. Further, controls should be done when it is likely that pathologic changes can be revealed radiographically. This is due to the fact that pathologic changes have to develop to a certain critical size (usually larger than 0.6 mm) before they can be visualized radiographically.

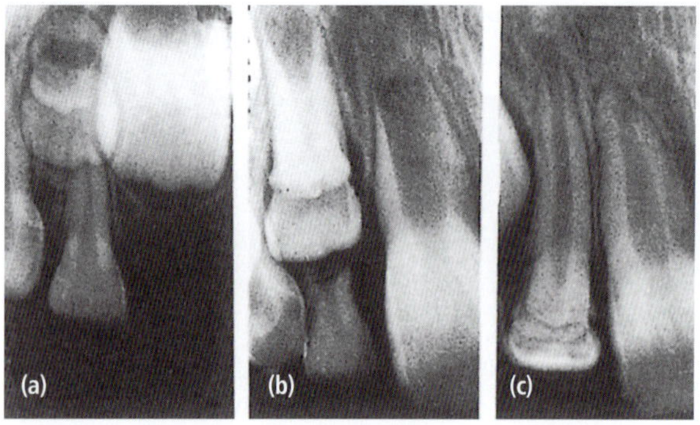

Figure 19-4 Severe malformation of permanent lateral incisor following intrusive luxation of predecessor at the age of 2 years. (a) Condition 1 year after trauma. (b, c) Further development of deformed incisor and uncomplicated eruption, respectively.

Primary teeth: follow-up and prognosis

If it is decided to preserve a traumatized primary tooth, it should be carefully observed for clinical and radiographic signs of pulpal or periodontal complications. Radiographs are also examined closely to disclose any damage to the permanent successor (Fig. 19-4). The intervals between re-examinations depend on the type of injury, the expected type of complication, and the age of the child. It may be necessary to see the child once a week for the first 3–4 weeks. Thereafter, re-examinations should take place at 3–6-monthly intervals for the first year, and then annually until the primary tooth is shed and the permanent successor is in place.

Pulpal and periodontal complications following trauma to primary teeth

Pulp necrosis

Pulp necrosis is the most common complication. All traumatized teeth should therefore be carefully observed for clinical or radiographic signs of pulpal death. In evaluating pulpal status in primary teeth, sensitivity testing is of limited value, due to the difficulty in obtaining adequate cooperation from the child. Most often, diagnosis of necrosis is based on inspection of tooth color, response to sensitivity testing, and radiographic observation of the periapical condition.

Discoloration of the tooth crown is an important sign of the condition of the pulp. It is observed that traumatized teeth with a normal color only rarely develop periapical inflammation. A discolored tooth, on the other hand, is not necessarily indicating the necrotic state of the pulp. A grayish discoloration recorded shortly after a trauma frequently reflects intrapulpal bleeding. On further examination, the gray hue may gradually fade, and return to normal or almost normal. In this case, the pulp will retain its vitality. However, if the grayish color persists, necrosis should be suspected, and the tooth examined radiographically at 3-monthly intervals to disclose any periapical inflammation as soon as possible.

Information on the pulpal condition can also be obtained by evaluation of the size of the pulp cavity. If pulp death has occurred, normal physiologic reduction in size will not take place. At the first sign of periapical inflammation, i.e., formation of a periapical radiolucency (Fig. 19-5), extraction is the treatment of choice to prevent possible sequelae to the permanent successor.

Pulp canal obliteration

Obliteration of the pulp chamber and canal is a frequent reaction to trauma. The radiograph reveals either partial or total mineralization of the pulp cavity (Fig. 19-6). Clinically, the tooth crown gradually assumes a yellowish hue. In the majority of cases, obliterated teeth remain unaffected up to the time of shedding. However, since a small percentage may develop periapical inflammation indicative of necrosis, radiographic examination should be performed once a year.

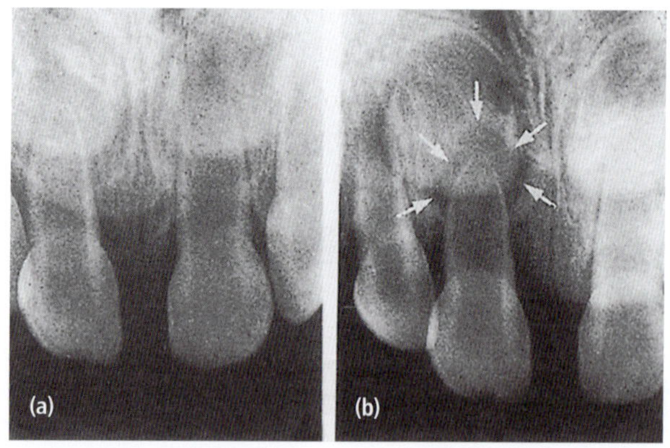

Figure 19-5 (a) Radiograph taken 1 week after slight intrusive luxation of right central incisor. (b) Three months after the trauma there is marked periapical inflammation (arrows).

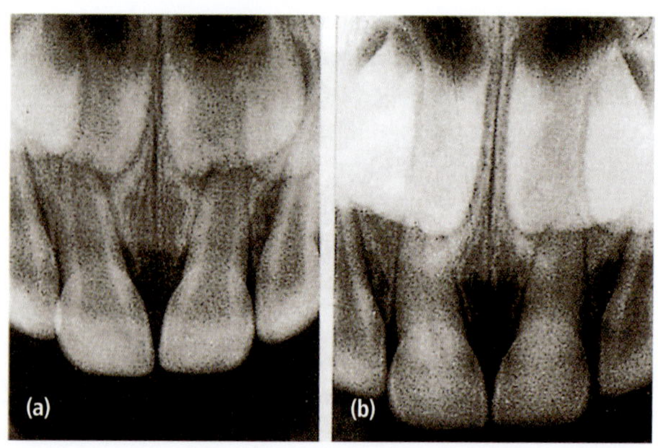

Figure 19-6 Subluxation of both central incisors leading to pulp canal obliteration. (a) At time of injury. (b) Two years later, there is almost total obliteration of the pulps.

Root resorption

The etiology and pathogenesis of root resorption in primary teeth are identical to root resorption in traumatized permanent incisors. External infection-related root resorption is usually seen after intrusive luxation, whereas internal resorption may develop as a result of both subluxation and luxation injuries. Extraction is the treatment of choice with all types of pathologic root resorption.

Injuries to developing permanent teeth

It is well documented that trauma to a primary tooth is easily transmitted to its permanent successor (7,8). The highest and lowest frequencies of developmental disturbances are found after intrusions and subluxations, respectively. In this connection, it is emphasized that avulsion of a primary incisor may also disturb further growth and development of the underlying permanent successor. The explanation for this is probably that a primary tooth is avulsed, with a movement of the apex in the direction of the permanent tooth germ.

Most disturbances occur when the apex of the primary tooth directly traumatizes the permanent tooth bud (Fig. 19-7). However, periapical inflammation of the primary tooth may also have harmful effects. The type and severity of disturbances found among permanent incisors are also closely related to the age at the time of injury. A tooth germ is especially vulnerable during its early developmental stages. Thus, the most serious disturbances are seen when the damage occurs before the age of 3 years. Changes in morphology or mineralization of the crown of the permanent incisor are the most common types of complications. These lesions range from small enamel opacities to severe malformations. In case of displacement of a primary tooth directly into the follicle of the permanent successor, dislocation of the mineralized part of the tooth may occur in relation to the soft part of the tooth germ whereby a *crown dilaceration* will occur (Fig. 19-4). A frequent finding is a yellow–brown discoloration, localized on the buccal surface, with or without hypoplasia of the enamel. In these cases it is essential that a hypoplastic area is restored with composite in order not to lead to a caries lesion (Figs 19-8 and 19-9). Trauma may also interfere with root formation, leading to bending of the root or partial arrest of the development.

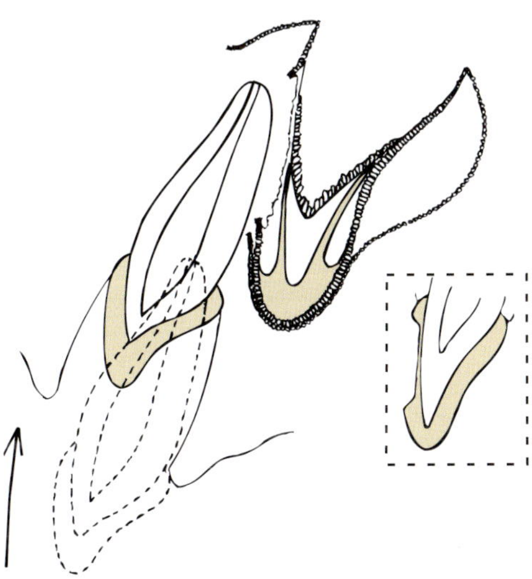

Figure 19-7 Disturbance of development of permanent tooth bud due to intrusion of primary incisor. Due to laceration of the follicle, disturbances in enamel formation will develop.

Permanent teeth: follow-up and prognosis

The initial treatment phase is followed by a period of observation. Due to the variance of dental tissue involved, each specific injury has a specific prognosis (Table 19-1). Trauma cases should therefore be recalled often enough to disclose any complication as soon as possible in order to intervene at the right time. The intervals between re-examinations should be individualized depending on the severity of trauma, the expected type of complication and the age of the patient. Most complications are observed within the first year of the trauma. However, the follow-up evaluation of permanent teeth should continue until treatment of all complications is completed, or until a lost or extracted permanent tooth has been adequately replaced. The following time schedule may serve as a guide for trauma types with moderate or high frequencies of complications: 1 week, 3 weeks, 6 weeks, 8 weeks, 3, 6, and 12 months. Thereafter, once a year for 5 years.

The follow-up examinations should include testing of pulp sensitivity, percussion and mobility, and inspection of the tooth color.

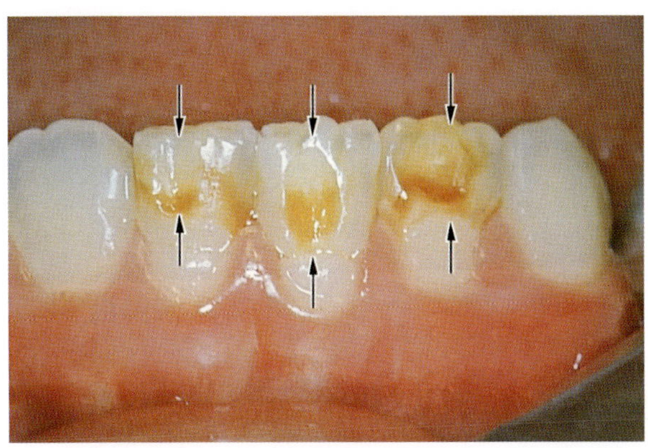

Figure 19-8 Enamel defects in three mandibular incisors (arrows) resulting from avulsion of corresponding predecessors at the age of 2 years.

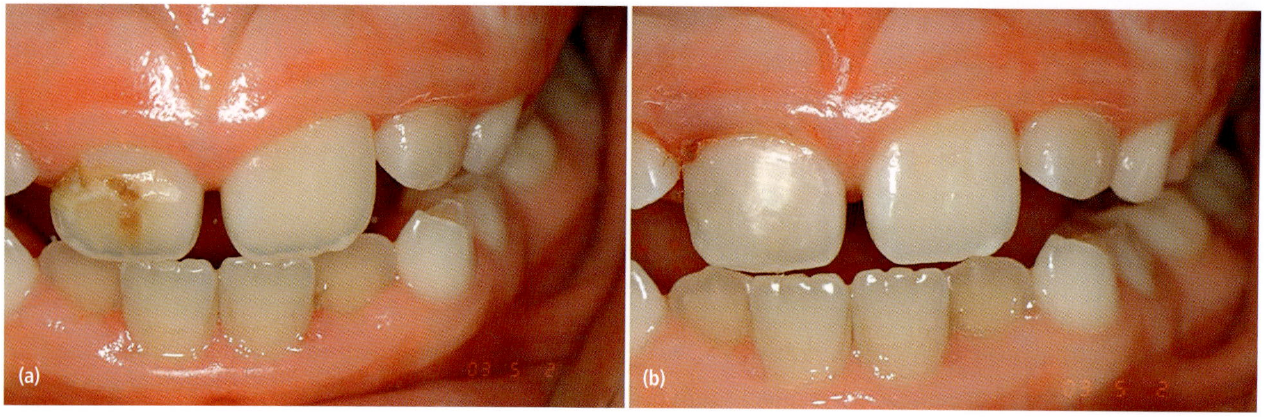

Figure 19-9 External enamel hypoplasia of right central incisor caused by intrusion of predecessor at the age of 18 months. The hypoplastic area is covered with composite.

Radiographs should be examined with respect to the periradicular condition and changes within the pulp cavity.

Prognosis following infraction and uncomplicated crown fracture

Teeth without associated periodontal injuries are followed by remarkably few complications (Table 19-1). High-risk teeth with respect to pulp necrosis after crown fractures appear to be those with untreated deep corner fractures.

A negative response to the electric pulp test must be accompanied by other clinical and/or radiographic signs before pulp necrosis can be diagnosed. With infractions and uncomplicated crown fractures, either periapical inflammation or a grayish discoloration should be

Table 19-1 Frequency of pulp and periodontal healing complications in traumatized permanent teeth [after (1)]

		Pulp necrosis	Pulp canal obliteration	Inflammatory resorption	Ankylosis resorption	Marginal attachment loss
Uncomplicated crown fracture	Immature	0%	0%	0%	0%	0%
	Mature	0%	2%	0%	0%	
Complicated crown fracture	Immature	5%[a]	0%	0%	0%	0%
	Mature					
Root fracture	Immature	0%	73%	0%	0%	0%
	Mature	31%		2%	0%	
Concussion	Immature	0%	3%	0%	0%	0%
	Mature	4%	6%	0%	0%	
Subluxation	Immature	0%	11%	0%	0%	0%
	Mature	14%	8%	1%	0%	
Extrusion	Immature	7%	60%	6%	0%	6%
	Mature	35%	18%	5%	0%	
Lateral luxation	Immature	10%	71%	3%	0%	7%
	Mature	79%	9%	3%	1%	
Intrusion	Immature	63%	25%	38%	13%	31%
	Mature	100%	0%	38%	32%	
Avulsion	Immature	66%	34%	37%	43%	7%
	Mature	100%	0%	28%	61%	

[a] Partial pulpotomy.

expected as the definite sign of pulpal death. Most cases of pulp necrosis can be disclosed within 3 months after the accident. Treatment of uncomplicated crown fractures in childhood often consists of composite using dental bonding (see Chapter 18). This procedure usually represents only a semipermanent solution, whereas a definitive restoration with porcelain laminates onlays or jacket crowns normally has to wait until adult age has been reached.

Prognosis following a complicated fracture

The two standard treatments – pulp capping and partial pulpotomy – appear to result in successful healing in more than 90% of cases (see Chapters 12 and 18).

Prognosis following crown-root fracture

No studies have compared the results of the different treatment procedures described in Chapter 18. It appears, though, that orthodontic extrusion of apical root fragment leads to a stable periodontal condition, whereas surgical exposure of the palatal fracture site has been found to lead to chronic inflammatory changes within the palatel sulcus in some cases. After some time, this may result in slight migration of the restored tooth in a buccal direction. Surgical repositioning of an apical fragment has been found to have a very high long-term survival (16).

Prognosis following root fracture

In about 80% of all root fractured teeth the pulp remains viable or becomes revascularized, and repair occurs in the fractured area (1,14). In this regard, four main types of healing events have been found (Fig. 19-10 and Box 19-1).

Necrosis is the main obstacle to healing and is caused by an infected pulp in the coronal fragment. This condition is usually diagnosed within 3 months after injury. Severe dislocation of the coronal fragment and mature root formation at the time of injury significantly favors the development of pulpal death.

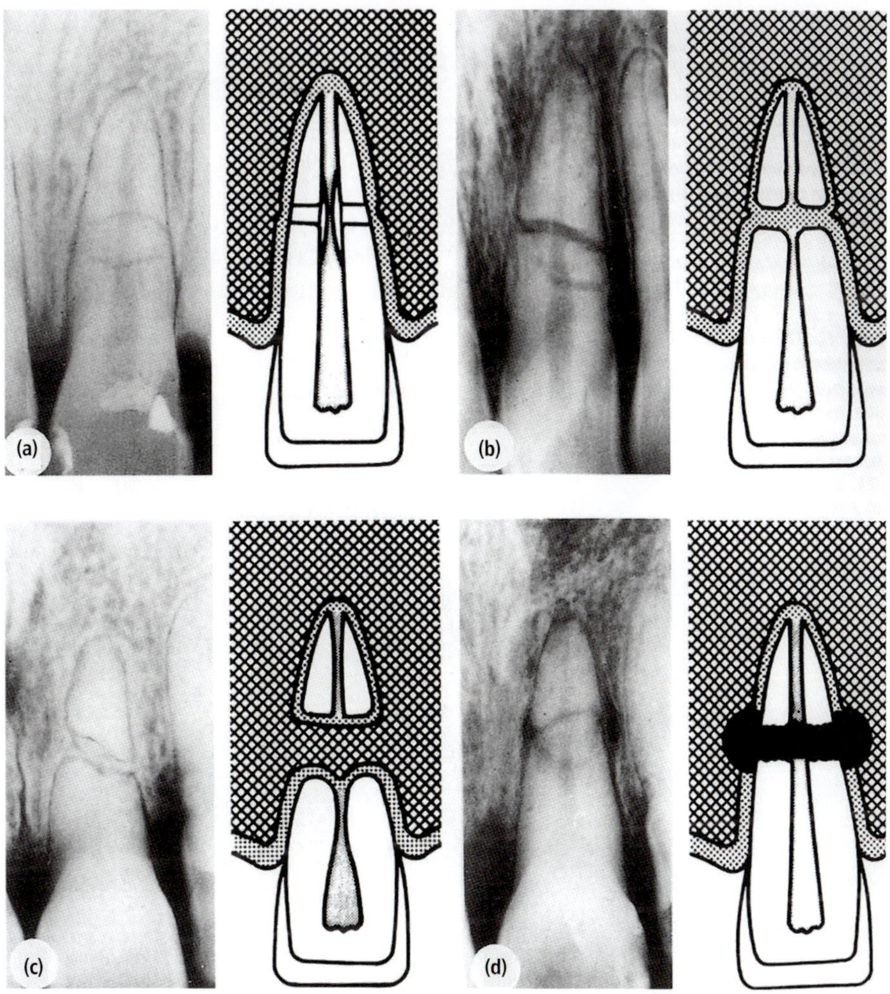

Figure 19-10 Radiographs and diagrams illustrating various modalities of healing after root fractures. (a) Healing with calcified tissue. (b) Interposition of connective tissue. (c) Interposition of bone and connective tissue. (d) Interposition of granulation tissue [from (1)].

Box 19-1 Situations following root fractures

Repair with calcified tissue
The fracture is united by hard tissue and the fracture line becomes either invisible or hardly discernible. The tooth has normal mobility.

Repair with connective tissue (PDL)
A narrow, radiolucent fracture line surrounds the fracture and there is peripheral rounding of the fracture edges. The tooth has increased mobility depending on the level of the fracture.

Repair with bone and connective tissue (PDL)
A bony bridge separates the two fragments. The tooth has increased mobility depending on the level of the fracture.

Pulp necrosis
A gradually widened gap between the fragments appears and radiolucencies appear adjacent to the fracture. The tooth shows increased mobility.

Concerning therapy, it is important to realize that the apical fragment almost always contains viable pulp tissue. In teeth with middle or apical third fractures, endodontic treatment can therefore usually be confined to the coronal fragment. After completion of endodontic treatment, repair between the two fragments with connective tissue (PDL) is a consistent finding (Fig. 19-11).

When teeth with fractures in the cervical third of the root develop necrosis, the following procedure should be considered: extraction of the coronal fragment with subsequent orthodontic extrusion of the apical fragment.

Irrespective of healing type, root fractured teeth have a reasonable good long-term prognosis, especially fractures located in the mid or apical position of the root.

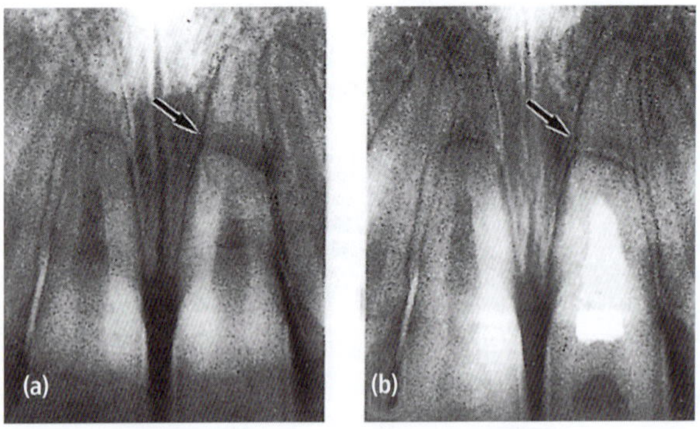

Figure 19-11 Root fractures of both central incisors. (a) Retained pulpal vitality and calcified tissue repair in the right incisor, whereas radiolucency corresponding to fracture line (arrow) indicates necrosis in the left incisor. (b) Two years after completed root filling of left incisor PDL union between segments is evident.

Prognosis following luxation injuries

Following the initial treatment, it is anticipated that pulpal and periodontal repair will take place uneventfully. However, a number of complications may develop (Table 19-1).

Pulp canal obliteration

Pulp canal obliteration is the term used to describe the progressive hard tissue formation within the pulp cavity. A gradual narrowing of the pulp chamber and root canal is observed on radiographs, leading to either partial or total obliteration (Figs 19-12–19-14). Because of the calcification, reduced electrometric response and even loss of sensitivity may be recorded. Another clinical observation is a yellowish color of the crown.

It is not fully understood what stimulates odontoblasts to start the formation of hard tissue on the root canal walls. Obliteration appears, however, to be significantly related to teeth with incomplete root formation. Obliteration is also more frequent after extrusion, lateral luxation, and intrusion than after concussion and subluxation, which indicates that the disturbance in dentin formation may be related to a pulp revascularization phenomenon (Table 19-1).

Although a radiograph gives the illusion of complete calcification of the pulp cavity, a minute strand of pulp tissue always remains. In about 13% of these teeth the pulp becomes necrotic and periapical inflammation develops. This is a late complication, usually seen 5–20 years after the injury (14). In a long-term follow-up study these pulp necrosis events were found to increase at about 1% a year. Endodontic treatment of these cases may be difficult on technical grounds. Therefore, prophylactic endodontic therapy of teeth showing progressive hard tissue formation has been recommended.

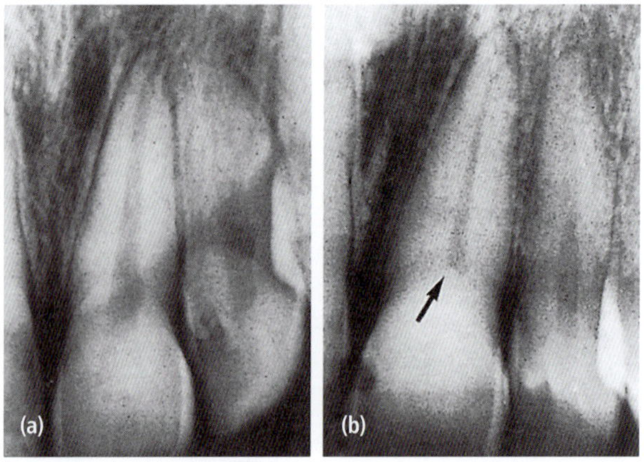

Figure 19-12 Partial pulp canal obliteration in left central incisor. (a) At time of injury. (b) Condition 15 years later. Pulp chamber completely obliterated and root canal slightly reduced in size (arrow).

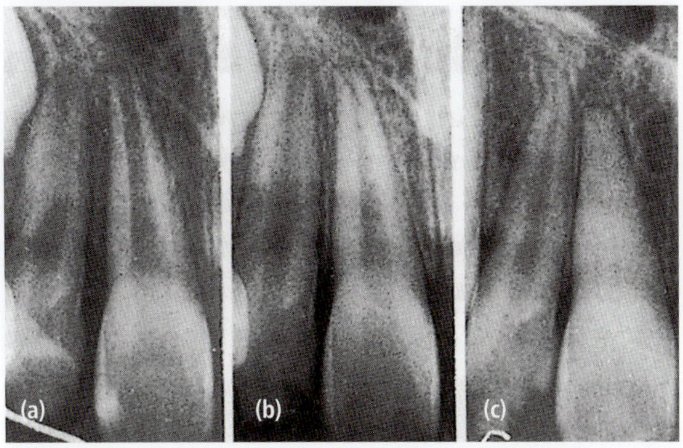

Figure 19-13 Obliteration after successful replantation of right central incisor. The tooth was replanted within a few minutes. (a) Normal findings 3 weeks later. (b) A radiograph taken 6 months later shows apical closure. (c) Seven years after replantation, there is total pulp canal obliteration and no sign of root resorption.

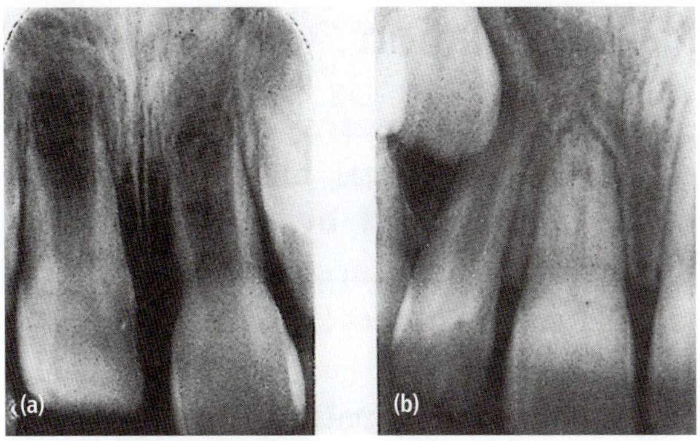

Figure 19-14 (a) Intrusive luxation of immature right central incisor. (b) Spontaneous re-eruption, closure of apical foramen, and pulp canal obliteration have occurred.

However, this does not seem reasonable, mainly due to the rather low frequency of a complicating necrosis. Furthermore, in spite of the excessive calcification, the root canal is nearly always accessible for conventional endodontic treatment and prognosis for such a procedure appears to be good (11).

Pulp necrosis

Necrosis is the most common post-traumatic complication (18,19). It is difficult to establish the extent of pulpal damage immediately after the injury and to predict in which cases pulp necrosis will occur. However, as shown in Table 19-1, the survival or death of the pulp tissue is primarily related to the severity of the periodontal injury, as implied by luxation injuries with displacement where the neurovascular supply to the pulp has been severed.

Several studies have also shown that necrosis occurs less frequently in immature teeth than in mature ones. With a large apical opening, slight movements of the apex can probably occur without disruption of the blood vessels. Furthermore, if circulatory disturbances do occur, the recovery capacity of a young pulp is very favorable (Fig. 19-14).

Diagnosis of necrosis. While most pulp necroses can be diagnosed within the first 3 months after injury, up to 2 years may pass before signs of necrosis become definitive. Diagnosing pulp necrosis usually implies the use of sensitivity electrometric testing, evaluation of color changes, and radiographic examination for signs of pathology such as periapical radiolucency and/or resorption.

Sensitivity testing. More than half of all subluxated and luxated teeth do not respond to electric stimulation at the initial examination. It is, however, documented that a large number of teeth with subluxation later regain their sensitivity. Although less frequent, a change in reaction from negative to positive may also take place in luxated and displaced teeth. A return to normal sensitivity is commonly found within the first 2–3 months. However, it has also been observed as late as 2 years after the accident. A negative test alone should, therefore, not be regarded as proof of necrosis and at least 3 months should elapse after injury before a negative sensibility testing can be relied on. Endodontic treatment should always be postponed until at least one other clinical and/or radiographic sign of necrosis appears (i.e., two out of three signs are present).

Tooth discoloration. An almost immediate pinkish discoloration indicates intrapulpal bleeding and not necessarily pulpal death. It is thought that injuries such as concussion and subluxation may sever or occlude the veins at the apical foramen. The arteries may not be disrupted, leading to continued blood flow into the pulp cavity and penetration of hemoglobin from ruptures in the subodontoblastic plexus into the dentin tubules. The immediate observation is a pinkish discoloration. There is a fair chance that the vascular system will repair. In this event, discoloration slowly disappears, and the pulp will retain its vitality (Fig. 19-15). However, if the tooth crown turns progressively gray, necrosis should be suspected. A grayish color that appears for the first time several weeks or months after trauma is regarded as a sign of necrosis. In this case, the gray color signifies decomposition of necrotic pulp tissue.

Radiographic signs of pulpal necrosis. To get maximum information from a radiographic follow-up it is mandatory that radiographs are obtained at periods where pathologic changes are diagnosable (i.e., more than 2–3 weeks after trauma) and that a standardized radiographic technique is used so that series of radiographs become comparable. For comparison, it is essential that follow-up radiographs are taken with the same angulation as the radiographs from the time of injury.

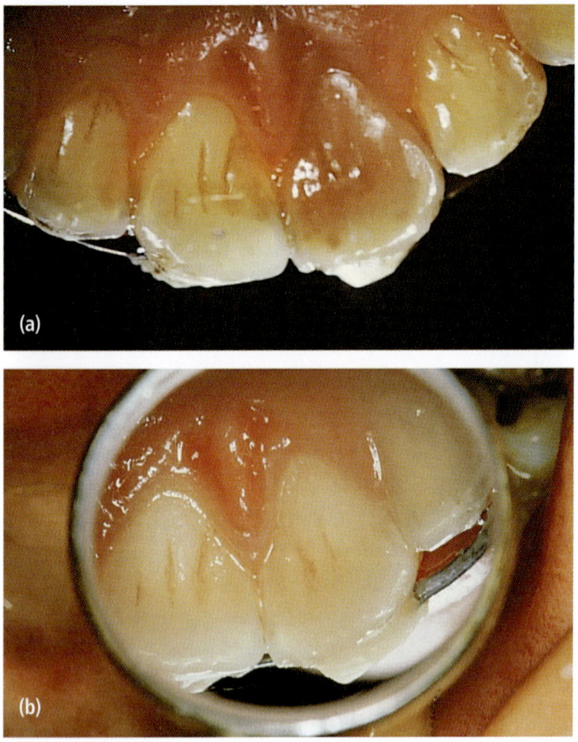

Figure 19-15 (a) Left central incisor in 10-year-old boy discolored within 1 week after subluxation injury. (b) Three months later. Discoloration has disappeared and the tooth responds normally to electrometric pulp testing.

Periapical inflammation. Periapical radiolucencies secondary to necrosis can be seen as early as 3 weeks after trauma, although, frequently, several months pass before an apical pathosis is evident.

Arrest of further root development. If necrosis involves the epithelial root sheath before root development is complete, no further root growth takes place. It should be borne in mind that necrosis may progress from the coronal to the apical part of the pulp. In this way, vitality may apparently persist for a while apically, resulting in the formation of a calcified barrier across the wide apical foramen (Fig. 19-16).

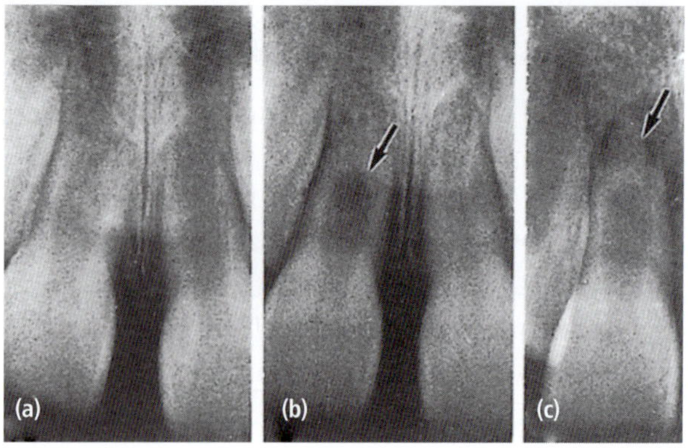

Figure 19-16 Pulp necrosis of right central incisor following intrusion. (a) Re-eruption took place 3 months after injury. (b) No further root development. Hard tissue formation (arrow) is found together with continued vitality. (c) Pulp necrosis is diagnosed from a periapical radiolucency (arrow), which developed 1 year after injury.

Cervical root fractures after endodontic treatment

Endodontic treatment of nonvital immature teeth is reported to be highly successful (see Chapter 12). However, it is important to realize that success refers to the primary goal: a tight seal apically. A point to remember is that necrosis in a developing tooth results in arrested dentin formation, leaving thin dentinal walls. These fragile walls are susceptible to fracture particularly in the cervical area (Fig. 19-17). The frequency of cervical root

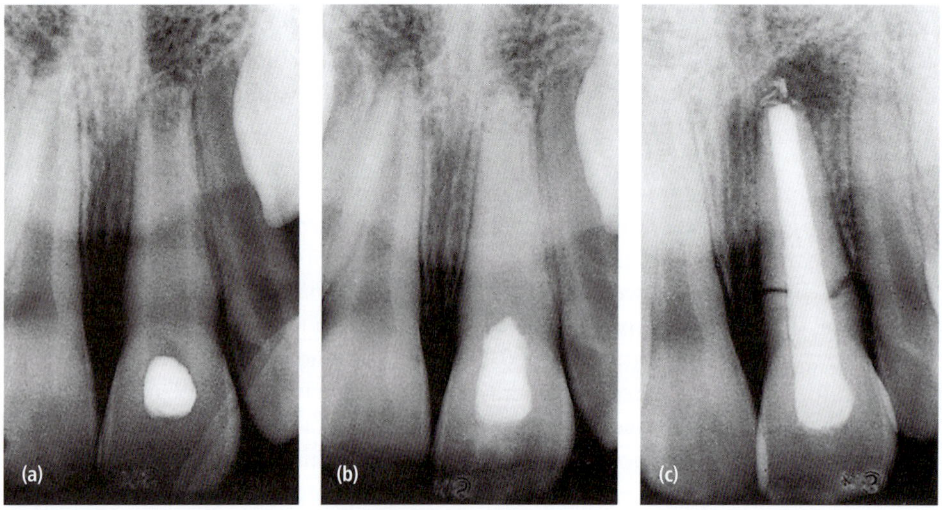

Figure 19-17 Spontaneous root fracture of nonvital immature central incisor. (a, b) During long-term treatment with calcium hydroxide. (c) The fracture was observed 1 year after completed endodontic treatment.

Box 19-2 The risk of cervical fractures decreases with increasing age at the time of the injury

Age	Frequency
6 years	77%
7 years	53%
8–9 years	43%
9–10 years	28%
>11 years	2%

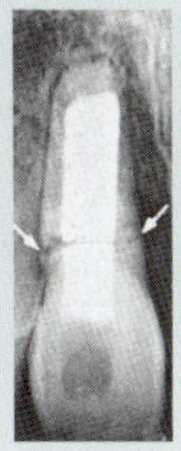

fracture is reported to range from 2% in an 11 year old to 77% in a 6 year old (Box 19-2) (13). The thin dentinal walls are the main reason for cervical fractures. However, it is reported that long-term use of calcium hydroxide in the root canals increases the risk of these cervical fractures. In a recent experimental study calcium hydroxide was kept in the canal for only 30 days followed by root filling with mineral trioxide aggregate (MTA), and no significant decrease was found in the strength of the root (6,12). This finding may lead to a shift in the endodontic procedure for teeth with immature root formation.

However, the prognosis should still be regarded as doubtful to poor with pulp necrosis in children 6–11 years of age, and a long-term treatment plan should always be made. This is of particular importance in malocclusion cases where extraction of premolars is part of the orthodontic treatment. The question is whether a nonvital immature incisor should be kept for as long as possible or whether the best treatment is to remove the tooth and close the space orthodontically or by a premolar transplantation.

Root resorption

Subsequent to luxation injuries with tooth displacement, root resorption is a very frequent complication (Table 19-1) (4,9,10). In this regard, three varieties of root resorption have to be considered.

Repair-related resorption (surface resorption). This resorption entity is characterized by small cavities on the root surface surrounded by a periodontal ligament space of normal width. In the case of multiple cavities affecting the root apex, repair-related resorption may appear as a shortening of the apex. This resorption type is self-limiting and requires no treatment. Repair-related resorption is especially frequent after luxation injuries with displacement (lateral luxations, extrusions).

Infection-related resorption (inflammatory resorption). Traumatic injuries with damage to the periodontal structure may cause progressive resorption of the root. Infection-related resorption is a common type of progressive root resorption and is most frequently seen after intrusive luxation and replantation (Table 19-1). The development is due to cell damage of the periodontal ligament and the cementum induced by the trauma, and the presence of infected necrotic pulp tissue. Bacterial products from the infected root canal will penetrate through the dentin tubules into the periodontal ligament. Thus, an inflammatory response is provoked, leading to further resorption of the root surface.

The diagnosis is made radiographically and this resorption appears as bowl-shaped areas of resorptions associated with radiolucencies in adjacent bone. Most frequently, infection-related resorption is identified in the middle or coronal third of the root (Figs 19-18 and 19-19).

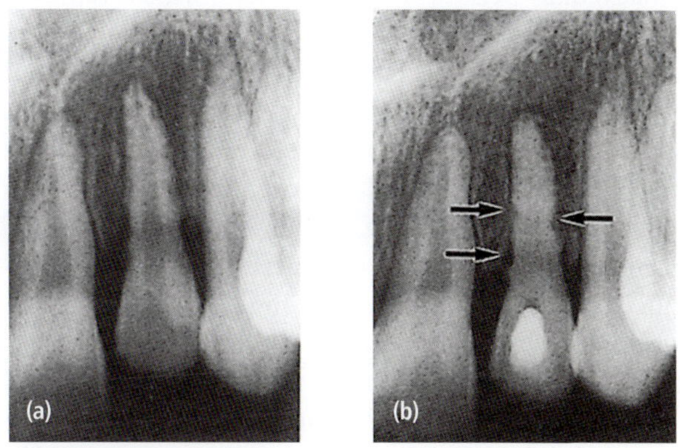

Figure 19-18 External infection-related root resorption along root surface of an intruded lateral incisor. (a) Six weeks after injury. (b) During endodontic treatment, the pulp cavity was temporarily filled with calcium hydroxide. Persistent defects are seen on the root surface (arrows), but no further progression has taken place.

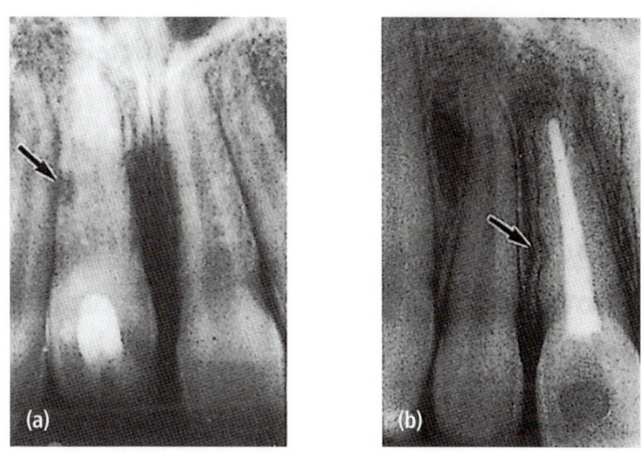

Figure 19-19 External infection-related root resorption following intrusive luxation of a right central incisor. (a) An area of resorption (arrow) was seen 8 weeks after injury. The pulp canal was temporarily filled with calcium hydroxide. (b) Two years later, there is a persistent defect (arrow), but no further progression of resorption.

The first sign of resorption can be seen as early as 3 weeks after trauma, and most cases are disclosed within 4 months. If not present within the first year after injury, infection-related resorption is unlikely to occur. If allowed to progress, the resorptive process may destroy the tooth completely within a few months.

The treatment of choice is immediate removal of necrotic pulp tissue, canal debridement, and treatment with calcium hydroxide followed by a guttapercha root canal filling or MTA filling (see below). In the majority of cases this arrests the process, and cement repair takes place in the resorption cavities (Fig. 19-19).

Replacement resorption (ankylosis-related resorption). This resorption is the most severe type of external root resorption and is significantly related to intrusions and replantation of avulsed incisors after an extended dry extraalveolar period, both instances which represent extensive damage to the PDL (Table 19-1). Replacement resorption is caused by extensive cell damage to the periodontal ligament and to the cementum. A bony union (ankylosis) is established between the alveolar socket and the root surface, followed by continuous resorption of cementum and dentin (Fig. 19-20). Radiographically, the normal periodontal space disappears and the tooth substance is gradually replaced by bone. Clinical examination may reveal this type of resorption before it can be seen on X-ray. A typical finding is a high, metallic percussion sound differing clearly from an uninjured tooth. It appears that most replacement resorptions are evident within 2 months to 1 year after the accident.

Unfortunately, there is presently no effective treatment for an ankylosed tooth, the ultimate result being complete resorption of the root However, the rate of progression is often very slow, and the tooth can be maintained for several years. It may take 3–7 years before the root is completely resorbed. This progession factor is strongly age related (Fig. 19-20).

A factor to consider is that ankylosis will disturb growth of the alveolar process in young patients due to infraposition of the tooth (Fig. 19-21). This may complicate further prosthetic solutions. For this reason a decoronation procedure is recommended. The treatment procedure is to separate the crown from the resorbed root at the bone level (decoronation procedure). The ankylosed root will then be gradually transformed to bone during the remodeling process and thereby keep the labial-lingual volume of bone. Furthermore the establishment of a periosteum on top of the left root will allow a regrowth of the height of the process (17). Both processes are essential for the later tooth replacement that being a conventional bridge, dental autotransplant or an implant. Concerning timing of the decoronation procedure it is essential that it is carried out when the

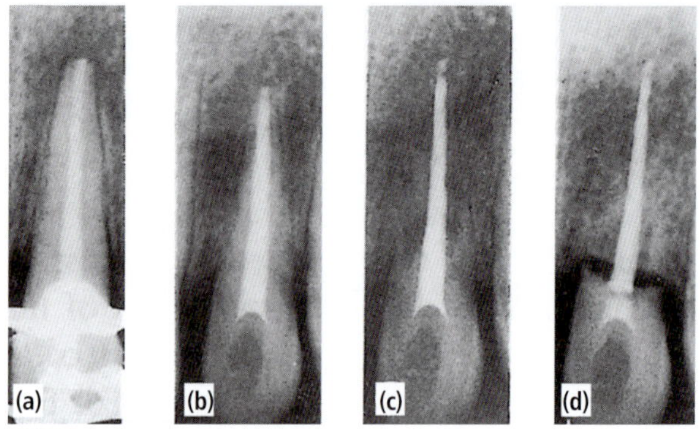

Figure 19-20 Progression of replacement resorption after avulsion and subsequent replantation of left lateral incisor. (a–c) Radiographs taken 6 months, 2 and 4 years after injury. (d) Condition at time of removal of lateral incisor 7 years after replantation.

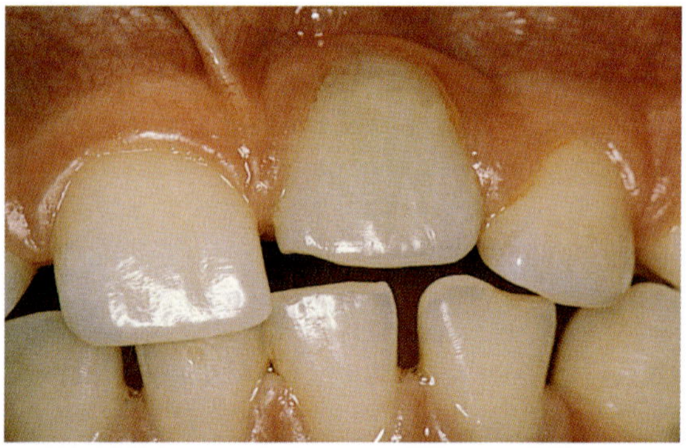

Figure 19-21 Infraposition of a left central incisor due to replacement resorption (ankylosis).

tooth has gone only 2–3 mm in infraposition and there is still more residual growth (and thereby infraposition) to be expected.

Root canal resorption (internal resorption). In addition to the post-traumatic complications listed in Table 19-1, internal root resorption is a possible outcome. This type of resorption is an infrequent pulpal complication and is probably caused by a chronic pulpal inflammation due to a partial pulp necrosis.

Internal resorption is usually present without clinical symptoms, and is first diagnosed radiographically. The process may progress very rapidly, and endodontic treatment should be started as soon as the diagnosis is made. If the involved tooth is treated before resorption becomes extensive, with perforation of the root surface, the treatment has a good chance of being successful.

In conclusion, the long-term prognosis of luxated teeth without displacement is very good, whereas lateral luxations show quite frequent complications, usually pulp necrosis. Intrusions represent a very severe injury type, which may lead to tooth loss due to progressive root resorption.

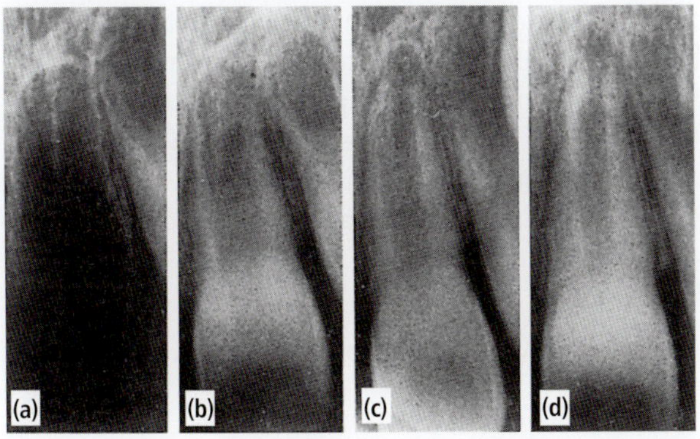

Figure 19-22 Successful replantation of a left central incisor (arrows). The tooth was stored in the mouth of the child's mother for 45 min. (a–c) Radiographs taken before, 12 days and 6 months after replantation, respectively. (d) One year after injury, with continued root development and narrowing of pulp canal.

Prognosis following replantation

The type and frequency of complications after replantation are shown in Table 19-1.

In teeth with a wide-open apical foramen, revascularization of the pulp may occur (Fig. 19-22). The pulp tissue of an avulsed tooth apparently has the potential to survive for up to 3 hours out of the socket. Therefore, in teeth replanted within 3 hours, endodontic treatment is postponed until pulp necrosis is evident. These teeth must be followed closely. With signs of necrosis, such as inflammatory root resorption, endodontic treatment should be started immediately. It is recommended that a replanted tooth with incomplete root formation is examined radiographically every second week until pulp necrosis is confirmed or until continued root formation is evident.

Pulp revascularization is not likely to take place in teeth with closed apical foramen, and endodontic treatment must be started within 1–2 weeks after replantation to prevent the onset of inflammatory root resorption. The canal should be filled temporarily with a paste of calcium hydroxide for 6 months.

Root resorption is very frequent following replantation, and all three types of resorption may occur (Table 19-1). Treatment consequences are the same as described for luxated teeth.

Treatment methods following loss of permanent incisors

When anterior tooth loss has occurred or is anticipated (e.g., due to progressive root resorption), the most important factors to consider with respect to treatment planning are:

- age of the patient
- anticipated vertical growth of the alveolar process
- space available between crowns and roots adjacent to the recipient site
- occlusal relations and condition of the alveolar process.

These factors usually determine the treatment of choice, whether orthodontic space closure, resin-retained or conventional fixed prosthetics, autotransplantation of premolars or implants. To aid in the choice between these treatment possibilities, study models and panoramic radiographs are essential.

Conventional fixed prosthetics usually have to wait until adult age, whereas resin-retained fixed prosthodontics (Rochette or Maryland bridges) can be inserted in growing individuals (see Chapter 13). Another treatment procedure that can be used in adolescents is autotransplantation of premolars to the region of the tooth loss. Due to the unique osteogenic capacity of a tooth graft, this procedure offers a treatment alternative in which both the lost tooth and the atrophied alveolar process can be replaced. Recent studies have demonstrated good long-term survival of these transplants, thus providing a realistic treatment alternative for tooth replacement in young individuals. The key to successful tooth transplantation has been shown clinically and experimentally to be proper selection of grafts with adequate root development as well as the design of a surgical techniques for atraumatic graft removal and graft donor site preparation.

Another procedure exists, namely, insertion of single standing implants. This treatment modality offers patients with completed jaw growth a unique treatment possibility whereby a biologic compatible material such as titanium serves as an osseointegrated root that is subsequently united with a porcelain crown (suprastructure).

In individuals where maxillary or mandibular vertical growth is not yet complete, the use of implants is contraindicated, as the osseointegrated implant will be maintained in its original position and progressive infraocclusion can be anticipated. This process is identical to that seen with progressive replacement resorption in growing individuals. However, if only 0.5–1 mm vertical growth of the alveolar process is expected (i.e., at the age of 18 years), implant treatment can be considered. The patient needs to be informed about the likelihood of later infraocclusion, which may lead to renewal of the suprastructure.

The choice between implantation and autotransplantation is thus influenced by the age of the patient. As autotransplants are generally indicated only in cases where teeth with incomplete root formation can be transplanted, this naturally limits the use of autotransplantation to young individuals with a suitable tooth to transplant. The morphology of the alveolar process at the recipient region is also of significance when the choice between implants and autotransplants has to be made, because bony reconstruction of the alveolar ridge (i.e., reduced height and sharp ridge) is a necessary part of the treatment with implant, a procedure with a very doubtful prognosis.

Predictors for healing complications

It is essential for proper treatment planning to have a realistic concept of the risk of healing complications such as pulp necrosis, root resorption, marginal bone loss, and disturbed root development. Recently an analysis was published on the relationship between healing complication after traumatic dental injuries and series of factors found to influence the healing pattern. These factors can be split into three groups (1):

- The first group of factors contains descriptive factors, for the patient, like stage of root development and age.
- The second group of factors are trauma-related factors describing the injury, e.g., extent and direction of tooth displacement, extent and location of tooth fracture, extra-alveolar time and storage medium (avulsion), etc.
- The third group contains treatment factors, e.g., optimal/nonoptimal replantation, choice of splinting type (flexible/rigid), and treatment delay.

The influence of all these factors has been evaluated for all types of traumatic dental injuries affecting the primary and the permanent teeth. This was done on the basis of statistical analysis of a large clinical database covering more than 2400 traumatic dental injuries with long-term follow-up (1). These studies indicate that the factors in the first and second groups have the greatest impact in relation to healing sequelae whereas the treatment factors in the third group only play a minor role.

Development of an interactive Internet-based dental trauma guide

Assessment of the risk of healing complications is an important part of picking the best possible treatment approach. Recently the work on establishing an interactive prognostic dental trauma base was initiated at the Trauma Center at the University Hospital in Copenhagen. The idea behind this interactive, web-based guide is to give the practitioners a possibility of having the latest treatment advice for a given trauma injury and, via an interactive database, to have a realistic evaluation of the chance for healing complications given the actual information. This database is expected to be operational in 2008 and will be hosted as part of the International Association for Dental Traumatology (IADT) website. The URL will be www.DentalTraumaGuide.org.

References

1. Andreasen FM, Andreasen JO, Andersson L, eds. *Textbook and color atlas of traumatic injuries to the teeth*, 4th edn. Oxford: Blackwell Munksgaard, 2007.
2. Andreasen FM, Andreasen JO, Cvek M. Root fracture. In: Andreasen JO, Andreasen FM, Andersson L, eds. *Textbook and color atlas of traumatic injuries to the teeth*, 4th edn. Oxford: Blackwell Munksgaard 2007; 337–71.
3. Andreasen FM. Pulpal healing after luxation injuries and root fracture in the permanent dentition. Thesis, Copenhagen University, 1995.
4. Andreasen JO, Andreasen FM, Bakland LK, Flores MT. *Traumatic dental injuries – a manual*, 2nd edn. Oxford: Blackwell Munksgaard, 1999.
5. Andreasen JO, Andreasen FM. Root resorption following traumatic dental injuries. *Proc Finn Dent Soc* 1991;**88**:95–114.
6. Andreasen JO, Løvschall H. Response of oral tissues to trauma. In: Andreasen JO, Andreasen FM, Andersson L, eds. *Textbook and color atlas of traumatic injuries to the teeth*, 4th edn. Oxford: Blackwell Munksgaard, 2007.
7. Andreasen JO, Munksgaard EC, Bakland LK. Comparison of fracture resistance in root canals of immature sheep teeth after filling with calcium hydroxide or MTA. *Dent Traumatol* 2006; **22**:154–6.
8. Andreasen JO, Ravn JJ. The effect of traumatic injuries to primary teeth on their permanent successors. II. A clinical and radiographic follow-up study of 213 injured teeth. *Scand J Dent Res* 1970;**79**:284–94.
9. Andreasen JO, Sundstrøm B, Ravn JJ. The effect of traumatic injuries to primary teeth on their permanent successors. I. A clinical, radiographic, microradiographic and electronmicroscopic study of 117 injured permanent teeth. *Scand J Dent Res* 1970;**79**:219–83.
10. Andreasen JO. Experimental dental traumatology: development of a model for external root resorption. *Endod Dent Traumatol* 1987;**3**:269–87.
11. Andreasen JO. Review of root resorption systems and models. Etiology of root resorption and the homeostatic mechanisms of the periodontal ligament. In: Davidovitch D, ed. *The biological mechanisms of tooth eruption and root resorption*. Birmingham: EBSCO Media, 1988; 9–21.
12. Cvek M, Granath L-E, Lundberg M. Failures and healing in endodontically treated non-vital anterior teeth with post-traumatically reduced pulpal lumen. *Acta Odont Scand* 1982;**40**:223–8.
13. Cvek M, Mejare I, Andreasen JO. Conservative endodontic treatment of teeth fractured in the middle or apical part of the root. *Dent Traumatol* 2004;**29**:261–9.
14. Cvek M. Prognosis of luxated non-vital maxillary incisors treated with calcium hydroxide and filled with gutta-percha. A retrospective clinical study. *Endod Dent Traumatol* 1992;**8**:45–55.
15. Jacobsen I, Kerekes K. Long-term prognosis of traumatized permanent anterior teeth showing calcifying processes in the pulp cavity. *Scand J Dent Res* 1977;**85**:588–98.

16. Jacobsen I. Traumatized teeth. Clinical studies of root fractures and pulp complications. Thesis. Oslo, 1981.
17. Kahnberg K-E. Surgical extrusion of root fractured teeth – a follow-up study of two surgical methods. *Endod Dent Traumatol* 1988;**4**:85–9.
18. Malmgren O, Malmgren B. Orthodontic management of the traumatized dentition. In: Andreasen JO, Andreasen FM, Andersson L, eds. *Textbook and color atlas of traumatic injuries to the teeth*, 4th edn. Oxford: Blackwell Munksgaard, 2007.
19. Robertson A, Andreasen FM, Bergenholtz G, Andreasen JO, Norén JG. Incidence of pulp necrosis subsequent to pulp canal obliteration from trauma of permanent incisors. *J Endod* 1996; **22**:557–60.
20. Robertson A. Pulp survival and hard tissue formation subsequent to dental trauma. *Swed Dent J* 1997; Suppl 125.

20

Oral mucous lesions and minor oral surgery

Göran Koch

Children and adolescents present a large variety of oral pathological conditions, such as lesions of the oral mucosa, bone lesions, cysts, and tumors or tumor-like lesions. Knowledge of such changes is a prerequisite for correct diagnosis and adequate treatment. This chapter will deal with the most common oral pathological conditions or changes in the oral mucosa found in children and adolescents. For more extensive knowledge of oral pathology in children the reader is referred to textbooks cited in the background literature list. Oral surgery in children and adolescents is, with few exceptions, similar to oral surgery in adults. However, there are some specific and common surgical procedures which, due to the special condition of a growing individual, are different to procedures performed in adults. The most common of such procedures will be presented in this chapter.

Oral mucous lesions

Herpetic gingivostomatitis

Herpetic gingivostomatitis is caused by herpes simplex virus (HSV) and communicated through personal contact, e.g., transmission via the saliva of the mother. Primary oral infection occurs following the first exposure to the virus. Studies have found antibodies to HSV in 40–90% of individuals in different populations, showing that HSV infection affects almost all individuals even if many of them only suffer the infection subclinically. The incidence of primary herpes simplex infection increases from the age of 6 months and reaches its peak at the age 2–4 years. The primary herpes simplex infection is therefore to be considered mainly a disease in children. The incubation period is 3–5 days. The primary infection is often manifested as an acute herpetic gingivostomatitis where the entire gingiva is red, edematous, and inflamed. The general symptoms are fever, headache, malaise, and pain. After 1–2 days small vesicles develop on the oral mucosa. They rupture, leaving painful ulcers with a diameter of 1–3 mm (Fig. 20-1).

Normally, the primary herpes simplex infection is self-limiting and the child will recover within a 10-day period. Treatment is primarily supportive, such as paracetamol for the pain and fever, fluid to maintain sufficient hydration and, if necessary, topical anesthetic ointments to facilitate eating. In severe cases, hospitalization and/or the use of antiviral agents is necessary.

It has been shown that recurrent herpes simplex infection originates from a reactivation of HSV, which

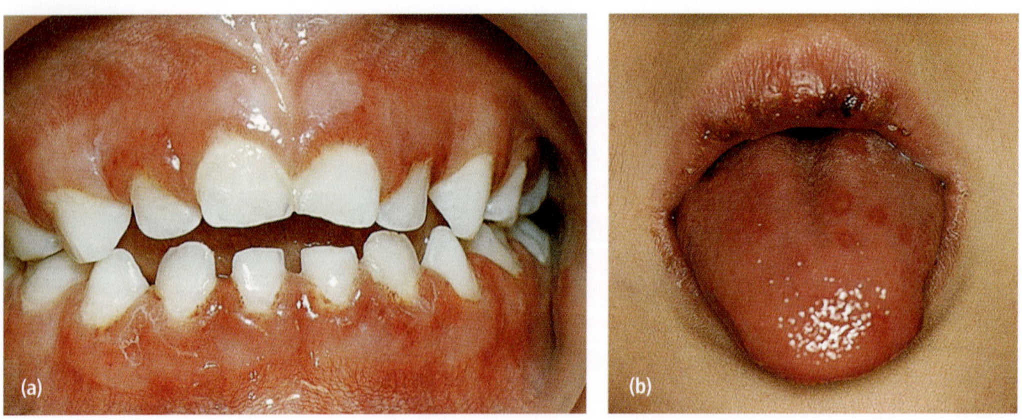

Figure 20-1 (a) Herpes simplex lesions spread over the alveolar mucosa (b) and the tongue.

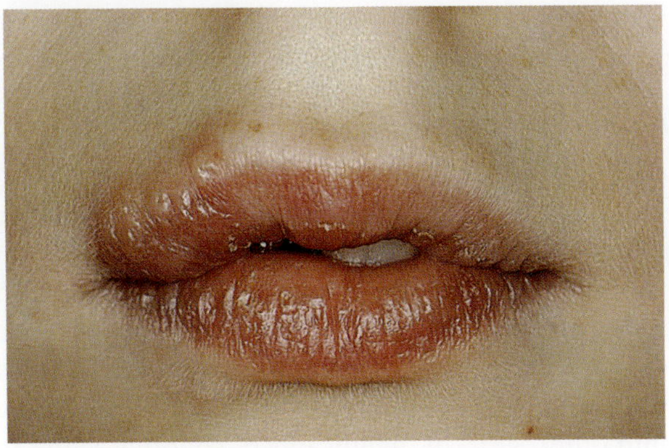

Figure 20-2 Herpes labialis.

remains dormant in nerve tissue between periods of excitation. Reactivation may be caused by injuries to the mucosa caused by sunlight, citrus fruits, or dental treatment, etc. Recurrent herpetic infection will develop in the same location at every excitation, e.g., herpes labialis (Fig. 20-2).

Differential diagnosis

Coxsackie virus infection, traumatic ulcerative gingival lesion (see Chapter 12), and impetigo contagiosa.

Impetigo contagiosa

This lesion is more common in children than adults. It is caused by streptococci and staphylococci and often affects the perioral area. The infection causes inflammatory vesiculobullous lesions that rupture, leaving secreting or crust-covered lesions (Fig. 20-3). The lesions will cause only a low sensation of pain. As the disease is contagious it can be spread within the family and between playmates. In the acute stage, dental treatment should be avoided. In most cases the lesions heal without complication after strict hygiene measures, but antibiotics are often recommended.

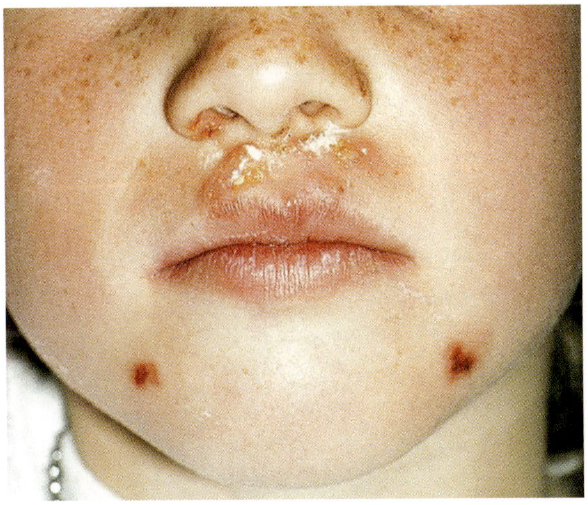

Figure 20-3 Impetigo contagiosa in a 7-year-old girl.

Aphthous ulcers

Recurrent aphthous ulcerations (RAU) or recurrent aphthous stomatitis (RAS) are the most common oral ulcerations seen in children. Studies indicate a prevalence of about 35% in adolescents. An altered immune defense system has been suggested as the main predisposing factor. This is confirmed by the frequent aphthous ulcers seen in children on immunosuppressive drugs and by their familiar occurrence. As a trigger factor, infection with specific oral streptococci has been suggested.

The lesions are most frequently localized to the nonmasticatory mucosa, e.g., the vestibulum and the tongue. The lesion starts as a small white papule which gradually ulcerates. The ulcers are 0.2–1 cm in diameter with the central part covered with a yellow–gray coating, and a crateriform base with raised reddened margins. The surrounding tissue shows a light swelling. The ulcers are extremely painful and may be of varying size and numbers (Fig. 20-4). The ulcers heal without scars in 1–2 weeks. The intervals between recurrent episodes may vary from a week to several months.

A variety of treatment modalities have been suggested. In general, the treatment has followed one or more of the following approaches:

- treatment of the oral microbiota (chlorhexidine, Aureomycin®, hydrogen peroxide-producing enzyme solutions)
- increasing the immunodefensive system (Longovital®)
- symptomatic treatment of the pain (etching solutions, topical anesthetics).

Differential diagnosis

Ulcers caused by trauma.

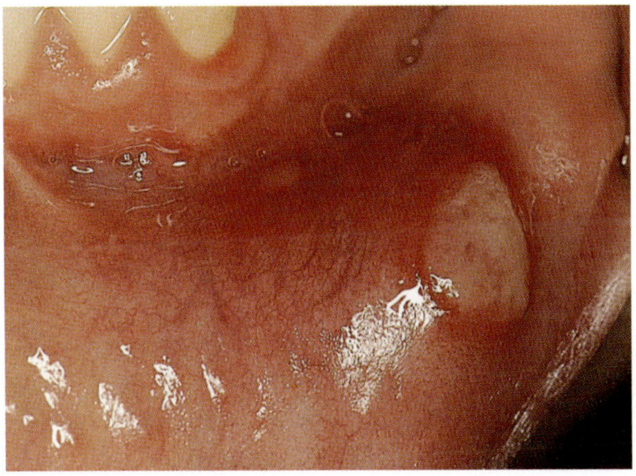

Figure 20-4 Aphthous ulcer.

Oral candidiasis

Oral candidiasis is caused by the fungus *Candida albicans*, which is normally found in the oral flora. The fungus invades the mucosa only when there is a change in the oral environment or a general impairment of the immunological or hormonal balance. Such changes can be brought about by the administration of antibiotics and immunosuppressive drugs, for example, and by the conditions of endocrinopathic syndromes. The clinical manifestations in the oral mucosa can vary. Pseudomembranous candidiasis (thrush) is the most common fungal infection in newborn children and in children with chronic disease. It is characterized by raised, pearly-white patches (Fig. 20-5) that can be rubbed off, leaving an erythematous or bleeding mucosa surface. The clinical manifestations can vary: acute, chronic atrophic, or hypertrophic forms can be found (Fig. 20-6). The treatment is medication with antifungal preparations such as nystatin, amphotericin B, or miconazole. Systemic administration or topical application by mouthrinses, sucking lozenges, and gels containing these preparations will be effective in most cases.

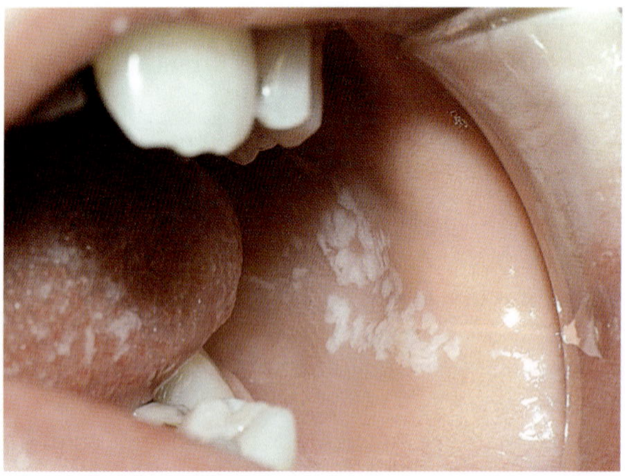

Figure 20-5 Candidiasis lesion in cheek mucosa.

Traumatic lesions

Traumatic irritation of the oral mucosa is occasionally seen in children. The most common situation is cheek or lip bites after dental local anesthesia. The clinical appearance is considerable swelling and bleeding followed by the development of a large, whitish pseudomembranous mucous lesion. The lesion is self-limiting and will heal within a week. Self-mutilation of the mucosa is most commomly seen in handicapped children with, for example, uncontrolled tongue movements. The irritation of the mucosa is caused by the child forcing the tongue out of the mouth and thereby injuring it on the mandibular incisors. Hyperkeratotic wounds may develop. Smoothing of the incisal edges of the incisors or an acrylic splint in the mandible may help to heal the lesion.

Bohn's nodules

Bohn's nodules (gingival cysts of the newborn) occur with high frequency up to the age of 3 months. The cystic formulations develop from epithelial remnants from the dental lamina and often appear in groups of four to six, situated on the buccal and lingual area of the dental ridge (Fig. 20-7). The nodules, which can be misinterpreted as early erupting primary teeth, need no special treatment as they will disintegrate spontaneously.

Mucous retention cysts (mucocele)

Mucocele occurs frequently in children, most frequently in the lower lip. It is caused by a trauma of the lip, resulting in an obstruction of the excretory duct of one of the numerous glands in the lip. It may lead to formation of an epithelium-lined mucous retention cyst. The clinical picture is often a smooth, painless, rounded swelling in

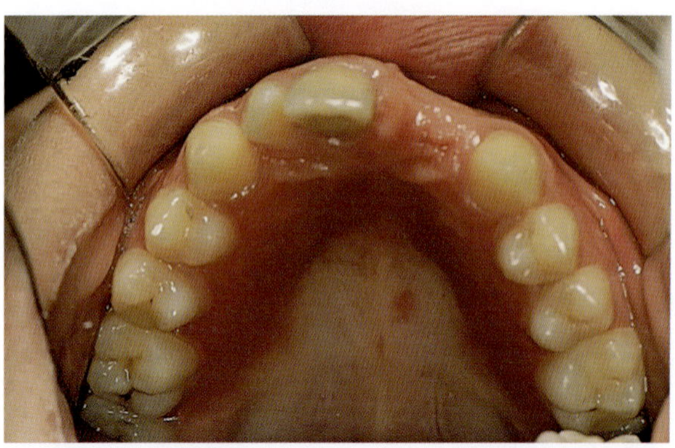

Figure 20-6 *Candida albicans* infection of the palatal mucosa in child with a partial denture.

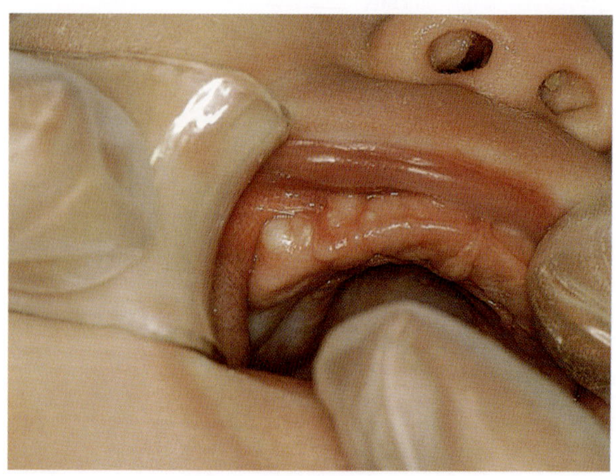

Figure 20-7 Bohn's nodules in an newborn baby.

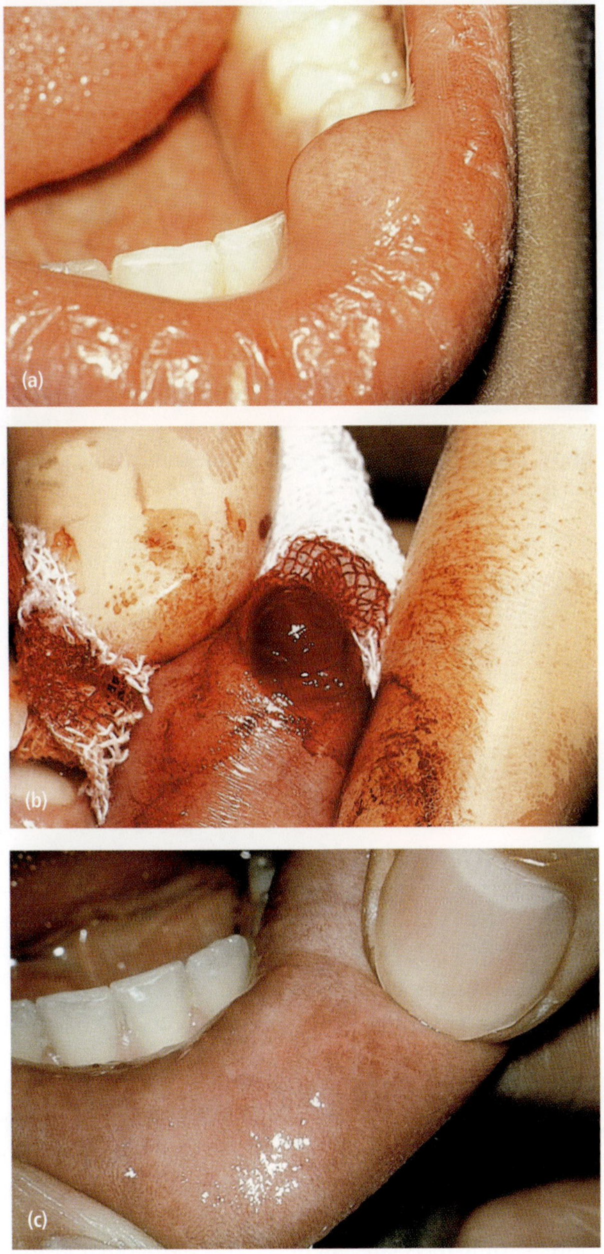

Figure 20-8 (a) Mucous retention cyst in the lower lip. (b) Surgical removal of the cyst. (c) Healing after 1 week.

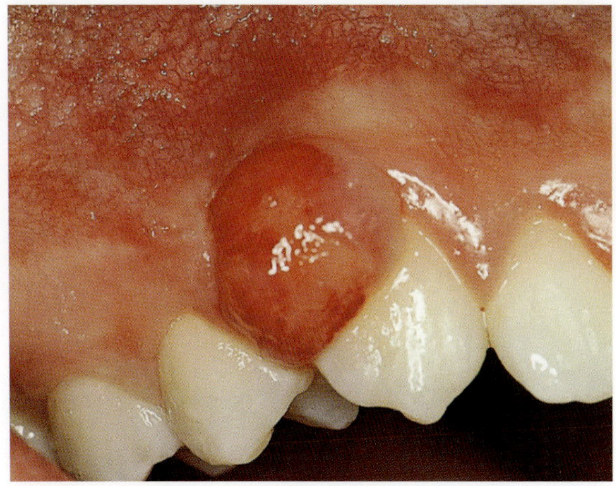

Figure 20-9 Peripheral calcifying granuloma.

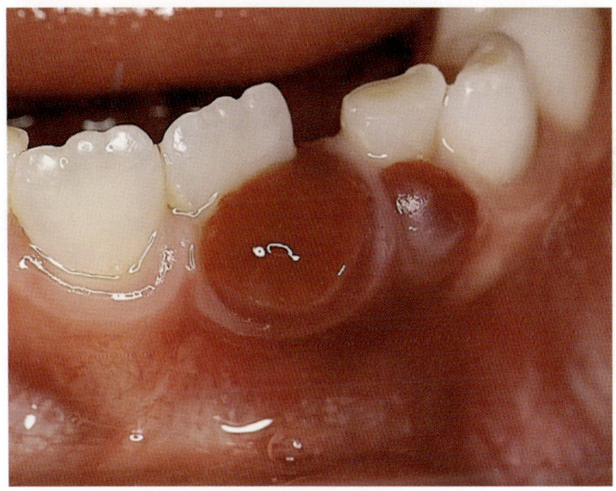

Figure 20-10 Peripheral giant cell granuloma.

the lip mucosa. The treatment is removal of the cyst and associated salivary gland (Fig. 20-8). Marsupialization often leads to recurrences.

Epulides

Epulides are by definition tumor-like hypertrophic tissue formations located on the gingival mucosa. The etiology is often trauma or irritation in connection with tooth eruption or exfoliation. The size may vary from some millimeters up to several centimeters in diameter. They differ in surface texture, consistence, and color, depending on tissue composition. Pyogenic granuloma, peripheral calcifying granuloma, and peripheral giant cell granuloma (Figs 20-9 and 20-10) are all examples of epulides. The treatment is excision and the final diagnosis is confirmed by histopathological analysis.

Hemangioma

Hemangioma is a relatively common hamartomatous tumor in children. Most of the lesions are present at birth. The most common location is the tongue, followed by the lips and buccal mucosa. Clinically, two different forms can be distinguished: the *capillary hemangioma* and the *cavernous hemangioma*. The former consists of a proliferation of tiny capillaries, often manifest as red birthmarks on the skin and oral mucosa (Fig. 20-11). The cavernous form is frequently situated more deeply and consists of large cavernous blood-filled vessels. The tumor often causes a compressible swelling

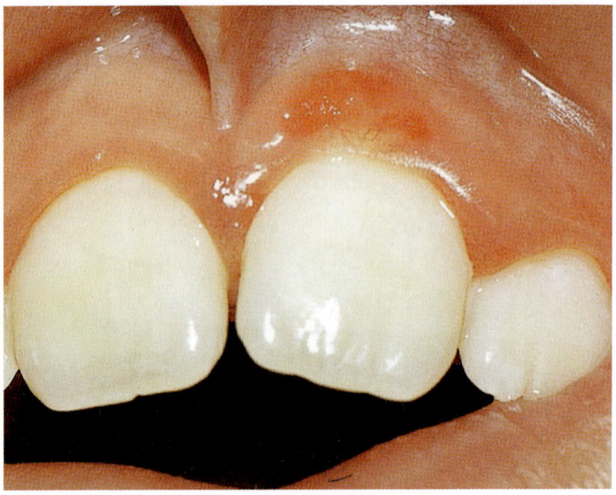

Figure 20-11 Capillary hemangioma.

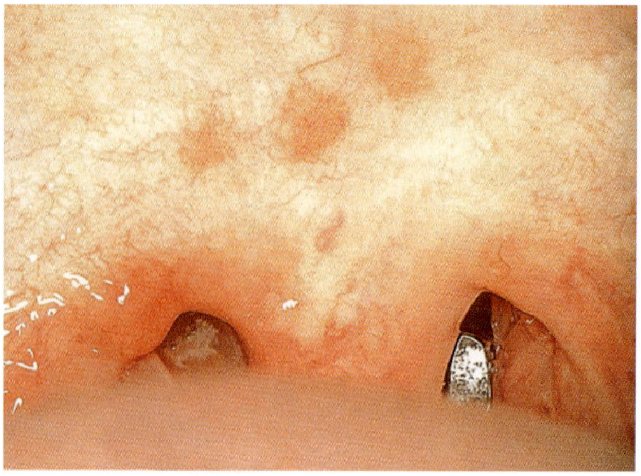

Figure 20-13 Forschheimer's spots on the soft palate in a child with rubella.

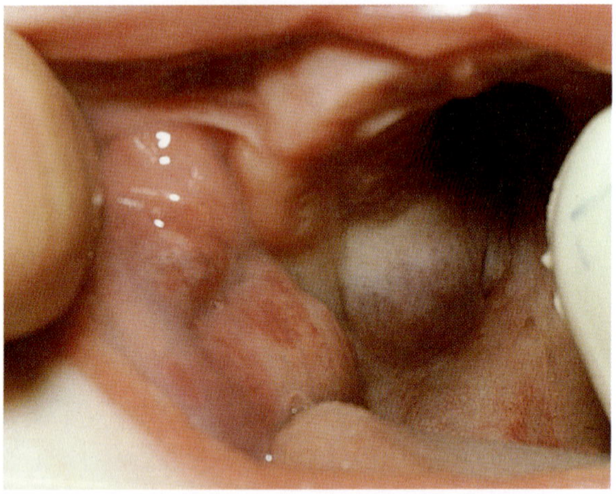

Figure 20-12 Cavernous hemangioma in the palate of a newborn. Note also the capillary hemangioma in the cheek.

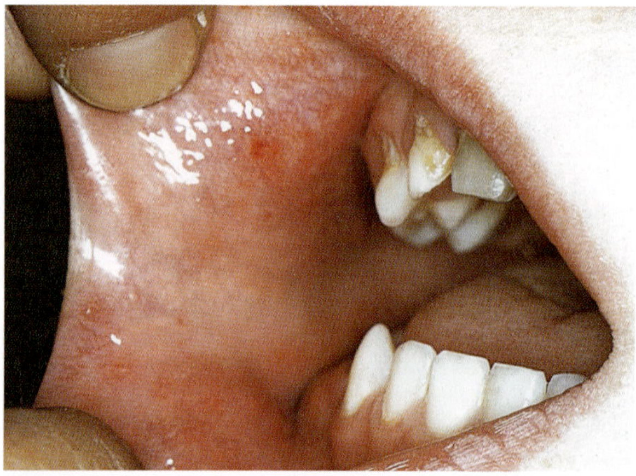

Figure 20-14 Koplik's spots in the cheek mucosa in a child with measles.

of the tissue affected and the color is frequently more bluish than the capillary hemangioma (Fig. 20-12). Fortunately, congenital hemangioma in the mucosa most frequently undergoes spontaneous regression.

Lesions connected with common infectious diseases in children

A number of common infectious diseases in children are manifested by oral lesions, apart from specific skin lesions. Unnecessary dental treatment should be avoided during the child's disease and the week following recovery due to risk of infectious transmission.

Rubella

Rubella is a virus infection characterized by light red macules on the skin. Occasionally, macules are also found on the soft palate: Forschheimer's spots (Fig. 20-13).

Measles

Measles is a viral disease. After an incubation time of 10–12 days the child will have a cough, fever, and photophobia. Some days later, light red maculopapular lesions develop all over the skin. The oral manifestations, Koplik's spots, occur on the buccal mucosa as prodromal grayish-white macules surrounded by a slightly erythematous zone some days before eruption of the skin lesions (Fig. 20-14).

Scarlet fever

Scarlet fever is a common disease in childhood caused by beta-hemolytic streptococci. The general symptoms are fever, tonsillitis, and lymphadenitis. A papular red skin rash will develop within a few days. The most characteristic oral manifestation besides swollen tonsils is the gradual change of the appearance of the tongue from a "strawberry" to a "raspberry" tongue. In the initial stage of the infection the white-coated tongue shows a scattered pattern of hyperemic fungiform papillae. Later, this coating is lost and the red edematous fungiform papillae dominate the clinical picture.

Varicella (chickenpox)

Varicella is a viral disease mostly seen in children. The general symptoms are fever, pharyngitis, and vesicular lesions on the skin, beginning on the trunk and then spreading all over the skin. The lesions have varying degrees of development. The oral manifestations are whitish vesicles surrounded by a red halo found mostly on the mucosa of the lips, bucca, and tongue (Fig. 20-15).

Mumps

Mumps is a viral infection affecting the salivary glands. The general symptoms are fever and pain from the infected glands. In cases where the parotitis is unilateral, difficulties in distinguishing the condition from a swelling of odontogenic origin may arise (Fig. 20-16).

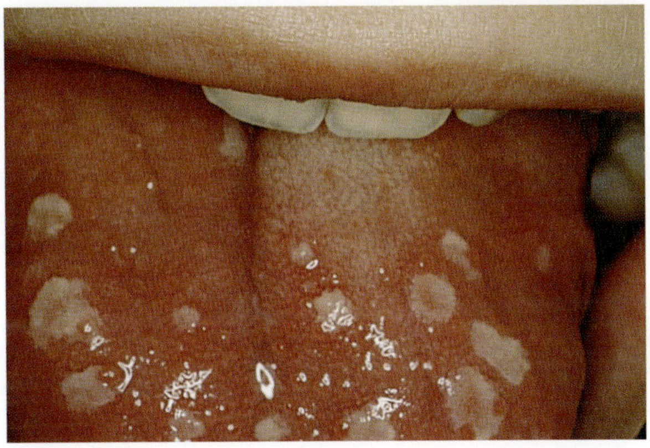

Figure 20-15 Vesicles on the mucosa of the tongue in a child with varicella.

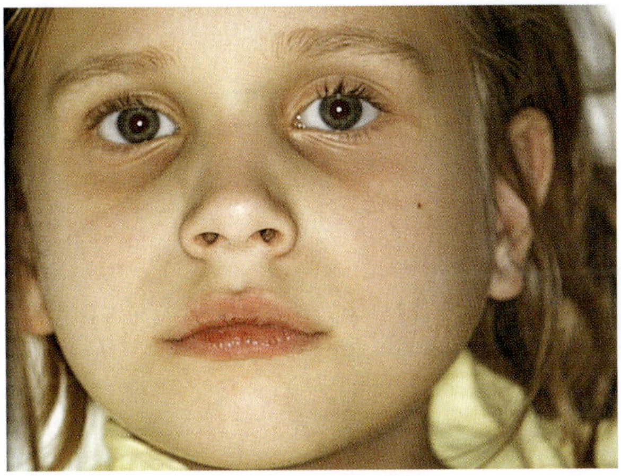

Figure 20-16 Child with unilateral parotitis (mumps).

Surgical procedures

Extraction of teeth

The indications, contraindications, and techniques at extraction of teeth in children are somewhat different compared to those for adults. In the primary dentition there may, for many reasons, be more extensive indications. Generally, necrotic teeth, ankylosed primary teeth without permanent successors, seriously carious teeth, especially with advanced root resorption, and primary incisors exposed to severe traumatic injuries should be extracted. The forceps for extraction of primary teeth are specially designed for the anatomical form and size of these teeth. The risk of root fractures during the extraction procedure is somewhat higher for primary molars than for permanent teeth due to the more slender and curved roots. Therefore, careful loosening of the tooth with a straight elevator is recommended before the forceps are applied. It is important to have a firm grip of the jaw in order to control the movement of the forceps more easily. Apply the working branches of the forceps steadily around the crown and neck of the tooth deep in the gingival pocket. The primary molars are extracted by slightly pressing the tooth down in the socket and slowly moving the tooth in a bucco-lingual direction to enlarge the socket before the tooth is lifted out. Incisors are extracted by a slight rotation of the tooth (Fig. 20-17).

In some cases the roots of the primary molar encircle the permanent tooth bud (Fig. 20-18). Before extraction it is therefore wise to cut the tooth into two halves with a diamond or fissure bur (Fig. 20-19) to avoid dislodging or avulsing the permanent successor. If a small root tip fractures, the best treatment is to leave it if it is not infected and does not interfere with eruption of the succeeding tooth. However, if the fragment is infected or nonvital it should be removed by using a sharp elevator or a root-reamer screwed into the root canal of the fragment.

Treatment of impacted teeth

The surgical treatment of impacted teeth will also be discussed in Chapter 15. Impacted primary teeth should generally be surgically removed. Permanent teeth with ectopic eruption position will usually be treated by surgical exposure often in combination with orthodontic treatment to guide the impacted tooth into its proper location. Such treatment is often used in cases with ectopic eruption of maxillary canines when risk for resorption of permanent incisors exists (Fig. 20-20). Impacted permanent teeth have to be surgically removed if they interfere with eruption of surrounding teeth, cause abnormal positions of erupted teeth, or develop pathological conditions in the region.

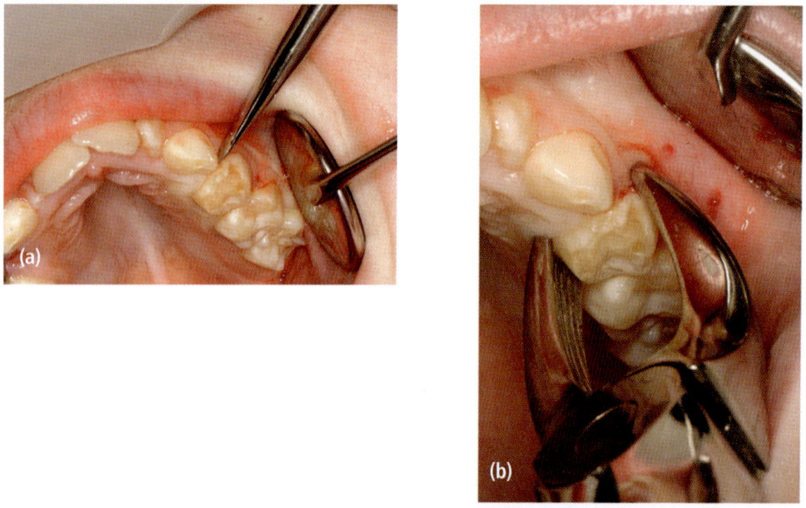

Figure 20-17 Extraction of primary teeth: (a, b) molars in upper jaw and (c, d) lower jaw – loosen the tooth carefully with an elevator, place the forceps around the tooth and apply apical pressure and buccal–lingual movements before the tooth is lifted out. (e–g) Incisors are extracted by slight apical pressure and rotary movement.

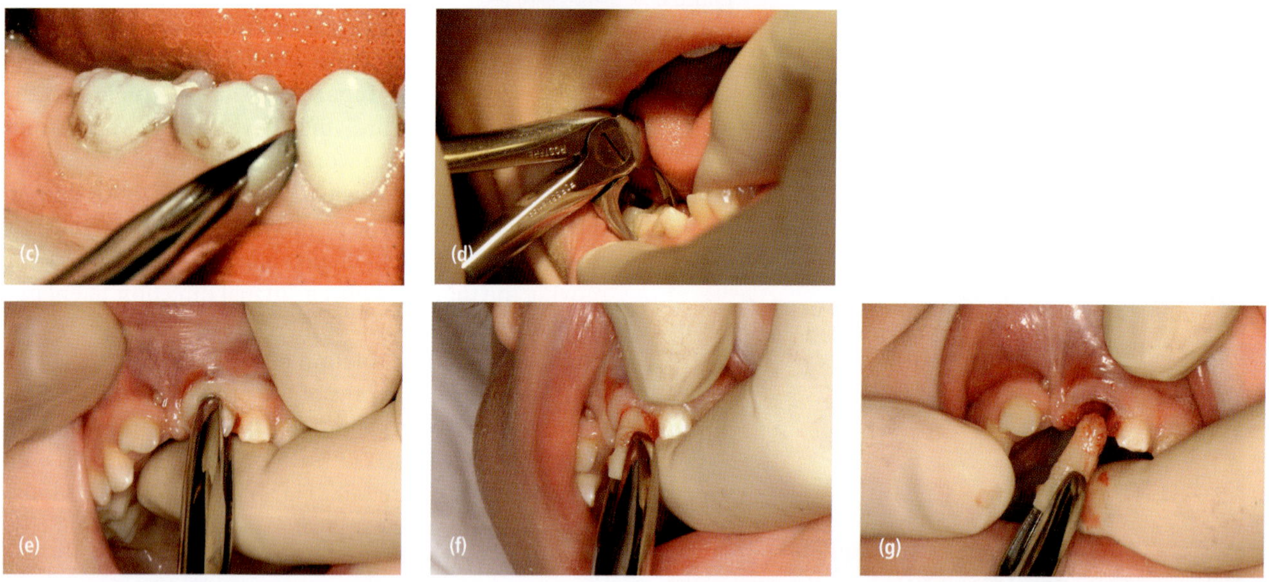

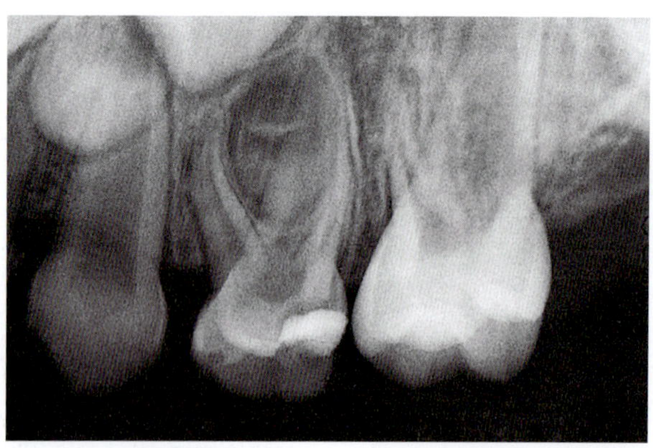

Figure 20-18 Primary first molar with pulpitis. Roots of the tooth encircle the permanent tooth bud.

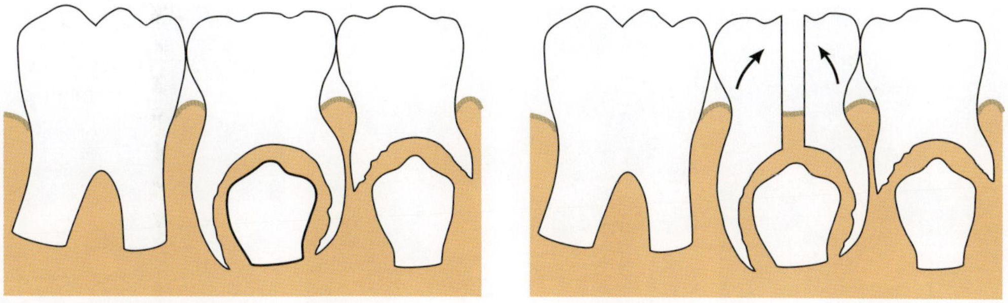

Figure 20-19 Primary molar cut into two halves before extraction.

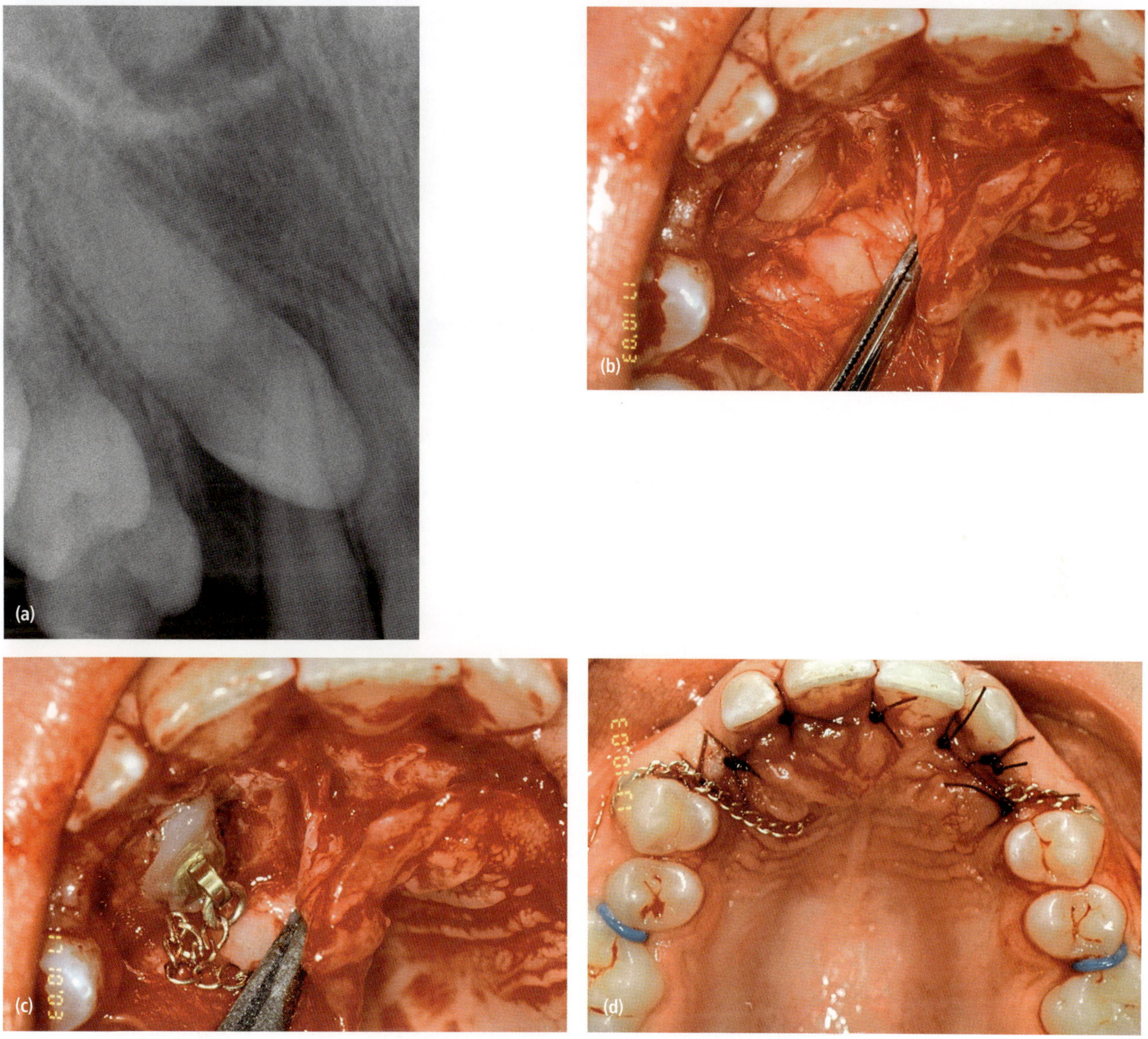

Figure 20-20 (a) Radiographs of upper right canine in palatinal ectopic position with risk for resorption of the permanent incisors. (b) After a palatinal mucoperiostal flap is raised and bone is removed the canine is exposed. (c) Brackets and gold chain are etched to the lingual surface of the canine. (d) The flap is sutured and the free end of the chain is temporarily fastened to a premolar. The contralateral canine was treated at the same session. The patient is now ready for the orthodontic treatment.

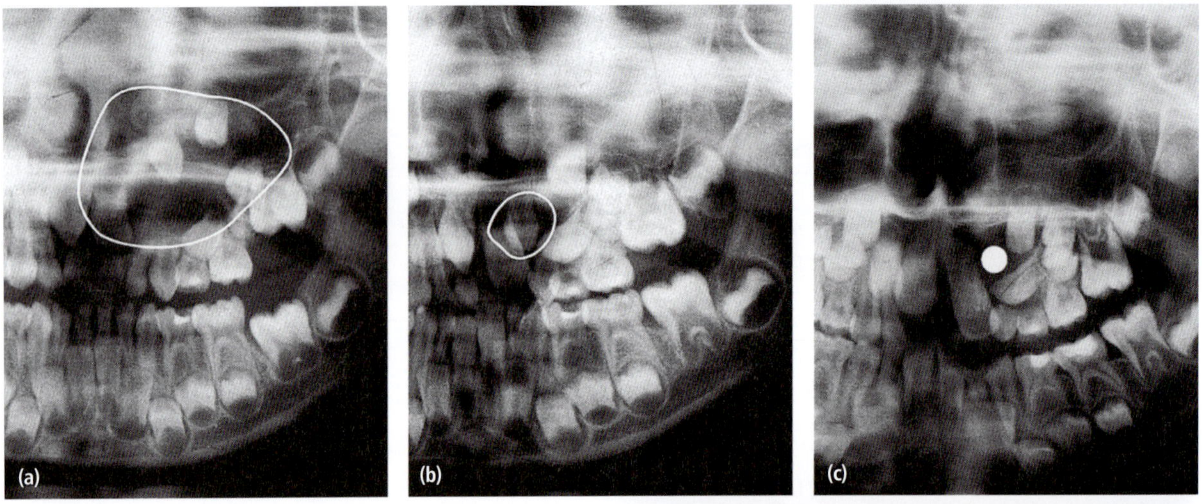

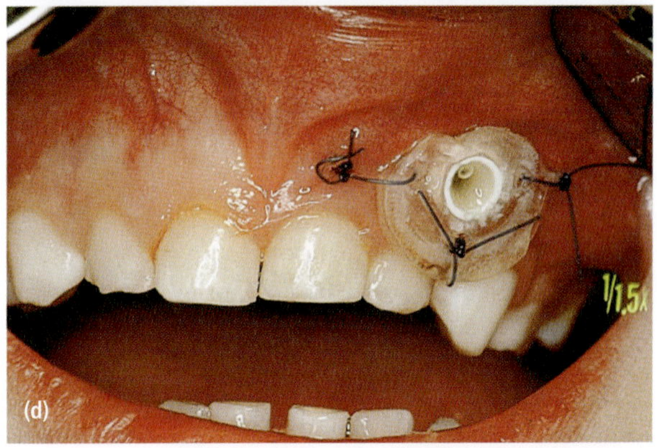

Figure 20-21 (a) Extensive follicular cyst in left maxilla emerging from a supernumerary tooth and displacing tooth germs and disturbing normal eruption in a 5-year-old girl. (b) Radiographic examination after 5 months revealed that the cyst had been reduced considerably and was now available for surgical removal without risk of disturbing the involved teeth. (c) After 4 months and surgical removal of supernumerary teeth and residual cyst tissues. (d) Obturator inserted to facilitate rinsings of the cyst. The obturator was removed after 6 weeks.

Cysts

Cysts in the jaws, and especially large follicle cysts emerging from nonerupted teeth, may displace tooth anlages and disturb tooth eruption (Fig. 20-21a–c). In children it is important not to remove the cysts surgically as a first procedure since this might damage a number of teeth and tooth germs. Instead, it is recommended in cases with large cysts that the cyst should be shrunk by use of rinsings with saline through an obturator introduced through the cyst wall (Fig. 20-21d). In young individuals the cyst will rapidly decrease and will be substituted by bone and often the dislocated teeth will spontaneously find their normal positions and eruption pathways.

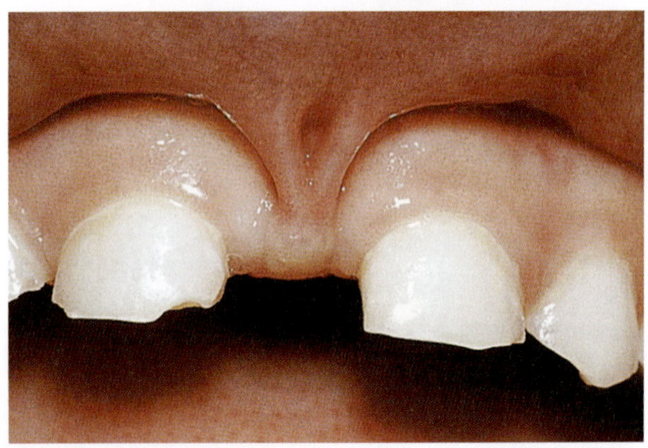

Figure 20-22 Fibrous frenulum causing bony defects in a 5-year-old girl.

Frenuloplasty

Frenulum labii superioris

Occasionally, the frenulum labii superioris has a broad attachment to the upper lip with a thick fibrous string attaching the frenulum to the incisive papilla. This strong fibrous part of the frenulum can cause "blanching" of the incisive papilla when forward tension is applied to the upper lip. A bony cleft or fissure can often be found between the central incisors in combination with an extensive diastema. In general, no treatment is necessary as most of these "abnormal" frenula and the diastema will normalize and disappear at the time of eruption of the permanent incisors and canines. However, if there is no spontaneous closure of the diastema, surgical intervention is recommended. In cases with very fibrous and extensive frenulum labii superioris causing deep bony defects between central incisors, the surgical treatment might be performed earlier (Fig. 20-22).

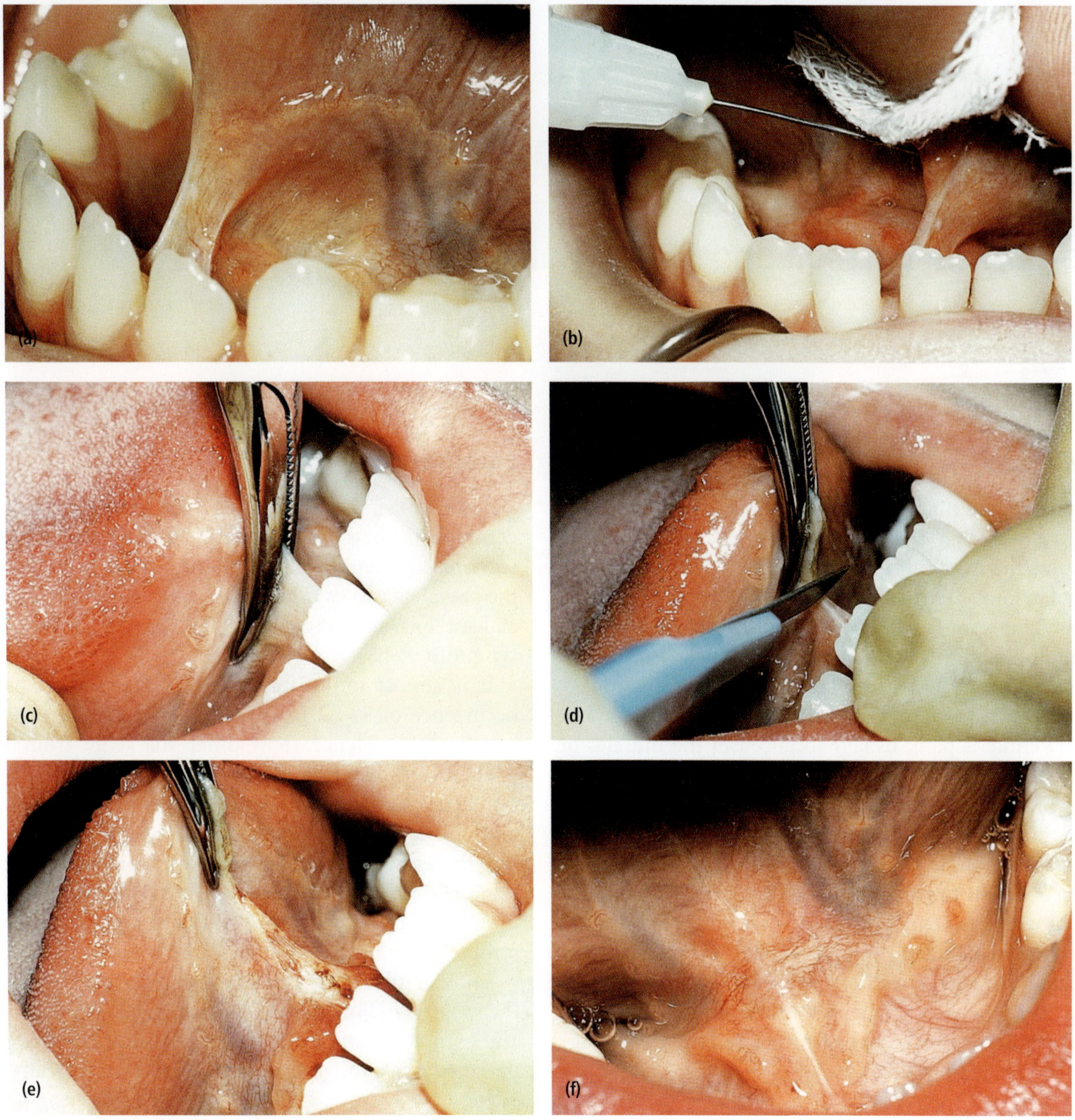

Figure 20-23 Lingual frenuloplasty. (a) Lingual frenulum restricting the movements of the tongue. (b) Local anesthesia. (c) Curved hemostat is placed close to the tongue. (d, e) Frenulum is cut. (f) Healing after 10 days.

Frenulum linguae

If a lingual frenulum is frequently traumatized by the mandibular incisors, causes retraction of the lingual gingiva or the mandibular incisors, or interferes with nourishment, speech development, or hygiene procedures it should be cut. It is vital to avoid two structures in this region: the submandibular duct and the sublingual vein. The dissecting cut is best made lingual to the caruncles, parallel to the undersurface of the tongue, taking care not to go too deep (Fig. 20-23).

Background literature

Hall RK. *Pediatric orofacial medicine and pathology*. London: Chapman & Hall, 1994.

Jones JH, Mason DK, eds. *Oral manifestations of systemic disease*. London: Baillière Tindal, 1990.

Pindborg JJ. *Atlas of diseases of the oral mucosa*. Copenhagen: Munksgaard, 1992.

Scully C, Welbury R. *Color atlas of oral diseases in children and adolescents*. London: Wolfe, 1994.

21

Temporomandibular disorders

Tomas Magnusson and Martti Helkimo

Definitions

Temporomandibular disorders (TMD) is a collective term embracing a number of clinical problems that involve the masticatory musculature, the temporomandibular joint (TMJ) and associated structures, or both (20). The term is synonymous with the terms craniomandibular disorders (CMD), functional disorders of the masticatory system, and mandibular dysfunction.

The most frequent reason for seeking treatment at a TMD clinic is pain, usually localized in the muscles of mastication and/or the TMJ. Typically the pain can be provoked and aggravated by chewing or by other jaw functions. TMD have been identified as a major cause of nondental pain in the orofacial region (20).

In addition to pain, limited or asymmetric mandibular movements, and TMJ sounds are commonly found in these patients. Common patient complaints also include jawache, earache, headache, and facial pain. Bruxism (jaw clenching and tooth grinding) and other oral parafunctions (e.g., nail-biting and gum chewing) may be related problems.

Epidemiology

Signs and symptoms of TMD seem to be relatively common in the general population of adults. In cross-sectional epidemiological studies of adult populations, the prevalence rates range from about 40 to 75% having at least one sign and about 35% having at least one symptom of TMD.

It is almost impossible to get a clear picture as to occurrence of TMD in children and adolescents. Estimates of prevalence rates differ markedly from one study to another (Fig. 21-1 and Table 21-1). This variation arises from a combination of factors such as inter- and intra-individual variations among examiners, differences in the composition of the study populations, examination methods, choice of variables as well as a multitude of incomparable definitions and criteria for symptoms and signs.

Another plausible, and often overlooked, reason for the great variation in the reported frequencies of signs and symptoms of TMD is that examination methods designed for adults have been applied uncritically on

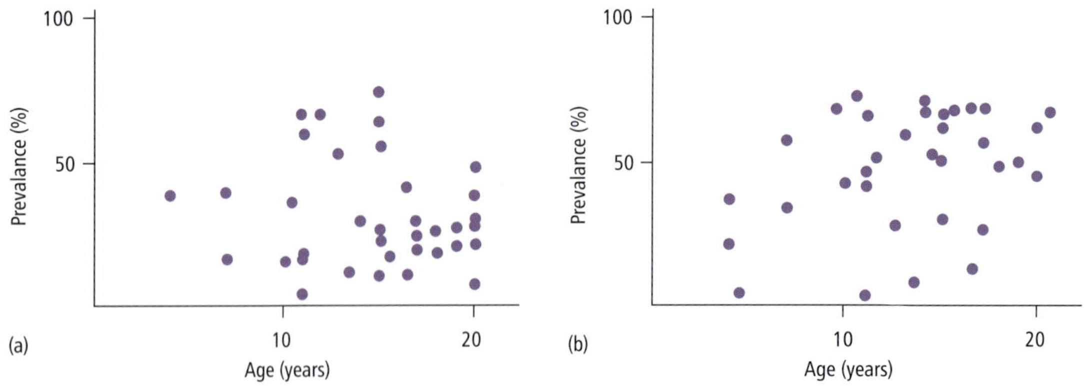

Figure 21-1 Diagrams showing prevalence of one or more (a) subjective symptoms and (b) clinical signs of TMD presented in different epidemiological studies of children and adolescents. The single dots represent the prevalence figure found in different studies. Note the wide variations within the same age groups, ranging from single percent to more than 70% [from Nydell *et al.* (18)].

Table 21-1 Range and median values for the prevalences of (a) subjective symptoms and (b) clinical signs of TMD in different epidemiological investigations [modified from Nydell *et al.* (18)]

	All reported data	
	Range (%)	Median (%)
(a) Subjective symptoms		
Tiredness or stiffness in the jaws	0–59	5.0
TMJ sounds	0–32	13.0
Pain on opening the mouth or other jaw movements	0.4–59	4.0
Pain in the face or jaws	0–19	3.0
Headache	1–88	13.2
Difficulties in opening the mouth	0–9	1.8
Locking or luxation	0.4–7	3.0
One or more subjective symptoms	3–74	26.2
(b) Clinical signs		
Impaired opening capacity	0–29	1.8
TMJ sounds	0–50	19.2
Deviation upon opening and closing the jaw	0–78	6.5
Locking or luxation	0–1	0.5
Tenderness on palpation of the TMJ	0–44	4.0
Tenderness on palpation of the masticatory muscles	1–68	21.2
Pain upon movement	0–18	2.5
One or more clinical signs	2–78	51.2

children without taking the age and cognitive development of the child into consideration (18).

In spite of the large volume of data from recent literature on the epidemiology of TMD, it is still not possible to make a conclusive statement as to the "true" prevalence of TMD signs and symptoms in children and adolescents, nor can we even say if these phenomena change with age. In longitudinal studies, symptoms and signs have shown a great fluctuation with time (12,23). Most signs and symptoms seem to come and go in an unpredictable way (8,17). In a 20-year longitudinal study, no significant progression of the signs and symptoms of TMD from childhood, through adolescence, to adulthood have been found (13). From the many epidemiological studies performed in this field, it can be concluded that signs and symptoms of TMD in children and adolescents are in most cases occasional and mild, except for some rare conditions and diseases such as juvenile idiopathic arthritis (Still's disease), which can be progressive and develop into severe functional limitation and pain in some few individuals.

Bruxism

Oral parafunctions include bruxism, lip-biting, thumb-sucking, and abnormal posturing of the jaw. In contrast to normal functional behaviors, such as chewing and swallowing, these parafunctional behaviors seem to have no obvious functional purpose.

Parafunctional activities are very common in all age groups, and only occasionally have significant negative effects on the structures of the masticatory system. As in adults, muscular pain, headache, and TMJ overloading may result also in children. In those cases, a protective bite splint may be indicated.

Nail-biting and excessive chewing on chewing gum are fairly common habits in children and adolescents, and can be as important etiological factors for TMD as tooth grinding and tooth clenching. Unphysiologic sleeping posture, e.g., belly sleeping, can also result in unfavorable loading of the TMJs and be a contributory factor to dysfunction of the joints.

In most cases, nocturnal bruxism in children does no harm. The patients and parents should be informed that, although very loud noises may occur, there is little evidence that permanent damage results from bruxism in childhood. The child will probably outgrow the behavior in time. It has even been suggested that bruxism in small children is a physiologic phenomenon necessary for a normal eruption of the permanent teeth.

TMD and orthodontics

The possibility that orthodontic treatment in childhood might be a risk factor for the development of TMD later in life has been an issue of great controversy in the dental literature for a long time. Several comprehensive review articles and meta-analyses have focused on this question (9,11,15,16). The conclusion from these studies is that there is no scientific evidence that orthodontic treatment increases the risk for development of TMD. On the contrary, there is some support for the conclusion that properly performed orthodontic treatment in childhood might have a positive effect on the functional status of the masticatory system later in life (22).

Taking the history in children and adolescents with suspected TMD

Taking the history in children entails several difficulties. For instance, many children try to please the questioner by giving the answer they believe is the desired one (5). Because of this, care must be taken to avoid leading questions as far as possible when reviewing the history (21). Another problem is that younger children cannot use language to express pain. Not until about the age of 12 years, at the end of the cognitive development and when the ability to think abstractly has developed, are children able to describe their pain verbally (10).

Bearing these limitations in mind, taking the history can be an important key to a correct diagnosis and a subsequent successful treatment. The history should be taken in a calm and confident atmosphere. The questions should be relevant and kept as simple as possible. Some examples of questions that should be included in the history are presented in Box 21-1.

As stated in the introduction of this chapter, pain in the face and jaws, as well as headaches, are fairly common symptoms in children and adolescents. In most cases, however, they occur only occasionally. Only if they are frequent complaints and only if they are associated with clinical signs do they merit TMD treatment. Asymptomatic joint sounds are not, with rare exceptions, an indication for treatment, but observation on recall is the proper course of action.

Clinical functional examination of the masticatory system

An important part of the functional examination is registration of pain reaction to palpation. Once again it is important to stress that for a child, pain can be more than the physiological experience of pain. The discomfort experienced during the examination, e.g., pressure during palpation, can be expressed as pain. Because of this, both reports of palpatory tenderness in masticatory muscles and/or TMJs, as well as reports of pain during mandibular movements should be interpreted with caution in young children.

Measurement of maximal jaw opening capacity is to be included in a functional examination of the masticatory system (Fig. 21-2). The individual vertical overbite should be included in the range of movement. The normal variation is large with slightly higher figures for boys, but the individual opening capacity is established in the early teenage years (Table 21-2). Impairment or improvement of the maximal jaw opening capacity is thus a significant clinical parameter of the functional status. If the individual opening capacity at health is unknown, an opening of 36 mm is an accepted minimum limit from the age of 6–7 years (1).

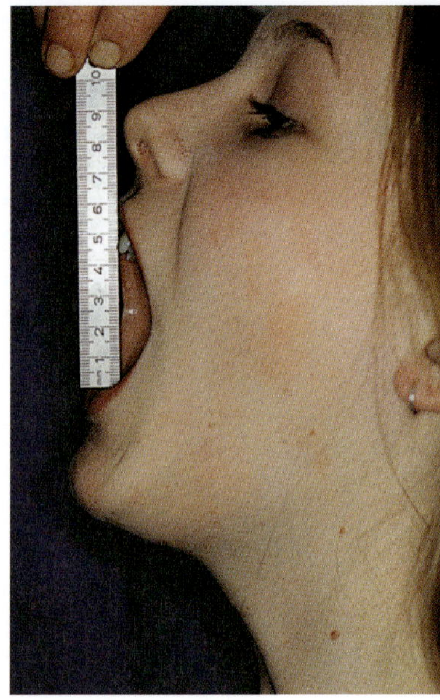

Figure 21-2 Measurement of maximal jaw opening capacity.

The lateral aspects of the TMJs are palpated bilaterally (Fig. 21-3) while the patient performs two or three maximal jaw openings. Pain on palpation, pain during opening, irregular jaw movement as well as TMJ sounds are recorded. The use of a stethoscope to record joint sounds is questionable, since it may reveal insignificant or normal joint sounds.

Palpation of the jaw muscles should be limited to a few, informative muscles. We recommend that the masseter and temporalis muscles are palpated bilaterally.

Box 21-1 Questions that should be included when taking a TMD history

- Do you feel pain in your face or jaws?
- Do you frequently suffer from headaches?
- Do you feel tired or have pain when chewing or when opening the mouth wide?
- Have you noticed TMJ sounds, and if so: are those sounds associated with pain?
- Do you clench or grind your teeth?
- Do you frequently bite your nails or use chewing gum?
- What is your favorite sleeping posture?

Table 21-2 Maximal mouth opening at different ages according to Agerberg (2)

Age (years)	Mean value (mm)	Range (mm)
1.5	38.4	32–44
6	44.8	33–60
13	53.9	41–73
16	56.0	39–82
20	56.0	42–77

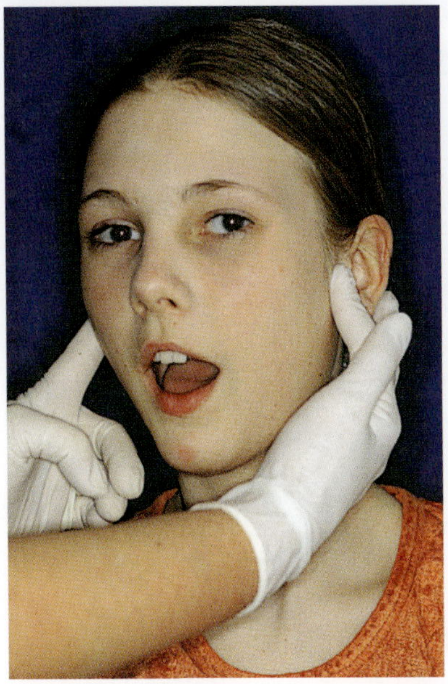

Figure 21-3 Bilateral palpation of the lateral aspects of the TMJs.

The anterior part of the superficial portion of the masseter muscle is easy to locate, and is palpated bidigitally from its origin on the zygomatic arch to the insertion on the mandible (Fig. 21-4). The large, fan-shaped attachment of the temporalis muscle can be palpated extraorally on the lateral part of the head, but more informative, and thus more important, is to palpate the insertion of this muscle on the medial part of the coronoid process.

A functional examination should also include an evaluation of the occlusion since it may act as a predisposing factor for TMD in the individual patient. It is, however, important to consider the extensive dynamics of the occlusion in children and adolescents due to exfoliation and eruption of teeth, as well as growth of the jaws. The role of occlusal factors in the etiology of TMD is controversial, but it seems that unilaterally forced cross bite might be of importance in this respect (7,19).

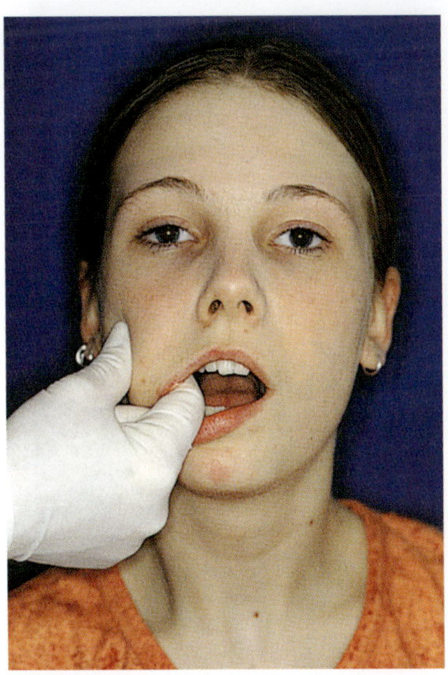

Figure 21-4 Palpation of the anterior part of the superficial portion of the right masseter muscle.

Radiographic imaging of the TMJs

Imaging is warranted when the clinical examination and/or the history indicate a recent or progressive pathological joint condition such as trauma, significant dysfunction, or limitation in movement, sensory/motor alteration, or significant change in occlusion (3) as well as in cases with general joint disease with suspected engagement of the TMJs. However, radiographic findings will rarely influence the initial, conservative treatment plan for TMD.

The most common radiographic projections and methods used are the oblique transcranial lateral projection, which may be supplemented by axial and frontal views, and tomography. The latter method has the greatest relevance concerning osseous structure and intra-articular skeletal relationships (6).

It is, however, of utmost importance to realize that each period in the growth of the child and adolescent has its own morphological character. The ever-changing normality criteria of the radiographic image of the TMJ are a complicating factor when information from the images is interpreted (6). There is a great risk of misinterpretation if criteria from images of adults are adopted without due consideration (Fig. 21-5).

Treatment of TMD in children and adolescents

With some exceptions, the TMD treatment concepts in children and adolescents are the same as for adults. In the following, we will focus mainly on these exceptions, but for details concerning the different treatment modalities, we refer to other current textbooks (4).

There is no scientific support for the opinion that TMD can be prevented with early treatment. Because of this, prophylactic intervention to prevent TMD is not indicated, with the possible exception of orthodontic treatment of laterally forced cross bites.

Only a few scientific data are available that support the need and efficacy of different treatment modalities of TMD in children and adolescents. Because of this, simple, conservative, and reversible treatments are strongly recommended. In the authors' opinion, such treatments have proved to be effective in reducing most TMD symptoms in children and adolescents.

When the history has been taken and the clinical examination performed, the patient, and *even more the*

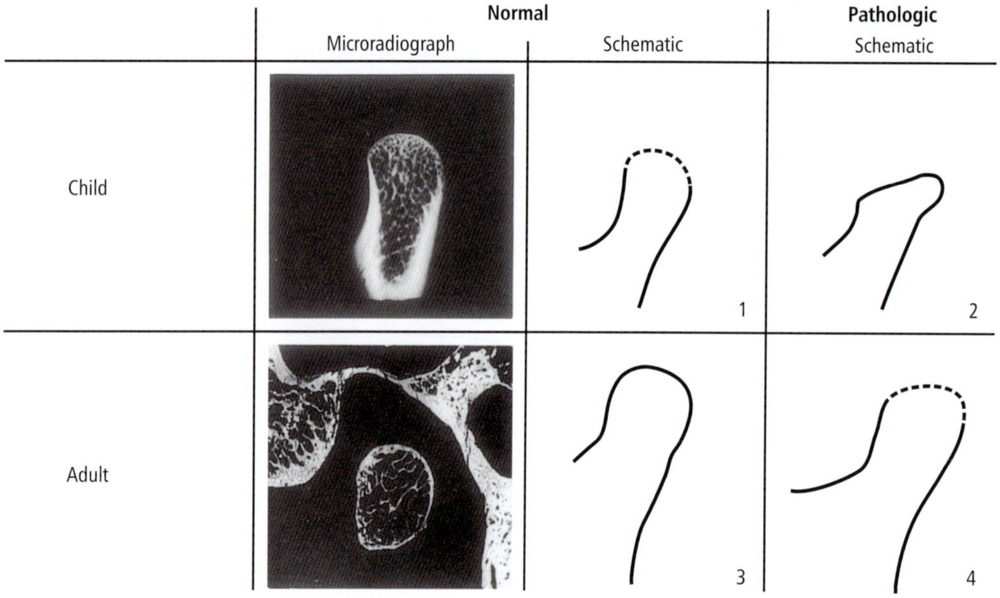

Figure 21-5 Figure from Eckerdal (6). Schematic illustration of the apparent paradoxical peripheral delineation of the condylar heads of normal and pathologic joints in the child and the adult. A normal delineation of the condylar head of a child (1) has characteristics in common with that of a pathologic adult TMJ (4) and the pathologic condylar head of a child (2) with that of a normal adult (3). (Reproduced with the permission of Förlagshuset Gothia.)

parents, should be reassured about the benign character of the condition, and the favorable prognosis of simple, conservative treatments should be stressed. It is also important to educate the patient to avoid unnecessary loading of the masticatory system such as by nail-biting and excessive use of chewing gum.

When treating TMD in adults, occlusal adjustments are often used as a part of the treatment. Due to the dynamics of the occlusion in children and adolescents, this treatment should be avoided or performed with great caution in these age groups, but minor adjustments can be made as well as smoothing ragged incisal edges.

Exercise therapy is an often effective treatment of TMD (14) that has been used for many years. This treatment also merits its place in the treatment of children and adolescents with TMD. Its mode of action is probably a combination of several muscle physiological

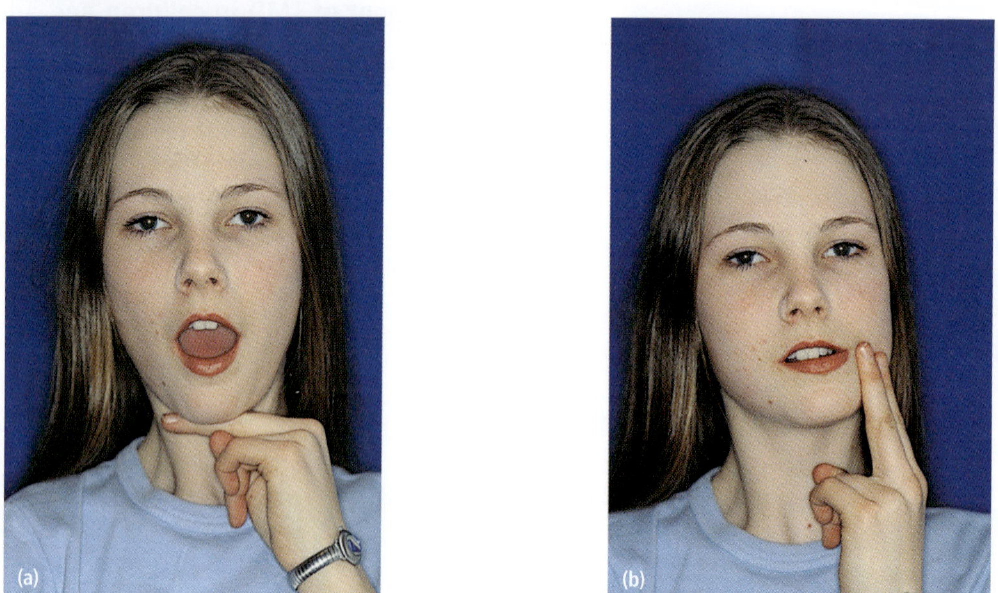

Figure 21-6 Examples of therapeutic jaw exercises. (a) Active jaw opening against a slight resistance. (b) Active lateral excursion to the left against a slight resistance.

mechanisms, such as proprioceptive neuromuscular facilitation, reciprocal inhibition, and stretching, but it is also a cognitive and behavioral treatment. The success of therapeutic jaw exercises depends on the motivation, cooperation, understanding, and compliance of the patient. Many different programs, as well as how they are to be performed (4), have been presented in the dental literature. To be successful with this treatment modality, it is important that the patient is thoroughly instructed in how the exercises are to be performed (Fig. 21-6).

Another reversible, conservative, and often effective treatment of TMD is interocclusal appliance therapy. To minimize the risk of negative effects on growth and development, a soft appliance placed in the mandible can be recommended as the appliance of first choice in children and adolescents (Fig. 21-7). Most patients in these age groups respond quickly and the appliance therapy can often be interrupted after 6–8 weeks. In single cases, where an appliance is needed for a longer period of time (more than 3 months), or when large forces from parafunction are exerted, appliances of hard acrylic are to be used. In these cases, however, it is important to consider the developmental stage of the dentition and the type of occlusion when the appliance is designed (Fig. 21-8), and the patients should be submitted to regular check-ups as long as the treatment continues. Not until the permanent dentition (excluding third molars) is developed (around the age of 14 years) is the appliance treatment of adolescents similar to the treatment of adults.

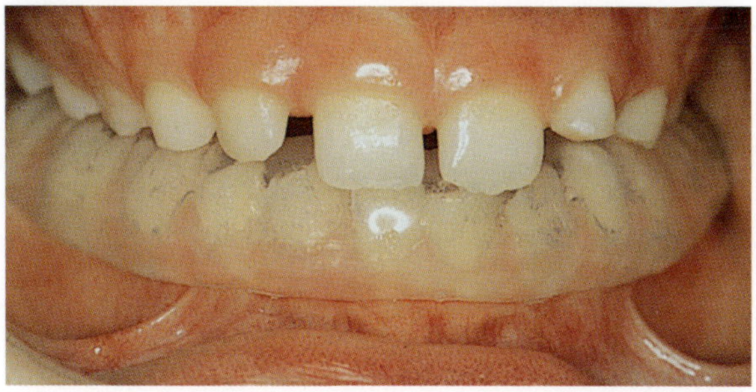

Figure 21-7 Soft interocclusal appliance placed in the mandible.

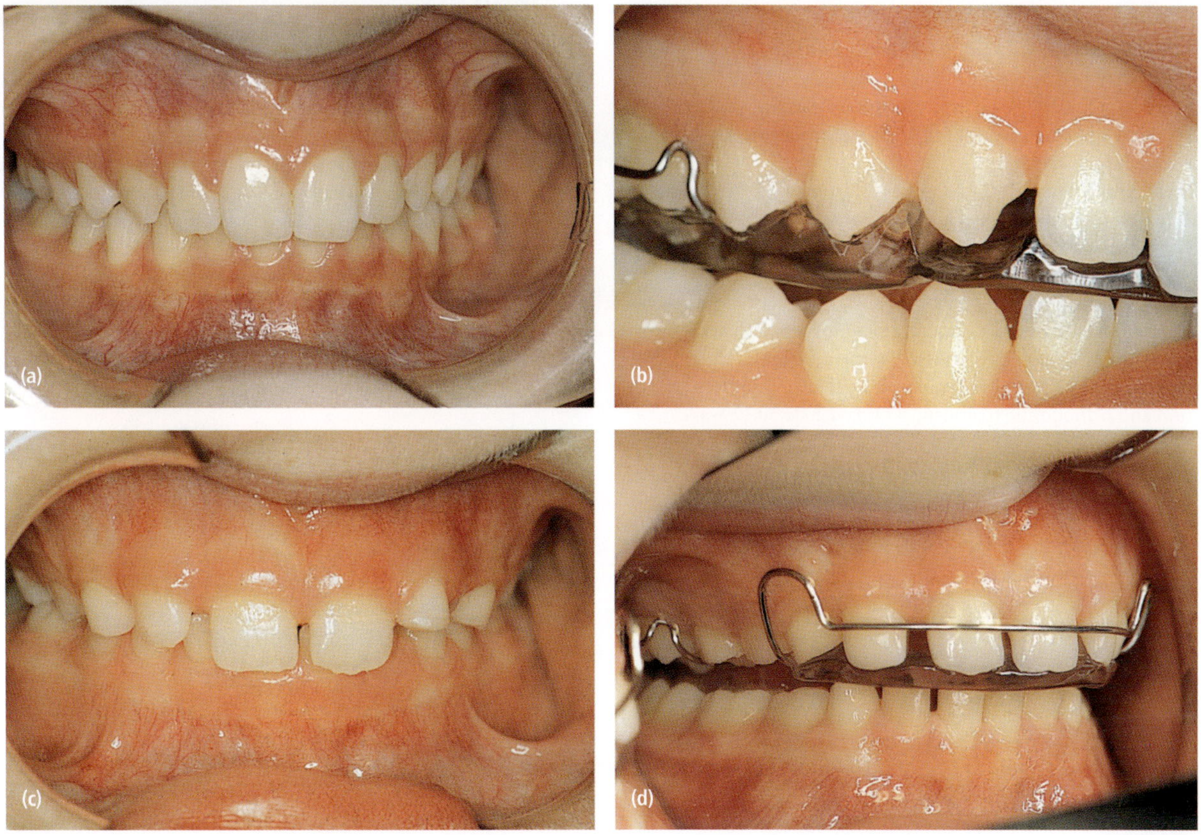

Figure 21-8 (a) A 12-year-old girl in whom the canines in the maxilla are not completely erupted. (b) She is provided with a hard acrylic appliance (Shore-plate), where the acrylic is removed in the region of the canines to allow further eruption. (c) A 7-year-old boy with a mixed dentition and a deep bite. Severe bruxism and frequent headaches. (d) He is provided with a hard acrylic bite-plate to prevent the teeth from further wear, to unload the jaw muscles, and eventually to decrease the deep bite.

Summary

Signs and symptoms of TMD are common in children and adolescents, but are in most cases mild and infrequent. When taking the history, the age and maturity of the patient must be considered. A functional examination of the masticatory system should comprise measurement of maximal mouth opening capacity, palpation of TMJs and a few informative jaw muscles, as well as an examination of the occlusion. Those patients who merit treatment mostly respond quickly to simple, conservative treatment methods such as therapeutic jaw exercises and/or interocclusal appliances.

References

1. Agerberg G. Maximal mandibular movements in children. *Acta Odontol Scand* 1974;**32**:147–59.
2. Agerberg G. On mandibular dysfunction and mobility. Thesis. University of Umeå, 1974.
3. American Academy of Pediatric Dentistry. Treatment of temporomandibular disorders in children: summary statements and recommendations. *J Am Dent Assoc* 1990;**120**:265–9.
4. Carlsson GE, Magnusson T. Treatment of TMD. In: Carlsson GE, Magnusson T, eds. *Management of temporomandibular disorders in the general dental practice.* Chicago, IL: Quintessence, 1999; 87–121.
5. Doverborg-Österberg E, Pramling I. *Att förstå barns tankar. Metodik för barnintervjuer.* Stockholm: Liber Utbildningsförlaget, 1985.
6. Eckerdal O. *Radiologic reproduction of healthy and arthritic temporomandibular joints of children and adolescents.* Stockholm: Förlagshuset Gothia, 1997.
7. Egermark-Eriksson I, Carlsson GE, Magnusson T, Thilander B. A longitudinal study on malocclusion in relation to signs and symptoms of cranio-mandibular disorders in children and adolescents. *Eur J Orthod* 1990;**12**:399–7.
8. Heikinheimo K, Salmi K, Myllärniemi S, Kirveskari P. Symptoms of craniomandibular disorders in a sample of Finnish adolescents at the age of 12 and 15 years. *Eur J Orthod* 1989;**11**:325–1.
9. Henrikson T, Nilner M. Temporomandibular disorders, occlusion and orthodontic treatment. *J Orthod* 2003;**30**:129–37.
10. Jeans ME. The measurement of pain in children. In: Melzack R, ed. *Pain measurement and assessment.* New York: Raven Press, 1983; 183–9.
11. Kim MR, Graber TM, Viana MA. Orthodontics and temporomandibular disorders: a meta-analysis. *Am J Orthod Dentofacial Orthop* 2002;**121**:438–46.
12. Könönen M, Nyström M. A longitudinal study of craniomandibular disorders in Finnish adolescents. *J Orofacial Pain* 1993;**7**:329–6.
13. Magnusson T, Egermark I, Carlsson GE. A prospective investigation over two decades on signs and symptoms of temporomandibular disorders and associated variables. A final summary. *Acta Odontol Scand* 2005;**63**:99–109.
14. Magnusson T, Syrén M. Therapeutic jaw exercises and interocclusal appliance therapy. A comparison between two common treatments of temporomandibular disorders. *Swed Dent J* 1999; **23**:27–37.
15. McNamara JA, Seligman DA, Okeson JP. Occlusion, orthodontic treatment and temporomandibular disorders: a review. *J Orofac Pain* 1995;**9**:73–90.
16. McNamara JA, Turp JC. Orthodontic treatment and temporomandibular disorders: is there a relationship? Part 1. Clinical studies. *J Orofac Orthop* 1997;**58**:74–89.
17. Nilner M, Kopp S. Distribution by age and sex of functional disturbances and diseases of the stomatognathic system in 7–18 year olds. *Swed Dent J* 1983;**7**:191–8.
18. Nydell A, Helkimo M, Koch G. Craniomandibular disorders in children. A critical review of the literature. *Swed Dent J* 1994; **18**:191–5.
19. Okeson JP. Temporomandibular disorders in children. *Pediatr Dent* 1989;**11**:325–9.
20. Okeson JP. In: Okeson JP, ed. *Orofacial pain: guidelines for assessment, diagnosis and management.* Carol Stream, IL: Quintessence, 1996.
21. Okeson JP, O'Donell JP. Standards for temporomandibular evaluation in the pediatric patient. *Pediatr Dent* 1989;**11**:329–30.
22. Olsson M, Lindqvist B. Mandibular function before and after orthodontic treatment. *Eur J Orthod* 1995;**17**:205–14.
23. Wänman A, Agerberg G. Two-year longitudinal study of signs of mandibular dysfunction in adolescents. *Acta Odontol Scand* 1986; **44**:333–42.

22

Children with chronic health conditions: implications for oral health

Göran Dahllöf and Luc Martens

The number of children with chronic health conditions (CHCs) has increased during the past few decades. With new technology, better drugs, and more efficient use of existing treatments an increasing number of children survive their CHCs. In industrialized countries, over 85% of children with CHCs will survive at least to 20 years of age. Other important changes are that children with CHCs are not institutionalized as frequently as in earlier times, they receive early stimulation, and they are usually integrated in the schooling system and attend outpatient medical and dental clinics.

Managed care protocols including oral care are at present being developed for several CHCs. For example, in programs for children undergoing bone marrow transplantation it is recommended that they should be referred to the dentist prior to the start of cytotoxic therapy for oral health information and evaluation of the oral health status, particularly the presence of infectious foci. In some instances, oral diseases and also dental care may be life-threatening to the child, e.g., surgical treatment in children with blood or bleeding disorders. A close collaboration with the medical treatment team is an integral part of the management of oral health care in children with CHC.

General dentists will increasingly meet children with CHC in their practices and up-to-date knowledge of how a CHC affects the oral health of a child is an important aspect of pediatric dental care.

Definition of CHCs

A modern definition of CHC in children focuses on the consequences of the disorder and is independent of diagnosis (15). Three elements must coexist for a child to be classified as having a CHC (Box 22-1). The duration of a condition can be difficult to predict, particularly when the onset is recent. Disease pattern is defined as the relative consistency or permanence of symptoms or consequences with time. Five patterns of disease have been identified (see Box 22-2 and Figs 22-1–22-5) (8).

Box 22-1 Definition of chronic health conditions

- Disorder on a biological, psychological or cognitive basis.
- Duration of at least 12 months.
- The consequences of the disorder are either:
  - functional limitations
  - reliance on compensatory mechanisms or assistance
  - service use beyond that which is considered routine.

CHCs in children have a variable expression. In order to give the best treatment to a child with such a condition it is important to identify the limitations and also the possibilities of each child. In Box 22-3, 13 different dimensions on a continuous scale used to describe a child with a CHC are presented. It should be observed that the definitions of CHC and impairment, disabilities, and handicap are related. They concentrate on the consequences for the individual rather than on the diagnosis (see Chapter 23, Box 23-1). The international classification of impairments, disabilities, and handicaps model proposes that there are three consequences of disease, impairment, disability, and handicap, and that they are sequentially related.

Prevalence

The prevalence of CHCs has been studied in different populations. Depending on the definition, estimates vary from less than 5% to more than 30% of children. It was found that 14.8% of children were diagnosed with a chronic health condition using a noncategorical definition with three different domains: (a) functional limitations, (b) dependence of compensatory mechanisms, and (c) service use beyond routine care for age (14). In a study of a total population in the south of Sweden in

Box 22-2 Five different patterns of chronic health conditions in children

Pattern	Definition	Example
Permanent condition	Manifests consequences in a consistent and unchanging way	Cerebral palsy (Fig. 21-1)
Recovery	The intensity and duration of symptoms and sequelae improve gradually or resolve	Asthma, epilepsy (Fig. 21-2a, b), leukemia in long-term remission
Deteriorating course	The condition deteriorates for years or decades	Aplastic anemia (Fig. 21-3a, b), cystic fibrosis, muscular dystrophy
Episodic	Recurrent periods of disease activity that alternate with periods of silence	Juvenile rheumatoid arthritis (Fig. 21-4a, b)
Diagnosed before symptoms	Conditions diagnosed long before symptoms are expressed	Cerebral palsy (Fig. 21-1), HIV infection (Fig. 21-5), hypercholesterolemia

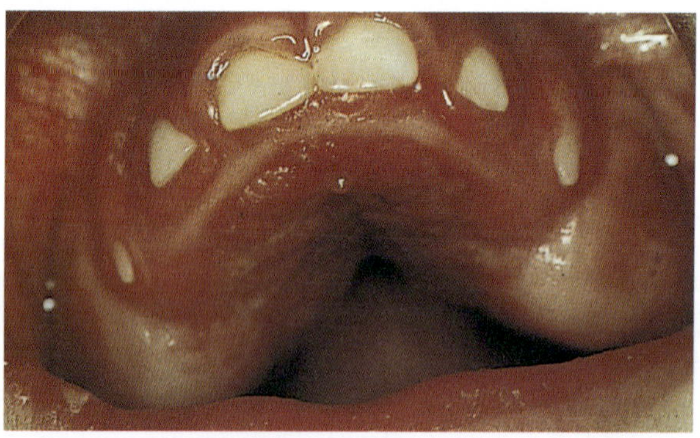

Figure 22-1 A 3-year-old boy with cerebral palsy and showing severe gingival overgrowth.

children aged 0–15 years, 8.4% were identified as having a CHC (16). There is a predominance of boys over girls: 9.2 vs 7.6%. Eight percent of children with CHCs needed extensive help with activities of daily life and/or had a bad prognosis concerning short-term survival, while 70% had only occasional limitations or needed regular medical treatment which did not interfere with normal activities.

Disabling atopic diseases such as dermatitis and hay fever were identified as the most common CHCs followed by bronchial asthma (Box 22-4). Multi-handicaps are common, particularly in children with mental retardation who exhibit additional diagnoses such as congenital malformation, epilepsy, vision impairment, and cerebral palsy. Among children with chronic conditions, approximately 70% have one diagnosis, 21% have two, and 9% have three or more. The prevalence of developmental delay, learning disabilities, emotional, and behavioral problems increases sharply with the number of chronic conditions in a child. The number of days in bed, school absences, and activity limitation also increased.

There are strong correlations between social disadvantage and child health. Overall, mortality throughout childhood and adolescence is increased among socially disadvantaged groups. In addition, survival of CHCs is worse in socially disadvantaged children. Factors apart from the material aspects are poorer social support, lifestyle factors such as smoking, poor dietary habits, lack of breastfeeding, and parenting style.

Despite obvious differences among the specific types of health conditions, important commonalties exist in the experience of children and families affected with various conditions. Among them are the need for a wide array of community and professional services, increased challenges to self-concept and optimal emotional development, extra financial hardship, and disruption of family and social activities (see also Chapter 23).

Increased risk for oral diseases in children with chronic health conditions (CHCs)

Children with CHCs have an increased risk of oral diseases due to consequences of the disease or the medication given. In Box 22-5, groups of children with CHCs who have an increased risk for oral diseases are presented (9). An important part of the general dentist's role is to maintain contact with the family and to initiate the necessary preventive measures and to refer the patients if the condition of the patient requires pediatric dentistry specialist care. An early diagnosis of oral diseases is also of major importance as well as knowledge of any changes in health condition and medication that may affect the dental treatment. The medical history should be examined very carefully covering the child's whole lifespan. It is of particular importance if local anesthesia and sedation are to be used that the child is classified according to anesthetic risk.

CHCs

Asthma

Asthma is one of the CHCs with an increasing prevalence in the Western world. It is a serious global health problem affecting more than 100 million people, and in most countries the prevalence has increased during the past two decades. In Sweden, 5–7% of the population has asthma. Chronic inflammatory mechanisms are

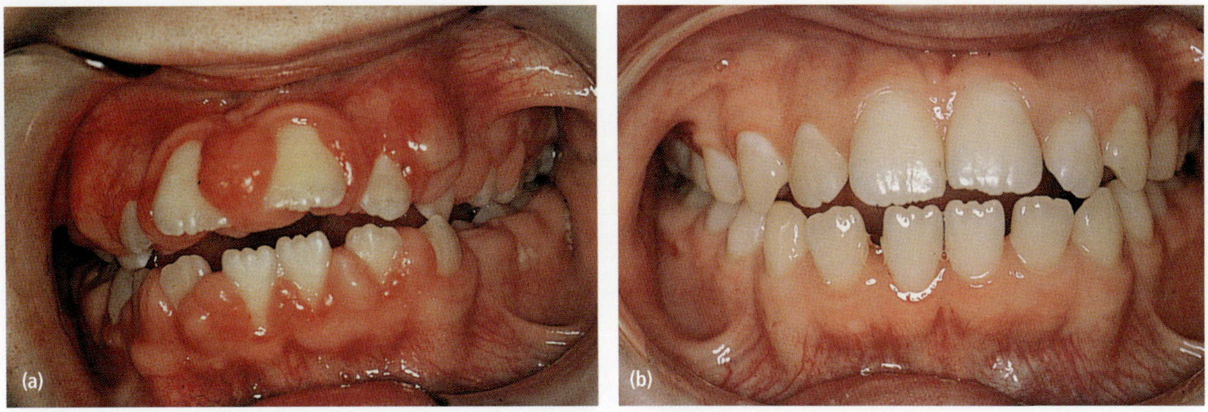

Figure 22-2 (a) A 10-year-old girl on phenytoin medication exhibiting severe gingival overgrowth. (b) At 13 years of age, exhibiting a normal gingival 1 year after gingivectomy and discontinuation of phenytoin medication.

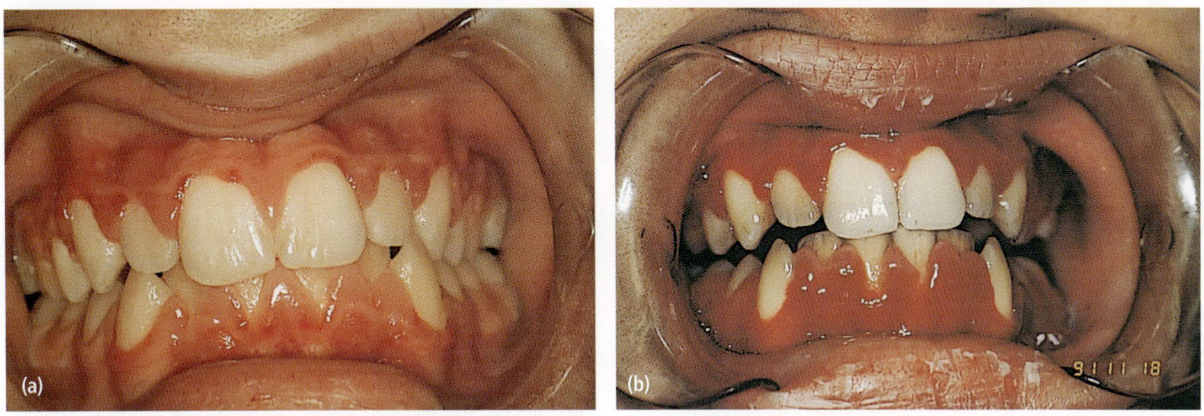

Figure 22-3 (a) A 15-year-old boy with aplastic anemia prescribed cyclosporine medication. (b) At 18 years of age, deteriorating gingival health coincidental with a haematological crisis.

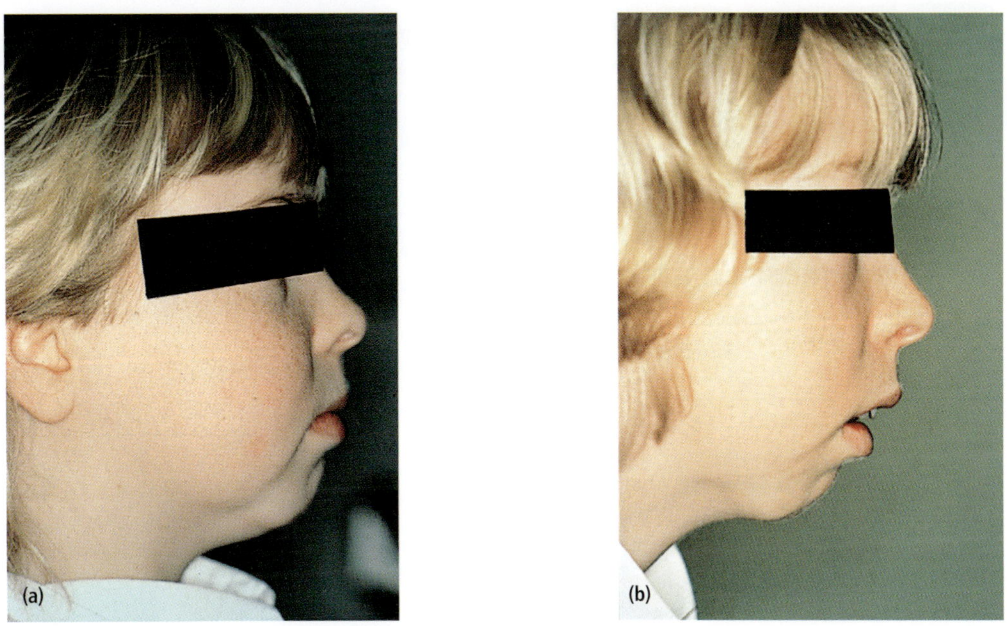

Figure 22-4 (a) A 13-year-old girl with juvenile chronic arthritis. (b) At 16 years of age, a reduced growth of the mandible is diagnosed (courtesy of L. Olsson).

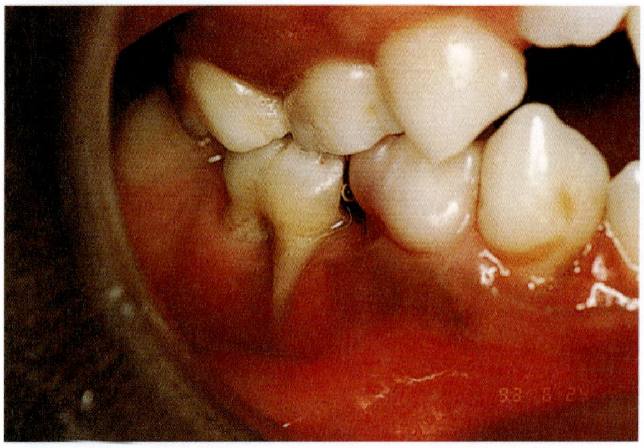

Figure 22-5 A 9-year-old boy with a congenital HIV infection exhibiting periodontal disease.

Box 22-3 Dimensions describing a child with a chronic health condition

Dimensions	Descriptions	
Duration	Brief	Lengthy
Age of onset	Congenital	Acquired
Limitations of age-appropriate activities	None	Unable to conduct
Visibility	Not visible	Highly visible
Expected survival	Usual longevity	Immediate threat to life
Mobility	Not impaired	Extremely impaired
Physiologic functioning	Not impaired	Extremely impaired
Cognition	Normal	Extremely impaired
Emotional/social	Normal	Extremely impaired
Sensory functioning	Not impaired	Extremely impaired
Communication	Not impaired	Extremely impaired
Course	Stable	Predictable
Uncertainty	Episodic	Predictable

important in the development of obstructive symptoms in asthma. Mild symptoms are treated with β_2-agonists and, when symptoms occur more frequently, treatment with inhalation steroids is instituted.

Implications for oral health. Children with asthma have an increased incidence of dental caries, particularly in the permanent dentition, gingivitis, calculus, and dental

Box 22-4 Prevalence of chronic health conditions[a] in a total child population, aged 0–15 years (12)

Diagnosis (ICD-8)		Prevalence per 1000
Infections and parasitic diseases		0.7
Neoplasms		0.8
Endocrine, nutritional and metabolic disorders:		5.3
Immune deficiency	1.8	
Obesity	1.3	
Diabetes mellitus	1.0	
Mental disorders:		18.3
Psychiatric disorders	3.3	
Speech disorders	7.4	
Mental retardation	5.4	
Diseases of the nervous system and sense organs:		21.5
Cerebral palsy	3.1	
Epilepsy	5.1	
Otitis media, recurrent	7.2	
Diseases of the circulatory system		0.2
Diseases of the respiratory system:		21.0
Asthma bronchiale	15.0	
Rhinitis allergica	9.2	
Diseases of the digestive system:		1.3
Allergic gastroenteritis	0.7	
Diseases of the genitourinary system:		1.8
Recurrent urinary tract infections	1.2	
Diseases of the skin and subcutaneous tissue:		19.6
Atopic dermatitis	18.1	
Diseases of the musculoskeletal system and connective tissue:		0.8
Juvenile rheumatoid arthritis	0.3	
Congenital malformations:		10.5
Heart and circulatory system	3.0	
Cleft lip–palate	1.0	
4-Mb Down	0.5	
Perinatal morbidity		0.5
Symptoms and ill-defined illnesses		0.3
Accidents, poisonings, and violence		0.5

[a] The definitions used were:

- a disorder which was disabling and obviously chronic and incurable,
- a disorder of at least 3 months' duration and interfering with daily life functioning and/or needing treatment or special aids during at least 3 months,
- a disorder requiring hospitalization for at least 1 month or at least three periods during 1 year.

Box 22-5 Examples of oral diseases in children with chronic health conditions

Chronic health conditions	Oral diseases
Asthmatic conditions	Increased caries risk Gingivitis Calculus Dental erosions Decreased salivary secretion rate
Childhood malignancies	Viral and fungal infections Mucositis Disturbances in dental development
Diabetes	Gingivitis Periodontitis
Hypophosphatasia	Premature exfoliation of primary teeth Alveolar bone loss
Immune deficiencies	Oral ulcerations Viral and fungal infections
Renal disorders	Disturbances in dental development Calculus

erosion as well as an altered salivary composition and flow rate (8). Although there are conflicting results in the literature regarding the effect on caries, most investigators suggest that children are at higher risk due to their pharmacotherapy as well as the duration of the disease (3). Contributing factors are the medication these children are taking in the form of inhalers and liquid medicine. A large proportion of inhaled drugs, up to 80%, is retained in the oral cavity. Since inhalation powder often contains sugars such as lactose, this may contribute to the increased caries prevalence. It is recommended that children rinse their mouths with water after each steroid inhalation. An increased consumption of sugar-containing beverages has also been reported.

The use of β_2-agonists is associated with a decreased salivary secretion rate. The mechanism involved is a down-regulation of β_2-receptors in the salivary glands, leading to a decreased secretory signal.

An increased incidence of gingivitis is also found in asthmatic children. This has been explained by an altered immune response and their tendencies to mouth breathe, particularly during an episode of rhinitis or acute asthmatic attack. Increased levels of calcium and phosphorus in parotid saliva may be associated with higher levels of calculus in asthmatic children. An increased level of erosive tooth loss is also found. A low salivary secretion rate, frequent consumption of acidic drinks and an increased incidence of gastroesophageal reflux are reportedly associated factors. Due to the risk of drug interactions and the risk of precipitating an attack, aspirin-containing medications and nonsteroidal anti-inflammatory drugs (NSAIDs) should be avoided. The dental treatment itself may cause a stress reaction that may precipitate an attack. Children are advised to bring their medication list to the dental office. Nitrous oxide/oxygen sedation should be used in preference to intravenous sedation if sedation is required. Due to increased risk of caries a regular preventive program should be instituted and the salivary secretion rate should be monitored.

Cardiovascular disorders

Almost all heart disease in children is congenital in origin, with a birth prevalence of eight per 1000 live births. The eight most common structural congenital heart diseases (CHDs) account for over 80% of the total; they are: ventricular septal defects, patent ductus arteriosus, atrial septal defects, tetralogy of Fallot, pulmonary stenosis, coarctation of the aorta, aortic stenosis, and transposition of the great arteries. Larger defects are closed surgically in the first years of life, and some defects may require complex surgery and eventually transplantation. Acquired heart diseases such as myocarditis and infective endocarditis are still a cause of death and disability in children. The incidence of rheumatic fever has fallen sharply.

Implications for oral health. Invasive dental procedures such as extractions, scaling, oral surgery, and endodontic treatment are likely to induce a transient bacteremia. It has recently been shown that all procedures involving the gingival tissues, even toothbrushing, induce a bacteremia (11). Antibiotic prophylaxis is given to patients listed in Box 22-6 who undergo any dental procedure that involves the gingival tissues and the

Box 22-6 Cardiac conditions for which antibiotic prophylaxis with dental procedures is reasonable (17)

- Prosthetic cardiac valve or prosthetic material used for cardiac valve repair.
- Previous infectious endocarditis.
- Congenital heart disease (CHD):
  - unrepaired cyanotic CHD, including palliative shunts and conduits
  - completely repaired CHD with prosthetic material or device, whether placed by surgery or by catheter intervention, during the first 6 months after the procedure
  - repaired CHD with residual defects at the site or adjacent to the site of a prosthetic patch or device.
- Cardiac transplantation recipients who develop cardiac valvulopathy.

periapical region of a tooth and for those procedures that perforate the oral mucosa. The following procedures and events do not need antibiotic prophylaxis: routine anesthetic injections through noninfected tissue, taking dental radiographs, placement of removable prosthetic or orthodontic appliances, adjustment of orthodontic appliances, placement of orthodontic brackets, shedding of primary teeth, and bleeding from trauma to the lips or oral mucosa. In this limited patient population, prophylactic antimicrobial therapy should be directed against viridans group streptococci (Box 22-7) (17).

In children with complex heart disease, problems with nutrition and vomiting are common during their first years of life. Frequent meals are necessary to ensure the caloric intake. In addition, some of the medications contain sucrose together with diuretics that can cause salivary dysfunction. Children with CHD are a risk group for caries development, particularly in the primary dentition. Children on digoxin therapy, administered with a sucrose-containing syrup, had increased caries prevalence (13). Children with CHD also have an increased prevalence of disturbances in enamel mineralization. As soon as a child is diagnosed with a significant cardiac problem he or she should be referred for dental evaluation. A preventive program including dietary counseling, fluoride therapy, fissure sealants, and oral hygiene instruction should be implemented.

Chronic renal failure

Chronic renal failure (CRF) is the result of progressive, irreversible damage to the kidney, as a consequence of reduction in glomerular filtration speed. Initially, CRF is treated with a protein-reduced diet supplemented with calories. Carbohydrates will deliver the necessary energy.

Box 22-7 Recommended antibiotic prophylaxis for patients with an increased risk of developing bacterial endocarditis

Patient	Antibiotic and dose
Adults	Amoxycillin 2 g single dose orally, 30–60 minutes before procedure
Children < 12 years of age	Amoxycillin 50 mg/kg body single dose orally, 30–60 minutes before procedure
If allergic to penicillin	
Adults	Clindamycin 600 mg single dose, single dose orally, 30–60 minutes before procedure
Children < 12 years of age	Clindamycin 20 mg/kg body weight, single dose orally, 30–60 minutes before procedure

Implications for oral health. Often, intake of softened food can lead to excessive calculus formation. Children suffering from CRF at young age show growth retardation and a delay in the development of the dentition. An early effect is enamel hypoplasia due to deficiencies in enamel development and mineralization. If the glomerular filtration is very low, 50% of the children show mineralization disturbances of the teeth. Despite the frequent intake of carbohydrates and a reduced secretion of saliva, the caries prevalence of CRF children does not seem to be higher than in healthy counterparts. This can be explained by an increased concentration of urea in saliva and, consequently, a higher saliva pH. Children with CRF experience significantly less gingivitis than healthy children due to immunosuppressive therapy, which leads to a depressed gingival response to inflammation.

The production of the vitamin D metabolite that is essential for calcium absorption is inhibited. Consequences include demineralization of the mandible and maxilla, loss of trabeculation, partial or total loss of the lamina dura, giant cell lesions, and metastatic calcification. Socket sclerosis is commonly seen and the prevalence of pulp calcification is very high in patients on haemodialysis, but less so following kidney transplantation. Calcification of the soft tissues and salivary glands and brown tumors have also been reported. On X-rays of CRF children one can find localized radiolucencies – comparable to cysts – in the jaws, as well as total or partial loss of lamina dura and/or bone demineralization (osteoporosis).

Renal transplant

In the case of complete loss of kidney function transplantation is the preferred therapy. After kidney transplantation, azathioprine and cyclosporine are used as immunosuppressive agents.

Implications for oral health. In these patients, who already have lowered host resistance, acute or chronic oral infections or bacteremia resulting from dental procedures may cause serious complications. For this reason it is recommended that any necessary dental treatment should be completed before transplantation. About 30% of the patients develop a dose-correlated gingival overgrowth after the use of cyclosporine. Replacement of cyclosporine with tacrolimus in organ transplant recipients who develop severe gingival enlargement, together with an extensive plaque-control program, provides an effective means with which to control gingival hyperplasia, with a minimal risk of graft dysfunction. Concomitant use of calcium channel blockers (nifedipine) and cyclosporine is a significant risk factor for severe gingival overgrowth.

As in all patients on immunosuppressive medication, fungal infections with *Candida albicans* may occur which require prompt antifungal treatment. There is some evidence that an extensive amount of secondary dentin formation along the pulp chamber walls and the root canal is present in renal transplant patients. Following successful kidney transplantation, the *Streptococcus mutans* counts are likely to increase compared to those of healthy children, implicating an increased caries risk.

Diabetes mellitus

Diabetes mellitus is a chronic metabolic disturbance characterized by a decreased production of insulin. In children, this is referred to as juvenile diabetes or type 1 diabetes. The lower insulin activity leads to a higher concentration of blood glucose. Diabetes is rare in infancy, but the incidence rises among school-age children. The treatment is based on the normalization of the blood glucose concentration. This is achieved using insulin treatment and strict dietary advice adapted to the physical activity of the child. A fat-reduced and fiber-rich diet is recommended. Three major meals and two/three in-between meals (snacks) constitute the recommended feeding pattern. Strict patient compliance is essential for effective treatment.

Implications for oral health. From several investigations, it is obvious that children with diabetes have a lower salivary secretion rate. Moreover, the concentration of glucose in saliva and in crevicular fluid is increased. The latter are caries-inducing factors. On the other hand, the lower frequency of carbohydrate intake helps prevent caries. Only children with poorly controlled diabetes who are not accepting the prescribed diet and who have a high variability of blood glucose can be considered a high caries risk group. In children with diabetes and poor metabolic control, increased levels of gingivitis have been found. The association between diabetes and periodontal disease has been under discussion for many years, with conflicting conclusions. Patients with non-insulin-dependent diabetes mellitus (NIDDM) have a higher prevalence and severity of periodontal disease than people without diabetes. Studies of patients with insulin-dependent diabetes mellitus (IDDM) have found an increased prevalence and severity of periodontal disease compared to controls. For both IDDM and NIDDM, there does not appear to be any correlation between the prevalence and the severity of periodontal disease and the duration of diabetes. Patients with well-controlled diabetes, as measured by blood glycated hemoglobin levels, have less severe periodontal disease than do patients with poorly controlled diabetes. The principles of treatment of periodontal disease in diabetic patients are the same as in non-diabetic patients. Plaque remains the etiologic factor. Extra periodontal prophylaxis, especially when children reach puberty, is strongly recommended. Dental appointments should be made during the morning when the blood glucose level is stable.

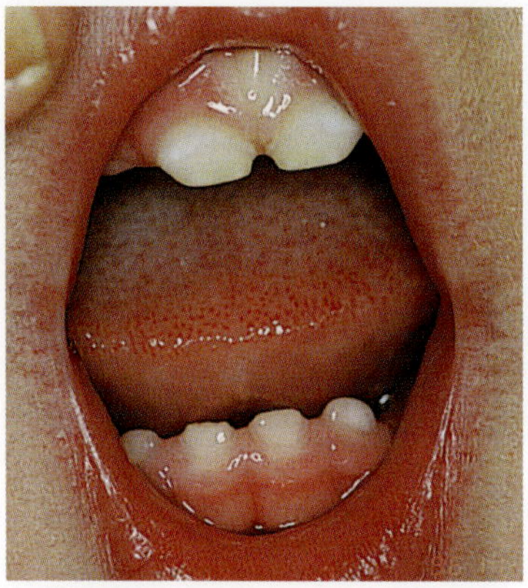

Figure 22-6 A 3-year-old boy with a malabsorption syndrome with daily vomiting and regurgitation. Note erosive change on anterior teeth.

Gastroesophageal reflux

Gastroesophageal reflux (GER) is the involuntary passage of gastric contents into the esophagus. It occurs where inappropriate relaxation of the lower esophageal sphincter results in reflux of stomach contents back into the esophagus. Long-term GER is associated with failure to thrive, feeding problems, esophagitis, and aspiration pneumonia and esophageal stricture. It is particularly frequent in children with cerebral palsy, asthma, bronchitis, and other respiratory disorders.

Implications for oral health. Gastric acidity ranges in pH from 1 to 3, and regurgitation or vomiting of gastric acid into the mouth has been linked to dental erosion. In recent studies, it has been found that erosion occurred in only 17% of children with moderate to severe GER disease. Tooth surface loss was diagnosed on primary molar teeth as well as on primary incisors (Fig. 22-6). This low prevalence is probably due to the fact that children with GER avoid acidic and carbonated foods and beverages, which are major contributing factors to dental erosion.

Eating disorders

Severe obesity

Obesity is an excess of body fat frequently resulting in a significant impairment of health. About 40–50% of men and 25–40% of women have a body mass index (BMI = weight in kg/height in m^2) over 25. Severe obesity (BMI > 30) affects up to 10% of the adult population. Childhood obesity is also widespread, affecting as many as 10–15% of children. Obese children who become obese adults are at greater risk of developing heart disease, diabetes, high blood pressure, high cholesterol, and arthritis at a younger age. Weight gain among children is probably due to a combination of factors including family lifestyle, socioeconomic status, and ethnicity.

Implications for oral health. Dietary habits promoting the development of cardiovascular disease have been documented in studies of children and adolescents with high caries prevalence.

Obese children with high caries prevalence exhibit more risk factors for cardiovascular disease at 15 years of age (Fig. 22-7). With regard to periodontal disease, there is increasing evidence the adipose tissue is secreting proinflammatory cytokines such as tumor necrosis factor α and interleukin-6. An increased prevalence of sites with increased probing depth has been reported with increasing BMI, as well as an increased prevalence of periodontal disease. Among individuals aged 17–21 years, the risk of periodontitis increases by 6% with every kilogram of weight gain (11).

Dietary counseling to adolescents with a high caries score or periodontal disease in combination with obesity should not be restricted to reduction of fermentable carbohydrates but aim also to reduce risk factors for cardiovascular disease (3).

Anorexia nervosa

The diagnostic criteria for anorexia nervosa are presented in Box 22-8. Two subtypes have been identified: with or without binge-eating or purging behavior (self-induced vomiting). Comorbid conditions such as depression, obsessive compulsive disorders, and social phobia are particularly common. The incidence is seven per 100,000. Eating disorders occur predominantly in young women with the male-to-female ratio being approximately 1:10. The median age of onset is about 17 years.

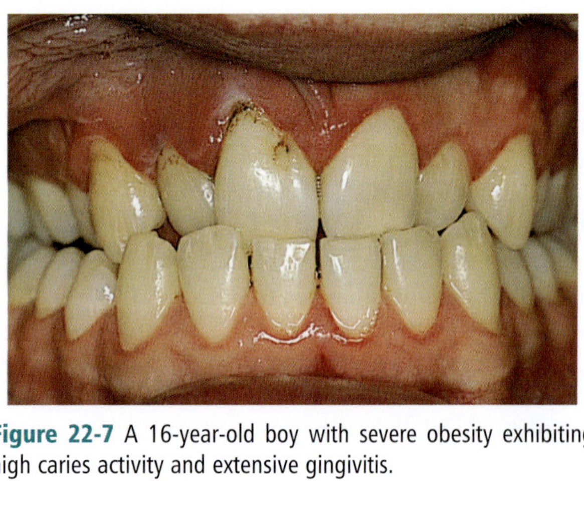

Figure 22-7 A 16-year-old boy with severe obesity exhibiting high caries activity and extensive gingivitis.

Box 22-8 Diagnostic criteria for anorexia nervosa

- Refusal to maintain body weight at or above a minimally normal weight for age and height (i.e., body weight <85% of normal).
- Intense fear of gaining weight or becoming fat.
- Disturbances in the way which one's body or shape is experienced.
- Amenorrhea in postmenarchal females.

The median duration of the illness is up to 6 years with a significant mortality from medical complications and suicide.

Implications for oral health. Erosion is the oral manifestation most often reported in patients with anorexia nervosa, particularly on the palatal surfaces of the maxillary anterior teeth. An increased frequency of erosion is found in subjects with self-induced vomiting but there is no linear association with the frequency and duration of self-induced vomiting or the total number of vomiting episodes. Other factors may be involved, such as oral hygiene practices and the intake of low pH beverages and fresh fruit.

Patients with eating disorders are recommended to reduce the intake of acidic drinks, fresh fruits, especially citrus fruit, and alcohol. They should also rinse their mouths with water or chew gum and, in severe cases, rinse with an antacid preparation in order to increase pH after self-induced vomiting. Toothbrushing may be performed after self-induced vomiting, using a gentle brush and bicarbonate-containing toothpaste. An evaluation of salivary secretion rate should also be performed if the medication list includes medications that cause nausea or dry mouth.

Malabsorption

Malabsorption is the inability to absorb dietary foods. It may be caused by maldigestion (deficiency or inactivation of pancreatic enzymes and bile salts) or by a disease of the small intestine that results in a mucosal barrier to absorption. Patients with the malabsorption syndrome (MAS) may have symptoms of general malabsorption or symptoms caused by the deficiency of a specific substance such as vitamin A, D or K, calcium, magnesium, iron, or folate. The patient with MAS classically has bulky, oily, malodorous stools associated with significant weight loss, muscle wasting, weakness, edema, anemia, ecchymoses, abnormal bleeding, a smooth tongue, hyperkeratosis of the skin, skeletal pain, and even tetanus.

Implications for oral health. The oral manifestations of malabsorption occur when vitamin deficiencies are part of the clinical presentation. These may include reddening and ulceration of the oral mucosa (stomatitis), swelling and burning of the tongue (glossitis), and fissuring of the corner of the mouth (cheilosis), all of which are associated with vitamin B deficiencies. If vitamin B_{12} deficiency is prominent, atrophy of the tongue may be present.

In patients with MAS or patients receiving long-term antibiotic therapy, the bacteria in the intestine that produce vitamin K may be affected adversely. The patient's physician should be consulted regarding the patient's health and bleeding status before surgery.

Celiac disease

Celiac disease or gluten-induced enteropathy is a genetic, immunologically mediated disorder of the small intestine caused by intolerance to the gliadin fraction of gluten which is one of the protein fractions of wheat, barley, rye, and oats.

Prevalence data indicate that symptomatic and latent celiac disease is present in one in 300 children. The age of onset ranges from infancy to old age. It is characterized by degenerative changes in the mucosa (villous dystrophy), resulting in a chronic malabsorption with abdominal distension, pale, bulky, foul-smelling stools, wasting of muscles, anemia and retarded growth, and weight gain. Diagnosis can be confirmed by a biopsy of the jejunum, which shows flattened mucosa with lack of villi therefore resulting in malabsorption. The villi return to normal following the elimination of gluten from the diet.

Implications for oral health. Hypoplasia of the permanent dentition may occur in those teeth forming at the time solids were first introduced into the diet. Symmetrically and chronologically distributed enamel defects have been reported to be associated with celiac disease. The severity of the hypoplasia probably depends on the severity of the celiac disease and the time that elapsed between the onset of symptoms and the initiation of treatment.

Cystic fibrosis

Cystic fibrosis is an autosomal recessive disorder of the exocrine glands and occurs in approximately one in 2000 births. All the mucus-producing glands produce thick mucus that causes obstruction of the flow secretions from the ducts. The pancreas as well as the lungs are involved. The lungs are invariably involved and there is a nonproductive cough that leads to acute respiratory infection, bronchopneumonia, bronchiectasis, and lung abscesses.

Implications for oral health. Patients with cystic fibrosis may show occlusion of the nasal cavity and maxillary sinus after recurrent infections. This results in chronic mouth breathing and a higher incidence of open bite and a high palatal vault.

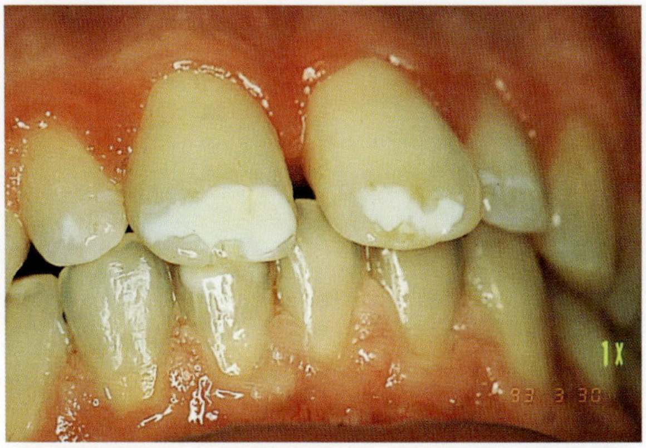

Figure 22-8 Discoloration and enamel hypomineralization in a 14-year-old boy with cystic fibrosis.

The teeth of patients with cystic fibrosis are often discolored. The discoloration is more pronounced at the cervical and middle third of the clinical crown and is first seen at the cementoenamel junction, where the enamel layer is the thinnest. Tetracycline administration has been implicated as a cause of the staining, since the drug has often been used to combat recurrent pulmonary infections. In addition to a relatively high prevalence of tetracycline discoloration, enamel defects have been found in approximately 10% of these patients (Fig. 22-8). The prevalence of dental caries is not significantly elevated. There are indications, however, that adolescents and adults with cystic fibrosis can show high caries rates. In recent studies, it was shown that although cystic fibrosis homozygotes potentially have a high caries risk due to their essential sugar-rich diet, they do not have a significantly higher caries experience compared to their heterozygote counterparts or healthy controls (1). As patients with cystic fibrosis nowadays survive into their 20s and early 30s, assessment of caries risk is important.

The dentist must avoid exacerbating the underlying disease in patients with cystic fibrosis. High flow of gases such as oxygen or nitrous oxide can dry out respiratory secretions. This can lead to further plugging and infection. Rubber dam should be used to decrease the possibility of aspiration from dental hand-piece aerosols.

Primary and secondary immunodeficiency states

Immunodeficiency states may be primary or secondary (Box 22-9). Primary immunodeficiency syndromes vary in incidence from the relatively common, such as selective immunoglobulin A (IgA) deficiency with a prevalence of about one in 600 of the population, to the

Box 22-9 Immunodeficiency states

Primary
- Selective IgA deficiency.
- Immunoglobulin G subclass deficiencies.
- Cyclic neutropenia.
- Agammaglobulinemia (X-linked).
- Severe combined immunodeficiency syndrome.

Secondary
- AIDS.
- Chemotherapy for cancer.
- Anti-rejection treatment for transplants.
- Steroid treatment.

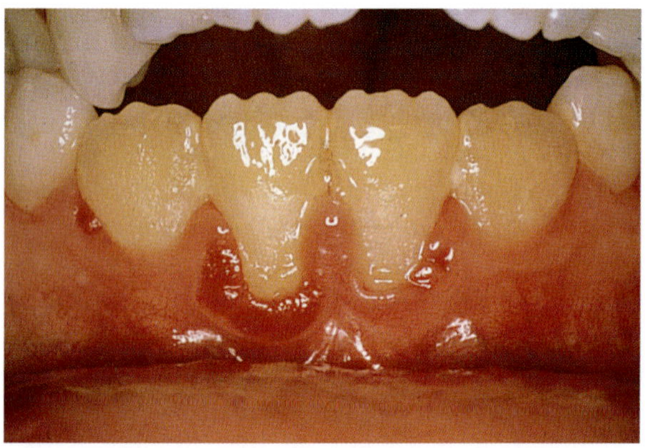

Figure 22-9 A 12-year-old boy with immunoglobulin A and G deficiency exhibiting ulceration of the marginal gingiva.

extremely rare. Four main components of the immune system may be affected: (a) phagocytosis (both granulocytes and macrophages), (b) immunoglobulins, (c) cellular immunity, and (d) the complement system.

Implications for oral health. Candidiasis and herpetic infections are common in children with T-cell deficiencies, while children with B-cell deficiencies are most susceptible to bacterial infections (Fig. 22-9). Periodontitis and candidiasis are found in some but not all phagocyte deficiencies (1).

HIV infection/AIDS

Globally, acquired immunodeficiency syndrome (AIDS) is one of the five leading causes of death among children. Antiretroviral drugs reduce viral replication and can reduce mother-to-child transmission of human immunodeficiency virus (HIV). In Western countries the vertical transmission rates are around 1–2%, but highly active antiretroviral therapy (HAART) is not yet available in low and middle income countries. The use of HAART has reduced the mortality and increased the life expectancy in children with HIV infection.

Implications for oral health. HAART has also reduced the incidence of oral lesions in both children and adults. The median age of children at AIDS diagnosis is 12 months, and the oral manifestations are the first sign of infection in about half of all infected children. The oral lesions are associated with immune suppression. Oral *C. albicans* infection, in particular, is associated with immune suppression.

The incidence of pseudomembraneous candidiasis has been reported to be about 10% in a pediatric population. Other common oral lesions are parotid enlargement, herpes simplex gingivostomatitis, cytomegalovirus-induced lesions, aphthous ulcers, and angular cheilitis.

Periodontal disease is a late manifestation of HIV infection. Periodontal disease is the most frequently diagnosed oral lesion in African HIV-positive children (Fig. 22-5). Delayed tooth eruption had been reported to occur in HIV-infected children. A preventive program for HIV-infected children should include a careful oral examination at regular intervals to ensure early detection of and intervention for pseudomembranous candidiasis and other oral lesions.

Neutropenia

Blood leukocyte counts normally range between 5000 and 10,000 cells/mm^3 with a predominance of neutrophils. Although a reduction in circulating neutrophils usually leads to a decline in the total leukocyte count, such values are not meaningful unless a differential count is performed and the absolute numbers of each cell type are calculated. In healthy individuals, the total neutrophil counts range between 1800 and 7200 cells/mm^3. Thus, neutropenia is defined as a decrease in the neutrophil count below 1800 cells/mm^3. The disease may occur as an isolated finding or may be associated with a variety of underlying disorders, which may cause anemia and thrombocytopenia.

Implications for oral health. Oral lesions are common and often severe in patients with neutrophil dysfunction syndromes. Three findings repeatedly reported are severe gingivitis, rapidly advancing periodontal disease, and oral ulcers. Since periodontal disease is caused by a chronic bacterial infection, it is not surprising that an increased level of periodontal breakdown accompanies disorders of neutrophils (Fig. 22-10). In Kostman's disease, chronic severe neutropenia, the bacterial infections are treated with granulocyte-macrophage colony stimulating factor with good results, but this therapy has no effect on periodontal disease progression. It is speculated that deficiencies in the innate immunity contribute to the susceptibility to periodontal disease.

Patients with abnormal neutrophil function should be under the close supervision of a dentist to minimize

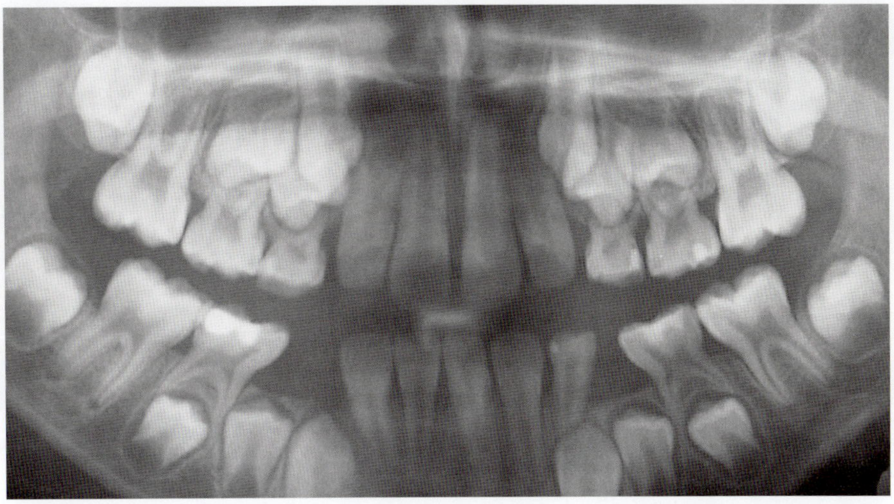

Figure 22-10 Panoramic radiograph showing severe periodontal breakdown in a 6-year-old boy with cyclic neutropenia.

local inflammatory factors causing periodontal disease, dental caries, and oral ulcers. Patients should follow a strict oral hygiene regimen and have periodic dental examinations. When extensive dental treatment is performed in susceptible patients, broad-spectrum antibiotic coverage should be considered. If surgical procedures are necessary or oral bacterial infection develops, granulocyte transfusions may be necessary.

Juvenile chronic arthritis

Juvenile chronic arthritis (JCA) is defined as an inflammatory arthritis occurring before the age of 16 years. It may be the result of infection or it may be due to an autoimmune reaction. This condition has a prevalence of approximately one in 10,000. Fever, skin rash, lymphadenopathy, and inflammatory arthritis, usually affecting four or more joints, characterize JCA. There is a chronic nonsuppurative inflammation of the synovium. The joints become swollen, warm, and tender to touch and painful to move.

Implications for oral health. In the polyarticular type, 20% have temporomandibular joint (TMJ) disease (4). The most common radiographic finding is flattening of the condyle heads, but sclerosis of the condyle surface is also noted bilaterally in 10% of the cases. This plays a significant role in the development of the facial morphology and also contributes to the facial heterogeneity among children with JCA. The chewing movements in children with JCA are restricted by the disease and by the presence of these condylar lesions. In children with JCA, TMJ involvement may lead to disturbance in dentofacial growth and mandibular function (Fig. 22-4). The dentofacial morphology in children with JCA is characterized by a smaller, more retrognathic and more steeply inclined mandible compared to that of healthy children with normal occlusion. Oral hygiene measures are extremely important as many children take drugs in syrup form. There may be involvement of the TMJ, resulting in restricted opening.

Epidermolysis bullosa

Epidermolysis bullosa comprises a number of genetically determined skin conditions in which the skin and mucous membrane blister as a result of mechanical trauma.

Basement membrane and cellular defects characterize the condition as well as skin fragility and variable extracutaneous involvement. Clinically, two main types were originally described: the simplex type, in which mucous membranes are rarely affected and scarring does not occur, and the dystrophic type, in which scarring occurs (Fig. 22-11a). Blistering occurs within the epidermis, within the basement membrane or beneath the basement membrane, respectively, in epidermolysis bullosa simplex, epidermolysis bullosa dystrophica, and junctional epidermolysis bullosa.

Implications for oral health. The simplex and dominant dystrophic epidermolysis bullosa groups have DMFS levels similar to those in healthy children. Individuals with recessive dystrophic epidermolysis bullosa have the most severe oral blistering and scarring (Fig. 22-11b) and do not have generalized enamel hypoplasia. In contrast, junctional epidermolysis bullosa is always associated with generalized enamel hypoplasia, but the intraoral blistering rarely involves scarring. Rampant caries afflicts many individuals with junctional or generalized recessive dystrophic epidermolysis bullosa. Although systemic treatment remains primarily palliative, it is possible to prevent destruction and subsequent loss of the dentition through appropriate interventions and dental therapy. Even the most severely affected

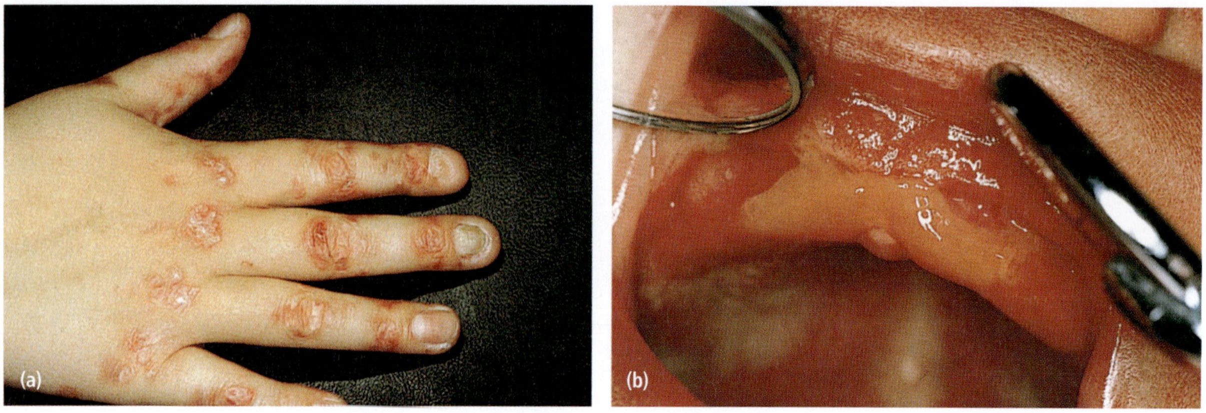

Figure 22-11 (a) Blistering of hand and fingers in a 10-year old boy with dystrophic epidermolysis bullosa. (b) Oral blistering and scarring in a 1-month-old boy with dystrophic epidermolysis bullosa (courtesy of G. Koch).

individuals with epidermolysis bullosa can retain their dentition through the use of modern dental restorative techniques delivered using general anesthesia. Preventive advice regarding a noncariogenic diet is essential. Advice should be given on the use of a soft toothbrush to maintain oral hygiene and chlorhexidine mouthwashes to prevent the accumulation of plaque. Cleaning with sponges or cotton wool buds may also be beneficial.

Bleeding disorders

Hemophilia A and B

Hemophilia affects all races and is inherited as an X-linked recessive factor. Because it is transmitted on the X-chromosome it affects only males; females, having two X-chromosomes, are protected. The incidence in males is one in 10,000. Hemophilia A is caused by a lack of factor VIII and hemophilia B by a lack of factor IX. Female carriers of hemophilia B also have a tendency to bleed.

Von Willebrand's disease

Von Willebrand's disease is another condition in which abnormal bleeding occurs and it is probably the second most common form of hereditary clotting disorder. The condition affects both males and females and is inherited as a dominant trait. Those affected have large tortuous capillaries and low levels of factor VIII and the condition may simulate hemophilia. These patients also have defective platelets, which do not adhere to each other. Bleeding from the gingiva, the mucosa of the nose, and the gastrointestinal tract is common and there is prolonged bleeding following trauma or surgery.

Patients should carry a hemophiliac card, which records details such as factor deficiency and level, the presence or absence of inhibitors, and the telephone number of their hemophiliac center.

Implications for oral health. The bleeding disorders in themselves do not affect dental health, but preventive treatment is extremely important, including regular dental examinations. Each patient should be given an individualized program including fluoride supplements and topical fluoride applications. Bitewing radiographs should be taken at regular intervals in order to detect caries at an early stage. With regard to management, pulp treatment of primary molars is preferred in order to avoid extractions. Extractions require admission to a hospital or special care center and there must be adequate replacement therapy and careful monitoring of factor VIII levels. Routine therapy with the anti-fibrinolytic agents, tranexamic acid, or epsilon aminocaproic acid prior to and for a few days following the procedure will significantly reduce the requirement for replacement of factor VIII.

Primary teeth when shed in the normal way cause little or no hemorrhage. However, if very mobile, extraction may be necessary because constant movement may cause trauma of the soft tissues and bleeding. With regard to local anesthesia, inferior dental nerve blocks should be avoided, since bleeding in the pterygomandibular region may result in asphyxia. Medications containing aspirin (salicylates) should not be prescribed as they may cause gastric bleeding, whereas paracetamol and NSAIDs can be used safely. In view of the large numbers of hemophiliac patients who are now affected with HIV and hepatitis virus, it is essential that appropriate precautions are taken to prevent cross-infection.

Idiopathic thrombocytopenic purpura

Idiopathic thrombocytopenic purpura (ICP) is a relatively common disorder in which isolated thrombocytopenia occurs in otherwise healthy individuals. Two clinical forms of the disease are recognized: acute and chronic. Acute ICP is seen most frequently in children but may occur at any age. The onset is usually sudden, with thrombocytopenia manifested by bruising, bleeding, and petechiae a few days to several weeks after an otherwise uneventful viral illness. Acute ICP is a self-limiting disease that generally remits permanently without sequelae.

Implications for oral health. Oral manifestations of ICP may represent its initial signs. Purpura, the most common oral sign, is defined as any escape of blood into subcutaneous tissues and includes petechiae, ecchymoses, hemorrhagic vesicles, and hematomas. These may appear on any mucosal surface and are often first seen on the tongue, lips, and occlusal line of the buccal mucosa. They are often secondary to some minor trauma. Initially, the color may be bright red, resembling vascular dilation. Other oral signs include spontaneous gingival hemorrhage and prolonged bleeding following trauma, toothbrushing, extractions, or periodontal therapy.

Spontaneous gingival bleeding can usually be managed with oxidizing mouthwashes, but platelet transfusions may be required to stop the bleeding. Good oral hygiene and conservative periodontal therapy help to remove the plaque and the calculus that potentiate the bleeding. Platelet levels of 50,000/mm^3 are desirable before dental treatment and further transfusion should be given as needed postoperatively to maintain hemostasis.

Block injections should not be given when the platelet count is less than 30,000/mm^3 because of the possibility of hematoma formation and airway obstruction. Aspirin-containing analgesics are contraindicated because they may potentiate bleeding.

Malignant disease in children

The incidence of cancer during childhood is very low. The incidence rate in the Nordic countries is increasing slowly and is now 17.3 in 100,000 children per year. Acute leukemia, lymphoma, and central nervous system (CNS) tumors represent the three largest diagnostic groups. Unlike the majority of adult cancers, most pediatric tumors are curable. In 1999, the 5-year survival rate was over 80% among children diagnosed with acute lymphoblastic leukemia. For each diagnosis, a treatment protocol is established according to international guidelines. The treatment is separated into an induction period of 4–5 weeks aiming at achieving remission, followed by a consolidation period and finally a maintenance period of up to 30 months. The treatment for most hematological malignancies consists of a protocol combining cytotoxic drugs with different modes of action. In children with CNS tumors the therapy comprises radiation therapy, surgery, and cytotoxic drugs. In patients with high-risk disease and relapse, bone marrow transplantation (BMT) may be considered. BMT often includes total body irradiation.

Implications for oral health. Oral complications following antineoplastic therapy can be divided into two groups, the acute complications that occur as a direct consequence of the cytotoxic or radiation therapy given and the long-term complications such as disturbances in dental development, craniofacial growth, and salivary dysfunction.

Cytotoxic drugs have effects not only on malignant cells but also on normal cells with rapid turnover such as the hematopoietic cells in the bone marrow and epithelial cells in the gastrointestinal tract and the oral mucosa. The direct effects of cytotoxic therapy are mucositis involving atrophy, desquamation, and ulceration of the mucosa (Fig. 22-12), which increase the risk for local and systemic infections, cause pain and discomfort for the patient, and impair peroral nutrition. Septicemia with oral streptococci is common during the induction period.

During cytotoxic therapy a transient reduction of salivary secretion is diagnosed, which then attains normal values after completion of therapy. Children treated with cytotoxic drugs only experience a catch-up growth with no disturbances in dental and craniofacial development.

BMT often comprises a combination of cytotoxic drugs and 10–12 Gy total body irradiation (TBI). In these children a permanent reduction of salivary secretion rate below 0.5 ml/min is found in approximately 50% of the patients when examined 4 years after BMT. Impaired root development is seen in all children treated with TBI. Other disturbances diagnosed are enamel hypomineralization and hypoplasia, microdontia, and aplasia (Fig. 22-13) (10).

During antineoplastic therapy, also for extended periods after completion of therapy, children are diagnosed with high counts of mutans streptococci and lactobacilli.

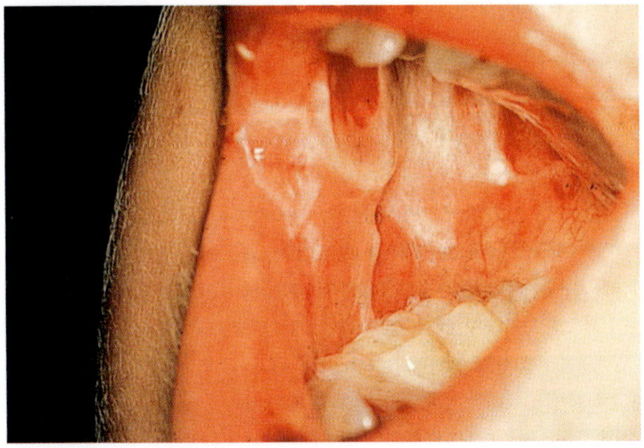

Figure 22-12 Severe oral ulceration in a 5-year-old boy during induction chemotherapy for acute lymphoblastic leukemia.

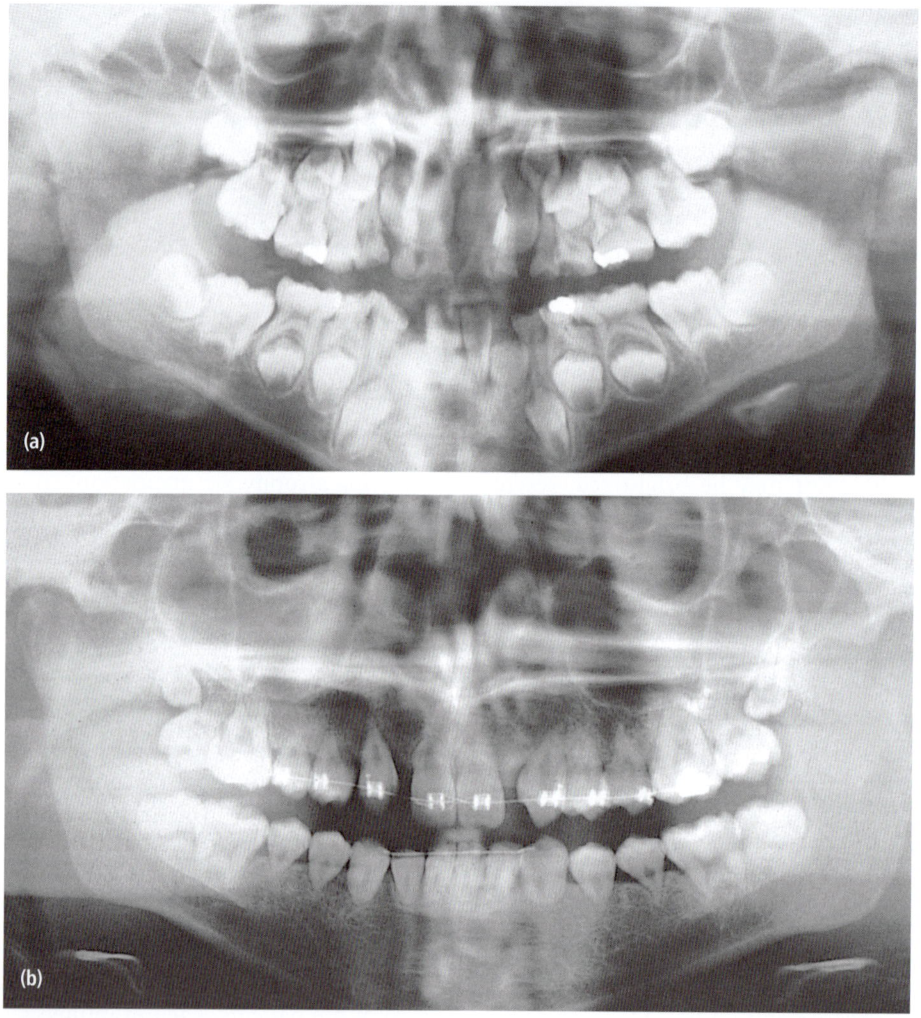

Figure 22-13 (a) Panoramic radiograph showing premature apical closure of permanent first molars in an 8-year-old boy treated with 10 Gy total body irradiation at 5 years of age. (b) At 17 years of age, all permanent teeth exhibit short V-shaped roots.

There is also a rapid recolonization of oral streptococci after chlorhexidine therapy. Children subjected to oral preventive programs during antineoplastic therapy do not exhibit an increased caries incidence. The preventive program for children can be divided into three phases:

- Before the start of cytotoxic therapy the aim is to treat all existing oral diseases and to educate children and parents on oral complications and how to perform oral hygiene.
- During active cytotoxic therapy the patients are instructed to use a soft toothbrush and toothpaste that does not contain sodium lauryl sulfate. During periods of increased bleeding and infection risk, mouthrinses with chlorhexidine 0.1% are recommended.
- During the long-term follow-up, special attention should be paid to patients receiving radiation therapy. Evaluation of salivary secretion rate and levels of oral microorganisms is important. Caries development is extremely rapid in children with poor compliance to preventive measurements. Attention should also be directed towards evaluation of disturbances in dental and craniofacial development.

Epilepsy

Epilepsy has a tendency to recurrent seizures. About five children in 1000 have epilepsy. Most of these will have primary or idiopathic epilepsy (i.e., no underlying cause will be evident), but some will have secondary epilepsy due to a cause such as head injury, meningitis, or birth asphyxia. The international classification of epileptic seizures divides the epilepsies into those that are generalized, where the whole brain is involved, and the partial seizures, where the aberrant activity involves only a part of the brain. Prognosis in the childhood epilepsies is very variable. Most of the refractory epilepsies are found in children who have multiple disabilities.

Box 22-10 Preventive strategies in children with chronic health conditions (CHCs)

Diagnosis of CHCs	Referral for dental evaluation (if congenital before 1 year of age).
Risk assessment	Impact of the CHC (see Box 21-3). Socioeconomic status. Specific dietary requirements. Canceled appointments. Evaluation of salivary secretion rate. Risk factors for caries and periodontal disease.
Preventive program	Dietary counseling. Oral hygiene instruction. Fissure sealants. Chlorhexidine if oral hygiene cannot be performed. Reinforcement of preventive regimen and strict evaluation of compliance.
Risks for general health	Contact with responsible physician. Susceptibility to infection and bleeding. Drug interactions. Cross-infection.
Referral	Early referral to specialist pediatric dentistry clinic when appropriate.
Long-term follow-up	Compliance. Evaluation of salivary secretion rate. Risk factors for caries and periodontal disease. Effects on growth and development.
Examples of managed care protocols	Oral motor function and periodontal disease in children with Down syndrome. Prevention of phenytoin-induced gingival overgrowth in children with epilepsy. Management of children with childhood malignancies.

Implications for oral health. Children who are given phenytoin medication exhibit gingival overgrowth to a varying degree (see Fig. 22-2a). Also sodium valproate and carbamazepine have symptoms, but less pronounced. The reaction begins as a diffuse swelling of the interdental papillae, which enlarge and coalesce. Clinically significant overgrowth occurs in approximately 50% of patients (4). The incidence and severity of overgrowth is greatest on the labial surfaces on maxillary and mandibular anterior teeth. The development of phenytoin-induced gingival overgrowth requires gingival inflammation, and can therefore be minimized by plaque control. A program including frequent sessions of professional tooth cleaning should be instituted before the start of medication. If it is not possible to maintain optimal oral hygiene, a rather conservative approach to surgical removal of gingival overgrowth is recommended because of the high risk of reccurrence. Six months after withdrawal of phenytoin medication, the gingival tissues return to a normal state.

Preventive strategies in children with CHCs

There are many CHCs that can directly influence dental care and some where the consequences of dental disease and also dental treatment may have life-threatening consequences. Unfortunately, there exist barriers to access dental care. Many children and adolescents with CHCs require frequent and sometimes prolonged hospitalizations that separate them from their home environment. This could result in frequently missed appointments. Parents may also be reluctant to once again review the history of the child with the dentist or may not understand the need to share this information. Knowledge and skills among dentists may also not be adequate to treat children with severe CHCs.

Box 22-10 summarizes preventive strategies that can be implemented in children with CHCs.

Early professional intervention is particularly important to provide examination, risk assessment, and information and guidance to parents so that oral diseases can be prevented.

References

1. Aps J, Van Maele G, Martens L. Caries experience and oral cleanliness in cystic fibrosis homozygotes and heterozygotes. *Oral Surg Oral Med Oral Pathol Oral Radiol Endod* 2002;**93**:560–3.
2. Atkinson JC, O'Connell A, Aframian D. Oral manifestations of primary immunological diseases. *J Am Dent Assoc* 2000;**131**: 345–56.
3. Eloot AK, Vanobbergen JN, De Baets F, Martens LC. Oral health and habits in children with asthma related to severity and duration of condition. *Eur J Paediatr Dent* 20045;**5**:210–15.
4. Kjellberg H. Juvenile chronic arthritis. Dentofacial morphology, growth, mandibular function and orthodontic treatment. *Swed Dent J Suppl* 1996;**115**:1–45.
5. Larsson B, Johansson I, Weinehall L, Hallmans G, Ericson T. Cardiovascular disease risk factors and dental caries in adolescents: effect of a preventive program in Northen Sweden (the Norsjö project). *Acta Paediatr* 1997;**86**:63–71.
6. Lucas VS, Roberts GJ. Oro-dental health in children with chronic renal failure and after renal transplantation: a clinical review. *Pediatr Nephrol* 2005;**20**:1388–94.

7. Marshall RI, Bartold PM. Medication induced gingival overgrowth. *Oral Dis* 1998;**4**:130–51.
8. McDerra EJC, Pollard MA, Curzon MEJ. The dental status of asthmatic British schoolchildren. *Pediatr Dent* 1998;**20**:281–7.
9. Modéer T, Dahllöf G, Storhaug K, Svendsen P. Allmänpraktikerns roll vid odontologiskt omhändertagande av kroniskt sjuka barn. *Tandlaekartidningen* 1998;**90**:53–60 (English summary).
10. Näsman M, Forsberg CM, Dahllöf G. Long-term dental development in children treated for malignant diseases. *Eur J Orthod* 1997;**19**:151–9.
11. Roberts GJ. Dentists are innocent! Everyday bacteremia is the real culprit: a review and assessment of the evidence that dental surgical procedures are a principal cause of bacterial endocarditis in children. *Pediatr Cardiol* 1999;**20**:317–25.
12. Reeves AF, Rees JM, Schiff M, Hujoel P. Total body weight and waist circumference associated with periodontitis among adolescents in the United States. *Arch Pediatr Adolesc Med* 2006;**160**: 894–9.
13. Stecksén-Blicks C, Rydberg A, Nyman L, Asplund S, Svanberg C. Dental caries experience in children with congenital heart disease: a case–control study. *Int J Paediatr Dent* 2004;**14**:94–100.
14. Stein RE, Silver EJ. Operationalizing a conceptually based noncategorical definition: first look at US children with chronic conditions. *Arch Pediatr Adolesc Med* 1999;**153**:68–74.
15. Stein REK, Bauman LJ, Westbrook LE, Coupey SM, Ireys HT. Framework for identifying children who have chronic conditions: the case for a new definition. *J Pediatr* 1993;**122**:342–7.
16. Westbom L, Kornfält R. Chronic illness among children in a total population. *Scand J Soc Med* 1987;**15**:87–97.
17. Wilson W, Taubert KA, Gewitz M, Lockhart PB, Baddour LM, Levison M, *et al.* Prevention of infective endocarditis. Guidelines from the American Heart Association. *Circulation* 2007;**116**: 1736–54.

23

Dental care for the child and adolescent with disabilities

June Nunn and Gunilla Klingberg

Context

Disability is a term that evokes different images for readers, depending on their cultural background, their personal experiences of disabling conditions, and the norms of the society in which they live. In recent years there has been a move away from the fairly narrow definition imposed by the medical model, with its emphasis on an individual's impairment "handicapping" that person. For example, a child with Down syndrome is disabled by being intellectually impaired and unable to keep up educationally with his or her peers. Pressure, largely from advocates for people with disabilities and parent support organizations, has led to a more inclusive definition that places an emphasis on an individual's ability, rather than what they cannot do. This is in part captured in the social model where it is society that disables an individual with an impairment, rather than the other way round. For example, a flight of stairs into a dental surgery disables a person who has quadriplegic cerebral palsy and so needs to use a wheelchair to move around.

More recently, the World Health Organization's International Classification of Functioning and Health (ICF) (30) seeks to stress the health status of the individual rather than their potential *dis*ability. This latter classification is based on a biopsychosocial model that aims to integrate the medical and social models referred to above. Functioning and disability are defined in relation to the outcomes between the health condition(s) of the person and the context in which he or she operates. This context is defined at three levels of functioning, at the level of a body part, at the level of the whole individual, and lastly, functioning that occurs at the level of society. These occur within domains as in Table 23-1.

Clearly, this framework opens up the possibility of refining the definitions of, for example, which children

Table 23-1 ICF defines functioning and disabilities in relation to outcomes between the health conditions of a person and the context in which they operate. This context is defined at three levels of functioning, at the level of a body part, at the level of the whole individual, and the functioning that occurs at the level of society. This table shows the domains in which these occur and the definitions

Domain	Defined as
Body functions	Physiological or psychological functions of body systems
Body structures	Anatomical parts of the body
Impairments	Problems with body function/structure, such as significant loss
Activity	The carrying out of a task or an action by the person
Participation	Involvement in daily activities
Activity limitations	Difficulty experienced by the person in carrying out task/actions
Participation restriction	Problems experienced by the person in involvement in activities of daily living
Environmental factors	The environmental context in which people live their lives

it is considered need special care dentistry and which do not. Examples of this are given in Table 23-2 (9). In both these examples, the need for specialist facilities such as expert knowledge about different conditions, conscious sedation, or wheelchair-accessible dental surgeries may mean that special dental care is required.

The ICF complements the World Health Organization (1993) ICD-10 codes (31), which is an international statistical classification of diseases and health-related problems. The latter system will identify people with an intellectual impairment, for example, and divide them into four categories of intellectual functioning based on intelligence quotient (IQ), with people with an IQ < 70 classified as having mental retardation and those with an IQ < 50 having severe mental retardation.

Prevalence

For the reasons outlined in the preceding section, the definitions of impairments may vary so that determining accurate prevalence figures for some disabling conditions can be difficult. In a review of disability in children

Table 23-2 ICF structure and domains applied on example patients, a child with Asperger syndrome and a child with quadriplegic cerebral palsy and epilepsy (9)

Domain (*examples*)	Example 1: child with Asperger syndrome	Example 2: child with quadriplegic cerebral palsy and epilepsy
Body function (*physiological and psychological functions of body systems*)	Global mental functions (e.g., global psychosocial functions) Specific mental functions (e.g., emotional functions)	Control of voluntary movement functions Involuntary movement functions
Body structures (*anatomical parts of the body*)	Structure of the brain	Structure of upper extremity Structure of lower extremity
Impairments (*significant deviation or loss of body function or structure*)	Impaired ability to sustain attention Impaired control of voluntary movements Delayed acquisition of the mental functions of language Impaired psychosocial functions	Impaired involuntary movement reaction functions (e.g., posture) Impaired control of voluntary movements and functions Impaired involuntary movement functions (e.g., involuntary muscle contraction)
Activity (*the execution of a task or action*)	Undertaking single or multiple tasks Handling stress and other psychological demands	Undertaking single or multiple tasks
Participation (*involvement in a life situation*)	Maintaining one's health	Maintaining one's health
Activity limitations (*difficulty in executing activities*)	Difficulty in completing a given task, e.g., simple dental instruction	Difficulty in washing oneself Difficulty in caring for teeth
Participation restrictions (*problems in involvement in life situations*)	Problems with seeking care and accepting dental treatment	Problems with cooperating with dental treatment due to movement disorder
Environmental factors (*physical, social and attitudinal environment*)	Support given by health professionals Attitudes of health professionals, health services	Support given by health professionals Attitudes of health professionals, health services
Environmental facilitators	Well-informed and understanding dental team Appropriate adaptation of dental services (e.g., assimilation of patient's routine) Additional services (e.g., use of conscious sedation)	Well-informed and understanding dental team Appropriate adaptation of dental services (e.g., wheelchair access, nonflickering lighting) Additional services (e.g., use of conscious sedation)

conducted in 2004, the prevalence of all disabilities in children varied between 5.8% in the USA and 9.8% in Finland (21). One finding from most prevalence studies is that there are more boys than girls affected, with respiratory disorders (e.g., asthma) being the most frequently occurring impairment. In the USA, children living in poverty or whose parents had little formal education were at greater risk of disability (1). Adolescents with disabilities were three times more likely to visit a doctor each year and nine times more likely to have hospital visits annually compared with their nondisabled peers.

As in some other countries, Denmark has a birth cohort of children that are being followed longitudinally. Of the 9125 children born, some 673 did not survive beyond the first 28 days of life (25). Many of these babies will have had impairments that were not compatible with life. Of the survivors, 11.2% were diagnosed with a disability. In Sweden, a survey of 10-year-old children concluded that 26% had health problems that significantly impacted on the child's day-to-day functioning (18). Physical disorders were the most frequent, occurring in 11.7% of the sample of children. What is notable for children with disabilities are the consequences: in the UK there are approximately 17,000 families who have one or more disabled children (24). Some 6500 families care for two or more severely disabled children. Such families are more likely to be single parents, less likely to be in paid employment but if they are, for them to be in semi-skilled or unskilled jobs. They are thus families who are reliant on state aid and less likely to own their own homes. A hidden group of children are those who, because of chronic physical or mental illness, may be in health care settings for prolonged periods and thus not accessible to, or looked after by, dental services. In one study in England over a year, children aged between birth and 19 years occupied two million "bed days" because of such complex needs (16).

Survival from life-threatening illnesses is increasing among children and adolescents; those with, for example, cystic fibrosis have improved their median survival from 14 years in 1969 to 32 years in 2000. The median life expectancy of a baby with cystic fibrosis now is 40 years. Cancer, although rare in children in that it represents only 0.5% of all cancers, accounts for 20% of deaths in the 1–14-year-old age group. Its incidence has changed little over the past 40 years. Approximately one-third of all cancers in childhood are leukemias, 25% of brain and spinal cord, and 15% embryonal (neuroblastoma, retinoblastoma, Wilm's tumor). Lymphomas account for 10% of childhood cancers. However, survival is good: in 1971 only 100 adult survivors were over 30 years of age compared with 7000 (>45%) in 2000 (19).

Unlike other conditions in which there would appear to be an increased incidence, perhaps because of better reporting, the occurrence of cerebral palsy has actually decreased among babies born prematurely (between 20 and 27 weeks and between 500 and 1249 g) to 19 per 1000 live births.

Oral health and disability

Impairments tend to occur more commonly in boys, in those from low-income families, and in school-age children. Their health needs, including oral and dental, are frequently unmet. Oral and dental diseases may be more prevalent in children and adolescents with impairments because of the potential for increased risk. Some countries have undertaken national surveys of children with disabilities, others have taken samples of children with different types of impairments and compared the data collected with those from a nondisabled population.

Most of these national or local studies report similar findings; while the numbers of children with impairments who are caries-free may be higher than for nonimpaired children, the management of dental disease is different. Children with impairments are more likely to have untreated dental caries and where it is managed, this has in the past been by extraction rather than restoration. However, as dental care is developing with improvements in both oral health and management/treatment techniques there is a chance that these differences will diminish. Preventive dental services vary in different countries. In some places prevention is provided and well organized while in others it is only accessible for a minority of the patients.

Despite overt needs, there is a lack of awareness among medical professionals of the oral and dental needs of their child patients with impairments and dentists express an unwillingness to treat because of uncertainty, as well as a lack of commitment, to such groups in the population. Families often experience severe financial hardships in obtaining necessary dental care for their children, although in Scandinavian countries, comprehensive dental care is free from birth to 18 or 19 years.

Children with impairments are more likely to use publicly funded services and increasingly, to access those services that can provide care under sedation or general anesthesia. In those countries where people with impairments are still in residential care in large units, there are reports of poorer oral hygiene and worse dental health.

There are risk factors that are more prevalent in children with impairments, compared with the rest of the child population. Many more children with impairments will be taking sweetened liquid oral medicines over the long term with consequences for poor dental health including dental caries and possibly erosion. The prevalence of another form of tooth wear, bruxism, is more frequently seen in children with disabilities. Periodontal health is often poorer in children who are impaired because of underlying host factors, as in Down syndrome, as well as poor manual dexterity and inefficient plaque removal.

However, it is aspects of oral health and function, as depicted in the earlier discussion of the World Health Organization's ICF classification, that often concern parents and carers, namely drooling, grinding, and feeding problems, not necessarily dental caries and periodontal diseases. This should be acknowledged. However, it is important that dentists also pay attention to the dental and gingival health in these patients and encourage the parents and family to be committed to the prevention of these diseases. If not, there is a risk that, for example, dental caries is overlooked.

Consent

As for any child, parents or legal guardians are the only people entitled to give consent for dental care. In some countries this will be until the age of 16 years, in others, 18 years. In a number of countries, adolescents, if they are judged to have the maturity to give their consent, or indeed to withhold their agreement for a dental procedure, will be able to make that decision without the need for parents to give their consent. However, many young people who have a communication disorder and especially those with a learning disability may never develop the capacity to give consent, verbal or written, for dental procedures. It will be for the members of the dental team to decide if the person has the capacity to consent and if not, to work with the legislation in their country to manage issues of consent for the adolescent near or above the usual age of consent. Capacity will vary from day to day and depending on the nature of the procedure. Regardless of this, the patient should always receive individually tailored information about treatment and be given the opportunity to assent.

Neuropsychiatric disorders

Neuropsychiatric disorders constitute a substantial group of diagnoses, for example, autism spectrum disorders, autism, Asperger syndrome, attention deficit hyperactivity disorder (ADHD), and Tourette syndrome. It has been estimated that at least 5% of the child population may have a neuropsychiatric disorder. The diagnoses are based on a specific set of symptoms describing the main domains of problems experienced by the individual person. A person's diagnosis may change over time, as problems and symptoms change with individual development (13).

Autism spectrum disorders: autism, Asperger syndrome

An estimated prevalence for the entire autism spectrum has been suggested as six per 1000 people (11). Autism spectrum disorders include a number of diagnoses, for example, autism (sometimes referred to as autistic syndrome) and Asperger syndrome. Autism is a behavioral expression of neurobiological dysfunction. The prevalence varies, but is approximately one to three per 1000, and some increase in prevalence has been noted since the 1990s. This is probably due to more knowledge about the diagnoses leading to higher ascertainment rates. More boys than girls are affected (13). Three criteria, known as Wing's triad, need to be fulfilled in order to make the diagnosis:

- severe abnormality of reciprocal social relatedness
- severe abnormality of communication development, regularly including spoken language
- restricted, repetitive, and stereotypical patterns of behavior, interest, and imagination.

Additional problems that may affect some individuals include hyperactivity, sleeping problems, and abnormal and strong reactions to perception (hearing, sight, physical contact). Up to 50% of people diagnosed with autism never achieve spoken language. They also have problems with social interaction and communication including difficulties in using and understanding eye contact, facial expressions, and gestures, as well as in understanding, especially language's deeper meaning. Children and adolescents with autism are often engaged in a restricted range of behaviors, interests, and activities; repetitive and stereotypic behaviors are common. Comorbidity, that is having one or more diagnoses in addition to the main diagnosis, in this case autism, is frequently seen. In particular, there is an increased risk of epilepsy. Autism and autism spectrum disorders occur more frequently in individuals with, for example, some syndromes and in persons with learning disorders/cognitive disabilities. It is important to recognize that autism spectrum disorders have a very wide range in phenotype, i.e., there are large variations between individuals.

Asperger syndrome represents a high functioning autism with a prevalence of three to five per 1000 people, and affects boys more often than girls; the disorder can range from mild to severe. People with Asperger syndrome usually have a normal or above normal IQ and many exhibit exceptional skills or talents in specific areas. At the same time they have significant deficiencies regarding social skills and can be preoccupied with their special interests. Although having a rich vocabulary, the patient may sound like a "little professor" and the language development may appear normal on the surface, but there are often deficits in pragmatics and prosody.

Autism spectrum disorders are lifelong disabilities but many children can develop considerably provided early and individually tailored educational input is provided. It is important to help the child with tools for communication, and in the structured training for daily living different pedagogic concepts have developed. It is also important to provide good information and education to parents and family and to establish a trusting relationship between the family and the educational system. Depending on the individual's deficits, the need for assistance varies considerably between people with autism spectrum disorders. Some may be in need of assistance full time, while others only require help in organizing their studies or for some special activities.

Oral health considerations

As many patients with autism are dependent on others for their daily life, risk factors may be different from nonaffected children. Providing there is no other underlying medical condition, the literature reports no differences in caries prevalence. This is probably due to family or caregivers being able to provide a good diet for the child, with a low intake of cariogenic items. On the other hand, there are reports of a higher prevalence of plaque and gingivitis compared with healthy children. Again the reason may relate to family/caregivers' influence as many children and adolescents are dependent on help from others to carry out oral hygiene procedures and brushing the teeth of, for example, a teenager with autism is often difficult.

Special considerations for dental care

People with autism need help to understand and focus on dental treatment. Often several appointments are required just for an introduction to dentistry. It is important for the patient to meet the same dentist and preferably the same assistant or dental hygienist in order to get to know the personnel and be able to trust them. If the dental team knows beforehand that a patient has an autism spectrum disorder or autism it is advisable to contact the family by phone in advance. It is useful to get as much information about the patient as possible from this telephone interview: focusing on her or his strengths, what the child likes, what rewards are appropriate, does the child speak and if not, the best way to communicate, does the child have fears of particular things like noise or strong light, etc. Often, people with autism are overly sensitive to sounds, tastes, smells, and sights. Sometimes it is good for the parents or carers to visit the clinic beforehand without the child in order to get to know the facilities, where to park, what door to enter, who to meet, and so on.

The introduction to examination or treatment can be carried out over a number of appointments scheduled just one or a few days apart, or as several short appointments sequentially on the same day. It is usually possible to carry out a good examination with mirror and probe and to perform preventive items such as toothbrushing, polishing, and applying topical fluorides, after this kind of special introduction to dental care. However, exposing radiographs or carrying out treatment such as fillings often requires general anesthesia. Therefore, to reduce the need for general anesthesia it is very important to emphasize prevention of oral/dental disease. The preventive care may be carried out by a dental hygienist or a trained dental nurse, but regular appointments with short intervals in between, in order to maintain contact and ensure a successful experience for the child, are vital.

Many children and adolescents with autism use pictures or photographs as an aid in communication. Today, modern techniques with digital cameras and high-quality printers have made it easy for the dentist to create this kind of individually customized help. Photos of the dental clinic and the dentist and staff the patient will meet, should be included. Also, photos of an open mouth symbolizing "open your mouth", a toothbrush, equipment for polishing, mirror, operatory lamp, and dental chair are useful (Fig. 23-1). The pictures or photographs can be put in the sequence the patient will see them at the appointment in a photo album. This can be used both at home when preparing for the visit, and during the appointment as a help to remember and understand what is going to happen. This kind of aid is

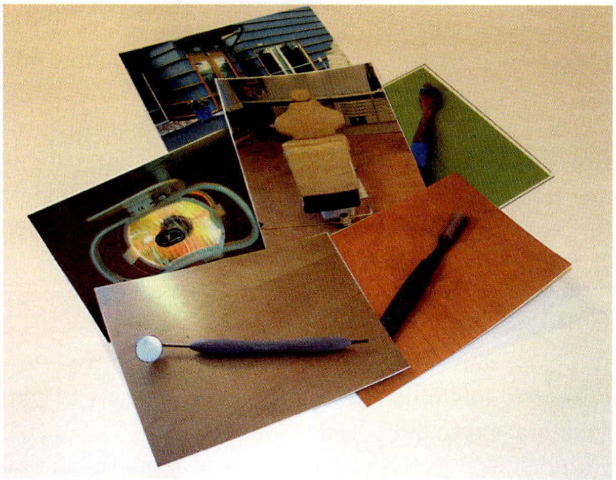

Figure 23-1 Examples of photographs that can be used as pedagogic tools in patients with neuropsychiatric disorders. Based on individual needs: pictures showing the main entrance, the dental chair, the operatory light, and a toothbrush, chosen and put in sequence in a photo album.

useful also when treating other patients, such as patients with ADHD, learning disabilities, or even young or anxious children (3, 26).

Communication with a patient with autism should be very clear and objective as he or she understands you literally and will have a great deal of difficulty reading nonverbal cues (body language). Tell the patient what you want and avoid "small talk". This will help the patient to focus on the dental treatment. See further under ADHD below.

Attention deficit hyperactivity disorder

ADHD is a common disorder affecting 3–7% of children and adolescents and thus something that all dental health care personnel working with young patients are likely to meet. Knowledge about the condition is therefore important. ADHD is caused by neurobiological dysfunction. There is evidence of a genetic background affecting the frontal lobe and dopamine and norepinephrine neurotransmitters, although the etiology is not fully understood. The main problems in ADHD are displayed as inattention, hyperactivity, and impulsivity. The diagnosis can be either of a combined type (most common) where the individual exhibits symptoms in all domains, or inattentive, or hyperactive–impulsive type, depending on the main grouping of impairments. The prevalence varies considerably between different studies, mainly due to differences in definitions applied, but also due to differences in ascertaining study populations. Boys are diagnosed more often than girls, who are supposed to be underdiagnosed. The reason for this is likely to be that girls present with fewer observable impairments such as hyperactivity. Many of the problems in ADHD are persistent as the individual grows older, and many of the patients have difficulties as adults. These include higher frequencies of alcohol or drug abuse and psychiatric disorders.

Therapy for ADHD includes the use of psychoeducative strategies with educational programs for parents and teachers. Medication, mainly with methylphenidate or amphetamine, aimed at inhibiting dopamine transport has been shown to be effective in many patients.

Oral health considerations

It is likely that children with attention disorders of various types, and difficulties adjusting their activity level to situational demands, have more problems complying with dental care. There are reports of more behavioral management problems during dental care in patients with ADHD, and probably a risk of more dental anxiety. Many patients with ADHD behave and function at a lower age level in the dental setting. With respect to oral health, dental caries studies have reported somewhat contradictory results, but on balance there would appear to be an increased risk. Children with ADHD have also been reported to have poorer oral health behavior in terms of higher frequency of food and beverage intakes and a lower frequency of toothbrushing (6).

Special considerations for dental care

Prevention of oral health problems should be the main target together with promoting a positive attitude and acceptance of dental care. Many patients with ADHD have problems in concentrating and focusing on the dental treatment. In order to help the patients, disturbing visual and auditory noise should be reduced. For example, there should be no radio on, the door to the treatment room should be closed to reduce disturbance, and visual distractions such as toys or books should be kept to a minimum in the room. Communication should focus on clear information to the child about what will happen during treatment, who will be involved, how long the procedure will last, and what to do afterwards. Direct and objective guidance during the treatment can help the patient to focus; for example, directions like "Sit in the chair" rather than "Would you like to sit in the chair?" (6). As for many other children with neuropsychiatric disorders pictures or photos can be used as pedagogic tools to provide a "travel plan" of the appointment. Pictures can also be used as tools and aids for toothbrushing at home. Praising is essential as in all dental care for children, and should come directly when the child is cooperating instead of summing up at the end of the appointment.

Tourette syndrome

Tourette syndrome is defined by multiple involuntary motor and vocal tics, present for more than a year. The prevalence is approximately 1% and boys are affected three to four times more often than girls. The motor tics may be complicated, involving the entire body, such as kicking and stamping. The verbal tics include making sounds like grunting, throat clearing, shouting and barking, and may also be expressed as coprolalia (involuntary use of obscene words or sentences). Associated conditions can include ADHD and obsessive compulsive disorder. Therapy includes, apart from psychoeducative strategies, cognitive behavior therapy and in case of obsessive compulsive disorder medication often with selective serotonin reuptake inhibitors.

Oral health considerations

Children and adolescents with Tourette syndrome have more difficulties complying with dental care. This probably leads to an increased risk of both dental behavior management problems and also in the long term dental anxiety. The oral health considerations are similar to those of patients with ADHD.

Special considerations for dental care

See under ADHD.

Other disorders

Learning disability/mental retardation

Learning disability/mental retardation is a deficiency in theoretical intelligence and social functioning acquired before adulthood. The term mental retardation is primarily used in North America, while the term learning disability is used in the UK and most of Europe. One definition used encompasses psychometric measures where an IQ < 70 is a definition for learning disability/mental retardation, and an IQ < 50 denotes severe mental retardation. Learning disability affects approximately 2.5–3% of the population, and 0.6% have severe mental retardation. Learning disabilities can be caused by genetic or congenital factors or acquired at an early age. There is a wide range in how the individual is affected. Some individuals with a mild learning disability may need very little support and go to normal schools, while those with a profound learning disability will need full-time support in all types of activities. Comorbidity is common and includes for example physical, behavioral, and sensory impairments, syndromes, congenital heart defects, and epilepsy. Examples of conditions where learning disability are frequent are Down syndrome, fragile X syndrome, and 22q11 deletion syndrome.

Oral health considerations

Children with learning disabilities generally have the same prevalence of dental caries and periodontal problems as others. However, there are reports of more oral/dental disease in older people, maybe due to difficulties in carrying out treatment, which results in untreated disease that progresses. As with patients with autism, many patients with learning disabilities are dependent on help from others to carry out toothbrushing; poor manual dexterity or lack of motivation often leads to poor oral hygiene if the person has to carry out this task for themselves. However, the use of powered brushes for those who have the motivation but who may lack dexterity, can impact positively on gingival health (8).

Special considerations for dental care

Children and adolescents with learning disabilities accept dental treatment, but it has to be tailored to the individual person's capacities and needs. Very much depends on the individual's degree of understanding of the treatment as well as on age. Local analgesia is, for example, abstract and involves aspects that can be fear-provoking in a patient with learning disability as in any other patient. In some cases a strong negative reaction can be expected after the injection, mainly due to the feeling of numbness. The patient could hurt herself or himself by biting because of the lack of sensation in the anesthetized part. It is still important that pain-free treatment is provided in these patients and the use of periodontal ligament injections or mepivacaine can be helpful. As when treating patients with neuropsychiatric disorders, introduction and appropriate communication are important in these individuals. Introduction using tell–show–do is often effective and can be accompanied by use of photos or pictures as pedagogic tools. Competence regarding communication varies considerably and the dentist should be prepared to use body and even sign language. Children and adolescents with learning disabilities need time to feel comfortable in the dental setting, and effort has to be invested in these patients. These patients also benefit from meeting the same dental team during dental visits.

22q11 deletion syndrome

The 22q11 deletion syndrome is one of the most common multiple anomaly syndromes with an incidence of approximately one per 4000 newborns. The syndrome has previously been described as DiGeorge syndrome or velocardiofacial syndrome. It has an autosomal dominant inheritance, but for 80–90% of the patients the deletion occurs *de novo*. The clinical appearance varies considerably and several patients show a complex medical picture. Characteristic features that may be present include congenital heart defects, velopharyngeal insufficiency with or without cleft palate, frequent infections due to thymic hypoplasia or aplasia, feeding difficulties, hypocalcemia/hypoparathyroidism, learning disabilities, and behavioral abnormalities.

Oral health considerations

There are reports of a high prevalence of dental caries in patients with 22q11 deletion syndrome. This may be explained by a low saliva secretion rate, altered properties of saliva, and high levels of cariogenic bacteria. In addition, problems related to frequent infections (foremost in the preschool age) and feeding difficulties increase the risk of more frequent meals and probably also the intake of food and beverages containing sucrose. Dental aberrations, primarily enamel hypoplasia and hypomineralization, hypodontia, and late eruption of teeth, may occur (17).

Special considerations for dental care

Dental care for patients with 22q11 deletion syndrome

should focus on prevention. Many patients have difficulties related to neuropsychiatric problems and mild learning disability and the treatment should be modified according to individual needs. However, most patients accept dental treatment if this is preceded by introduction and sufficient time is allocated for the appointment. Several patients have problems keeping appointments, and there are often frequent cancellations because of illness and infections in young children or the plentiful medical appointments. In cases of congenital heart defects, endocarditis prophylaxis should be considered according to national guidelines.

Fragile X syndrome

Fragile X syndrome is caused by an unstable DNA fragment on the X chromosome. Approximately one in 5000 boys and one in 4000 girls are affected, but only 20–30% of the girls present with symptoms as they have a second X chromosome that usually functions well. Common features include learning disability, autism spectrum disorders, attention deficit disorders, speech disturbances, low muscle tone, and connective tissue problems. Many children and adolescents with fragile X are very shy and stressed in novel situations.

Oral health considerations

Apart from problems related to autism and learning disability it is common to find feeding difficulties. There are also reports on higher frequencies of malocclusions.

Special considerations for dental care

The dental care should have focus on prevention. The treatment should be modified with regard to the individual patient's problems related to any autism or learning disability.

Down syndrome

Down syndrome is the commonest chromosomal syndrome and cause of diagnosed learning disability. There are three different types of Down syndrome: trisomy 21, mosaicism, and translocation. Trisomy 21 occurs when there is an extra chromosome 21 and this form accounts for the majority of cases. In mosaicism (2–5%), the person has a mix of some cells containing 46 and some 47 chromosomes. The person affected will have some of the usual characteristics of the syndrome, depending on the number of cells involved, and which they are. In the translocation type of Down syndrome, part of chromosome 21 becomes detached and is attached to another chromosome. Thus, genetically they have 47 chromosomes. The prevalence of this condition is in the range of one in 800–1000 live births, and even higher in mothers older than 40 years. Approximately 25% of all babies born with Down syndrome are born to mothers over 35 years of age.

Specific comorbid features associated with Down syndrome are a learning disability, neuropsychiatric disorders and behavioral problems (20–40%), congenital cardiac anomalies, thyroid problems, seizures, hearing and visual impairments, early onset dementia (Alzheimer-like), frequent infections, hepatitis B carriage, especially in countries where people with disabilities may still live in residential care with suboptimal standards of hygiene, and leukemias.

The general features of Down syndrome are: short stature, tendency to obesity, muscle hypotonia, atlanto-axial mid-face hypoplasia, slanting palpebral fissures, prominent epicanthic folds, and simian palmar creases (10).

Specific intraoral features seen in Down syndrome are a mouth-open posture, sometimes accompanied by drooling, a protrusive tongue often with deep fissuring (Fig. 23-2), which can be a challenge for oral hygiene, a relative prognathism, hypodontia, microdontia, enamel hypoplasia, aggressive periodontal disease, delayed eruption in both dentitions, and delayed exfoliation of primary teeth.

Oral health considerations

Unlike unaffected children of a similar age, many young people with Down syndrome may not ever be able to consent to more invasive dental procedures although they may have capacity to consent for less invasive preventive care, such as fissure sealants and topical fluoride therapy. Increasingly, experts are becoming more aware of a premature disintegrative disorder that manifests in adolescence and may be the precursor to dementia, especially of the Alzheimer type. Young people who are affected suddenly start to lose skills and become introverted and seemingly depressed.

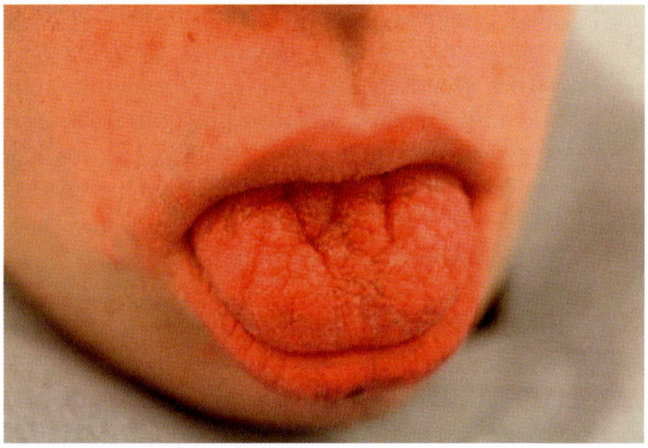

Figure 23-2 Large, fissured tongue of a boy with Down syndrome.

Significant sensory problems, as a barrier to oral care, do not become obvious until adulthood although hearing may be impaired early on. Visual disturbances are seen initially as a consequence of cataract formation but later, other visual disturbances impair the person's ability to read instructions and to visualize toothbrushing.

Although in the past, caries prevalence has been reported as low in a child with Down syndrome, this may be a false picture since by comparison with nonaffected peers, there may be fewer teeth erupted for dental caries to affect. Enamel hypoplasia and spacing may make children more or less prone to dental caries, respectively. However, use of sweetened medicines for seizure control or infection management may predispose to dental caries as will a dry mouth induced by some medications, especially those drugs used to manage mood swings. The literature supports the theory that secretion rates, as well as quality of saliva, may be reduced in young people with Down syndrome. Because of a compromised immune system, in particular, impaired phagocytosis together with altered cell-mediated but especially humoral immune responses, children with Down syndrome may develop a severe form of periodontal disease, similar to localized aggressive periodontitis in that it mainly affects the lower incisor area (22). Regular reviews and professional tooth cleaning of young people with Down syndrome have been shown to be effective in slowing the progression of destructive periodontal disease.

Special considerations for dental care

Despite the assumed picture of amiable, lovable children, a proportion of children with Down syndrome will have a significant degree of intellectual impairment together with behavioral problems. These may mean that dental treatment needs to be provided under sedation, or possibly general anesthesia. For any dental care, consideration needs to be given to the use of antibiotic prophylaxis, where there is a significant cardiac condition requiring this, according to national guidelines.

Where dental care needs to be delivered with the aid of sedation or general anesthesia, care in handling is required where atlanto-axial instability is known or suspected. Sedation is preferable to general anesthesia, where difficulties in intubation because of a retrusive maxilla and propensity to develop chest infections make this a more hazardous procedure.

In many countries, orofacial regulation therapy is employed to train and stimulate the tongue and lips. This is carried out in collaboration with a speech-language pathologist (see further page 346).

Cerebral palsy

Cerebral palsy is the commonest cause of significant childhood disability. It is characterized as a nonprogressive disorder of the brain stem which results in varying impairment of motor activities. The defect occurs as a consequence of some form of insult (trauma, infection) prenatally, perinatally, or postnatally. Cerebral palsy presents as four main types: spastic (muscle stiffness), atheotid (slow, writhing movements), ataxic (rarer type affecting balance, coordination), and mixed. Frequently there is comorbidity in the form of intellectual impairment and/or epilepsy (27). A consensus conference in 2004 questioned the traditional classification of cerebral palsy and has proposed a new classification which excludes those children who have no motor defect and places more emphasis on the accompanying nonmotor, neurodevelopmental impairments of performance and behavior, consistent with the ICF classification outlined above. The prevalence of cerebral palsy is of the range 1.5–2.5 per 1000 live births and in Sweden, as in other countries, has been declining (14).

Oral health considerations

Children who have impaired mobility might be expected to have an increased prevalence of trauma and the literature would support this theory. The altered muscle control produces two other oral effects in these children. One is an increase in malocclusions and the second is the greater prevalence of drooling (Fig. 23-3). Most studies involve too few children to indicate the type of malocclusion, but in those that have been reported, an increased overjet and a tendency to an Angle Class II malocclusion is seen.

Drooling occurs for a number of reasons. Children with cerebral palsy often have poor head control and together with an inadequate lip seal, gravity results in pooling of saliva at the front of the mouth and drooling or sialorrhea. The dysfunctional second stage of swallowing also adds to the problem. Most of the resting saliva in the mouth comes from the submandibular

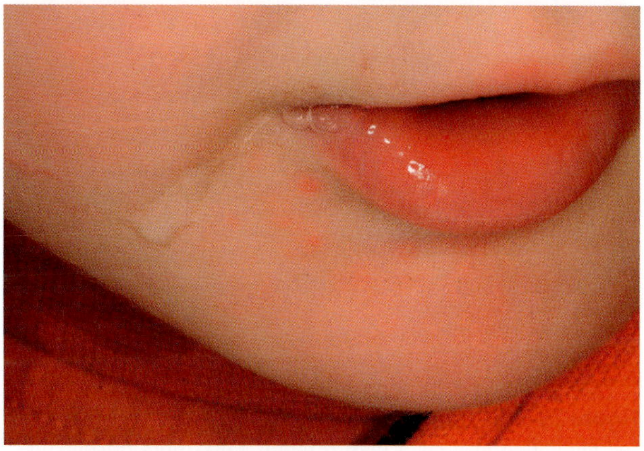

Figure 23-3 Drooling in a child with cerebral palsy.

glands. The management of this includes behavioral, pharmacological, and oral motor therapy. In special cases where this is not sufficient, surgical treatment to reroute submandibular ducts to the oropharynx is carried out. This treatment may increase the risk for dental caries.

Tooth wear is commoner in children with cerebral palsy. This may result from factors such as gastroesophageal reflux disease (GERD/GORD) that is seen in these children and which often comes under control after a gastrostomy procedure (e.g., via a percutaneous endoscopic gastrostomy, PEG) to aid feeding. Another dental feature of children who are PEG-fed is that once all oral feeding ceases, there is a tendency to accumulate greater quantities of calculus (Fig. 23-4). Dentists may be the first people to notice the signs of reflux, from evidence of wear to, usually, palatal surfaces of maxillary teeth and occlusal/buccal surfaces of lower posterior teeth, although the child may have had symptoms from the GERD/GORD for many years. Such symptoms may lead to self-inflicted injury, because of the inability to communicate the pain and distress of reflux. The other main cause of tooth wear seen in children and young people with cerebral palsy is bruxism.

Enamel hypoplasia as well as hypomineralization occur more frequently in children with cerebral palsy and are caused by a systemic upset where amelogenesis is disrupted. Dental development may be delayed in children with cerebral palsy but the prevalence of dental caries is usually higher than for their normal peers. This may be related to the increased prevalence of enamel defects, poor oral hygiene, and often hyperplastic gingival tissue. In addition, some studies have shown that these children have higher counts of mutans streptococcus and lactobacillus as well as diminished salivary flow, buffering, and lower pH levels as compared with non-impaired groups. In those children with cerebral palsy and drooling that has been managed by saliva gland removal, and even saliva duct rerouting, a rampant form of dental caries may develop, particularly in the lower incisor teeth.

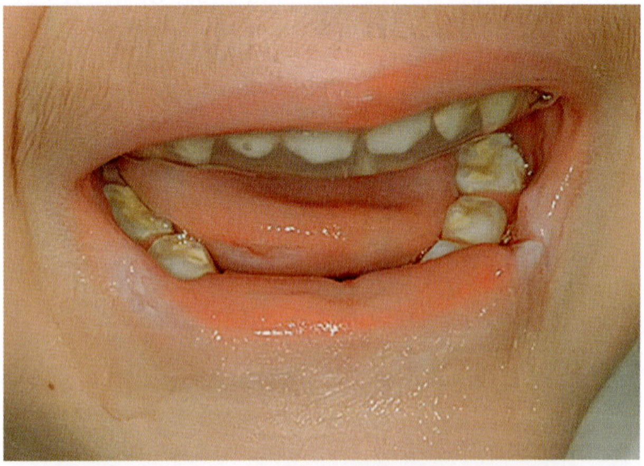

Figure 23-4 A vacuum-moulded splint in place to prevent further self-mutilation in a child with cerebral palsy (note calculus as a consequence of nil-by-mouth PEG feeding).

Special considerations for dental care

As with all children with impairments for whom the risk of developing dental disease and/or its treatment may pose significant hazards for their general health and well-being, prevention of oral and dental disease is a priority (see below). Some children with severe mobility impairments may have difficulty accessing dental care, which in turn results in neglect and more advanced disease on presentation.

The unpredictable movement disorders may mean that parents/carers have difficulty initiating and maintaining good oral hygiene and need practical demonstrations and support from the dental team. Appropriate seating to maintain comfort and security for disabled children can be achieved by maintaining children in their own wheelchairs for those who need this form of aid, on a special ramp, or using the support of cushions in a normal dental chair.

Such movement disorders may necessitate the use of conscious sedation to control these nonpurposive movements during dental treatment. This is especially true in a child who has a normal intellect and for whom the desire to cooperate is confounded by movement that is worse the greater degree of control they attempt to exert. In these instances, the use of nitrous oxide sedation is beneficial. A prop (Fig. 23-5a, b) may be helpful to make dental treatment more comfortable for the child and safer for the dentist or hygienist.

Good assistance to aspirate away secretions and dental debris is necessary during dental treatment since many children with cerebral palsy have dysphagia. This is especially important in children who are PEG-fed and accumulate large deposits of calculus that need to be removed frequently.

For children with self-inflicted injury, referral to a specialist is necessary. Management usually consists of identifying the cause and treating it; for some the trigger may be teething, in others it may be undiagnosed pain. In the short term the fitting of a vacuum-formed splint may break the habit and allow the lesion to heal (Fig. 23-4). For other children, a longer term solution is to correct their malocclusion. Only as a last resort are teeth extracted.

Spina bifida

Spina bifida is one of the commonest birth defects. The incidence varies: in Sweden it is one per 2000 live births

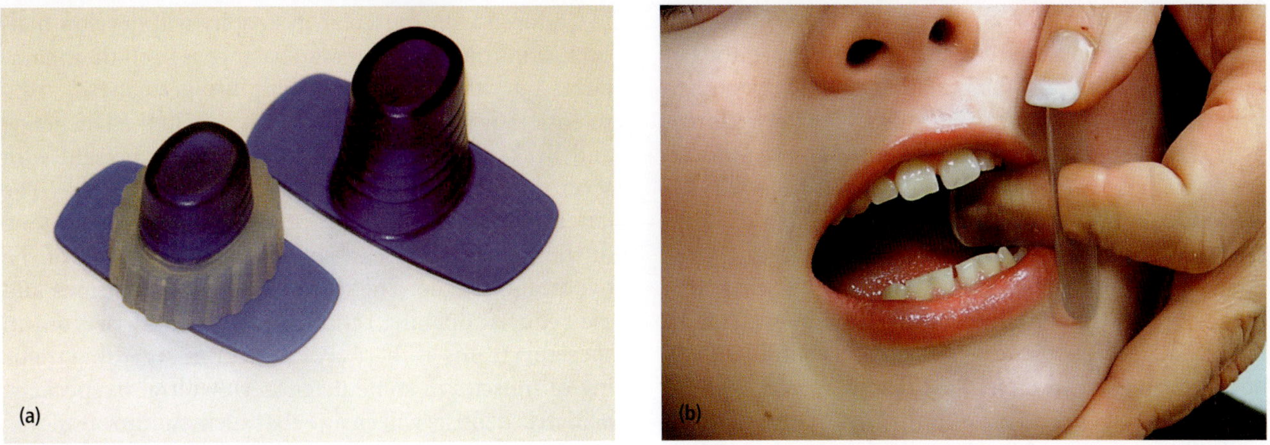

Figure 23-5 (a) A prop, with and without an occlusal "guard", and (b) in use.

and in Celtic areas (Wales and Ireland) may be as high as three to four per 1000 live births.

The cause of spina bifida is unknown but may be due to both genetic and environmental causes; supplementation of the diets of women of child-bearing age with folic acid preconception can reduce the risk by up to 70%. Affected families are at greater risk of having a second affected child.

The impairment in spina bifida is an incomplete spinal cord and a defect, predominantly in the lumbar or sacral region, in the overlying vertebrae. It occurs as a result of failure of the vertebrae to fuse, usually within the first month of embryonic development. There are three main manifestations: spina bifida occulta, which is a defect of the spinal cord but with no external signs, apart from occasional dimpling and/or a collection of hairs over the affected part. There are usually no symptoms. In meningocoele, the vertebrae are defective and part of the meninges protrudes through the opening but without any spinal cord involvement. Symptoms are usually not evident early in life.

The most severe form of spina bifida is a myelomeningocoele or spina bifida cystica. In this form, the spinal cord and covering meninges protrude through the defective vertebrae. Because the nerve supply to this region is affected, there is accompanying paralysis at and below this level. Consequently there will be paralysis of the legs, a paraplegia, and loss of bladder and bowel control. In some children with spina bifida there is an accompanying malformation of the cerebellum, which is pushed out through the base of the skull. This produces a hydrocephalus as fluid builds up in the ventricles, because the exit channels are blocked by the displaced cerebellum. Occasionally, hydrocephalus spontaneously arrests. For most, fluid needs to be drained from the ventricles with a shunt, usually into the peritoneum (ventriculo-peritoneal shunt). In older patients, the shunt may be directed to the right atrium (ventriculo-atrial shunt).

Oral considerations

There is very little reported in the literature with respect to oral health in spina bifida. The oral health will be affected by consideration of the degree of physical impairment and use of liquid oral antibiotics for persistent urinary tract infections.

Special considerations for dental care

A significant, potential problem for the delivery of dental care is the increased likelihood of an allergy to latex seen in children with spina bifida (5). This occurs because of the frequent catheterizations as a result of the neuropathic bladder and with the placement of shunts to manage any hydrocephalus. In addition, patients who have a ventriculo-atrial shunt will usually require antibiotic prophylaxis prior to invasive dental care. However, most children will now be fitted with a ventriculo-peritoneal shunt, which will not require antibiotic cover. The majority of patients with spina bifida will use a wheelchair and so will require to be treated in a unit that has a modification to accept a wheelchair or to employ some means of manually handling the patient from wheelchair to dental chair with a slide.

Because of the potential to develop latex sensitivity or true allergy, it is advisable to restrict the latex load as much as possible. Such patients should therefore be managed in a unit that is latex safe, and first thing on a Monday morning when the latex load in the atmosphere is at a minimum. Prevention is a key to the management of these children so that they do not require dental treatment.

Muscular dystrophy

Muscular dystrophies are a group of genetic disorders caused by mutation in the gene for the dystrophin protein, that results in progressive muscle weakness, principally affecting voluntary muscles but smooth muscles are also affected, for example in the gut. Muscle fibers are gradually replaced by fat and fibrous tissue. There are 30 conditions under the term muscular dystrophies, but nine major categories. The three most prevalent groups are Duchenne muscular dystrophy, which is an X-linked condition clinically manifest predominantly in boys (the most common muscular dystrophy with an incidence of one per 3500 newborn boys), Becker (which is a milder version of Duchenne muscular dystrophy), and a group of conditions based on the muscle groups affected, for example, fascioscapulohumeral.

The general presentation of the condition is in muscle weakness, difficulty walking, and reliance, by early adolescence, on the use of a wheelchair. Children tend to fall easily and have an awkward gait. As time goes on they develop muscle contractures, scoliosis, and deterioration in respiratory muscles in the Duchenne type. These patients will need medication, ventilatory support, or even assisted ventilation. With modern treatment and medication the lifespan of these patients has increased and now there are individuals surviving into their 40s. Cardiac myopathies occur in up to 50% after the age of 12 years.

Oral considerations

Dentally, such children present with wide-spaced arches because of the relative hypotonia so that teeth are not in the usual soft tissue balance. Shedding of primary teeth may be delayed in widely spaced arches (12).

If the child requires ventilatory support, this can affect facial growth. The muscle effects are also seen in a reduction in bite force and hand grip, the latter potentially making mouth cleaning a problem. There is also a decrease in opening capacity occurring mostly in older teenagers.

Special dental considerations

Preventive dental care is the number one priority for these patients. Because heart muscle may be affected, patients pose an anesthetic risk because of abnormal reactions to smooth muscle relaxants, made more complex by the effects on involuntary respiratory muscles. Children are sensitive to succinylcholine and volatile anesthetic gases and these should be avoided. Such patients can be at risk of sudden cardiac death because of conduction disturbances and may have pacemakers fitted electively. Local analgesia must be used with caution as tolerance is lower than for the general population.

Children with muscular dystrophy will develop malocclusions but the soft tissue balance is such that maintaining tooth movements, without permanent, fixed retention, is impractical. Children will, in the Duchenne and Becker types of muscular dystrophy, present with severe, skeletal open bites, and posterior cross bites. The latter occurs as a consequence of the relative lack of tone of the masseter muscles and the increased bulk of the hypotonic tongue. The treatment of malocclusions and the reduced opening capacity should be carried out in specialist teams as there are restrictions regarding training of muscles in some diagnoses. Referral to specialist pediatric dentists will ensure that such multiprofessional care is provided.

With decreasing muscle function, plaque control becomes more difficult and, especially associated with the open-mouth posture, leads to gingivitis. Macroglossia due to hypotonia and tongue thrusting are also features.

Breathing difficulties, ventilatory support systems, and difficulty in stabilizing the head and neck for patients in advanced stages of Duchenne muscular dystrophy require special dental care for the individual. All treatment has to be carried out with patients in their wheelchairs and there is a risk of aspiration of, for example, water.

Cleft lip and palate

This is a congenital anomaly that occurs in one in 800 live births worldwide although there is wide cultural variation: 0.9–1.9 per 100 live births (7).

Children may have a cleft of the lip alone, palate, or lip and palate. In addition, the defects may be bilateral. Approximately 70% of cases are isolated clefts of the lip or palate. Isolated clefts especially are associated with syndromes, in up to 20% of cases.

The etiology is unclear but is thought to be multifactoral with environment playing a big part. Coexisting morbidity in the mother, like diabetes, folate deficiency, anticonvulsant drugs, and alcohol, have all been implicated as causative factors. A genetic trait consisting of variations in the DNA of susceptible families, called single nucleotide polymorphisms, associated with the IRF6 gene, increases the risk of cleft three-fold.

The timing of surgical correction varies from country to country but usually approximates to the "rule of tens" – that is 10 weeks in age, 10 kg in weight, and a hemoglobin of 10. The first procedure is usually to repair the lip. Thereafter, before speech is developed the palate is repaired, both primary and secondary. Children with velopharyngeal insufficiency may require further surgery to prevent nasal escape causing hypernasal speech.

Some centers provide palatal plates in the neonate to encourage the segments to approximate to aid the surgical correction, as well as a subsidiary effect in supporting feeding. Most infants with clefts are fed with the aid of special bottles, for example, Rosti or Haberman that reduce the effort required by the child to feed. Such bottles make it easier to achieve an oral seal and avoid the build-up of negative pressure.

Oral considerations

Children with a cleft may have delayed dental development as well as disorders of eruption and missing teeth and/or enamel hypoplasia. Teeth adjacent to the cleft may fail to erupt, especially canine teeth. In such children, bone grafting between 9 and 10 years of age, carried out prior to tooth eruption, encourages the eruption of the canine.

Special dental considerations

With a cleft of the palate, the surgical repair often results in a narrowed arch. Orthodontic treatment consists of arch expansion prior to alignment and so caries prevention is paramount in these children who frequently undergo extensive orthodontic treatment. Ectopic eruption of first permanent molars is seen much more commonly, in up to 10% of children, who have clefts (4). This is associated with crowding, as a result of the maxillary arch constriction.

Poor self-esteem may demotivate children so that oral hygiene is poor. Frequent ear infections because of the intimate relationship between the muscles in the oropharynx that operate the Eustachian tubes and which are defective in a child with a palatal cleft, are treated with antibiotics. In the young child these factors may lead to an increased prevalence of dental caries.

Preventive dental care

Preventing dental disease is important for everyone but especially so for children with disabilities, whose general health may be put at risk from the presence of untreated oral/dental disease and/or for whom the treatment of such disease may put the child at risk. Which particular preventive strategy is adopted as optimal, both clinically and cost-effectively, will depend on the level of provision: at the individual or community level and on the personnel available to deliver a particular program.

Diet

Children with disabilities may not achieve developmental milestones at the same time as their normal peers and may retain infant feeding practices for longer. These can be potentially damaging, for example, the prolonged use of bottle feeding or even breastfeeding after 12 months of age, given the higher lactose content of human milk.

Frequent infections in early childhood, which are commoner in children with disabilities, are often managed by the use of liquid oral medicines, some of which will still be sweetened with sucrose. For example, the child with a cleft palate may have middle ear infections and have regular courses of antibiotics. In addition, depending on dose form, the risk for dental erosion may be greater. Children with renal disease may take some of their medication in an effervescent form that contributes to tooth wear because of its low pH and high titratable acidity. Discussion with the medical team caring for the child will find ways of delivering necessary medication in a safer way, for example, if liquid, by syringe via the retromolar area or in tablet rather than liquid form. Alternatively, sugar-free medication may be available to prescribe.

Failure to thrive is a feature of some impairments and after a period of parenteral feeding, such children may progress to being fed directly through a PEG. This may resolve reflux, a common finding in some children with cerebral palsy, which also contributes to dental erosion. Children who are PEG-fed exclusively develop greater amounts of calculus than usual.

Children who have difficulties in feeding because of dysphagia or other aspects of disordered oromotor function may have food liquidized since they cannot tolerate food of normal texture, especially lumps. Sometimes, liquidized food is high in sugars and/or is retained around the oral cavity for prolonged periods, leading to dental caries. Other children, for whom calorie-dense food supplements are required, may be more vulnerable to dental caries because of the high burden of sugars contained in such products. However, the dental team have to be realistic and it is more important that the child survives and thrives, not that they have perfect teeth! Ways need to be found of working around these challenges.

Fluorides

The appropriate use of fluorides is important in the prevention of dental caries in patients with disabilities, and many of the strategies used for the child population in general are relevant (20). However, owing to the disability or medical condition the patients are often regarded as high risk for dental caries. As many patients with disabilities have difficulties rinsing with fluorides, sucking on fluoride tablets, or chewing fluoride chewing gums, a preventive home care regime where the teeth are brushed twice a day using fluoride toothpaste needs to be combined with regular chair-side prevention. This should include professional cleaning and topical application of fluoride, carried out at intervals appropriate for the individual child's risk situation. These preventive strategies must be emphasized in the treatment plan for patients with disabilities. See further Chapter 9.

Pit and fissure sealants

Published evidence suggests that fluoride varnishes are more effective in caries prevention if susceptible tooth sites also have sealants applied. Conventional pit and fissure sealants can be difficult to apply in some disabled children; these children often object to the aspiration of water to wash away the etchant gel and/or to the taste of the etchant. In addition, some children object to the noise of the whole procedure. An alternative is to apply a fluoride-rich glass ionomer cement, which is moisture tolerant and does not require pre-etching.

Oral hygiene aids

Children's teeth should be cleaned on eruption. Initially this might be with a piece of gauze wrapped around a finger. The use of a smear of toothpaste is advocated. The fluoride content will depend on the child's risk for caries and level of impairment, which may be difficult to determine at this stage of development, approximately 6 months of age (see above, toothpaste use).

Once teeth erupt, a parent can be guided on the use of a suitable tooth-cleaning aid. This may be with a finger brush or baby's toothbrush (Fig. 23-6). The former gives the parents more confidence as they not only worry less about the child clamping down on their fingers as they brush, but they feel they are less likely to damage soft tissues as with a conventional brush.

As the child develops more teeth, a powered brush may be helpful although many children object to the sensation and noise of such brushes. An alternative is the "Superbrush"® that has three sets of bristles arranged so that the occlusal as well as buccal and lingual surfaces can be brushed simultaneously (8). A Collis Curve® performs a similar task (Fig. 23-7). Sometimes a prop can be helpful to maintain the mouth open so that the parent or carer can brush one side effectively (Fig. 23-8).

For children with significant dysphagia in whom aspiration may be a risk, special aspirating mouth cleaners are available, which clear oral secretions as well as tooth-cleaning products.

Chlorhexidine

Chlorhexidine products (chlorhexidine gluconate) have been advocated for use with people with disabilities when mouth cleaning is challenging because of poor or noncooperation by the child. This can be either swabbed around the mouth on gauze, touchettes, or sponge sticks (Fig. 23-9), as a rinse or spray (28). They are also available as gels that can substitute for toothpaste and as varnishes for professional application. Chlorhexidine does have side-effects, most notably for the patient as tooth staining and alteration in taste. Some patients

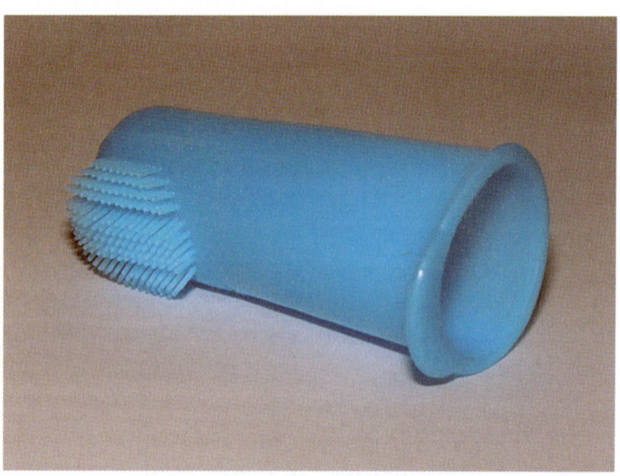

Figure 23-6 A finger brush that can be used for gentle cleaning of the child's teeth and/or for oral motor stimulation.

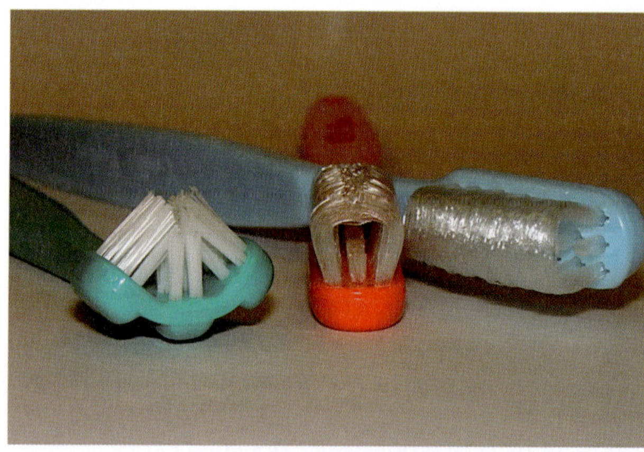

Figure 23-7 A "Superbrush"® on the left and two Collis Curve® brushes on the right.

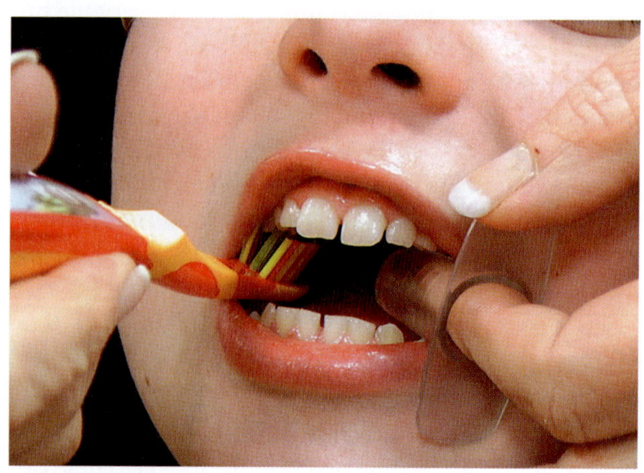

Figure 23-8 A prop to facilitate brushing.

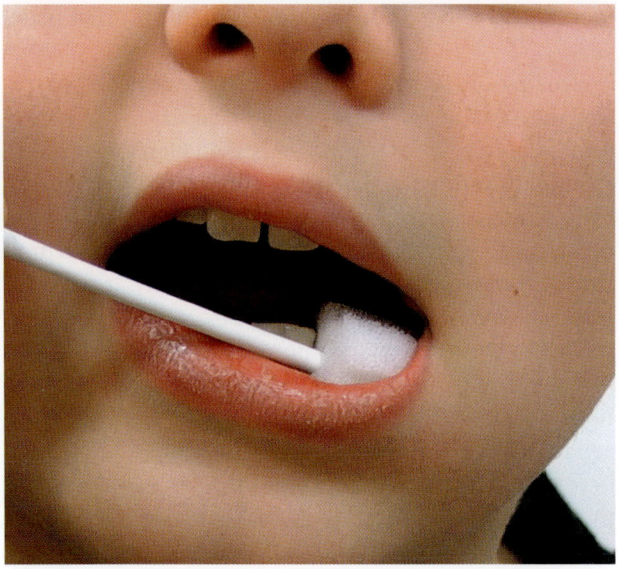

Figure 23-9 A "touchette" or sponge stick for cleaning mouths.

experience swelling of the parotid glands. In children with very sore mouths, such as those with chemotherapy-associated mucositis, 2% chlorhexidine can be diluted 1:1 with water. Where a patient is really very uncooperative, chlorhexidine can be used in a spray form (conventional or mint flavor), or applied as a gel on a finger directly or with a finger brush. The use of chlorhexidine products should be based on risk assessment and part of a treatment strategy. There is the potential for patients to develop resistance towards chlorhexidine. The agents are usually used for certain periods of medication or when the child has an infection. For children with progressive terminal conditions, chemical plaque control with use of chlorhexidine is an important substitute to traditional oral hygiene.

Dental visits

It is crucial that children with disabilities are made known to the dental team at the earliest possible opportunity. Ideally a country should have a reporting mechanism in place so that all health care professionals involved with children who have an impairment are notified, with the consent of the family, about the child. By such means, appropriate support and interventions can be designed around the child and the family.

Behavior management

As in any other patient, the dental treatment for children and adolescents with disabilities should be based on a thorough examination and treatment planning. The dental treatment itself is essentially the same, but it has to be carried out in a way that is modified, depending on the patient's specific diagnosis and individual needs. Treating children and adolescents with disabilities involves a triangle of people. First, the young patient, second the parents and family, and third the dental health care personnel. In many cases the patient may also be accompanied by assistants. Having a disability or a chronic disease implies going through numerous visits to different health care facilities every year, which is why it is important that the dental visits are well organized in advance. This preparation includes learning more about the patient's diagnosis and its implications for oral health and dental treatment, preferably before the visit. This signals interest and knowledge, which patients, as well as parents, express as important in order to have confidence in the dentist and the dental treatment (15,29). Today there are many reliable sources of knowledge about even rare diagnoses to be found on the Internet, e.g., OMIM which can be accessed via PubMed. In addition, the dentist should plan for continuity of care by means of assuring that the patient will meet the same dentist at the dental appointments.

The ability to cope with dental treatment varies in children and adolescents with disabilities. The main reason for this lies in the degree of disability, and is related to factors such as cognitive and behavioral factors. Physical disability, body posture, and medication will also affect the treatment. Apart from this, it is important to acknowledge that patients with disabilities may, in addition, have behavioral management problems related to dental fear and anxiety. The basis for the patient's willingness to undergo treatment relies on having established a good relationship with the dental team, an enhanced feeling of control in the patient, and treatment carried out in a way that minimizes pain. For some patients sedation with nitrous oxide/oxygen or benzodiazepines can be helpful, and should follow the normal guidelines. This is covered in Chapters 4 and 5. One difference, however, when treating patients with a disability is the greater need to customize the experience for them, which requires time. It is therefore wise to allocate some extra time for the appointments. Some patients may still be difficult to examine or treat, or have a medical condition that requires specialist treatment. In such cases referral to specialized pediatric dentistry clinics are advocated. It is important that patients with disabilities are ensured good oral health and dental treatment and that the disability or medical condition does not constitute a barrier to this. For some patients general anesthesia is required to fulfill these needs. Thus, the indications for treatment under general anesthesia may be wider than for healthy patients. This is usually a specialist treatment, but it should be pointed out that there is need for these facilities (23).

Body posture

High-quality treatment and good management of the patient are facilitated if the patient is able to relax in the dental chair. It is easier for the dentist to perform good examination or treatment when the patient is seated in the dental chair. For patients using wheelchairs it is usually possible to move the patient to the dental chair with a lift or special equipment for sliding the patient over to the dental chair. Most dental chairs are constructed to fit a full-length body, and they are often uncomfortable for young patients to lie on. In these situations it is also difficult for the dentist to work in good ergonomic positions. For many young patients this can be improved by using cushions for the child to sit on in the chair. In a hypotonic patient, specially designed cushions (Fig. 23-10) can be used to further support the body posture in the chair. In the case of spasticities, such cushions are used to flex knees and hip joint and to incline the head to a chin to chest position, which can reduce spastic problems and help the patient to relax (23).

Oral motor function

The oral cavity is more than teeth, something that is very obvious when meeting children and adolescents with disabilities. Often the patient has problems related to communication, nutrition (eating, drinking, sucking, swallowing), perception or breathing. The etiology of these problems can be a combination of deviations in anatomy, sensation, oral motor function, and also the underlying medical condition and environmental aspects play a part. The handling of oral motor problems mainly concerns multiprofessional teams, including specialist pediatric dentists, in collaboration with a speech-language pathologist, but it is essential that the general dentist is familiar with the management of these issues (23).

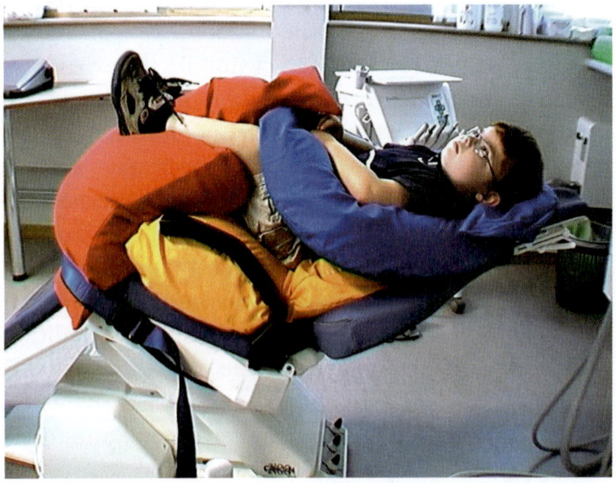

Figure 23-10 Body cushions to give support to a child during treatment.

Feeding disorders (difficulties in eating, drinking, sucking, swallowing) are often seen in, for example, infants born preterm, in patients with clefts, neurological or neuromuscular disease, or congenital heart defects. For some reason, sucking and breastfeeding have been unsuccessful and many children need artificial nutrition through a nasogastric tube or a gastrostomy. If the child is not fed by mouth, this will interfere with the development of oral sensory and motor skills. The oral cavity often becomes hypersensitive, making it difficult to touch the mouth or to brush the teeth. A vicious circle can be established where the child does not tolerate food or liquid in the mouth, and will thus not exercise or use the oral sensory systems or motor functions, leading to difficulties in terminating tube feeding. There are different strategies and techniques to break this pattern, all within the competence of the speech-language pathologist. However, for the dentist it is important to know that while doing this, offering small portions of foods and drinks with different tastes (including sweetened products) usually on frequent occasions throughout the day is often recommended and has proved to be efficient. In these cases the dentist is advised not to interfere with these recommendations even though they are potentially damaging dentally. Instead, the dentist should provide extra help with check-ups and chair-side prevention. Once the feeding problems are resolved there will be time for more conventional dietary counseling from the dentist. Liaison with the dietician is helpful in these situations.

Many children and adolescents with hypersensory problems will not tolerate toothbrushing or the dentist checking the teeth. The acceptance of objects in the mouth has to be built up step by step; again an area of multiprofessional collaboration. What the dentist can suggest is introducing cleaning of the mouth from an early age, either with the help of gauze wrapped around the index finger or by use of a special finger toothbrush (see Fig. 23-6). In older children an electric toothbrush can be helpful as the vibrations help to stimulate and give rise to tactile sensations in the oral cavity.

In order to train and exercise the oral motor complex, new methods are constantly being developed and evaluated. For example there are massage techniques where the sensorimotor stimulation can affect muscle tone and improve motility. One particular method has been developed by Argentinian neurologist Rodolfo Castillo Morales and includes working on body posture, use of massage, and use of palatal plates or other oral devices. Poor lip closure combined with hypotonic muscles often results in drooling. To improve the function there are

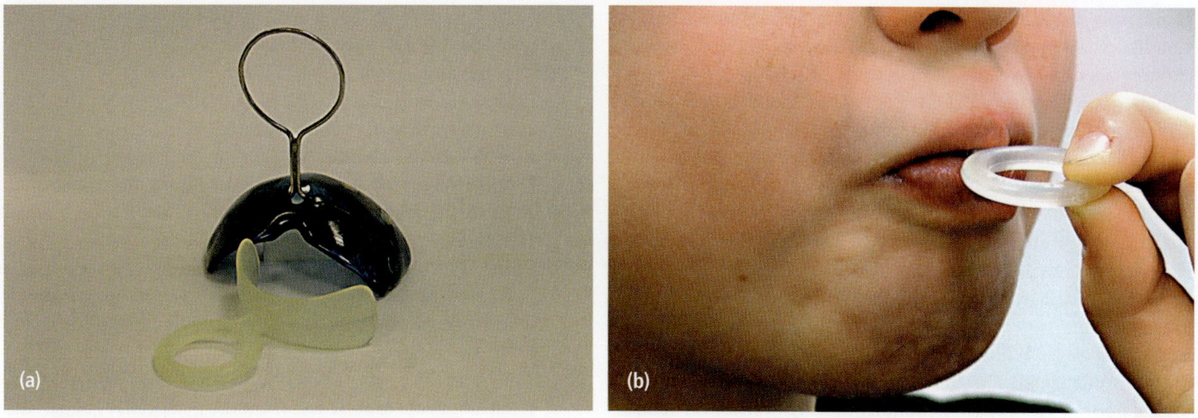

Figure 23-11 (a) An oral screen; (b) a patient training with an oral screen by straining lip muscles and pulling the screen out with a light, balanced force.

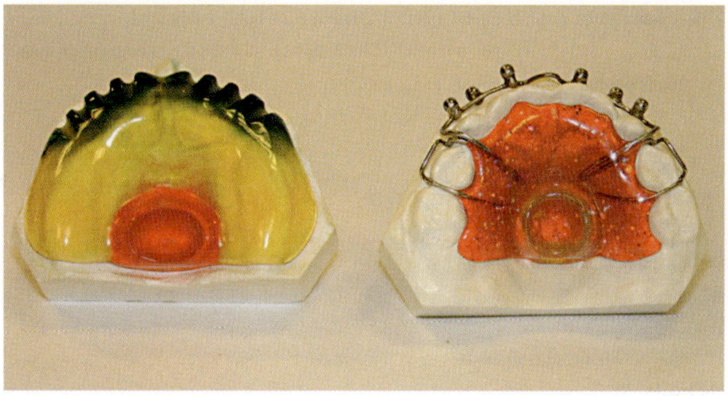

Figure 23-12 Palatal plates used for oral motor training in children.

exercise programs and the patient can also train with an oral screen device (Fig. 23-11a, b). There are individually fabricated palatal plates (Fig. 23-12) to be used for specific training stimulation of, foremost, the tongue. Some results from studies in patients with Down syndrome indicate that training with palatal plates has a positive effect on oral muscle function and speech development (2). Palatal plates can also be used to train children in overcoming articulatory problems. For this purpose the plate is individually designed with a fixed or mobile object inserted into the plate in the region where the child is supposed to put the tongue, in order to produce the correct sound. The use of different appliances should be based on multiprofessional assessments and evaluations. While the training is usually supervised by a speech-language pathologist, the appliances require the taking of impressions for casts and this, as well as the regular supervision of the plate or oral screen, has to be managed by the dentist.

References

1. Altarac M, Saroha E. Lifetime prevalence of learning disability among US children. *Pediatrics* 2007;**119** Suppl 1: S77–83.
2. Bäckman B, Grevér-Sjölander AC, Bengtsson K, Persson J, Johansson I. Children with Down syndrome: oral development and morphology after use of palatal plates between 6 and 48 months of age. *Int J Paediatr Dent* 2007;**17**:19–28.
3. Bäckman B, Pilebro C. Visual pedagogy in dentistry for children with autism. *ASDC J Dent Child* 1999;**66**:325–31.
4. Bjerklin K, Kürol J, Paulin G. Ectopic eruption of the maxillary first permanent molars in children with cleft lip and/or palate. *Eur J Orthod* 1993;**15**:535–40.
5. Bernardini R, Novembre E, Lombardi E, Mezzetti P, Cianferoni A, Danti DA, *et al.* Risk factors for latex allergy in patients with spina bifida and latex sensitization. *Clin Exp Allergy* 1999;**29**:681–6.
6. Blomqvist M. Oral health and behavior in children with Attention Deficit Hyperactivity Disorder. Thesis. Stockholm: Karolinska Institutet, 2007.
7. Calzolari E, Pierini A, Astolfi G, Bianchi F, Neville AJ, Rivieri F. Associated anomalies in multi-malformed infants with cleft lip and palate: an epidemiologic study of nearly 6 million births in 23 EUROCAT registries. *Am J Med Genet A* 2007;**143**:528–37.
8. Doğan MC, Alaçam A, Aşici N, Odabaş M, Seydaoğlu G. Clinical evaluation of the plaque-removing ability of three different toothbrushes in a mentally disabled group. *Acta Odontol Scand* 2004;**62**:350–4.
9. Faulks D, Hennequin M. Defining the population requiring special care dentistry using the International Classification of Functioning, Disability and Health – a personal view. *J Disabil Oral Health* 2006;**7**:143–52.
10. Fiske J, Shafik HH. Down's syndrome and oral care. *Dent Update* 2001;**28**:148–56.
11. Fombonne E. Epidemiology of autistic disorder and other pervasive developmental disorders. *J Clin Psychiatry* 2005;**66** (Suppl 10):3–8.
12. Ghafari J, Clark RE, Shofer FS, Berman PH. Dental and occlusal characteristics of children with neuromuscular disease. *Am J Orthod Dentofacial Orthop* 1988;**93**:126–32.
13. Gillberg C, Coleman M. *The biology of the autistic syndromes*, 3rd edn. London: MacKeith Press, 2000.
14. Hagberg B, Hagberg G, Beckung E, Uvebrant P. Changing panorama of cerebral palsy in Sweden. VIII. Prevalence and origin in the birth year period 1991–94. *Acta Paediatr* 2001;**90**:271–7.
15. Hallberg U, Klingberg G. Giving low priority to oral health care. Voices from people with disabilities in a grounded theory study. *Acta Odontol Scand* 2007;**65**:265–70.

16. Henderson J, Goldacre MJ, Fairweather JM, Marcovitch H. Conditions accounting for substantial time spent in hospital in children aged 1–14 years. *Arch Dis Child* 1992;**67**:83–6.
17. Klingberg G, Lingström P, Óskarsdóttir S, Friman V, Bohman E, Carlén A. Caries-related saliva properties in individuals with 22q11 deletion syndrome. *Oral Surg Oral Med Oral Pathol Oral Radiol Endod* 2007;**103**:497–504.
18. Kornfält R, Köhler L. Physical health of ten-year-old children. An epidemiological study of school children and a follow-up of previous health care. *Acta Paediatr Scand* 1978;**67**:481–9.
19. McGregor LM, Metzger ML, Sanders R, Santana VM. Pediatric cancers in the new millennium: dramatic progress, new challenges. *Oncology (Williston Park)* 2007;**21**:809–20.
20. Marinho VC, Higgins JP, Sheiham A, Logan S. Combinations of topical fluoride (toothpastes, mouthrinses, gels, varnishes) versus single topical fluoride for preventing dental caries in children and adolescents. *Cochrane Database Syst Rev* 2004;(1):CD002781.
21. Merrick J, Carmeli E. A review on the prevalence of disabilities in children. *The Internet Journal of Pediatrics and Neonatology* 2003;**3**(1).
22. Morgan J. Why is periodontal disease more prevalent and more severe in people with Down syndrome? *Spec Care* 2007;**27**: 196–201.
23. Nunn J, ed. *Disability and oral care.* London: FDI World Dental Press, 2000.
24. Office for National Statistics. *The health of children and young people. 2004.* http://www.statistics.gov.uk/children/ (accessed August 2007).
25. Olsen J, Melbye M, Olsen SF, Sørensen TI, Aaby P, Andersen AM, *et al.* The Danish National Birth Cohort – its background, structure and aim. *Scand J Public Health* 2001;**29**:300–7.
26. Pilebro C, Bäckman B. Teaching oral hygiene to children with autism. *Int J Paediatr Dent* 2005;**15**:1–9.
27. Rosenbaum P, Paneth N, Leviton A, Goldstein M, Bax M, Damiano D, *et al.* A report: the definition and classification of cerebral palsy, April 2006. *Dev Med Child Neurol Suppl* 2007; **109**:8–14.
28. Stiefel DJ, Truelove EL, Chin MM, Zhu XC, Leroux BG. Chlorhexidine swabbing applications under various conditions of use in preventive oral care for persons with disabilities. *Spec Care Dentist* 1995;**15**:159–65.
29. Trulsson U, Klingberg G. Living with a child with a severe orofacial handicap: experiences from the perspectives of parents. *Eur J Oral Sci* 2003;**111**:19–25.
30. World Health Organization. *International classification of functioning, disability and health (ICF).* http://www.who.int/classifications/icf/en/ (accessed August 2007).
31. World Health Organization. *International statistical classification of diseases and related health problems,* 10th revision, version for 2007. http://www.who.int/classifications/apps/icd/icd10online/ (accessed August 2007).

Index

Note: page numbers in *italics* denote tables and figures